Handbook of
Behavioral Neurobiology

Volume 3
Social Behavior
and Communication

HANDBOOK OF BEHAVIORAL NEUROBIOLOGY

General Editor:
Frederick A. King
Yerkes Regional Primate Research Center, Emory University, Atlanta, Georgia

Editorial Board:
Vincent G. Dethier
Robert W. Goy
David A. Hamburg
Peter Marler
James L. McGaugh
William D. Neff
Eliot Stellar

Volume 1   Sensory Integration
             Edited by R. Bruce Masterton

Volume 2   Neuropsychology
             Edited by Michael S. Gazzaniga

Volume 3   Social Behavior and Communication
             Edited by Peter Marler and J. G. Vandenbergh

A Continuation Order Plan is available for this series. A continuation order will bring delivery of each new volume immediately upon publication. Volumes are billed only upon actual shipment. For further information please contact the publisher.

Handbook of
Behavioral Neurobiology

Volume 3
Social Behavior
and Communication

Edited by

Peter Marler

Rockefeller University
New York, New York

and

J.G. Vandenbergh

North Carolina State University
Raleigh, North Carolina

PLENUM PRESS · NEW YORK AND LONDON

Library of Congress Cataloging in Publication Data

Main entry under title:

Social behavior and communication.

(Handbook of behavioral neurobiology; v. 3)
Includes bibliographies and index.
1. Social behavior in animals. 2. Animal communication. I. Marler, Peter Robert. II.
Vandenbergh, J. G. III. Series.
QL775.S6   599'.05'9   79-308
ISBN 0-306-40218-1

© 1979 Plenum Press, New York
A Division of Plenum Publishing Corporation
227 West 17th Street, New York, N.Y. 10011

Printed in the United States of America

Contributors

NORMAN T. ADLER, *Department of Psychology, University of Pennsylvania, Philadelphia, Pennsylvania*

STEVEN GREEN, *Department of Biology, University of Miami, Coral Gables, Florida*

JOHN R. KREBS, *Edward Grey Institute of Field Ornithology, Zoology Department, Oxford University, Oxford, England*

PETER MARLER, *Rockefeller University, Field Research Center, Millbrook, New York*

WILLIAM MASON, *Psychology Department and California Primate Research Center, University of California, Davis, California*

SANDRA L. VEHRENCAMP, *Department of Biology, University of California at San Diego, La Jolla, California*

PETER M. WASER, *Department of Biological Sciences, Purdue University, West Lafayette, Indiana*

R. HAVEN WILEY, *Department of Zoology, University of North Carolina, Chapel Hill, North Carolina*

JAMES F. WITTENBERGER, *Department of Zoology, University of Washington, Seattle, Washington*

Preface

Other books in this series focus on behavior at the individual level, approached from the viewpoints of biochemistry, anatomy, physiology, and psychology. In this volume we show how the functioning nervous systems of interacting individuals are coordinated, with the ultimate creation of complex social structures. The intricacies of an individual's nervous system have been subject to intense inquiry, and research at the chemical, cellular, and organ levels has made remarkable progress. Work at the social level has been conducted somewhat independently, by way of behavioral phenomena and communicative interactions. With the emergence of a large body of information from neurobiology, the beginnings of an integrated approach are possible. New data on social functions are presented in the chapters to follow, and the forward-looking reader may wish to reflect on how they clarify understanding of interactions between two or more independent nervous systems. The outcome is harmonious social structure and improvement in the inclusive fitness of group-living individuals. We believe that there is in prospect a new way of looking at social function that will ultimately increase our understanding of the highest and most complex levels of neurobiology.

The modern approach to the study of social behavior involves more than the recording of interactions between animals. Each individual brings to the process of social interaction the implications of its prior genetic and experiential history. William Mason explores the ontogeny of social behavior from an evolutionary and theoretical perspective. Central to his treatment is the concept of the "schema." A schema denotes the "inherent species-characteristic modes of organizing experience and of acting on information received." This pivotal concept provides the basis for a synthetic treatment of behavioral ontogeny, bringing together newly emerging evolutionary concepts with a wealth of empirical data on experiential factors influencing behavioral ontogeny.

The interplay between genetic constitution and experience is an implicit theme in Norman Adler's contribution, in that he deals with the inherent physiological characteristics of species, and how these are expressed as a function of changes in the environment. With a focus on reproduction and aggression, he deals with the physiological basis for the expression of social behavior. From the work of Beach (1975), Lehrman (1964), and others, it is clear that physiological events are as much a consequence of behavioral interactions with the environment as behavior is a function of physiology. For example, processes that were thought to be quite immune to behavioral influences, such as the movement of sperm up the female reproductive tract after ejaculation, are now clearly shown to be affected by the copulatory activity of both partners.

All who write on modern biology owe an obvious debt to Charles Darwin, and the contributors to this volume all share in this debt. Rapid progress has been made in recent years in developing and expanding upon earlier Darwinian concepts of evolution. Some of these advances are explored in chapters in this volume, as they bear on social behavior. Darwin's concept of natural selection was derived from his encounters with the writings of Malthus. He thus saw the process of evolution as a struggle for survival. As biologists dealt with the growing body of information about the living world, they came to agree that differences between species must have a functional basis (Mayr, 1963). The increased reproductive success of individuals with certain traits lead to the maintenance and spread of these traits throughout a species.

In the course of new attempts to explain the complexities of group behavior, involving a reduction of reproductive success for certain individuals, new explanations arose (see Wynne-Edwards, 1962). The problem, simply stated, was: How could traits resulting in reproductive suppression be selected for if the driving force for evolution is the maximization of his or her reproductive output? Reproductive suppression has been noted among rodents as their populations reach a high density, presumably acting to prevent the population from breeding itself into extinction. Other phenomena of an "altruistic" nature have been described, but suppression of reproduction is perhaps the most clear-cut example. Wynne-Edwards (1963) suggested that social groups as such have important adaptive characteristics, and that selection can operate at the group as well as the individual level.

Many observations have demonstrated the differential survival of social groups. Such observations do not necessarily indicate that selection is operating at the group level. Maynard-Smith (1964) pointed out that selection operating within a group would eradicate any traits related to altruism by an individual, thereby eliminating group-specific traits upon which selection could act. There is, however, a kind of group on which selection can act: a group consisting of individuals sharing genes. Hamilton (1964) described how an altruistic trait could be selected for if its genetic basis was shared by other individuals in the group. In two brief but very influential papers he posited that an altruistic trait would be selected for if a sufficient number of relatives survived as a result of the altruism. Survival of these relatives would ensure maintenance of the trait in the population. If the proportion of relatives to altruists was high, the trait would spread. Thus, groups of a particular type, namely kinship groups, can be units of selection. This basic advance in evolutionary theory has been developed by several investigators, most recently in an important comprehensive synthesis by Wilson (1975).

We have outlined these evolutionary issues as they relate to social behavior because they arise either explicitly or implicitly in chapters in this volume. Within a comprehensive scheme for the analysis of animal communication, Steven Green and Peter Marler consider topics with direct evolutionary implications, such as the role of signal familiarity in the discrimination of close from distant kin. The main focus in their treatment, however, is upon mechanisms, both behavioral and psychological, in harmony with recent exhortations from cognitive ethology not to eschew mental processes in theorizing about animal behavior (Griffin, 1978). Their notion of "assessments" made by animals in the course of signal perception and production is essentially a psychological concept, having much in common with Mason's exploitation of the idea of schemata as vehicles for organizing experience and acting upon it (Mason, 1976). Considerations of mechanism and function are also interwoven in the chapter by Peter Waser and R. Haven Wiley on animal spacing. Current research at this interface between ecology and ethology has presented a wealth of new data. An earlier, seminal review of patterns of distribution of animals in space ended by expressing the hope that "the study of spacing may rapidly develop into a theoretically rigorous and more experimentally oriented science" (Brown and Orians, 1970). The present treatment is a significant step in that direction. It presents new approaches to the description of spacing and its underlying social interactions and relates species differences in spacing to the availability of ecological resources.

All animals must feed to survive, and John Krebs discusses one specific mode of acquiring food, namely prey capture on the basis of the theory of natural selection. His approach is theoretical in that he examines how the rules of predation, as derived from principles of optimization, are borne out by observation and experiment. A similar approach is taken by James Wittenberger in examining vertebrate mating systems and their evolution. Just as food is essential for the survival of individuals, reproduction is essential for survival of populations. It is here that the role of altruism is best exemplified. The differentiation and specialization of the two sexes result in conflicts which shape the structure of animal mating systems. Such interactions between the sexes provide excellent models for clarifying the ways in which evolution has modeled individual nervous systems to achieve the cooperation that sexual reproduction requires. Following these considerations of the elemental needs of sustenance and reproduction, Sandra Vehrencamp describes the factors that shape the evolution of social systems. The relative roles of all three selection pressures at the level of the individual, kin, and the group, are appraised, culminating in development of the viewpoint that altruism is an unnecessary postulate for the evolution of societies.

It is our hope that this volume will provide the neurobiologist with not only a description of the more significant findings and theories about social behavior, its evolution and modes of operation, but also a framework in which knowledge about the neural functions of the individual can be integrated with those of others with which it interacts. We thank the authors for their cooperation and forbearance in the gestation process. Of many colleagues who have aided us in its preparation, we are especially indebted for help and advice to Myron C. Baker, J. Bruce Falls, Michael Gochfeld, Margaret McVey, William Searcy, George Williams, Larry Wolfe, and Ken Yasukawa.

PETER MARLER

J. G. VANDENBERGH

REFERENCES

Beach, F. A. Behavioral endocrinology: An emerging discipline. *Am. J. Sci.*, 1975, *63*, 178–187.
Brown, J. L., and Orians, G. H. Spacing patterns in mobile animals. *Annu. Rev. Ecol. Syst.* 1970, *1*, 239–262.
Griffin, D. R. Prospects for a cognitive ethology. *Behavioral and Brain Science*. 1978, 1–31.
Hamilton, W. D. The genetical evolution of social behavior. I and II. *J. Theor. Biol.* 1964, *7*, 1–52.
Lehrman, D. S. Control of behavior cycles in reproduction. In W. Etkin (ed.), *Social Behavior and Organization Among Vertebrates*. University of Chicago Press, Chicago, 1964, pp. 143–166.
Mason, W. A. Environmental models and mental modes. *Am. Psychol.* 1976, 284–294.
Maynard-Smith, J. Group selection and kin selection. *Nature*, 1964, *201*, 1145–1147.
Mayr, E. *Animal Species and Evolution*. Belknap Press, Harvard University Press, Cambridge, 1963.
Wilson, E. O. *Sociobiology*. Belknap Press, Harvard University Press, Cambridge, 1975.
Wynne-Edwards, V. C. *Animal Dispersion in Relation to Social Behavior*. Oliver and Boyd, Edinburgh, 1962.
Wynne-Edwards, V. C. Intergroup selection in the evolution of social systems. *Nature*, 1963, *200*, 623–627.

Contents

CHAPTER 1

Ontogeny of Social Behavior 1

William Mason

    Two Perspectives toward Development 2
    Developmental Plasticity 5
    The Evolution of Immaturity 7
    Development in a Social Context 16
    Summary and Conclusions 23
    References 25

CHAPTER 2

On the Physiological Organization of Social Behavior: Sex and Aggression . 29

Norman T. Adler

    Introduction 29
    On the Mechanisms of Sexual Behavior 31
      Introduction 31
      The Choice of Mate 32
      Proper Time and Place 37
      Mechanisms of Copulation 40
      Behavioral Induction of Pregnancy 44
    Some General Properties of Social Behavior and Its Mechanisms 51
      Motivation 53
      Hierarchical Organization 54
    Aggression 56
      General Properties 56
      Neural Organization and the Kinds of Aggression 57

Relation of Aggression to Other Motivational Systems 58
Neurally Defined Components of the Aggressive Response 59
Responses to Aggression 60
References 64

CHAPTER 3

The Analysis of Animal Communication 73

Steven Green and Peter Marler

Introduction 73
Signal Production, Transmission, and Reception 76
   The Sender 76
   The Receiver 77
   Signal Direction 78
   Noise 80
   Transmission and the Environment 82
Internal Transformations in Signal Processing 83
   Transformation Rules 83
   Generality of Transformations 84
   Specificity of the Transformation 86
   Unique Determination by the Transformation 87
   Uniqueness and Specificity 88
Signal Variation 89
   Stereotypy and Variability 90
   Categories of Signaler Output 91
   Receiving Animals: Input 95
   Digital versus Analog Coding in Signals 96
   Arbitrariness versus Iconicity 97
   Categorical and Continuous Perception 99
   Discrete and Graded Communication Systems 103
   Open and Closed Systems 106
The Heredity and Ontogeny of Communication 107
   Signaling, Sensation, and Perception 108
   Shared Procedures for Production and Perception 109
   Birdsong: Production and Perception 110
   The Motor Theory of Speech Perception 112
   Sensory Templates and Schemata 113
Signal Structure and Function 114
   The Importance of Context and Past Experiences 114
   An Unidentified Signal 115
   Identifying Signaler Species 116
   Signal Species-Specificity 117
Further Recognition of Signaler Identity 120
   Individual Recognition 120
   Discrimination of a Familiar from Others 121
   Strangeness, Familiarity, and Kin Recognition 122

Birdsong Dialects 124
Sex and Age 124
The Signal Address 125
Deictic Signals 125
Selective Addressing 125
Signals and External Referents 127
Affect plus Indexing 127
Enemy Specifications 127
Arousal, Emotion, and External Referents 129
Food Specification 130
Symbolic Signaling: Alarm Calls 130
Artificial Communication Systems 133
Signals and Internal Referents 134
Internal and External Triggering 135
Communicative Familiarity and Social Organization 136
New Directions 137
Signaling: Specification of Conditions for Signal Production 138
Signal Form: Selective Pressures and Description 138
Correlations between Signal Perception and Production 139
Responses: Effects of Signal Perception on Behavior 140
References 143

CHAPTER 4

Mechanisms and Evolution of Spacing in Animals 159

Peter M. Waser and R. Haven Wiley

Quantitative Description of Spacing Patterns 161
Activity Fields and Movement Patterns 161
Spatial Relations between Individuals 167
Behavioral Mechanisms of Spacing 173
Reactions to an Opponent's Proximity 174
Variation in Agonistic Tendencies with Location: Aggression Fields 177
Individual and Population Differences in Agonistic Tendencies 182
Categories of Individuals That Engage in Spacing Behavior 187
Conclusion 191
Communication of Advertisement or Threat 191
General Considerations 192
Channels for Spacing Signals 193
Adaptations of Signal Structure 194
Evolution of Spacing Behavior 196
Costs and Benefits of Spacing 197
Analysis of Contingencies in Social Interactions 199
Spacing in Relation to a Resource: Individuals with Bases of Operation 200
Spacing in Relation to Resources: A General Perspective 203
Spacing in Relation to Resources: Examples 206
Other Influences on the Evolution of Spacing Behavior 209

Conclusion 210
Appendix 210
References 212

CHAPTER 5

Foraging Strategies and Their Social Significance 225

John R. Krebs

Introduction 225
Allocation of Foraging Time between Areas 228
   Simple Rules of Allocation 228
   Optimal Time Allocation: Theory 231
   Optimal Time Allocation: Evidence 234
   Group Foraging and Time Allocation 241
   Time Allocation without Prey Depletion 245
Search Paths 246
   Optimal Search Paths 246
   Modification of Search Path through Experience 248
   Optimal Return Times 250
The Choice of Prey Types 254
   Optimal Choice: Theory 254
   Optimal Diets: Evidence 255
   Discussion 259
Sampling and Optimal Foraging 259
The Cost of Alternative Foraging Activities 260
Specialists and Generalists 261
Feeding Dispersion: Cost-Benefit Analyses 262
Conclusions 265
References 266

CHAPTER 6

The Evolution of Mating Systems in Birds and Mammals 271

James F. Wittenberger

Introduction 271
Male Competition and Female Choice 273
Female Competition and Male Choice 274
Terminology 276
Territorial Polygyny 278
   Theory 278
   Effects of Polygyny on Male Parental Behavior 282
   Evidence for the Polygyny-Threshold Model 284
   Colonial Rodents 288
   Other Mammals 292
   Passerine Birds 295
   Exceptions to the Polygyny-Threshold Model 303
Harem Polygyny 304

Polyandry 305
   Polygynous–Polyandrous Systems 305
   Simultaneous Polyandry 309
Promiscuity 311
   Theory 311
   Mammals 312
   Precocial Birds 314
   Altricial Birds 317
   Leks 321
Monogamy 323
   Theory 323
   Altricial Birds 324
   Precocial and Semiprecocial Birds 326
   Mammals 328
Conclusion 331
References 332

CHAPTER 7

The Roles of Individual, Kin, and Group Selection in the Evolution of
Sociality 351

Sandra L. Vehrencamp

Introduction 351
Individual, Kin, and Group Selection Defined 352
   Individual Selection 354
   Kin Selection 356
   Group Selection 360
Indices for the Relative Importance of Individual, Kin, and Group
Selection 362
   Individual versus Kin Selection 363
   Individual versus Group Selection 366
Evolutionary Routes to Sociality 367
   Spiders 369
   Insects 371
   Birds 373
   Mammals 376
Role of Environmental Factors 379
   Factors Affecting Group Stability 379
   Factors Leading to Cooperative Behavior 380
   What Cooperative Behaviors Are Most Likely to Lead to a Reproductive
   Division of Labor? 381
   How Much Skew Is Possible? 382
   The Effects of Cooperation and Manipulation among Kin 384
   Ecological Factors Affecting Group Selection 388
References 389

Index 395

Ontogeny of Social Behavior

WILLIAM MASON

Social ontogeny is the process of becoming social. If all organisms sprang into the world Minerva-like, complete and fully equipped with adult forms and functions, social ontogeny as a discipline could not exist. If all organisms moved from conception to maturity as though every detail in their individual careers was determined from the outset by the inexorable unfolding of some grand primordial plan, it would exist as a legitimate field of inquiry, but one that held little interest for the behavioral scientist. All is not ordained, however. What makes the study of social ontogeny an absorbing and challenging field for behavioral research is the presence of ordered variability in process and outcome. Becoming social is a matter of individual history—part of the unending dialogue between the organism and its environment that is characteristic of all life processes. More than that, it is the development of competences and skills, of deficiences and aberrations, the realization of potentials whose nature can be discerned only after the fact.

The special features of social development have to do, on the one hand, with sources of developmental change and, on the other hand, with the form and functional properties of developmental outcomes. In other words, what distinguishes social ontogeny as a field of inquiry from other investigations of behavioral development is the nature of the independent and dependent variables. The decision to define these variables in exclusively social terms is always somewhat arbitrary, a fact that is probably recognized by every serious student of the subject. Nevertheless, the data on social development are so voluminous that most writers tend to treat it as though it was a field sufficient unto itself and independent of

WILLIAM MASON   Psychology Department and California Primate Research Center, University of California, Davis, California 95616. Preparation of this article was aided by National Institutes of Health Grants HD06367 and RR00169.

broader developmental issues. For this reason, I have chosen in this essay to consider social ontogeny within a larger conceptual framework. The first section presents two general perspectives toward development; the next section deals with some general issues relating to developmental plasticity. The third section attempts to integrate variations in plasticity and developmental rates within an evolutionary framework. The final section examines some of the special problems and possibilities that are created when development occurs within a social milieu.

Two Perspectives toward Development

The fact that behavior develops is beyond dispute. What is made of this fact, however, depends on one's point of view. There are two major perspectives toward development, the organismic and the mechanistic. These views are based on different metaphors or models of what the world is like, and they are associated with different assumptions about what behavior is and how it should be approached scientifically (Langer, 1969; Reese and Overton, 1970; Overton and Reese, 1973). My preference, like that of most animal behaviorists, is for the organismic perspective. It is, in my opinion, more complete and comprehensive than the mechanistic view and more fully articulated with evolutionary theory, and it will in the long run prove more fruitful of hypotheses and explanations; that point of view pervades this essay. Nevertheless, it will be useful to present both perspectives, not only because the juxtaposition will sharpen the distinctive features of each, but also because the mechanistic approach, emphasizing, as it does, methodological rigor and theoretical parsimony, is a cogent reminder of some enduring scientific virtues. The distinguishing features of behavior from each perspective are presented in Table I.

The mechanistic perspective approaches the world as though it is a gigantic machine in which each part, in principle, bears a determinant relation to every other part, the whole being nothing more than the sum of its parts. Although this model can be traced back at least as far as Democritus, and owes much to Descartes and Locke, it received its primary scientific impetus from Newtonian physics.

In behavioral science, the mechanistic view is represented most clearly by the radical behaviorists. Individuals are reactive. They are incapable of spontaneity, lack autonomy, do not initiate behavior, and act only when acted upon. Because behavior is closely tied to external causes, the environment (conceptualized in terms of eliciting and supporting stimuli and reinforcing events) is emphasized as the primary determinant of the nature and direction of behavioral change. The chief mechanism for bringing this about is associative learning. Changes not attributable to experience (the environment) are ascribed to maturation (heredity).

In practice, the mechanistic approach to behavior is also characterized by its lack of systematic concern with evolution and species differences, and by a strong positivistic or operationalist tone, reflected in a passion for experimenter control over independent and dependent variables and a general aversion toward hypothetical structures and inferred processes, particularly those with mentalistic connotations. Behavioral development is conceptualized as continuous, incremental, and quantitative—the result of maturation and the steady accretion of stimulus–response associations. Qualitative differences are reducible in principle to quantitative variations (e.g., Baer, 1970; Bijou, 1968; Skinner, 1966).

The organismic alternative to the mechanistic view also has roots in the philosophy of the ancient Greeks; in more recent times, it was influenced by Leibniz, Kant, and Hegel. It received its major scientific impetus, however, from Charles Darwin. It views the world in terms of process and change. Individuals are active, self-regulating, organized wholes in continuous interchange with the environment. The living system is greater than the sum of its parts, and each part derives its meaning from its place within the whole.

This perspective inevitably has a strong teleological or teleonomic flavor. The living system is a system for living (Weiss, 1973). Organisms are viewed in terms of functions and the "purposes" or "vital ends" these functions serve. However, modern biological thought rejects the idea that such ends are necessarily recognized or sought by the individual or serve as the effective causes of its behavior. Instead, it is accepted that organisms *seem* to behave purposively, and this is a fact that needs to be explained (Nagel, 1957; Beckner, 1968; Pittendrigh, 1958).

TABLE I. PERSPECTIVES TOWARD DEVELOPMENT[a]

Mechanistic	Organismic
1. Reactive organism model of behavior.	1. Active organism model of behavior.
2. Organism is a collection of elements (elementarism) that cannot combine to yield emergent properties.	2. Organism is organized totality— each part derives its meaning from the whole.
3. Analysis based on antecedent–consequent relations—not structures, but causes and effects; not functions, but contingent relations.	3. Defining functions or goals and investigating the structures or means that serve them is a major task.
4. Behavior changes during development.	4. Structures and functions change during development.
5. All change is continuous; emergent qualitative differences are only apparent; emergence is predictable from the history of the organism.	5. Changes in parts or in the organization of parts result in a whole with new systemic properties.
6. Types of causes required for a complete explanation: (a) genetic and maturational (material) causes (b) interact with physical and social environment (efficient causes) (c) to produce behavioral change.	6. Types of causes required for a complete explanation: (a) phylogenetic programs (genetic, maturational = material causes) (b) interact with physical and social environment (efficient causes) (c) to produce or modify a series of structures (formal causes) (d) which result in functional changes.
7. One-way causality between environment and organism.	7. Reciprocal action or interaction between organism and environment.

[a]After Overton and Reese (1973); Langer (1969).

Darwin's contribution, of course, was to provide a conceptual framework in which apparent purpose is explained in principle without recourse to supernatural agents or forces. Natural selection accounts only for the possibility of purpose, however; it does not explain how purpose is built into the living system; it cannot identify the proximate causes of purposive behavior; it gives no clue as to how an adaptive outcome is actually achieved by a given individual, or to the conditions in which this will not occur. These are empirical questions and they constitute a major task for ontogenetic studies—as indeed they do for all behavioral research. Tolman (1932) recognized this many years ago, but the necessary conceptual tools for dealing with purpose have been much expanded and refined since his time, notably by developments in cybernetics and general systems theory (e.g., Bertalanffy, 1968; Rosenblueth, Wiener, and Bigelow, 1968; Bowlby, 1969).

For both perspectives, the relationship between the organisms and the environment is a central concern. In contrast to the mechanistic view, however, which considers the contributions of heredity and environment to development additive, the organismic model rejects the idea that ontogenetic determinants can be neatly partitioned into *innate* and *acquired;* opinions among organismic theorists differ chiefly regarding whether, or in what sense, these terms retain any scientific utility. A few ethologists in the classic tradition, such as Lorenz (1965), Eibl-Eibesfeldt (1970), and Hess (1970), still claim that it is useful to dichotomize specific patterns of behavior as innate or acquired, although they believe that gross behavior most often consists of an interweaving of these elements. The more popular position, however, is that the interpenetration of genetic and environmental influences is complete at all levels of function, and during all phases of ontogenetic development. Different degrees of openness, plasticity, or susceptibility to environmental influence are recognized, but these are regarded as phenotypic–functional properties of biological systems, with no direct bearing on the (unanswerable) question of whether the source of these properties is attributable primarily to genome or environment (Lehrman, 1970; Mason, 1970; Wilcock, 1972; Weiss, 1973; Mayr, 1974).

In any event, adherents of the organismic perspective agree that the organism's relations with the environment are selective and transactional. Reciprocity is the rule. At every stage in its development, the individual is an organized entity— an ongoing enterprise with established needs and functions, constrained by its existing organization—in active commerce with its environment. It selects from what it encounters in its surround, altering both itself and its environment as a consequence. Such transactions are characteristic of life processes at every level. At the level of behavioral development, they are the primary agents of organizational change. In the course of development, specific behaviors are brought into new working relationships within established action systems, existing systems acquire new functions, and new "higher-order" systems emerge (e.g., Schneirla, 1966; Bruner, 1967–1968; Kuo, 1967; Mason, 1970; Piaget, 1971; Wapner, Kaplan, and Cohen, 1973; Wertheim, 1975).

Implicit in this orientation is the idea that developmental changes are always guided by and occur within the framework of existing systems. These systems are inferential or hypothetical, of course, and various terms have been used to identify them. The term I will use is *schema*. Schemata are considered to be inherent species-characteristic modes of organizing experience and of acting on information received (Vernon, 1955; Flavell, 1963). They play a major role in the performance of biologically essential tasks, such as mating, caring for young, forming filial bonds, reacting to predators, and capturing prey. These performances are not based on a single schema, however, but on multiple schemata, usually organized hierarchically in ascending levels of complexity and control. In this form, they provide the basic ground plan within which behavioral development proceeds (Mason, 1968).

DEVELOPMENTAL PLASTICITY

Although these systems buffer, channel, and constrain development, they are also undergoing change as they do so. The essential idea is contained in Piaget's complemental concepts of assimilation (input from the environment is taken up and processed within existing systems) and accommodation (the systems are altered as a consequence of this activity).

The susceptibility of schemata to modification by experience is referred to as *openness*. Openness is always relative, a matter of degree. For example, the schema activated by a rapid increase in the size of an image on the retina (*looming*, or the visual equivalent of an impending collision) appears to be relatively closed, as compared to the schema elicited by the inverse stimulus, contraction of the image. The stimulus of looming produces persistent fear and withdrawal in rhesus monkeys, regardless of their age or previous experience, whereas the contraction of the stimulus apparently produces no stereotyped reaction, although it evokes signs of "interest" or "curiosity" (Schiff, Caviness, and Gibson, 1962).

Three different aspects of openness can be distinguished on logical grounds and are readily demonstrated empirically. They relate to the effective stimulus, to the flexibility and versatility of motor acts, and to what goes on between receiving and acting (decision making, the processing of information). It is safe to assert that, in general, openness is greater for the input than for the output or response-generating components of schemata. This is not to say that the normal development of motor patterns is independent of use, of course. On the contrary, numerous examples, covering a variety of species, from monkeys to salamanders, indicate that the effective application of motor patterns requires some degree of practice, or *tuning*, particularly where close and precise coordination with environmental structures is involved. For instance, Held and Bauer (1967, 1974) have shown that infant macaque monkeys raised from birth in a situation that prevented them from seeing their own hands were inferior to age-matched controls in accuracy of reaching toward a visible object. Nevertheless, the basic schema for eye–hand coordination was present, as evidenced by the fact that reaching in the general direction of the object occurred almost from the beginning, and by the finding that with opportunity for rehearsal and "self-instruction," the accuracy of performance improved noticeably within a matter of hours. In contrast to this rather modest degree of plasticity on the motor side of schemata, the vast literature on conditioning and discrimination learning attests to great plasticity on the input side.

Even so, it must be recognized that even here openness is not unconstrained. From the very beginning of receptor-guided interactions with the environment, stimuli are responded to selectively. Whether the schemata are concerned with the imprinting of the following response, the acquisition of song, or the selection of mates, there exist species-characteristic predilections for certain sensory modes, stimulus attributes, classes, or configurations. For example, rhesus monkeys during their first encounters with solid food (banana, variously colored with food dyes) showed a preference for orange over blue and green (Mason and Harlow, 1959). Likewise, certain colors and shapes are differentially effective in eliciting pecking by chicks and ducklings. Similar predilections have been described for the imprinting of the filial following response (Gottlieb, 1973; Hess, 1973).

The most significant, complex, and elusive aspect of openness concerns the central processing of information, what goes between receiving a stimulus and producing a response. Included here are the capabilities for putting together information from different modalities or from the same modality at different points in time and for abstracting, generalizing, and forming rules, strategies, and sets. What makes these higher-order functions possible is by no means certain. What is established beyond reasonable doubt is that they are not restricted to man and his closest biological kin (for they have been demonstrated in a variety of mammalian and avian species) and that their development is critically dependent on prior experience. For example, young socially sophisticated rhesus monkeys in competitive and agonistic situations display a number of social strategies that allow them to gain an advantage beyond any directly determined by their individual standings in the status hierarchy. They have knowledge of the power structure of the group and can apply this knowledge to their own advantage. Monkeys that have had no prior experience with group life lack these higher-order skills, and for such individuals, successes and failures are directly related to their ability to dominate other members of their group (Anderson and Mason, 1974; Anderson and Mason, 1978).

As a general rule, openness is greatest during the time when a system is undergoing rapid development, and, of course, this is most characteristic of the early phases of the life cycle. A useful distinction, suggested by Callaway (1970), is between general plasticity and special sensitivity.

The concept of special sensitivity is the easiest to illustrate, for the phenomenon is widespread and has been investigated extensively. The essential idea is that there exists a more-or-less circumscribed stage in the development of a system, often called the *critical period* or *sensitive period,* when the system is maximally susceptible to environmental influences (Scott, Stewart, and DeGhett, 1974). The concept does not imply that the period of special sensitivity is necessarily sharply circumscribed in time, or that the initial response to the environment is nonselective, or that experiences obtained during the sensitive period cannot under any circumstances be overridden by subsequent events. How these parameters are expressed very much depends on the species and on the particular functional systems.

The classic examples of age-related openness are filial imprinting of the following response in precocial birds and the acquisition of song in some altricial avian species. There are ample grounds, however, for supposing that analogous conditions exist in the development of other functional systems for a variety of species. Food preferences, for instance, appear to be established by the earliest feeding experiences in some reptiles (snapping turtles, diamond-back terrapins), birds (gulls, domestic chickens, finches), and mammals (some rodents, carnivores, primates). The early establishment of abiding preferences has also been reported for habitat selection in various species of fish, amphibia, birds, and rodents; for host preferences in parasitic birds and insects; and for mate selection in birds. (For reviews see Gibson, 1969; Hinde, 1970; Hess, 1973; Brown, 1975; Immelmann, 1975; and Galef, 1976.)

General plasticity refers to a feature of development that is undeniably of the first importance, even though it presents formidable practical as well as theoretical difficulties. General plasticity is closely akin to adaptability. It implies the potential for many different outcomes, only some of which are actually achieved by any given animal. For example, when comparing the same individual at different periods in its life cycle, or animals from the same species raised in radically different environments, or subjects from the different species across a variety of environments, it is clear that gross differences exist in the extent to which the individual is able to modify its behavior in response to changing environmental circumstances. In other words, general plasticity varies in relation to age, prior experience, and phylogeny.

The evidence in support of a concept of general plasticity for all these factors is abundant. With respect to changes with age, the most persuasive findings are at the level of the nervous system. As Jacobson (1969) put it, "During ontogeny, there is evidence of a progressive reduction of the capacity to form new neuronal connections and to modify existing ones." The thesis that within-species variations in general plasticity can be produced by environmental conditions is supported by a huge literature on the effects of early environmental enrichment and deprivation, handling, nutrition, and the like. The evidence for phylogenetic contrasts in general developmental plasticity is most persuasive for species that are widely separated—for example, amphibians versus birds versus mammals—but there is reason to suppose that more refined analyses will reveal reliable differences between orders, between genera, and, possibly, even between species.

The Evolution of Immaturity

I am uncomfortably aware at this point that the major concepts discussed in the previous section—schemata, openness, developmental plasticity—have been developed only sketchily. My aim, however, has been to suggest a way of looking at the phenomena of behavioral ontogeny rather than to proffer explanatory concepts. I have been more concerned with describing what needs to be explained than with offering explanations. The aim of the present section is more ambitious. It will attempt to link broad variations in ontogeny, particularly in the length of the prereproductive period, with the evolution of plasticity and of life-history patterns.

Accordingly, it will be useful to recall at this point that ontogeny, strictly speaking, is a continuous process, extending from conception to senescence, and is subject to natural selection from the beginning to the end of the life cycle. It is the organism's entire life history that evolves. If we tend to lose sight of this obvious fact, it is chiefly because adult animals are usually singled out for special attention in discussions of evolution. This is merely expedient, however, for the adult is only a practical and convenient unit for describing evolutionary change. The adult is the product, after all, of its developmental history.

Phylogeny, in fact, is most properly viewed as a succession of complete ontogenies across many generations, during which certain developmental patterns become progressively more frequent within a population. To be sure, in the final analysis it is gene frequencies that change, but as Waddington (1954) points out, "Changes in genotypes only have ostensible effects in evolution if they bring with them alterations in epigenetic processes by which phenotypes come into being." Modification of developmental patterns through natural selection may thus be regarded as the major source of evolutionary novelty and the primary phenotypic expression of evolutionary change (Waddington, 1954; de Beer, 1958; Beckner, 1968).

Despite the continuous nature of ontogeny, it is obvious that the amount of an individual's resources in time and energy devoted to development varies with particular periods in the life cycle; and as we have seen, ontogenetic changes (and developmental plasticity) are most prominent in the early stages of development. This is the so-called formative period, when the changes are many, are occurring rapidly, and are laying down the groundwork for important adult functions. For our purposes, it may be assumed that this period usually draws to a close at about the same time that the individual achieves reproductive maturity.

Species differ in the length of this period, both in absolute terms and in relation to the total life span. There is no obvious reason that they should do so. In fact, if production of offspring is accepted as the primary measure of evolutionary success, every species should be under strong selection pressure against the evolution of immaturity. Personal resources in time and energy devoted to development during the prereproductive period must be reckoned a "cost" in the currency of fitness. If immaturity has become established by natural selection in spite of this cost, it follows that the disadvantages must be overbalanced by a net gain in fitness. But how does this come about? And what are the advantages of immaturity? Several possibilities have been suggested:

Growth—the laying on of tissue, the building up of reserves—is one obvious benefit that could lead to the prolongation of immaturity beyond the time required for the creation of essential morphological structures. By devoting energy early in life to physical growth, at the expense of reproduction, an individual could become better equipped to exploit vital environmental resources, or to deal with predators, or to compete with its own kind. For example, a male that defers sexual competition until relatively late in life can avoid costly contests that he is likely to lose (perhaps with ruinous consequences) while he builds up the strength to compete later with better chances of success. This may be one reason that the males of many mammalian species in which intermale competition for mates is the norm achieve full sexual maturity later than females. Similarly, the female might improve her lifetime reproductive success by deferring conception until she establishes the physical resources that are called upon for the production and care of offspring. This may be a factor in the widespread phenomenon of adolescent sterility in female mammals (Montagu, 1957).

Another type of benefit that could lead to the prolongation of immaturity is the ability to exploit some resource that is not available to the adult form. This is most clearly the case in species with complex life cycles (Istock, 1967). For example, tadpoles have specialized filter-feeding adaptations that allow them to utilize a transient high-energy resource (plankton suspended in water) that is not available to the adult frog (Wassersug, 1975). It seems unlikely, however, that such benefits have played a significant role in the evolution of immaturity in birds and mammals. Although the young of these species show many distinctive behavior patterns that contribute directly to their survival—for example, gaping, rooting-and-sucking, freezing, following, distress vocalizations—these are more properly viewed as specialized adaptations to the particular conditions of immaturity than as explanations for its existence.

Finally, immaturity may contribute to improved reproductive success by allowing a period for the acquisition of knowledge and skills. This is the most common explanation for the prolonged immaturity of simian primates and man; the gist of the argument is that more time is provided for learning to occur during a period in which the individual enjoys a protected and privileged status, relatively free from the demands that are placed on an independent and self-sustaining adult. There is no reason to suppose that this benefit does not apply as well to other slowly maturing animals.

These are only plausible possibilities, of course, not complete explanations. Obviously, prolonged immaturity is not characteristic of all species, and the hypothesized benefits are evidently contingent on other factors that have yet to be mentioned. What might they be?

What is missing from these explanations is some indication of where immaturity fits into the total life-history pattern. The problem with the potential benefits we have considered is that they are not automatic, self-evident, and universally applicable. Even the hypothesized benefit of "more time for learning" is unsatisfactory in spite of its beguiling simplicity and intuitive appeal.

In the first place, there is no reason to believe that "more learning" is necessarily beneficial to an individual. Assumptions to the effect that learning is always and obviously a "good thing" and the "more learning the better" are plainly anthropocentric. For the majority of animals, learning is pragmatic and utilitarian.

Implicit in the notion that all learning is beneficial is the idea that the ability to learn is a unitary trait, that learning processes are entirely general and universally useful. This idea is at variance with the growing evidence that there are different kinds of learning, that learning varies not only with species but with situations and with phases within the life cycle. (For reviews see Hinde and Stevenson-Hinde, 1973; Warren, 1973; Bolles, 1975; Bitterman and Woodward, 1976; Brookshire,

1976.) These findings are consistent with the view advanced earlier to the effect that acquisition of knowledge and skills is directed and constrained by species-typical characteristics and is articulated within the individual's total life-history pattern. Furthermore, if the advantages of having more time for learning were as uncomplicated and generalized as is commonly supposed, all organisms would be under strong selection pressure to extend the period of immaturity. How then are we to account for the fact that broad differences in developmental rates exist, even (as we shall see) between closely related species?

Another deficiency of the knowledge-and-skills explanation of immaturity is that it does not spell out the functional connections between "more immaturity" and "more learning." The usual argument emphasizes that the immature individual, being buffered and protected by adults, can devote most of its waking hours to the acquisition of knowledge and skills. The presumption is that extending the period of immaturity provides more time for this sort of knowledge building to take place. There are at least two problems with this view. First, it is not at all clear how much more "free time" is available to the immature animal than to the adult or what proportion of it is actually involved in activities that contribute to the acquisition of knowledge and skills; second, there are strong indications that the immature organism, in spite of its greater plasticity, is a less efficient all-around learner than the adult on standardized learning tasks. It would be curious indeed for natural selection to create a special period in life for the acquisition of knowledge and skills and at the same time to produce an organism that did not reach the peak of its learning abilities until it had gone beyond this period; yet this seems to be the case. For the learning-and-skills hypothesis to remain credible, it must deal with this apparent paradox.

The point, then, is that none of the explanations offered to account for the prolongation of immaturity are adequate in their simple form. More is required than a mere enumeration of plausible possibilities. To appreciate the biological meaning of immaturity, it is necessary to recognize that the prereproductive period is only a segment in the total life cycle, one element in a broader adaptive strategy, whose evolutionary significance must be sought in terms of its place within the total pattern and its contribution to the whole.

As it happens, there is one rather common life-history pattern that holds a special interest for the present account. In this pattern, a relatively prolonged period of immaturity appears in association with several other traits, namely, small litter or clutch size, a wide interbirth interval, extended postnatal care, behavioral plasticity (expressed in playfulness, curiosity, "intelligence," lack of stereotypy in social relations, etc.), and a long life span. The correlations among these traits are far from perfect, but they occur together frequently enough and in a sufficient variety of disparate species to suggest that they are elements in a general adaptive strategy. For example, some of the largest raptorial birds, such as the Andean condor or the crowned eagle, do not reach sexual maturity until 4 years of age or older (much longer than the time required by most birds); they lay only one or two eggs per clutch; they feed their young for a year or more; and in contrast to the general pattern, they have nesting cycles that cover considerably more than one year (Amadon, 1964; Lack, 1966). Moreover, "play" behavior is often seen in the juveniles of such species (Ashmole and Tovar, 1968). A similar syndrome is displayed by the Olympic marmot, as compared to related species of *Marmota*, such as the woodchuck or the yellow-bellied marmot. Olympic marmots breed only in alternate years, the young live in their mother's burrow throughout their first year, and they take more than twice as long as the woodchuck to reach sexual maturity; they are also more socially tolerant and playful than members of the other *Marmota* species (Barash, 1974).

Two kinds of interpretations have been offered to account for the evolution of this syndrome. One, the "goodness-of-fit" interpretation, emphasizes the correlation between the trait pattern and specific, measurable features of the habitat (e.g., predation pressure and the amount, distribution, and stability of essential resources) in which the species is currently found (and in which it has presumably lived for many generations). The other, the "adaptive-potential" interpretation, regards the trait pattern as the expression of a change in the organization of behavior and emphasizes its general utility as a means of coping with environmental variability. Although the two interpretations are not fundamentally incompatible, they have developed more-or-less independently and focus on different aspects of the evolutionary process. The aim of this account is to describe the salient features of each interpretation, their similarities, and the contrasts between them.

The goodness-of-fit orientation toward development is characteristic of the ecologist or the population biologist. The focal question is what sort of environment is most likely to give rise to prolonged immaturity and its associated life-history traits. The usual answer is an environment that is heterogeneous, yet fairly stable (i.e., not subject to catastrophic variation), and in which essential resources are relatively scarce or can be utilized only by means of specialized skills or capture techniques. The population is near the environment's carrying capacity, and mortality is more likely to depend on the density of the population than on climatic factors or violent fluctuations in the level of vital resources. These are essentially the conditions that MacArthur and Wilson posit as leading to *K*-selection (Pianka, 1970; Wilson, 1975). Under such conditions, competition is keen and "the optimal strategy is to channel all available energy into maintenance and production of a few extremely fit offspring" (Pianka, 1970). In other words, selection favors quality over quantity—fewer offspring, which are more carefully nurtured and protected over a longer period of time and which are better prepared to cope with changing circumstances. This line of reasoning has been most persuasive in accounting for variations in developmental rates when the comparison species are closely related and the environments they currently occupy differ in precisely those ways that underscore the utility of the syndrome (e.g., Amadon, 1964; Ashmole and Tovar, 1968; Barash, 1974; Brown, 1974; Richardson, 1975). For example, Barash (1974) shows that the period of immaturity, the interval between births, and the degree of parental tolerance of maturing young are least in marmot species occupying temperate environments and increase progressively in higher latitudes as the habitat becomes more rigorous.

The adaptive-potential orientation is concerned with the proximal mechanisms that produce the immaturity syndrome and with the functional characteristics that make it an effective strategy. This approach shares with the goodness-of-fit interpretation the view that the immaturity syndrome provides a selective advantage in environments that are relatively unpredictable or place unusual demands on the organism. Instead of focusing on the syndrome strictly as it relates to contemporary environmental conditions, however, this orientation assigns the syndrome a broad and recurrent role in vertebrate evolution. Most habitats, after all, are characterized by some degree of uncertainty and change. No doubt, this is the reason that the overall trend in vertebrate evolution conforms to the K-selection model. Nevertheless, as Pianka (1970) has pointed out, K-selection and r-selection (which favors rapid growth, early reproduction, and large numbers of offspring) can be viewed as opposite ends of a continuum rather than as categorical alternatives. It seems likely that an evolving population shifts toward one end or the other of this continuum in response to enduring changes in the environment.

How do such shifts come about? It seems likely that the principal means of producing movement toward either end of the continuum in relatively few generations and without the need for radical structural change is through a modification in developmental schedules. What is accomplished by such shifts? The answer depends on whether one adopts a goodness-of-fit or an adaptive-potential orientation.

According to the goodness-of-fit interpretation (at least within the r- and K-selection framework), emphasis is placed on the characteristics and requirements of the current environment. Short-lived, fluctuating habitats favor low parental investment per offspring and the production of numerous progeny, at least some of which will have a chance to move into new and potentially more propitious habitats. This outcome is accomplished by a shift toward rapid individual growth, early reproduction, and high reproductive rates (r-selection). More stable environments, less subject to wide swings in available resources, favor greater parental investment per offspring and production of progeny with superior competitive skills. This outcome is accomplished by more extended parental care, wider interbirth intervals, and the other characteristics of the immaturity syndrome (K-selection).

The adaptive-potential interpretation places greater emphasis on niche characteristics than on gross features of the habitat, and it views the immaturity syndrome as being especially advantageous for individuals adapted to a broad niche and occupying a habitat that is necessarily heterogeneous in space or variable over time (Klopfer, 1962). In other words, according to this view, the most significant consequence of the immaturity syndrome is increased adaptability, the chief expression of which is behavioral plasticity.

To appreciate the interrelations between the habitat, behavioral flexibility, and the nature of the ecological niche, recall that the problem of adaptation to the environment always presents two facets, one relating to short-term survival and the other to more long-term evolutionary prospects. Every successful individual must adapt to a particular set of environmental circumstances, characteristic of a specific time and place. This adaptation to contemporary conditions is short-term, for the obvious reason that no environment remains completely constant for very long. Hence, members of a successful species must also possess a measure of adaptability, or the capacity to adjust to change. Although both requirements must be met in some degree by members of any viable species, the emphasis varies. Individuals of some species are best equipped to deal with a narrow niche in a habitat where the conditions essential to life are relatively stable; individuals of other species are adapted to a broader niche and can accommodate to a much broader range of environmental variation. In fact, there are reasons to suppose that these two modes of adaptation are in some degree opposed (Gause, 1942; Thoday, 1954).

The source of this antagonism can be clarified by considering the familiar distinction between the "specialist" and the "generalist." The specialist, it is often said, does one thing very well. It is best equipped to function within a narrow niche, in an environment that is relatively constant. On its own ground, it can compete effectively against a more opportunistic intruder, precisely because of its specialized traits. If the environment does not change appreciably over many generations, the expected trend is for the genotype of such a species to change progressively in ways that reduce both genetic and phenotypic variability, because variability in such circumstances is more likely to detract from adaptedness than to improve it. Phenotypically, this means that individuals in a population moving toward increased specialization become ever more finely tuned to specific features of the habitat until, in due course, the population reaches an adaptive plateau. At this point, the individual's early development is expected to be strongly channelized or homeostatic, firmly buffered against deflection by minor perturbations in the environment; its behavior will likewise be relatively impoverished in resources for coping with novelty and change. In effect, the population has moved toward the r end of the r- and K-continuum.

For the generalist, such a high degree of closed programming is clearly contrary to basic adaptive strategy. "Goodness-of-fit" within a particular environment is always desirable, of course, but only when this is compatible with preserving adaptability. The opportunist operates within a broad niche; heterogeneity is its forte; like Heraclitus, it carries the motto "Perpetual change." For such an individual, phenotypic flexibility is the mainstay of evolutionary success.

How is such flexibility achieved? I am proposing that one way that has been taken repeatedly by various species is by prolonging immaturity. The mere fact that an animal takes longer to achieve adult status is no reason to suppose that flexibility will be increased, of course, but as we have seen, the immaturity syndrome encompasses more than a mere prolongation of the prereproductive period; it is a constellation of traits. The present thesis is that this constellation reflects fundamental changes in the way behavior is organized, the major result of which is increased adaptability throughout the life cycle. In short, the immaturity syndrome offers, in Hardy's (1963) phrase, an avenue of "escape from specialization."

In what way does the syndrome lead to this outcome? Consider a prototypic specialist, well adapted to a relatively narrow and homogeneous niche. Such an individual, like all behaving organisms, deals with information. I have suggested that the processing of information occurs within organized systems or schemata.

The expected trend is for the specialist to move toward schemata that are relatively closed. The reasons must be sought in the advantages provided by closed schemata. The major ones are: they are not easily deflected during development by chance variations in the environment; they can develop as rapidly as possible within the limits set by structural growth (because they depend upon no specialized environmental inputs or opportunities); and they are unlikely to make costly mistakes, at least in the ecology in which they evolve. The real-life counterparts of this hypothetical prototype are those creatures whose early development and mature behavior is described as "rigid," "stereotyped," "prewired," or "innate."

But suppose the habitat were to shift in a direction that was disadvantageous to a relatively specialized population, for example, by becoming somewhat less stable and predictable? The adaptive problem becomes one of moving from a rigid pattern of behavioral organization toward a form that is more responsive to variations in the environment, is more capable of adjusting to change, and yet preserves as much of the existing behavioral repertoire and organization as possible. To dispense with schemata altogether is unthinkable. The *tabula rasa* would be as disastrous for behavior as for any other biological system. A more workable solution is to maintain the basic structural features of available schemata, while making them more open to immediate environmental influences.

I suggest that a first step toward accomplishing this solution is to retard the rate at which these functional systems develop, to maintain them in a somewhat immature and hence incomplete state. As a consequence, sensitive periods should become less prominent and sharply defined, and plasticity should become more generalized and prolonged. Presumably, this outcome could be brought about by changes in the regulatory functions of the genome, probably acting through the endocrine system. It would be advantageous to the individual if retardation could be achieved selectively, so that he reached reproductive maturity as close to the normal age as possible. This would enable him to derive the benefits of increased plasticity, while losing nothing in reproductive potential.

In the classic examples of neoteny among invertebrates and amphibians, the significant feature appears to be a retardation in the rate of somatic growth, relative to that of the reproductive glands; seemingly this retardation is achieved without delaying the onset of reproductive maturity. In birds and mammals, however, the critical factor is retardation in the rate of behavioral development rather than somatic growth, and in this case, selectivity is apparently no more than partial. Thus, in the best-documented examples, such as the nonhuman primates, the trend is for all aspects of development to undergo some degree of retardation. Even so, the physiological capabilities for reproduction may be present at earlier ages than is usually supposed. De Beer points out that the ovary of humans, the slowest-developing primates, attains its full size at the age of about 5 years (de Beer, 1958). Although this development does not imply that the reproductive system is functionally complete at this age, there are many authenticated cases of children as young as 8 or 9 years of age bearing children, and at least one documented example of a child of 5 years 8 months giving birth to a normal and viable infant (Montagu, 1957). There are other indications of dissociation between the physiological capabilities for reproduction and the onset of reproductive behavior in slowly maturing birds and mammals. Some condors, for instance, do not begin to lay until they are 9–12 years old, even though they are fully grown and independent of the parents by the end of their second year of life (Amadon, 1964); male macaque monkeys are capable of fertile mating at 3.3 years, less than half the age of full physical and social maturity for these primates (Maple, Erwin, and Mitchell, 1973).

The generalized openness that presumably results from an overall retardation of behavioral development achieves nothing unless means are available to ensure that schemata achieve some degree of functional integrity before they are called upon to regulate vital transactions with the environment. Moreover, open schemata are expected to reflect more accurately the particular structure, special features, or specific demands of the developmental environment (which could vary significantly from one generation to the next) than do more closed systems, and to preserve a greater degree of plasticity throughout the life cycle. It follows that those organisms that are moving in the direction of greater developmental openness and behavioral flexibility encounter strong selection pressures toward increased capacities for picking up, processing, and storing information.

These increased capacities imply a trend toward the elaboration of various "experience-producing" activities, such as play, exploration, manipulation, and the like (Hayes, 1962). As between two related taxa, individuals from the more open and slowly maturing species are expected to spend more time in the waking day engaged in experience-producing activities, to show a greater variety of them (or display them in less stereotyped form), and to engage in them during a relatively longer portion of the total life cycle. An anticipated corollary to this development is an improved capacity for incidental learning, and in fact, substantial correlations have been reported between curiosity and learning ability (Lester, 1974). Most learning during ontogeny is presumably guided by nascent schemata at the same time that it contributes to their development, as reflected in the phenomena of play at "fighting," "prey capture," "mating," "mothering," and "nest building" and the frequent appearance of the biting, chewing, and tasting of all manner of objects by the immature of many mammalian species. This is not to say that all incidental learning is necessarily constrained by major functional systems, but for the majority of species, a reasonable view is that most of it is.

The pressures that lead to an increased capacity for picking up, processing, and storing information should also lead to changes in the brain, the organ chiefly responsible for these functions. The significant changes will be functional, of course, but one might expect correlated changes in size (or brain–body ratios), differential growth in various regions of the brain (particularly those subserving "reversible" functions—such as attention, motivation, and learning—that mediate most directly between the organism and environmental variations), and a relatively longer period of brain growth. With respect to the latter, it is significant that data on neonatal brain and body weight and on gestation times for more than 90 mammalian species indicate that fetal brain growth is the major variable associated with increased gestation time (Sacher and Staffeldt, 1974). Moreover, in many animals, the growth of the brain continues after birth and is definitely influenced by the postnatal environment (e.g., Rosenzweig, 1966; Sperry, 1968; Callaway,

1970). It is also significant that species producing young with larger brains tend to have smaller litter size and a longer life span (Sacher, 1959; Sacher and Staffeldt, 1974). Thus, there is reason to expect that changes in the brain figure prominently in the evolution of the immaturity syndrome.

These data suggest that species tending toward longer life spans and smaller litter size also tend to have longer gestation times and to produce young with larger neonatal brains, which presumably continue to develop for a longer period after birth and are more open to postnatal environmental influences. The associations among at least some of these traits have been established by comparative correlational studies; others exist only as testable possibilities. Although there is no reason to suppose that all traits of the immaturity syndrome are tightly joined, it seems likely that given sufficient time, they will co-evolve. Thus, from a microevolutionary point of view, a population undergoing selection in the direction of greater openness may display strongly only a few traits of the immaturity syndrome, as compared to closely related species. From the macroevolutionary standpoint, however, the syndrome can be seen as a recurrent theme that waxes and wanes as a population shifts toward a relatively narrow niche (a move that is most likely to be adaptive in a relatively stable environment) or toward a broader niche (for which a variable or heterogeneous environment is required). We may suppose, however, that under all conditions, the amount of environmental variability is such that the syndrome retains some utility and therefore is never abandoned entirely. In fact, because the long-range advantage seems to lie in the direction of increased plasticity, it is easy to appreciate why the dominant trend in mammalian evolution has been toward the K-selection pattern.

Development in a Social Context

Openness, whether it relates to general plasticity or to more circumscribed sensitive periods, entails some obvious developmental risks. Chicks and ducklings can form filial attachments to balloons or flashing lights, and monkeys, to terry cloth towels; kittens accustomed to nursing from an artificial feeder will reject their real mother, even when she is the only source of food available; sparrows that have had no opportunity to hear other sparrows sing fail to develop the normal song pattern. And examples could be multiplied manyfold.

What usually prevents these atypical outcomes, of course, is that the newborn enters an environment for which it has been shaped by evolution. It is prepared to accommodate to and function within a limited range of circumstances, to encounter an environment that is so structured as to make the likelihood of "mistakes," such as those I have mentioned, extremely remote.

For the young of all mammals and the vast majority of birds, this environment includes other members of the same species—most often parents and siblings. Like other aspects of the environment, they may be considered potential resources for the developing individual. Presumably, they play a significant part in its development. But what do they contribute? And how are these contributions made? These questions provide the primary focus of this section.

The potential contributions of the social environment to development may be considered to fall within two broad classes: trophic and informational. Trophic resources consist of the energy and materials that are essential to sustain life, and, of course, specialized systems have evolved for making use of them. Informational resources are distinguished by the fact that their primary effect is to produce or control changes in organization; they too are handled by specialized systems, chiefly the sense receptors. Information derived in this fashion may be regarded as the primary external source of knowledge about the environment and of skills in dealing with it (Orians, 1969; Jander, 1975).

It is reasonable to assume that meeting the trophic requirements of the young has played a primary part in the evolution of parental behavior and that it occupies the central place in the relations between parent and young in vertebrate species. Indeed, one can imagine a species in which the parents are never in direct contact with their young but, nevertheless, make a vital trophic contribution to their welfare by locating them in a suitable site, protecting them against predation, and providing them with an adequate supply of food. In fulfilling these requirements, the parents virtually guarantee that the offspring will develop normally, along species-typical paths, in spite of the fact that physical separation between the generations is complete.

The more usual pattern for the warm-blooded vertebrates, of course, and the more interesting one for our purposes, is for such functions to be performed by the parent in the presence of the young, thereby creating the possibility of an informational as well as a trophic contribution. The point, however, is that the nature and extent to which the social environment contributes an informational component to development can vary across a broad range, from essentially no contribution, as in our imagined species, to one that is considerable.

As a *potential* source of information, the social environment is unusually rich, having all of the characteristics of the physical environment plus some very special features. In common with the objects of the physical realm, social agents reflect light and they produce thermal, chemical, and mechanical energy, all of which can serve as information sources. They are generally more mobile than the objects of the nonsocial world, of course, which means that they are more changeable stimuli, more capable of presenting novelty, of provoking attention, and of creating problems from the standpoint of identification or recognition. Such problems may be ameliorated considerably, however, by the presence of a large measure of redundancy and invariance. Multiple stimulus attributes from the same social object are likely to covary, to begin and end together, and thus to provide many potential bases for discrimination (Gibson, 1966).

Social agents are also able to act upon their surroundings, and this ability creates another potential source of information of a special sort. By handling objects, making them do things, and altering the environment in various ways, they are able to direct the young animal's attention to particular features of its surroundings, thereby selectively influencing how it perceives and relates to the world.

What distinguishes the social environment above all as a potential source of information for the developing organism is the fact that social agents are themselves information-processing systems. They not only provide information but are capable of receiving it as well. They can act upon others on the basis of information received, and they receive further information on the social consequences of their acts. Immediate social feedback and mutual stimulation permit the development of the most characteristic feature of social life. They are the basis for reciprocity, complementarity, interdependence, and cooperation—phenomena that are seen at all levels of complexity: in discrete two-step communicative acts, in coordinated chains and lengthy sequences of interactions, and in multifaceted relationships that endure over long periods in the developing individual's life cycle.

But if social objects often become the focus of many different activities, touching on various functional systems, they are also variable, capricious, "moody," and generally less predictable than the objects of the inanimate world. A monkey's favorite rock or tree is unlikely to shake him off, to "refuse" him his customary resting place, whereas analogous surprises are not at all uncommon in its social world. The social environment epitomizes Brunswik's (1956) "semierratic medium . . . no more than partially controlled and no more than probabilistically predictable." Coping effectively with such a world can place special demands on information-processing skills.

At the same time, however, prediction is possible. Behavior is orderly in some degree; patterns recur; situations repeat themselves. To the extent that the young animal's behavior contains potential information as to what he is about to do, it provides others with a basis for prediction and control. Among other possibilities, this information places his companions in the peculiar position of being able to "short-circuit" his behavior by responding to probable, rather than actual, consequences of his acts. For example, during the weaning period, a mother might respond punitively to subtle behaviors of her offspring that merely suggest a certain likelihood that it is seeking the nipple, rather than delaying her reaction until the indications are unequivocal that it is actually attempting to nurse. By the same token, she might also act to forestall consequences that might be harmful to the infant or to cause it discomfort or distress.

It will be evident that these are only possibilities, of course. They have been considered in the spirit of Gibson's (1966) "*opportunities* for perception . . . *available* information . . . *potential* stimuli." And as he pointed out, not all opportunities are grasped, not all information is registered, not all stimuli excite receptors. The social environment affords opportunities; it admits possibilities; it creates occasions. But it does not determine whether they will be effective or what effects will be produced.

We know, however, that the social environment is an important information source for many species and that the spectrum of developmental outcomes it affects is exceedingly broad and varied. Many of these effects have been mentioned. They include the choice of parental figures, of sexual partners, and of food; the quality of mothering; the organization of mating and other social skills; and the formation of rather generalized tendencies or predispositions—such as aggressiveness, timidity, and curiosity—that influence response toward other animals or the world at large. (For reviews, see Glass, 1968; Newton and Levine, 1968; Denenberg, 1972.)

This brings us to our second question. How are these effects brought about? A complete answer to this question is not possible at this point, in spite of the abundance of detailed information on the consequences of social experience for a host of species. This is not altogether surprising, for the question really calls for a complete theory of socialization, and, of course, we are still some distance from this goal. Nevertheless, a general outline of the kind of paradigm that is likely to serve is already clear. In fact, it was described earlier as "the organismic perspective."

An important feature of this perspective is that it combines an evolutionary approach to development with the orientation of general systems theory. The latter provides a set of carefully defined terms and explicit concepts that are particularly well suited to handle the organization and behavior of complex biological entities (Ashby, 1958; Bertalanffy, 1968; Weiss, 1973). Two examples of the explicit application to this perspective to the early development of social relationships can be found in Bowlby (1969) and Bischof (1975), but examples of less systematic or complete treatments within a similar conceptual framework abound (e.g., Sackett, 1970; Mason, 1971; Cairns, 1972; Hoffman and Ratner, 1973).

In all such approaches, it is taken for granted that the organism from birth responds selectively to the environment. Selectivity is evident in all major components of information-processing sequences or schemata. It influences the kinds of stimuli that are effective in eliciting a response, the types of response that are elicited, and the *valence,* or *hedonic tone,* that accompanies different kinds of stimulation, including that produced as proprioceptive or environmental feedback from different response patterns. Thus, from the beginning, behavioral development proceeds within the framework of existing structures or functional systems.

The elaboration and refinement of this model so as to take into account the detailed and complex changes in the actual development of living animals observed in real situations have taken a variety of forms. This diversity partly reflects conceptual differences among theorists, but the more significant factor, I believe, has to do with such matters as the range of species that the model is intended to cover, the particular developmental phenomena that it seeks to explain, and the level of analysis that is selected. In other words, differences relate more to scope and emphasis than to matters of principle. For example, Lehrman's (1970) analysis indicates that seemingly irreconcilable theoretical differences between the views of ontogeny advocated by Lorenz and Schneirla relate in large part to the different meanings these authors assign to key terms such as *experience, innate,* and *learning,* as well as to the particular stages of ontogeny that are their focal concern. Schneirla's interest encompasses the earliest stages of behavior development—the embryology of behavior—whereas Lorenz's principal concern is with behavior patterns that have already reached the stage where they can be seen as modes of adaptation to the environment.

To be sure, some conceptual issues remain controversial, but it appears that the most pressing questions of the day relate less to the relative merits of competing conceptualizations than to the lack of precision in the concepts that are available. And such precision can be achieved only as a result of additional empirical research. The two most important issues, in my opinion, concern how we characterize the environmental sources of developmental change and the developmental mechanisms through which such changes are brought about. These issues are obviously interrelated if one accepts an epigenetic view of development, because one cannot fully accomplish the first task without also dealing with the second. Precise description of the effective environmental variables requires comparably precise descriptions of the developmental processes they influence (Gewirtz, 1969).

Such a program focused specifically on the phenomena of socialization involves two essential prerequisites: first, a description of the organization of behavior in the newborn individual, including those propensities that lead it to respond selectively to its surroundings; second, a clear description of the various developmental outcomes or end points that characterize species-typical performance of the normally socialized, biologically competent adult. These descriptions (which are basically normative in character) bracket the temporal domain of the developmental inquiry, and they establish the level of discourse that will guide it. Intervening between these two points and connecting them causally are the environmental sources of change and the mechanisms through which such changes are brought about.

The question is, How can these intervening factors be characterized most usefully? There is no certain answer. However, it is clear that great latitude is possible with respect to the description of both environmental variables and developmental mechanisms. For example, at one extreme, the effective social environment is sometimes described in terms of gross demographic variables, such as *mothers, fathers, siblings, age-mates,* and the like, in spite of the evidence that these social agents present multiple attributes, enter into many different kinds of social activities and relationships, and are likely to produce overlapping developmental effects. At the other extreme, the social environment seems sometimes to be treated as though it were a kind of homogeneous learning medium, a mere generator of eliciting and discriminative stimuli, rewards and punishments, and contingencies of reinforcement, whose effects are largely independent of species-specific characteristics or the particular individuals or circumstances in which they are produced. Similar variations exist in the way that developmental processes are described—all the way from a holistic emphasis on "orthogenesis" expressed in progressive increases in "differentiation" and "integration," to a particulate concern with the formation of functional relations between discrete stimuli and topographically distinct responses.

Characterizations of environmental variables and developmental mechanisms in most contemporary approaches to socialization fall somewhere between these extremes. Although one cannot claim anything like a consensus, it does seem possible to extract from current efforts some indication of the kinds of problems that must be confronted in studies of socialization and of the sorts of solutions that are likely to lead to some advance. The following suggestions are offered in this spirit:

1. *Field orientation.* The effective environment (*Umwelt*) is a multivariate field in which certain objects or events may stand out as figure against ground. The effects of these focal objects are always influenced by the total setting or context in which they occur (Brunswik, 1956; Kantor, 1973). Characterizing this field in behaviorally relevant terms is one of the central tasks for behavioral-psycho-ecology. We may presume that the more closely related two species are, the greater the correspondence in the general features of their *Umwelten*. The details of the effective field will vary not only with the species but also with the developmental status of the individual and his personal history.

With respect to socialization, a field orientation implies that demographic categories will be accompanied by descriptions of the developmentally relevant "profiles" of various classes of individuals, including those attributes that are shared by several classes, as well as those that are peculiar to just one class. As a first step, it would be useful to look at similarities and differences in the interchanges between the developing individual and other animals in its environment and at their interchanges with each other. What I am suggesting here is rather like what Bernstein has accomplished for various primate species, although with a concern more focused on behaviors relevant to socialization (Bernstein and Mason, 1963; Bernstein and Sharpe, 1966; Bernstein, 1971).

2. *Multiplicity of stimulus effects.* That the contributions of experience to development can take many forms is too obvious for comment. In spite of the fact that many different functions of stimulation are recognized, however, few of these have been analyzed systematically, and almost never, so far as I know, have they been ordered within a comprehensive taxonomic scheme. On the basis of his researches into the embryology of behavior, Gottlieb (1976) suggested three functions of experience that appear to be generic categories applicable to all aspects of behavioral development, including socialization, and to all developmental phases. Gottlieb's functions include *maintenance* (preserving the integrity of completely formed systems), *facilitation* (modifying thresholds of responsiveness or rates of change in developing system), and *induction* (channeling development in one direction rather than another). These categories are not mutually exclusive, and it must be presumed that the same experience may simultaneously affect several functions.

With respect to socialization, maintenance functions are most clearly reflected in the earliest and most commonplace aspects of maternal behavior—suckling, grooming, retrieving, and the like—which serve not only to preserve intact the developing individual but also to maintain the ongoing relationship with the parent. Facilitative effects are seen in such areas as weaning from the nipple and the transition to solid foods and in modifications of interactions with objects in the social and nonsocial environment (social facilitation). Although the parent is characteristically in a strategic position to provide facilitation, it is clear that siblings and age-mates can also serve this function in a variety of ways. Inductive functions include the various phenomena described in traditional learning theory—classical conditioning, instrumental conditioning, generalization–transfer, reinforcement and extinction—although these are probably more properly viewed as generalized, operationally defined descriptions of the conditions for producing certain types of behavioral change, and the kinds of changes that are produced, than as labels for universal "laws" or inviolable "principles" (Bitterman and Woodard, 1976; Malone, 1975). Other examples of inductive functions are the formation of social strategies (Anderson and Mason, 1978) and the phenomena of perceptual learning, incidental learning, observational learning, imitation, and the like. For present purposes, the question of the nature of the specific processes underlying these behaviors may be left open, although its final resolution will obviously have an important impact on our views of the socialization process (Gewirtz, 1971). At the moment, however, a more important requirement is for a better understanding of the social conditions under which these changes occur most readily in various species and of their long-range developmental consequences. A related issue concerns the sources of developmental plasticity and the nature of species-typical constraints on the inductive functions of experience, as discussed earlier in the context of evolutionary aspects of ontogeny.

A systematic treatment of stimulus effects must also be prepared to deal with the problems of specificity–generality and persistence of developmental changes. As Bateson (1976) pointed out, a decision whether to classify a change as specific or general depends on the behavioral units that are considered, and these will vary with the kinds of questions that are being asked. Similar reasoning governs decisions concerning the question of persistence of developmental changes. In socialization research, such decisions reflect the fact that the developmental end points of ultimate concern are functional patterns with fairly obvious adaptative implications: the competences and achievements of the mature animal. Effects that are detectable only in a narrow aspect of adult performance are, from this point of view, "specific" (which says nothing about the causal nexus that produced them). Likewise, effects of early social experience that do not significantly impair or enhance adult performance are not considered enduring. The presumption is that suitable criteria are available for assessing the adequacy of adult performance. Although it is true that many useful criteria are available, it is also the case that in a strict sense, the adaptive potential of the normal adult of any species is not fully known; the point, then, is that any conclusions regarding the nature and persistence of the effects of early social experience must be relative to the circumstances in which the assessment is made.

3. *Taxonomy of transactions.* Interaction and interdependence are the hallmark of social life. What A does to B not only affects B's behavior in general but is also likely to affect what B does to A, and so on and on. In much research in animal behavior, such exchanges are described according to the formula "Who does what to whom." This is an incomplete description, of course, because only the first part of the interchange is included; however, by applying the same formula to the "whom" side and hooking up these elemental units, one might, it seems, come out with a reasonably faithful description of a social episode. Actually, this is possible only for the simplest forms of social interaction.

A more generalized and useful procedure is to start with the episode itself. All but the simplest interchanges have a beginning, a middle, and an end; they relate to some issue of importance to at least one of the participants; and they terminate with that issue either resolved to the satisfaction of one or both of them or left hanging. In any event, the outcome may carry important consequences not only for each individual but for the future of the relationship. In other words, the "natural" unit of social intercourse is a transaction, and transactions can be characterized by their content, by their structure, by their component processes, and by their outcome, all of which are subject to operational definition and empirical investigation.

As yet, we lack an adequate taxonomic scheme for dealing with social transactions in animals other than man, although a promising beginning has been made (Hinde, 1976; Anderson and Mason, 1974, 1978). It seems likely that apart from the light it will shed on social relations among adults, a workable taxonomy of transactions will reveal aspects of social development and the socialization process that would otherwise remain either undetected or apprehended only intuitively. For example, it may be possible to compare mothers with respect to their skills in avoiding conflictual transactions, or to compare infants with respect to their developing abilities to resolve conflictual transactions in ways that are favorable to themselves.

SUMMARY AND CONCLUSIONS

This essay has approached social ontogeny as one aspect of the general problem of behavioral development. Of the two major perspectives toward development, the mechanistic and the organismic, the latter was favored on the grounds of greater utility in dealing with questions of evolutionary origins, adaptive significance, and phyletic contrasts. The newborn individual was viewed as an ongoing enterprise with established needs and functions, constrained by its organization, in continuous commerce with its surround, and undergoing continuous change as a consequence of these transactions. Implicit in this orientation is the idea that developmental change is always guided by, and occurs within, the framework of existing functional systems.

The degree to which changes in these functional systems can be brought about by experience varies with the particular system, with developmental status, and with species characteristics. Generally speaking, the period of greatest plasticity or openness to environmental influence occurs before the onset of reproductive maturity. In some species, the period of immaturity is long, whether it is measured in absolute terms or relative to the total life span.

There is no obvious reason that species should differ in this respect. In fact, if production of offspring is accepted as the primary measure of evolutionary success, then every species should be under strong selection pressures against the evolution of immaturity. And yet it is obvious that large differences exist. What then are the advantages of immaturity?

Several advantages might be considered. This account focused mainly on one particular constellation of traits: the immaturity syndrome. This syndrome is most likely to emerge under ecological conditions that place a premium on behavioral flexibility. Its major adaptive consequence is that it tends to create openness in information-processing schemata and to encourage the intensification of curiosity, play, and exploration—activities that require time to achieve their purpose, which is to provide specific information that helps to round out these systems, to make them functionally complete. This process in turn creates selection pressures toward improved information-processing skills, leading to functional and structural changes in the central nervous system.

The immature individual of an open species does not merely develop more slowly than a member of a relatively closed species. It also differs in the way its behavior is organized. In many respects, it is a less complete and efficient organism, particularly in the earliest phases of its development. Although it benefits from openness by a gain in adaptability, it is also more vulnerable to developmental perturbations, for these are but different sides of the same coin. Consequently, the open organism requires more extensive and more extended parental care. This can be provided because the same openness that leads to inefficient behavior in the neonate allows the parent a greater degree of flexibility in coping with variability in the behavior of its young.

The potential contributions of the parent to the development of the young fall into two broad classes: trophic and informational. Trophic contributions consist of energies and materials that are necessary to sustain vital processes; informational contributions perform an organizational function. The degree to which parents or other social agents actually make an informational contribution (beyond that provided in the genome) varies widely among species.

Potentially, however, the social environment is an unusually rich information resource, and, in fact, we know that it makes important contributions to development in most avian and mammalian species. The question of how these effects are brought about identifies the general problem of socialization.

Although a detailed and coherent theory of socialization is not yet possible, the organismic perspective appears to provide a suitable paradigm, and it is gaining currency. The major issues that remain to be resolved relate more to the precision of available concepts than to their fundamental validity. In particular, there is a need for a more refined characterization of the effective elements in the social environment and of the kinds of effects they produce.

To this end, three areas are considered that would seem to repay systematic study and clarification:

1. *Field orientation.* Although it is generally recognized that the social environment constitutes a context or stimulus field for the developing individual, the current tendencies are to characterize this field in terms of classes of individuals (rather than their developmentally relevant attributes) or to treat individuals as though they were "de-naturized" sources of eliciting and discriminative stimuli and contingencies of reinforcement.

2. *Multiplicity of stimulus effects.* In spite of the fact that many different stimulus functions are recognized, a useful scheme for describing these effects within a common framework is not available. Following Gottlieb, it was suggested that three functions of stimulation that are broadly relevant to developmental pro-

cesses, including socialization, are *maintenance* (preserving the integrity of an existing system), *facilitation* (modifying thresholds or rates of change), and *induction* (channeling development in one direction or another). These functions are not mutually exclusive, and the same experience may be reflected in more than one of them. The concepts of traditional learning theory are regarded as generalized, operationally defined descriptions of some of the conditions that produce certain kinds of change and of the changes so produced.

3. *Taxonomy of transactions.* All but the simplest forms of social interaction require something more than a description of who does what to whom. Social interchanges are often episodic and thematic; they exhibit a structure and a content. An adequate taxonomic scheme for dealing with these properties will very likely lead to a different and more refined understanding of the ways in which social experience contributes to the achievement of adult accomplishments and skills.

Acknowledgments

I thank the following friends for their helpful comments and suggestions: D. M. Fragaszy, M. Kenney, P. S. Rodman.

REFERENCES

Amadon, D. The evolution of low reproductive rates in birds. *Evolution,* 1964, *18*, 105–110.
Anderson, C. O., and Mason, W. A. Early experience and complexity of social organization in groups of young rhesus monkeys (*Macaca mulatta*). *J. Comp. Physiol. Psychol.,* 1974, *87*, 681–690.
Anderson, C. O., and Mason, W. A. Competitive social strategies in groups of deprived and experienced rhesus monkeys. *Dev. Psychobiol.,* 1978, *11*, 289–299.
Ashby, W. R. General systems theory as a new discipline. *General Systems: Yearbook of the Society for General Systems Research,* 1958, *3*, 1–6.
Ashmole, N. P., and Tovar, H. Prolonged parental care in royal terns and other birds. *Auk,* 1968, *85*, 90–100.
Baer, D. M. An age-irrelevant concept of development. *Merrill-Palmer Q.,* 1970, *16*, 236–245.
Barash, D. P. The evolution of marmot societies: A general theory. *Science,* 1974, *185*, 415–520.
Bateson, P. P. G. Specificity and the origins of behavior. In J. S. Rosenblatt, R. A. Hinde, E. Shaw, and C. Beer (eds.), *Advances in the Study of Behavior,* Vol. 6, Academic Press, New York, 1976.
Beckner, M. *The Biological Way of Thought.* University of California Press, Berkeley, 1968.
Bernstein, I. S. Activity profiles of primate groups. In A. M. Schrier, H. F. Harlow, and F. Stollnitz (eds.), *Behavior of Nonhuman Primates,* Vol. 3. Academic Press, New York, 1971, pp. 69–106.
Bernstein, I. S., and Mason, W. A. Activity patterns of rhesus monkeys in a social group. *Anim. Behav.,* 1963, *11*, 455–460.
Bernstein, I. S., and Sharpe, L. G. Social roles in a rhesus monkey group. *Behaviour,* 1966, *26*, 91–104.
Bertalanffy, L. von *General System Theory.* George Braziller, New York, 1968.
Bijou, S. W. Ages, stages, and the naturalization of human development. *Am. Psychol.,* 1968, *23*, 419–427.
Bischof, N. A systems approach toward the functional connections of attachment and fear. *Child Dev.,* 1975, *46*, 801–814.
Bitterman, M. E., and Woodard, W. T. Vertebrate learning: Common processes. In R. B. Masterton, C. B. G. Campbell, and N. Hotton (eds.), *Evolution of Brain and Behavior in Vertebrates.* Lawrence Erlbaum, Hillsdale, N.J., 1976, pp. 169–189.
Bolles, R. C. *Learning Theory.* Holt, Rinehart and Winston, New York, 1975.
Bowlby, J. *Attachment.* Basic Books, New York, 1969.
Brookshire, K. H. Vertebrate learning: Evolutionary divergences. In R. B. Masterton, M. E. Bitterman,

C. B. G. Campbell, and N. Hotton (eds.), *Evolution of Brain and Behavior in Vertebrates*. Lawrence Erlbaum, Hillsdale, N.J., 1976.

Brown, J. L. Alternate routes to sociality in jays—With a theory for the evolution of altruism and communal breeding. *Am. Zool.*, 1974, *14*, 63–80.

Brown, J. L. *The Evolution of Behavior*. W. W. Norton, New York, 1975.

Bruner, J. S. *Processes of Cognitive Growth: Infancy*. Eighth Annual Report, Harvard University Center for Cognitive Studies. Cambridge, Mass., 1967–1968.

Brunswik, E. Historical and thematic relations of psychology to other sciences. *Sci. Monthly*, 1956, *83*, 151–161.

Cairns, R. B. Attachment and dependency: A psychobiological and social-learning synthesis. In J. L. Gewirtz (ed.), *Attachment and Dependency*. V. H. Winston, New York, 1972, pp. 29–80.

Callaway, W. R., Jr. *Modes of Biological Adaptation and Their Role in Intellectual Development* (PCD Monograph Series, Vol. 1, No. I), 1970.

de Beer, G. *Embryos and Ancestors* (3rd ed.). Oxford University Press, London, 1958.

Denenberg, V. H. (ed.). *The Development of Behavior*. Sinauer, Stamford, Conn., 1972.

Eibl-Eibesfeldt, I. *Ethology: The Biology of Behavior*. Holt, Rinehart and Winston, New York, 1970.

Flavell, J. H. *The Developmental Psychology of Jean Piaget*. Van Nostrand, Princeton, N.J., 1963.

Galef, B. G., Jr. On the social transmission of acquired behavior: A discussion of tradition and social learning in vertebrates. In J. S. Rosenblatt, R. A. Hinde, E. Shaw, and C. Beer (eds.), *Advances in the Study of Behavior*, Vol. 6. Academic Press, New York, 1976.

Gause, G. F. The relation of adaptability to adaptation. *Q. Rev. Biol.*, 1942, *17*, 99–114.

Gewirtz, J. L. Levels of conceptual analysis in environment–infant interaction research. *Merrill-Palmer Q.*, 1969, *15*, 7–47.

Gewirtz, J. L. Discussion of Professor Bandura's paper: The roles of overt responding and extrinsic reinforcement in "self-" and "vicarious-reinforcement" phenomena and in "observational learning" and imitation. In R. Glaser (ed.), *The Nature of Reinforcement*. Academic Press, New York, 1971.

Gibson, E. J. *Principles of Perceptual Learning and Development*. Appleton-Century-Crofts, New York, 1969.

Gibson, J. J. *The Senses Considered as Perceptual Systems*. Houghton Mifflin, New York, 1966.

Glass, D. C. (ed.). *Environmental Influences*. Rockefeller University Press and Russell Sage Foundation, New York, 1968.

Gottlieb, G. Neglected developmental variables in the study of species identification in birds. *Psychol. Bull.*, 1973, *79*, 362–372.

Gottlieb, G. Conceptions of prenatal development: Behavioral embryology. *Psychol. Rev.*, 1976, *83*, 215–234.

Hardy, A. C. Escape from specialization. In J. Huxley, A. C. Hardy, and E. B. Ford (eds.), *Evolution as a Process*. Collier, New York, 1963, pp. 146–171.

Hayes, K. J. Genes, drives and intellect. *Psychol. Rep.*, 1962, *10*, 299–342.

Held, R., and Bauer, J. A., Jr. Visually guided reaching in infant monkeys after restricted rearing. *Science*, 1967, *155*, 718–720.

Held, R., and Bauer, J. A., Jr. Development of sensorially guided reaching in infant monkeys. *Brain Res.*, 1974, *71*, 265–271.

Hess, E. H. Ethology and developmental psychology. In P. H. Mussen (ed.), *Carmichael's Manual of Child Psychology*, Vol. 1. Wiley, New York, 1970, pp. 1–38.

Hess, E. H. *Imprinting*. Van Nostrand, New York, 1973.

Hinde, R. A. *Animal Behaviour: A Synthesis of Ethology and Comparative Psychology* (2nd ed.). McGraw-Hill, New York, 1970.

Hinde, R. A. On describing relationships. *J. Child Psychol. Psychiatry Allied Discip.*, 1976, *17*, 1–19.

Hinde, R. A., and Stevenson-Hinde, J. (eds.). *Constraints on Learning*. Academic Press, New York, 1973.

Hoffman, H. S., and Ratner, A. M. A reinforcement model of imprinting: Implications for socialization in monkeys and men. *Psychol. Rev.*, 1973, *80*, 527–544.

Immelmann, K. Ecological significance of imprinting and early learning. *Ann. Rev. Ecol. Syst.*, 1975, *6*, 15–37.

Istock, C. A. The evolution of complex life cycle phenomena: An ecological perspective. *Evolution*, 1967, *21*, 592–605.

Jacobson, M. Development of specific neuronal connections. *Science*, 1969, *163*, 543–547.

Jander, R. Ecological aspects of spatial orientation. *Ann. Rev. Ecol. Syst.*, 1975, *6*, 171–188.

Kantor, J. R. System structure and scientific psychology. *Psychol. Rec.*, 1973, *23*, 451–458.

Klopfer, P. H. *Behavioral Aspects of Ecology*. Prentice-Hall, Englewood Cliffs, N.J., 1962.

Kuo, Z-Y. *The Dynamics of Behavioral Development: An Epigenetic View*. Random House, New York, 1967.

Lack, D. *Population Studies of Birds*. Oxford University Press, London, 1966.

Langer, J. *Theories of Development*. Holt, Rinehart & Winston, New York, 1969.

Lehrman, D. S. Semantic and conceptual issues in the nature–nurture problem. In L. R. Aronson, E. Tobach, D. S. Lehrman, and J. S. Rosenblatt (eds.), *Development and Evolution of Behavior*. Freeman, San Francisco, 1970, pp. 17–52.

Lester, D. A cross-species study of exploration and learning. *Percept. Mot. Skills*, 1974, *39*, 562.

Lorenz, K. *Evolution and Modification of Behavior*. University of Chicago Press, Chicago, 1965.

Malone, J. C., Jr. The "paradigms" of learning. *Psychol. Rec.*, 1975, *25*, 479–489.

Maple, T., Erwin, J., and Mitchell, G. Age of sexual maturity in laboratory-born pairs of rhesus monkeys (*Macaca mulatta*). *Primates*, 1973, *14*, 427–428.

Mason, W. A. Early social deprivation in the nonhuman primates: Implications for human behavior. In D. Class (ed.), *Environmental Influences*. Rockefeller University Press, New York, 1968, pp. 70–101.

Mason, W. A. Early deprivation in biological perspective. In V. H. Denenberg (ed.), *Education of the Infant and Young Child*. Academic Press, New York, 1970, pp. 25–50.

Mason, W. A. Motivational factors in psychosocial development. In W. J. Arnold and M. M. Page (eds.), *Nebraska Symposium on Motivation*. University of Nebraska Press, Lincoln, 1971, pp. 35–67.

Mason, W. A., and Harlow, H. F. Initial response of infant rhesus monkeys to solid foods. *Psychol. Rep.*, 1959, *5*, 193–199.

Mayr, E. Behavior programs and evolutionary strategies. *Am. Sci.*, 1974, *62*, 650–659.

Montagu, M. F. A. *The Reproductive Development of the Female*. Julian Press, New York, 1957.

Nagel, E. Determinism and development. In D. B. Harris (ed.), *The Concept of Development*. University of Minnesota Press, Minneapolis, 1957, pp. 15–24.

Newton, G., and Levine, S. (eds.). *Early Experience and Behavior: The Psychobiology of Development*. Charles C Thomas, Springfield, Ill., 1968.

Orians, G. H. *The Study of Life: An Introduction to Biology*. Allyn & Bacon, Boston, 1969.

Overton, W. F., and Reese, H. W. Models of development: Methodological implications. In J. R. Nesselroade and H. W. Reese (eds.), *Life-Span Developmental Psychology: Methodological Issues*. Academic Press, New York, 1973, pp. 65–86.

Piaget, J. *Biology and Knowledge*. University of Chicago Press, Chicago, 1971.

Pianka, E. R. On *r*- and *K*-selection. *Am. Nat.*, 1970, *104*, 592–597.

Pittendrigh, C. Adaptation, natural selection, and behavior. In A. Roe and G. G. Simpson (eds.), *Behavior and Evolution*. Yale University Press, New Haven, 1958, pp. 390–416.

Reese, H. W., and Overton, W. F. Models of development and theories of development. In L. R. Goulet, and P. B. Baltes (eds.), *Life-Span Developmental Psychology: Research and Theory*. Academic Press, New York, 1970, pp. 115–145.

Richardson, B. J. *r* and *K* selection in kangaroos. *Nature*, 1975, *255*, 323–324.

Rosenblueth, A., Wiener, N., and Bigelow, J. Behavior, purpose, and teleology. In W. Buckley (ed.), *Modern Systems Research for the Behavioral Scientist*. Aldine, Chicago, 1968, pp. 221–225.

Rosenzweig, M. R. Environmental complexity, cerebral change, and behavior. *Am. Psychol.*, 1966, *21*, 321–332.

Sacher, G. A. Relation of lifespan to brain weight and body weight in mammals. In E. W. Wolstenholme and M. O'Conner (eds.), *CIBA Foundation Colloquia on Aging*, Vol. 5. Churchill, London, 1959, pp. 115–141.

Sacher, G. A., and Staffeldt, E. F. Relation of gestation time to brain weight for placental mammals: Implications for the theory of vertebrate growth. *Am. Nat.*, 1974, *108*, 593–615.

Sackett, G. P. Innate mechanisms, rearing conditions, and a theory of early experience effects in primates. In M. R. Jones (ed.), *Miami Symposium on the Prediction of Behavior*. University of Miami Press, Coral Gables, 1970.

Schiff, W., Caviness, J. A., and Gibson, J. J. Persistent fear responses in rhesus monkeys to the optical stimulus of "looming." *Science*, 1962, *136*, 982–983.

Schneirla, T. C. Behavioral development and comparative psychology. *Q. Rev. Biol.*, 1966, *41*, 283–302.

Scott, J. P., Stewart, J. M., and DeGhett, V. J. Critical periods in the organization of systems. *Dev. Psychobiol.*, 1974, *7*, 489–513.

Skinner, B. F. The phylogeny and ontogeny of behavior. *Science*, 1966, *153*, 1205–1213.

Sperry, R. W. Plasticity of neural maturation. *Dev. Biol. Supp.*, 1968, *2*, 306–327.

Thoday, J. M. Components of fitness. *Symposia of the Society for Experimental Biology*, 1954, *7*, 96–113.

Tolman, E. C. *Purposive Behavior in Animals and Men*. Appleton-Century-Crofts, New York, 1932.

Vernon, M. D. The functions of schemata in perceiving. *Psychol. Rev.,* 1955, *62*, 180–192.

Waddington, C. H. Epigenetics and evolution. *Symposia of the Society for Experimental Biology,* 1954, 7, 186–199.

Wapner, S., Kaplan, B., and Cohen, S. B. An organismic–developmental perspective for understanding transactions of men in environments. *Environ. and Behav.,* 1973, *5*, 255–290.

Warren, J. M. Learning in vertebrates. In D. A. Dewsbury and D. A. Rethlingshafer (eds.), *Comparative Psychology: A Modern Survey.* McGraw-Hill, New York, 1973, pp. 471–508.

Wassersug, R. J. The adaptive significance of the tadpole stage with comments on the maintenance of complex life cycles in anurans. *Am. Zool.,* 1975, *15*, 405–417.

Weiss, P. *The Science of Life: The Living System—A System for Living.* Futura, Mount Kisco, N.Y., 1973.

Wertheim, E. S. Person–environment interaction: The epigenesis of autonomy and competence. II. Review of developmental literature (normal development). *Br. J. Med. Psychol.,* 1975, *48*, 95–111.

Wilcock, J. Comparative psychology lives on under an assumed name—Psychogenetics! *Am. Psychol.,* 1972, *27*, 531–538.

Wilson, E. O. *Sociobiology: The New Synthesis.* Belknap, Cambridge, Mass., 1975.

2

On the Physiological Organization of Social Behavior: Sex and Aggression

NORMAN T. ADLER

INTRODUCTION

This chapter treats the physiological bases of social behavior. Although the topic seems straightforward (albeit covering a vast area of research), there are several ways of relating biology and behavior.

There are the biological (physiological) mechanisms that produce behavior and that are affected by behavior. One can question the utility of these approaches, especially in a behaviorally oriented volume on social relationships. Experimental psychologists have been able to point out a large number of causal relationships between environmental contingencies and responses, without explicitly describing physiological factors. Similarly, classical ethology produced descriptions relating the occurrence of specific responses to species-specific signals. More recently, sociobiologists have devoted their attention to social structures' relationship to ecological and evolutionary strategies.

Given these multiple approaches, the study of the physiological causes of behavior seems to be an independent discipline, which could stand alongside other approaches to the study of behavior. There is, however, a more compelling reason that a chapter on physiological mechanisms should be included in a volume dealing with social behavior. While each of us devotes our attention to a specific problem or set of problems in the laboratory, or the field, our distal goal as scientists

NORMAN T. ADLER   Department of Psychology, University of Pennsylvania, Philadelphia, Pennsylvania 19104.

should be to provide a general, integrative framework for understanding behavior in its full biological context. The study of physiological mechanisms is part of this context.

Traditionally, there have been several separate but complementary questions that are to be answered in the study of behavior. First, we need to know the evolutionary–genetic causes of the behavior (Tinbergen, 1952). Second, we need to understand how a behavior pattern comes to develop. The temporal and causal gaps between the fertilized ovum and the behavior of an adult organism are filled in by a series of developmental interactions between the organism and its environment. Third, we can examine the proximal mechanisms (environmental, social, and physiological) that cause the genetically and ontogenetically prepared organism to perform in a certain way.

These three analyses of behavior are causal (Tinbergen, 1952). Genetic, developmental, and proximal mechanistic events lead to the production of the response. There is finally a fourth topic: the adaptive role of the behavior. In these analyses, we ask not what influences the behavior but rather what the behavior influences. This analysis, the functional, focuses not on the antecedents of behavior but on the consequences.

The copulatory behavior of a male cat, for example, has genetic (e.g., sex chromosome), developmental (e.g., neonatal hormone), and contemporary proximal causes (endogenous stimulation by androgen and exogenous stimulation by the female conspecific). However, it also has biological *consequences;* copulation leads to the release of ova in a female that would not ovulate without the behavior, and thus the behavior leads ultimately to an adaptive consequence, the production of progeny.

These four areas of inquiry are, of course, related. If a behavior is adaptive, the genes influencing this behavior will, other things being equal, be passed on to the next generation. These hereditary units will then serve as genetic–evolutionary causes for subsequent generations.

The point of view presented in this chapter is that the study of physiological variables is both an independent approach to the study of behavior and, perhaps even more importantly, a complement to the other approaches.

To cite one example of complementarity, experimental manipulations of the endocrine and nervous systems can lead to variations in behavior. These, in turn, can help the behaviorist "dissect" the responses into natural categories of behavior. Since evolved behavior patterns are often adaptive by virtue of their effects on other organisms (recall the example of induced ovulation in the cat), studying the neural events in the female cat is the study of the mechanism of the adaptation.

Because of this approach, there are two general purposes for this chapter. One is to provide a review of some physiological factors that influence behavior and that are influenced by behavior. This is the study of physiological psychology. The second purpose is to show how these analyses can facilitate the work of other behavioral scientists.

It is clearly impossible to present in one chapter a complete coverage of the physiological correlates of social behavior, especially if social behavior is broadly defined as all behavior involving the interactions of two organisms, a topic that could include courtship, copulation, maternal behavior, aggression, group foraging, group defense, and group migration, as well as patterns of social structure. Because of this open-ended nature of social behavior, I have chosen to deal with only two systems, in some depth. Sex and aggression will each be treated from the standpoint of their proximal causes and effects (and where possible, these will be related to evolutionary histories). By choosing an affiliative and an agonistic behavior, it should be possible to look for both similarities and differences in physiological organization.

On the Mechanisms of Sexual Behavior

Introduction

Let us start with some definitions. Sexual reproduction involves the coordination of two separate organisms interacting in such a way that progeny are produced. The purpose of this section is to discuss the mechanisms that produce sexual behavior in animals and to examine the way in which evolutionary processes have shaped these mechanisms.

Sexual behavior is that set of responses resulting in the reproduction of organisms by sexual means. In the phyletic history of reproduction, sexuality appeared as an adaptation with certain benefits accruing to those organisms that displayed that adaptation. One reason for the advantage of sexuality over asexuality is the richness of genetic permutations it promotes. Because of genetic segregation and recombination, the progeny from a sexual union display a great deal more genetic variability than do the progeny from asexually reproducing organisms (Crow and Kimura, 1970). Offspring from a sexual union can thus survive in a larger range of microenvironments (Wilson, 1975), and the genes of the sexually reproducing organisms that generate these offspring consequently enjoy a higher probability of being represented in the next generation.

Once sexuality has been adopted as an evolutionary strategy, however, there is immediately a set of problems that must be solved. These problems have to do with the synchronization of morphologically and behaviorally differentiated organisms. Sexuality requires differentiation of two sexual types, male and female, or other prototypes. At the most elementary level, there is a basic difference between male and female gametes: the female's egg is specialized to contain the basic nutritive elements for the embryo, while the male's sperm are specialized for motility (Trivers, 1972). This basic gametic difference between male and female becomes magnified as more and more of the organism's behavior and auxiliary reproductive physiology become specialized as secondary sexual adaptations. With even a moderate amount of genital specialization and differentiation, there is a problem of synchronizing the two animals' behavior so that gametes meet under appropriate conditions and lead to the production of viable young.

The problem of synchronization, which is fundamental to the organization of sexual behavior, is the basis of this chapter's discussion of the mechanisms controlling sexual behavior. In this essay, I discuss three general classes of synchronization involving the coordination of male and female reproductive behavior.

1. The first class deals with the establishment of a sexual bond between two appropriate organisms. Generally, appropriateness implies that the sexual partners are from the same species. In addition, they must be reproductively mature and competent to produce, and sometimes care for, offspring.

2. In addition to arranging for the right mate, sexual behavior helps ensure that reproduction occurs at the right place and the right time. Mating seasons and territories are biological phenomena that provide adequate climatic and geographical conditions for reproduction. The choice of a biotically adequate territory requires a way for the organism to evaluate the resources in an area and to gain social control of the chosen area. The occurrence of a breeding season often requires sexual behavior to be tied to a seasonally accurate "biological clock."

3. Once the place and partner are chosen, the more reflexological aspects of copulatory behavior lead to the induction of pregnancy. This is accomplished by four general sets of events: (a) the behavioral augmentation of reproductive motivation, so that the male and female are both willing to copulate; (b) the mechanical positioning of the male's intromittive organ into the female's vagina in those species where internal fertilization takes place; (c) the stimulation of ejaculation by the male; and (d) the alteration of the female's physiological status so that pregnancy can ensue.

The Choice of Mate

Intraspecific Selection of Mates: Sexual Selection and Male Attractiveness. Because of the great reproductive expenditure of the female, she must select the fittest mate *within* her own species (Williams, 1966). This selectivity of the female can lead to a competitive situation between the males of her species, and this competition among the males becomes especially intense in populations displaying polygamous mating systems and equal sex ratios (Wilson, 1975). In such populations, for every male that mates, there is another male that must, for a time, go without a female. The individual selection of males that occurs by virtue of the competition for available females leads to sexual selection (Campbell, 1972; Darwin, 1859, 1871; Fisher, 1958). This selective process leads to the evolution of behavior in the male the function of which is to attract females.

Morphological traits like the extravagant plumage of some birds and the "ritualized" courtship displays of males in many species are thought to reflect the results of sexual selection. Although the male may win a female by virtue of his individual display vis-à-vis a single female, there are additional behavioral mechanisms that can improve his chances in obtaining a mate. These mechanisms are discussed in the succeeding sections.

Intraspecific Selection of Mates: Male Aggression. Since, in polygamously mating species, a female is obtained at the expense of another male, a prospective male could indirectly compete for female attention by attacking and driving away his competition. To the extent that females prefer males that occupy nutritionally rich and/or reproductively appropriate mating-nesting areas (cf. dickcisssel, *Spiza americana,* discussed by Zimmerman, 1966, 1971), aggression, the basis of the establishment of the territories, serves a useful reproductive function for the male.

In several species of birds, the males congregate within one area (a lek). Within the total area, however, there are some subdivisions that are ecologically more advantageous than others. There is intense competition between males for preferred sites in the mating area, and highly elaborate competitive behavior patterns emerge. Male grouse strut about and vocalize loudly at their opponents (Kruijt and Hogan, 1967; Lack, 1968). A male that ultimately comes to occupy the preferred site may perform up to 70% of the matings (Robel, 1966, on *Tympanuchus cupido*; see Wittenberger on the evolution of polygyny, p. 278 this volume).

As the breeding season approaches, male red deer *(Cervas elephas)* round up harems of females. Males compete intensely among themselves, on the basis of their large body size and their head displays, which involve huge antlers. Males from which the antlers were removed in an experiment dropped in their position in the dominance hierarchy (Lincoln, 1972), thus decreasing their chances of obtaining females.

Part of the theory of sexual selection involves the premise that intermale competition for females is most intense in polygamous species. In these cases, some males mate with many females, and other males consequently receive less reproductive attention. Where stable monogamous pair bonds are set up (and assuming an equal sex ratio), there are enough females to go around; consequently, intermale competition, with its attendant behavioral and morphological ornamentation, is reduced (Selander, 1965). A comparison of the behavior of roe deer and red deer illustrates the behavioral consequences of polygamous mating systems (Darling, 1964). Unlike the red deer, which possess large antlers and are aggressive only during rut, the roe deer *(Capreolus capreolus)* is mainly monogamous and does not form harems. In this species, both the male's gross body size and his antlers are much smaller than in the red deer.

A conclusion from these selected examples is that the development of mechanisms for male aggressive behavior (especially in polygamously mating species) can be an important means of obtaining female sexual companions.

INTRASPECIFIC SELECTION OF MATES: MALE COOPERATION. There is a more cooperative element in the mechanisms by which males can obtain females. To the extent that a male's ability to attract a female is proportional to the quantity of stimulation he provides, there are likely to be cases in which groups of males *combine* their individual signals (Wilson, 1975). This device of combined signaling sometimes occurs in communal mating grounds (leks), in which males congregate into one general area during mating season. Hjorth (1970) showed that for grouse, the combined displaying and calling can be perceived from a much greater distance than would be the case for a single individual. There are even cases of active synchronization in the behavior of two males, as in the joint jumping displays of pairs of blue-backed manakins, *Chiroxiphia pareola* (Snow, 1963). Even when there are individual mating courts that are aggressively defended within the overall display ground, as in the black-and-white manakin, the resulting noise of simultaneously displaying males carries more than a hundred yards (Snow, 1956).

There are several mechanisms by which male–male behavior can be synchronized, but one of the most effective is through social facilitation. During mating season, male bullfrogs *(Rana catesbeiana)* aggregate in ponds (Capranica, 1965), where they emit a distinctive mating vocalization. One male calls. A second male responds to the call of the first male by calling back. The calling by the second in turn stimulates a third, and so on. This kind of social facilitation (or positive feedback) can generate a loud and frequent auditory signal that attracts females to the pond.

The advantage of male–male affiliative mechanisms' balancing aggressive ones is that males can reside sufficiently closely to one another to cooperate in attracting females. Collias and Collias (1969) have shown that more females *per male* nest in large colonies of the village weaver *(Ploceus cucullatus)* than in small ones. Just as the winning and the defense of individual territories requires an aggressive behavioral substrate, the combined displays require an affiliative system to operate. The integrated social structure of a particular species, then, reflects the balance of opposing agonistic and affiliative tendencies.

The conclusion from these studies of male courtship is that there are several kinds of behavioral mechanisms that promote the male's chances of obtaining a female: (1) the production of often exaggerated ("ritualized") displays that directly attract the females; (2) the development of aggressive mechanisms that serve to exclude competing males from the aggressor's area of reproductive activity; and (3) a balancing of the aggressive tendencies by affiliative patterns that allow males to combine their displays or signaling capabilities, the cumulative effect of which is to attract more females to the area. Although these three mechanisms are used to different degrees and in different combinations in different groups, the net effect of all of them is to increase the probability of the male's finding a willing mate. The first mechanism has to do with the male's relationship only with the female, while the second and third deal with male–male interactions.

INTRASPECIFIC SELECTION OF MATES: MALE RARENESS. There is a fourth mechanism by which males come to possess varying degrees of attractiveness; this mechanism simultaneously combines direct stimulating effects on the female with male–male interactions. This phenomenon, *frequency-dependent mating* (Petit, 1951; Ehrman, 1966), occurs when the number of successful matings of a particular genotype is inversely proportional to the frequency of the genotype in the potential mating pool. Also called *rare male advantage,* the genotype that is rare in a population tends to be favored at the expense of the common type. (Orange-eyed *Drosophila pseudoobscura* are preferred to purple-eyed males when the former are less frequent than the latter. When the orange-eyed males are more frequent, they are less preferred by the females; see Ehrman, 1970). One result of this kind of selection is to retain a balanced polymorphism in the population. Since the selective advantage of a gene increases as its frequency decreases, at low frequencies it is highly favored, and the gene is maintained in the population even if it is selected against at intermediate frequencies. This process provides a reservoir of genetic variation in the gene pool.

emphasis in this discussion so far has been on the characteristics of the male that
make him more attractive to the female. For sexual selection to operate, there are
also important properties of the female's behavior that are necessary for her to
obtain an optimal mate: she must be sensitive to the differences between conspecific males, she must consistently exert a preference, and her sensitivity–preference must have a heritable component. In a study by Ewing (1961) on artificial
genetic selection for changes in body length, consistent preferences of the female
Drosophila functioned as pressure for sexual selection.

In *Drosophila* the male courtship consists of four components: (1) orientation;
(2) wing vibration; (3) licking the female's genitalia; and (4) attempts at copulation.
In Ewing's study, the males selected for small size increased the proportion of
their courtship time devoted to wing vibration. Why should the smaller males
vibrate their wings more than the larger males? Since the smaller flies had smaller
wings, the stimulation from their vibrations was less intense than the vibratory
stimulation of the larger flies. The selection experiment had been performed by
placing 10 pairs of flies in a vial. Since there were presumably genetic differences,
which produced differences in the vibration rates of the flies in any given bottle,
there was an opportunity for the males to compete for the females on the basis of
this display. When the experiment of selecting for small body size was repeated,
with the variation of placing only a *single* pair of flies in each mating vial, there
were flies of decreasing body lengths over successive generations, but there was *no
concurrent increase* in vibration rates. After eight generations of selection with only
a single pair of flies per vial, Ewing returned to the procedure of placing 10 pairs
in each vial. The reintroduction of the opportunity for competition promptly
resulted in an increase in wing vibration rate over succeeding generations. This
experiment indicated that (1) females are sensitive to wing vibration as a courtship
display; and (2) given a competitive situation with the female acting as the agent
of natural selection, males with higher vibration rates are selected, resulting in an
increased mean vibration rate within the population.

In addition to possessing the ability to differentiate between the males' signals
related to their presumed sexual prowess, the female organism often possesses
auxiliary behavioral mechanisms for selecting her potential mate. She must often
be able to "remember" stimulation no longer present and be able to compare
displays from several males. This ability is especially important in the cases where
males are spread apart in separate territories and the female must pass through
several males' mating stations before choosing her partner. By attaching a telem-
etering device to female ruffed grouse *(Bonasa umbellus)*, Brander (1967) was able
to show that females visit most of the local males at their spatially separated display
grounds. By successively sampling the various males' displays, the female might
be able to store some representation of them and then could subsequently compare and choose among the males.

Another aspect of the female that may enhance her ability to obtain males is
her "novelty" as a sexual partner. In polygamously mating species (e.g., many
mammals), a given male stands a better chance of being represented in the gene
pool of the next generation by successively inseminating several different females

than by repeatingly copulating with the same female. In the rat *(Rattus norvegicus),* for example, a female will normally be impregnated following one ejaculatory series from a male (see sections below). In fact, further copulatory activities with that female can, under certain circumstances, disrupt the transport of his own sperm from the previous ejaculation (p. 49). Since a rested domestic rat can achieve up to seven ejaculations in one session (Larsson, 1956), he would be better off inseminating seven different females than concentrating on just one.

To support this notion that novel females are more stimulating than familiar females to the males of a polygamously mating species, there is a fair amount of evidence that male rats perform better sexually when they are offered a succession of different females than when they are repeatedly presented with the same female (Bermant and Davidson, 1974; Fisher, 1962; Fowler and Whalen, 1961; Wilson, Kuehn, and Beach, 1963). The increase in sexual performance with changing mates, termed the *Coolidge effect,* has also been demonstrated in male guinea pigs (Grunt and Young, 1952), rams (Beamer, Bermant, and Clegg, 1969), and bulls (Schein and Hale, 1965). These data imply that the period of sexual refractoriness that develops in a male following copulation with one female (Diakow, 1974) can be overcome by the introduction of a novel female, even one that has been previously mated to a second male (in rats, Hsiao, 1965). The strength of the effect varies across species (cf. Bermant and Davidson, 1974, for a review), and there are some contradictory comparative data (Dewsbury, 1975); however, for a normally polygamous or promiscuous male, the attractiveness of a new female would facilitate the spread of his genes among several different females.

Research on olfactory preferences in rodents provides several other examples of ways in which a novel female is more likely to attract a male. There are basic preferences in both male and female rats for olfactory cues from reproductively adequate mates. Sexually experienced male rats, for example, prefer the odor of an estrous female to that of an anestrous female (Carr, Krames, and Wylie, 1966); similarly, female rats prefer the odor of normal males to that of castrates. Within the class of stimuli elicited by reproductively adequate animals, there are, however, additional constraints that would support polygamous mating by males (but not polygamous mating by females). If an intact male rat has a history of mating with several different females, the odor of *novel females* is preferred (Carr, Krames, and Costanzo, 1970). (The preference for novel odors does not appear in inexperienced males.) His preference would lead a male to investigate, and consequently probably copulate with, different females. Conversely, the female rat, which becomes pregnant after one ejaculatory series, does not show a preference for new males. In fact, polygamously mated females preferred to approach the odor of a previous mating partner rather than that of a new one (Carr *et al.,* 1970).

In these studies of intraspecific mate choice, the behavior of species with polygamous mating systems (e.g., many mammals) were emphasized. By definition, no prolonged pair bonds were involved. In the case where a single male and female remained bonded for a period of time, other behavioral criteria were employed so that an individual selected an adequate partner with which to mate and to share parental responsibilities (Wilson, 1975).

LOCATIONS FOR BREEDING. Even if an appropriate male and female have chosen each other, viable offspring will not be produced unless there is an appropriate physical environment. The habitat available to most species is patchy, with variations in light, temperature, and food. Over large ranges in the physical environment (i.e., between latitudes), species may adapt with altered patterns of reproduction. With the variations inherent in smaller geographical ranges (i.e., the area occupied by a single population), a male can actively select the ecological context for breeding. For example, the selection and defense of a territory restricts breeding to a specific area. The combination of male territorial aggression and female selectivity results in two adapted organisms' residing in a niche that is suitable for the production of offspring.

TEMPORAL FACTORS: GENERAL. Even at a given location within the physical environment, conditions vary systematically as a function of time. (In Philadelphia, for example, there are approximately 9 hours 22 minutes of sunlight per day at the end of December, while, toward the end of June, there are 15 hours of light per day). Such seasonal variations in geophysical factors are critical for life processes. The annual changes in photoperiod produce fluctuations in mean monthly temperature (as much as 30°C in some boreal regions) and in rainfall—thereby influencing the ecosystems (Ricklefs, 1973, for review). In this section of the chapter, behavioral mechanisms are related to the synchronization of the organisms with respect to temporal variations in the physical environment.

TEMPORAL FACTORS: DAILY RHYTHMS. For many species, the primary environmental cycle is diurnal. Sexual behavior for some rodents follows a daily temporal pattern similar to that for eating, drinking, and general activity (Richter, 1965). Feral and domestic rats, for example, are sexually most active around dusk (Calhoun, 1962a; Kuehn and Beach, 1963). These species are nocturnal, and their optic apparatus is specialized for activity at night.

The restriction of sexual activity in rats to a limited time of day is controlled by a circadian biological clock (or clocks). Since much of the work concerning the timing of reproductive events has focused on female rats, the discussion that follows below is devoted to this organism.

The female rat comes into behavioral estrus once every four or five days (Long and Evans, 1922). Within this estrous cycle, active heat lasts for only about fifteen hours, corresponding to part of the evening on the day of vaginal proestrus.

By what mechanism is the female rat's mating behavior programmed to coincide with a particular time of day? At least part of the answer is that the occurrence of sexual behavior is tied to the female rat's ovarian cycle. From the classic work of Young and co-workers (Young, 1961), it is known that the ovarian hormones, estrogen and progesterone, lead to the occurrence of mating behavior. Estrogen, secreted over the four-day cycle of the female rat, reaches a peak on the day of proestrus (Smith, Freeman, and Neill, 1975). This background of estrogenic stimulation seems to be necessary for the subsequent appearance of sexual behavior on the evening of vaginal proestrus. Progesterone is secreted at low levels during most of the estrous (ovarian) cycle but begins to "surge" shortly before the onset of darkness on the evening of proestrus (Feder, Resko, and Goy, 1968). This surge of progesterone is followed quickly by an intensive interest in mating by the female rat.

If sexual behavior is facilitated by the estrogen peak during early proestrus, and the progesterone surge during late proestrus, what controls the timing of these hormones? The answer seems to be a surge of pituitary luteinizing hormone (LH) (Hoffman, 1973), which is in turn stimulated by a "neural clock" (Everett and Sawyer, 1950). The basic temporal organization of this clock is endogenous. Like other circadian rhythms, it is a self-sustaining oscillation. Placing the female rat in constant darkness often does not disrupt the continuation of estrous cycles at about four-day intervals (Hoffmann, 1967, 1969, 1970). However, as with most circadian clocks, environmental light cycles can entrain (synchronize) the endogenous periodicity: a phase shift in the day–night cycle of 12 hours is followed, after several cycles, by the estrous cycle's becoming synchronized with the new day–night rhythm (Hemmingsen and Krarup, 1937).

It seems, therefore, that the restriction of the female rat's mating activity to a particular time of day is due, in part, to the timing of pituitary–gonadal secretions. These secretions (e.g., the LH surge), in turn, are tied to a biological oscillator, the period of which is approximately 24 hours and which is entrained by the environmental lighting cycle.

The result of these neuroendocrine events is that mating behavior, in the nocturnal rat, occurs around dusk (its behaviorally most active time) on the day of vaginal proestrus. Later that night, ovulation occurs. This physiological event tends to occur toward the *end* of the night of proestrus (Young, Boling, and Blandau, 1941); like the surge of progesterone, ovulation is also triggered by the rapid, heightened secretion of pituitary LH. By the time ovulation has occurred, female receptivity has reached its peak (Young *et al.*, 1941; Kuehn and Beach, 1963), and mating will have occurred.

To summarize briefly: the temporal coordination of all of these biological events is dependent upon the operation of an endogenously organized biological clock (or clocks), the operation of which is translated into overt biological rhythms by hormonal mediators.

There are a number of adaptive features in the linking of several reproductive activities within an organism (e.g., receptivity and ovulation) to a circadian oscillation. The coupling of the several physiological and behavioral reproductive events to a common clock (or set of clocks) within the individual ensures that the neuroendocrine events required for reproduction will proceed in an orderly and integrated fashion. There is a second adaptive feature in the control of reproduction by biological clocks. Since reproductive behavior must, by definition, be social (at least two separate organisms must be coordinated), biological clocks can facilitate the necessary interorganismic integration. Because each animal's circadian rhythm can be entrained to a potent, stable geophysical variable like the light cycle, the biological periodicities of two organisms living in the same physical environment will come to have a common phase relationship to each other.

The importance of this rhythmic integration was highlighted by an experiment of Curt Richter (1970). A male and female rat were allowed to "free-run"; that is, their biological rhythms were not anchored to an environmental light cycle. Under their free-running conditions, their circadian ("about 24-hour") rhythms began to diverge from the precise 24-hour period that exists under entrainment by light, and the rats mated only when their activity rhythms overlapped.

TEMPORAL FACTORS: SEASONAL RHYTHMS. Because of the annual periodicity in their environments, many organisms display annual cycles in their reproductive performance.

As is the case for the circadian cycles of sexual behavior in female rats, annual cycles of reproductive behavior in some organisms are tied to hormonal cycles. The relation of circadian cycles to seasonal cycles is even more intimate than the analogy suggests; the mechanism controlling both may be a circadian clock (Elliott, Stetson, and Menaker, 1972).

According to the theory of *photoperiodism* (Bunning, 1973), the circadian clock can be used to measure day length. In Bunning's theory, there are two distinct effects of the external light cycle. The first is the process of "entrainment," by which the *approximately* 24-hour (circadian) rhythm inherent in the endogenous clockwork mechanism is tuned to a precise 24-hour rhythm (by the phase-shifting process underlying entrainment to the 24-hour solar light cycle). Once this endogenous rhythm is entrained to precisely 24 hours, it can itself act as a measuring device to determine day length. As a hypothetical case, assume that the 24-hour clock sequentially goes through two phases of 12 hours each. (Phase 1 is called a *photically noninducible phase;* Phase II is a *photically inducible phase*). In winter (or early spring), the day length is short; light stimulates the clock only during the first (noninducible) phase. As the duration of light per day increases during the approach of spring, light impinges upon the hypothetical organism during the second (photoinducible) phase of the clock's operation as well as during the first. This increasing imposition of light informs the organism that day length is increasing and activates the neuroendocrine system to resume reproductive activity.

The photoperiodic hypothesis may explain maintenance of the reproductive state in male hamsters. Gaston and Menaker (1967) found that testis growth was sensitive to environmental light cycles. Approximately 12.5 hours of light per day were required to maintain testis size; with less light, the testes regressed. To determine whether the photoperiodic hypothesis could account for these results, Elliot *et al.* (1972) performed the following experiment. After maintaining the subjects for 17 weeks in a control condition with 14 hours of light a day (LD 14:10), the animals were divided into several groups, each placed under a different lighting schedule. In each group, light was delivered in blocks of 6 hours each; however, there were different amounts of darkness between the 6-hour light periods. One group received a photoperiod of 6 hours of light followed by 18 hours of darkness (LD 6:18). The total photic day was therefore 24 hours. Another group received 6 hours of light followed by 30 hours of darkness (LD 6:30). This schedule corresponded to a photic cycle length of 36 hours.

The testes of the animals regressed under LD 6:18. These results support Gaston and Menaker's original finding that at least 12.5 hours of light per day are required for testicular maintenance, since the organisms in this group received only 6 hours of light per day. However, testis weight was *maintained* in the LD 6:30 condition. The results for this group support the photoperiodic hypothesis. Assume that at the start of the experimental light treatments, there is a circadian clock that is entrained so that Phase I (noninducible) coincides with the onset of light (Phase II begins 12 hours later). The circadian clock then makes one cycle, and Phase I starts again, this time 24 hours after the light came on. The second 6-hour block of light, however, came 36 hours after the first one started; by this time, the clock interprets the two short 6-hour blocks of light as being long (that is, able to stimulate both Phase I and Phase II). Consequently, the testes remain patent, a condition appropriate to long day-lengths. The biological clock has been "tricked" because Phase I was stimulated only in the first circadian day, while Phase II was stimulated only in the second circadian day.

Although the experimental procedure presented here is not to be found in an animal's normal environment, the results of these manipulations indicate that in nature, a circadian clock can be used to indicate that day length is increasing. To the extent that the appearance of sexual behavior is under the influence of endocrine events, the control of these humoral factors by a biological oscillator is an efficient way for sexuality to be tied to the season of the year. There may be, in addition, other mechanisms that would account for seasonality in some species (Rusak and Zucker, 1975).

One highly adaptive feature of tuning reproductive clocks to light is that relevant physiological states can begin to develop before the onset of the ecologically critical event (e.g., abundant food in late spring) and thus be ready for full operation by the time that the correct time for breeding approaches. Hamsters normally display testicular regression during the winter months. The gonads begin to grow considerably before the time when mating actually occurs (reviewed in Rusak and Zucker, 1975).

MECHANISMS OF COPULATION

Once an organism has selected an appropriate sexual partner, and the organisms are situated in a reproductively supportive physical and temporal environment, actual copulation can proceed.

The effective performance of copulation and the production of pregnancy require a finely tuned series of behavioral actions.

In the remainder of this section, I summarize research that deals with the mechanisms and function of copulatory behavior. Research in this field falls into three areas. First, there are studies on the way in which copulatory stimulation augments the reproductive motivation of the male and the female so that they are both willing to mate at the same time. Second, there is a good deal of work dealing with the more mechanical reflex coordination of the two animals' genital apparatus, so that sperm and egg can unite. Finally, a body of research is devoted to analyzing the ways in which behavior and behaviorally derived stimulation induce the physiological responses in the female that are necessary for her pregnancy.

AUGMENTATION OF SEXUAL MOTIVATION. As was discussed in the previous sections, sexual motivation (i.e., the readiness to mate) in females and males is not always at maximal levels. There are temporal fluctuations (seasonal cycles super-imposed upon the gonadal cycle), and full readiness for mating is sometimes real-ized only after initial sexual contact with the sexual partner. As female *Drosophila* mature, their receptivity increases rapidly between 24 and 48 hours after eclosion (Manning, 1967), probably as a function of endogenous changes in the secretory activity of the corpus allatum. Although their subsequent receptivity remains fairly constant thereafter, the females require some copulatory stimulation from males before they will accept the male. Analogously, domestic female rats come into heat as a function of their ovarian cycle; however, there is often an enhancement of mating behavior following initial copulatory stimulation from the male (Beach, 1948). Applying the "ecological method"—that is, comparing the responses of phylogenetically distant species to common environmental pressures (Lockard, 1971)—the copulation-induced augmentation of mating in *Drosophila* and rats has been found to have some common features. First, the increase in receptivity is a function of the kind of stimulation that a male of the species gives during copu-lation. Bennet-Clark, Ewing, and Manning (1973) found that female *Drosophila melanogaster* were more receptive to male courtship if immediately prior to the introduction of the males, the females were presented with an electronically sim-ulated analog of the courting song. Similarly, female rats showed an increased probability of presenting the receptive posture (lordosis) to male rats if they were first primed with two seconds of experimenter-delivered cervical stimulation. Cervical stimulation of this kind is the type that a male delivers during his copu-latory intromissions (Rodriguez-Sierra, Crowley, and Komisaruk, 1975).

These experiments demonstrate that female rats and fruit flies possess a kind of "reproductive memory" for stimulation; the effects of stimulation persist even after the stimulation itself has terminated. In the experiment on *Drosophila,* for example, the effects of five minutes of simulated courtship song exerted a facili-tating effect on mating for five minutes after the priming stopped. Thereafter, there was no effect of the premating stimulation. In the experiment in which mechanical stimulation of the cervix facilitated mating in female rats, the increase in receptivity lasted for several hours after the two seconds of vaginal stimulation had ceased (Rodriguez-Sierra *et al.,* 1975).

The mechanisms controlling the various classes of sexual responses, as well as the mechanisms controlling the more general "sexual drive," are complex. Female rodents, for example, are not simply "receptive" or "unreceptive" (Adler, 1974). In a variety of mammals, the female is currently thought to display several differ-ent kinds of sexual responses, relevant to her sexuality. The following terms and definitions describing a female's sexual behavior have been offered by Beach (1976, p. 105):

1. *Receptivity* is defined in terms of female responses "necessary and suffi-cient for the male's success in achieving intravaginal ejaculations."
2. *Attractivity* refers to the female's "stimulus value in evoking sexual responses by the male."
3. *Proceptivity* denotes "various reactions by the female toward the male which constitute her assumption of initiative in establishing or maintain-ing sexual interaction."

The notion that these three behavioral constructs are independent is supported by the fact that they can be experimentally separated. A female displaying spontaneously occurring constant vaginal cornification will often display lordosis in response to the experimenter's manual stimulation, while the probability of a male rat's eliciting lordosis can vary considerably; and even when a male can occasionally "force" a lordosis from one of these female rats, she will often emit rejecting behavior toward the copulating male (Adler and Bell, 1969).

In the experiments of Rodriguez-Sierra et al., (1975) described above, when the experimenter-delivered cervical stimulation increased the probability of a male rat's subsequently eliciting lordosis from the female, she sometimes went through several minutes immediately after the stimulation during which she fought off the male and rolled over on her back.

The sexual drive is not only complex, it is probably not a unitary construct (Hinde, 1959). It is known that a variety of exteroceptive stimuli (like mildly painful shock) can potentiate and/or accelerate a male rat's sexual behavior (Barfield and Sachs, 1968; Caggiula and Vlahoulis, 1974; Sachs and Barfield, 1974). This kind of stimulation does seem to motivate behavior and not merely evoke reflex-like components of the male's sexual response. In one study, the female was removed from the test cage after each series of mounts, and the male was required to press a bar to regain access to the female. Just as shock induces copulation in the presence of the female, in this study the shocks elicited the operant bar-pressing response, the reinforcement for which was the addition of the female to the cage (Sachs, Macaione, and Fegy, 1974). Peripheral shock therefore seems genuinely to "arouse" the animal and not simply to produce shortened reflex latencies.

Despite the evidence for a general motivational effect, however, such exteroceptive stimulation does not simply activate a specifically sexual drive state. When a female rat was not present, shocks increased general exploration and investigation of objects like food, pieces of wood, and water bottles in the test cage (Caggiula and Eibergen, 1969). General arousal is an important factor in sexual activity. Lethargic male rats can be induced to mate by peripherally administered electric shock (Crowley, Popolow, and Ward, 1973). There is, however, a fine balance between general and specifically sexual elements of behavioral activation. Too much general activity would decrease the male's tendencies to attend to the female and would thus diminish his sexual capacity.

Such a maladaptive increase in general activity seems to have occurred in selection studies with Drosophila melanogaster (Manning, 1961). In this experiment, Manning placed 50 pairs of flies in a vial and selected the 10 fastest-mating pairs and the 10 slowest. Continuing selection for 25 generations, Manning developed a line of "fast-mating" flies, a line of "slow-mating" flies, and an unselected control line that was intermediate in mating speed. After developing the two selected lines, he tested the activity of the flies by admitting them to an arena where the number of squares entered by a fly in a given time was scored. The flies from the slow lines had much higher scores on this measure of general activity than did the fast-mating lines. There were also differences between "fast" and "slow" males in more specifically sexual measures, like frequency of copulatory licking and latency for initiating courtship. The fast flies licked more and initiated courtship faster than the slow males. The fast-mating males thus had a higher level of sexual activity and a lower level of general activity than the slow-mating males. Under normal conditions, these two activities would presumably be coordinated at an optimum level. Unbalancing the coordination, as in artificial selection for the slow lines, disrupts overall sexual performance.

INTEGRATION OF COPULATORY REFLEXES. Even when the male and the female are at their respective peaks of sexual readiness, there are purely mechanical problems that must be overcome. Consider the mating sequence in rats. The female approaches the male from a distance and then quickly darts away (McClintock and Adler, 1978). The female's darting possibly represents a "soliciting pattern" (Beach, 1976), and if the cage is sufficiently large, the darting away is almost always followed by a male's pursuit and mount. Some of the mounts of the male rat are accompanied by a penile insertion (intromission), and the final insertion of a series is accompanied by the ejaculation of sperm and the seminal material that forms a vaginal plug in the female. The mount (with or without intromission) lasts for only a fraction of a second (Bermant, 1965); the period between successive copulatory contacts lasts a minute or more (Diakow, 1974).

Each of these phases of the complex coordinating of the genital apparatus of male and female rats has a function. The male rat's pattern of multiple intromissions preceding ejaculation is necessary for the induction of pregnancy (see below). For the male to be able to insert his penis into the vaginal orifice, however, the female must raise her rump and deflect her tail laterally (Diakow, 1975). The elevation of the female's rump and the deflection of her tail occur when she assumes the lordosis posture (the concave curvature of her back) indicating receptivity. Lordosis itself is a hormone-sensitive spinal reflex (Pfaff and Lewis, 1974). As is the case with the other sexual reflexes, there are supraspinal inhibitory influences on the spinal elements controlling lordosis. These inhibitory mechanisms are in turn disinhibited by the endogenous hormonal and exteroceptive behavioral stimuli associated with mating.

The behavior that supports the male's intromission also has a spinal reflexological component (Hart, 1968). In one experiment, male rats were spinally transected in the midthoracic region. After each animal recuperated from the operation, it was tested for the presence of genital reflexes. The rat was placed on its back in a restraining cylinder with the genital area outside the container. When the experimenter pulled back the preputial sheath over the glans, a series of genital "flips" occurred approximately every two or three minutes. The responses came in clusters, and although the specific responses that appeared in each cluster varied, there were only a few basic patterns. A typical response cluster included three or four erections, one to three quick flips of the penis, and one to four long flips of the penis. After the response cluster was completed, the animal remained completely quiet for at least two or three minutes, even though constant pressure was still being exerted on the penile area. Despite the constant stimulus to the penis and the presumable constant level of hormone circulating in the blood, the genital reflexes occurred periodically; the two or three minutes between clusters seemed programmed by the spinal cord itself.

The spinally programmed pacing mechanism for sexual reflexes is, however, modified by other neural control systems. (It is noteworthy that no one studying the spinal flips in transected male rats has ever observed ejaculation or even seminal emission.) Supporting the view that there are higher-order timing elements in the male rat's nervous system that affect copulatory pacing are the experiments that demonstrate the existence of "mount bouts" (Sachs and Barfield, 1970). The mount bout is a sequence of one or more mounts, with or without penile insertion, that is not interrupted by any noncopulatory behavior (except genital grooming or orientation of the male toward the female). If the pacing of the male's copulation were totally determined by spinal reflexes and if the elicitation of these reflexes was released by tactile stimulation, then males that did not receive penile stimulation should show grossly distorted pacing of the mount bouts. The model of copulatory behavior presented thus far is that there are spinal and supraspinal elements controlling the topography and timing of copulatory responses. These copulatory automatisms in male and female are effective only if they occur in a synchronized manner, with the male and female's genital apparatus positioned correctly with respect to each other. Painstaking analyses of high-speed film of rat copulation (Diakow, 1975; Pfaff and Lewis, 1974) have begun to unravel the complexity of the relation between mount, lordosis, and penile insertion.

In order to investigate the neurophysiological basis for copulatory reflexes, we have shown that there are at least three main sensory nerves in the genital region of female rats that may be involved in its mating sequence: the pelvic, the pudendal, and the genitofemoral nerves (Komisaruk, Adler, and Hutchison, 1972). One of these nerves, the pudendal, receives afferent input ipsilaterally from the perineal region surrounding the vagina. The sensory field of this nerve extends from the base of the clitoral sheath to the base of the tail in the midline, and laterally along the inner surface of the thigh.

There were two characteristics of this nerve's sensory field that are relevant to the occurrence of intromission. First, the total size of the sensory field was significantly greater (approximately 30%) in castrated females given exogenous estrogen injections than in uninjected castrate controls (Komisaruk et al., 1972). A similar increase in field size was found by Kow and Pfaff (1973–1974). Second, the most sensitive portion within the sensory field was not invariably the perivaginal area but a spot approximately 1 cm caudal to the tip of the clitoral sheath (Adler, Davis and Komisaruk, 1977). The enlarged estrous sensory field may facilitate a slightly misplaced penile thrust's activating the pudendal nerve, which is involved in orienting the female to the male. The "off-center" organization of the sensory field may also play a role in facilitating intromission: the most sensitive area of this field corresponds to a point on the female's perineum that the penis contacts during a mount with intromission. This perineal contact possibly facilitates the penis's "locating" the vaginal orifice (Adler et al., 1977; Adler, Komisaruk, and Davis, 1974).

BEHAVIORAL INDUCTION OF PREGNANCY

In this analysis of the functions and mechanisms of sexual behavior we have followed (1) the steps by which appropriate mates are selected from those available in the general environment; (2) how the sexual activities of these organisms are synchronized with the physical and temporal variations in that environment; and (3) how the pair's behavior becomes finely tuned enough to permit actual copulation to occur. This fine tuning encompasses several events, including the augmentation of sexual motivation and the coordination of the genital structures.

There is a final set of behavioral mechanisms involved in fine-grained integration that must be included in a description of sexuality. These are the responses that set up the physiological conditions necessary for the next stages of reproduction, pregnancy and parenthood. Behaviorally derived stimulation is especially important in this regard because the physiological processes of ovulation, fertilization, and pregnancy do not proceed automatically in all species. Behavior—and the stimulation derived from behavior—often plays a critical role in their induction. In this section of the chapter, we examine some specific effects of behavior on reproductive physiology and then analyze the mechanisms responsible for producing the behavior.

Although the ovarian cycle has a strong endogenous component, behavioral and social stimuli can modify a number of ovarian events. Consider the progression of events in the ovarian cycle of mammals. Data have been presented demonstrating an endogenous biological clock that controlled the timing of "spontaneous" ovulation in the rat. The event of ovulation is embedded in an ovarian cycle consisting of three main stages: (1) an initial follicular phase, during which the ovarian follicles grow; (2) ovulation, when the mature follicle releases the egg; and (3) the luteal phase, when the ruptured follicle is transformed into the corpus luteum, which in turn secretes progesterone. In different species, stimulation derived from behavior plays an important role in many, if not all, of these stages.

One of the most striking examples of behavioral control in the estrous cycle is seen in some species (e.g., cat, rabbit, ferret, mink, some species of mice, and perhaps three shrews) in which ovulation is not spontaneous but depends upon stimuli delivered by the male during courtship and copulation (Adler, 1974). In a broad and careful phylogenetic survey of muroid and cricetine rodents, Dewsbury and co-workers have related the patterns of copulatory behavior of male rodents with the induction of ovulation and pregnancy in the female (Dewsbury, 1975).

Behaviorally derived stimuli can even influence ovulation in species that normally ovulate spontaneously (Aron, Asch, and Roos, 1966). For example, in female rats displaying normal estrous cycles, copulatory stimulation can advance the time when ovulation will occur and can sometimes increase the number of eggs released (Rodgers, 1971; Rodgers and Schwartz, 1972, 1973). Behavioral stimuli exert an even stronger effect under some experimental conditions. In female rats, for example, ovulation can be experimentally inhibited by placing these animals under conditions of constant light (Brown-Grant, Davidson, and Grieg, 1973; Hoffman, 1973) or by injecting a number of pharmacological agents during a critical period of proestrus (Everett and Sawyer, 1950). Female rats thus treated become "induced ovulators": they do not ovulate spontaneously but will do so if they receive enough copulatory stimulation (Adler, 1974).

Although the female rat is normally a "spontaneous ovulator," she nonetheless possesses the neuroanatomical and neuroendocrine machinery for induced ovulation. This fact implies that the differences between various categories of reproductive function in related species (e.g., the difference between female rodents that are "induced" ovulators versus those that are "spontaneous" ovulators) can be attributed to slight quantitative differences in the neuroendocrine thresholds for triggering pituitary–ovarian events (Everett, 1964). The sufficiency of a female's endogenous endocrine cycles for inducing ovulation, independent of copulatory stimulation, determines the categorization of a species as "spontaneous" or "induced" ovulators.

BEHAVIORAL INDUCTION OF PROGESTATIONAL HORMONE SECRETION. In the mammalian ovarian cycle, once successful ovulation has occurred, either of two sequences can follow. A female can go through the luteal phase of the cycle and return to the start of another estrous cycle, or she can become fertilized and enter the prolonged luteal phase characteristic of pregnancy. In the females of some species (e.g., in some primates), the spontaneous luteal phase of each ovarian cycle is long, and there is enough progesterone to permit uterine implantation of a fertilized egg. If no egg implants, the uterus, which has been developing under the influence of progesterone, sheds its inner lining, the endometrium.

In the rat, the hamster, and several species of mice, however, there is no spontaneous luteal phase of any functional consequence; in these organisms, some aspect of the male's copulation triggers the progestational state underlying pregnancy (Adler, 1974; Dewsbury, 1975; Diamond, 1970; Diamond and Yanagimachi, 1968; McGill and Coughlin, 1970). In the remainder of this section I present data, primarily from our laboratory, on how the male rat's behavior facilitates the induction of pregnancy in the female, and I describe some of the mechanisms that produce these adaptive behavioral patterns. By concentrating on one species, an attempt will be made to integrate the behavioral and the physiological aspects of reproduction.

The copulatory behavior of the male rat consists of a series of mounts and dismounts from the female. On some of these mounts, penile intromission occurs, and on the final intromission, the male ejaculates sperm and seminal fluid, which form a vaginal plug. Following a period of behavioral inactivity (the postejaculatory interval), the male resumes copulating. The pattern of mount, intromission, ejaculation, and refractory period can be repeated several times in one session.

Since one of the most consistent features of this species' copulatory pattern is the series of multiple intromissions preceding each ejaculation (Dewsbury, 1975), the question arises: What function do these multiple intromissions have in successful reproduction? In several experiments, the probability of pregnancy was determined for females that received a normal complement of intromissions preceding the male's ejaculation (high-intromission group); these data were compared with the probability of inducing pregnancy in an experimental group of females that were permitted only a reduced number of preejaculatory intromissions (low-intromission group) (Adler, 1969; Wilson, Adler, and LeBoeuf, 1965). About 20 days after copulation, the females in both groups were sacrificed and their uteri examined for the presence of viable fetuses. In one study (Wilson *et al.*, 1965), approximately 90% of the females in the high-intromission group were pregnant, while only 20% of the females in the low-intromission group were pregnant. Thus, multiple intromissions appear to be necessary for the induction of pregnancy.

How do multiple copulatory intromissions stimulate pregnancy? Part of the answer is to be found in the organization of the female rat's four- to five-day estrous cycle. Unlike in most primates, the ovarian cycle of the female rat does not automatically go through a functional luteal phase. If the female is to become pregnant, some event must trigger the progestational state. Initially, we hypothesized that the stimulation derived from multiple intromissions triggers a neuroendocrine reflex that results in the secretion of progesterone.

To test this hypothesis, we compared the number of females in both groups that failed to show regular four-day estrous cycles (Adler, 1969; Wilson *et al.*, 1965). Almost 100% of the females in the high-intromission group ($n = 9$) failed to show four-day estrous cycles following stimulation, whereas only 22% of the females in the low-intromission group failed to show cycles ($n = 9$). Since cessation of behavioral cyclicity is one of the signs of progestational hormone secretion, we concluded that multiple intromissions stimulate the release of progesterone. Because the proportion of females in each group that stopped showing behavioral estrous cycles was approximately the same as the proportion that had developing pups in the previous experiment, multiple intromissions appeared to stimulate the induction of pregnancy by stimulating the secretion of gestational hormones. This interpretation was supported by progesterone assays (Adler *et al.*, 1970). Within 24 hours after mating, females in the high-intromission group had significantly more progesterone in their peripheral blood than did females in the low-intromission group. It is now known that cervical stimulation induces twice-daily surges of pituitary prolactin release and that this daily prolactin is necessary for secretion of the ovarian progesterone necessary for pregnancy (Smith, McLean, and Neill, 1976).

We wanted to study the dynamics of this behaviorally initiated neuroendocrine reflex. In one study, we found that with increasing numbers of intromissions (even without ejaculation), the proportion of females becoming progestational increased (Adler, 1969). With 4 or fewer intromissions, fewer than 10% of the females were progestational; with 13–16 intromissions, approximately 85% of the females became progestational. These data indicate that the occurrence of multiple copulatory intromissions is necessary and sufficient to trigger the hormonal state of pregnancy. We are now attempting to follow the behavioral stimulus through successive levels of the female's neuroendocrine system to determine the mechanism by which copulatory intromissions trigger the secretion of the gestational hormones. From the electrophysiological study of genital sensory processes, we determined that it was the pelvic nerve that innervated the vaginocervical area (Komisaruk *et al.*, 1972). These data support the hypothesis that the pelvic nerve is the afferent channel for the induction of progesterone secretion. Further evidence for this conclusion comes from experiments in which the pelvic nerves were cut. In these studies, the female rats did not become progestational after mechanical stimulation of the cervix (Kollar, 1953; Carlsson and De Feo, 1965; Spies and Niswender, 1971).

We are now attempting to trace the copulatory stimulus into the central nervous system components of the neuroendocrine reflex. Since a number of intromissions are required to trigger the progestational state, there must be some sort of storage mechanism by which the stimulation from each brief (250 msec) penile insertion is retained and combined with stimulation from succeeding intromissions.

To determine the limits of the storage capacity of this system, an experiment was performed in which the rate of stimulation was varied (Edmonds, Zoloth, and Adler, 1972). For a given group of females, both the number of intromissions permitted (2, 5, or 10) and the interval between intromissions varied: the interintromission-interval values ranged from the control rate of *ad libitum* copulation (approximately 40 sec) up to one hour.

With 10 intromissions, 100% of the females become progestational. This result is especially striking because the intromissions could be spaced one every half hour without a diminution in their effectiveness. The results for females receiving five intromissions also indicate that spaced intromissions are as effective as intromissions delivered at the control rate and, in addition, that intromissions at the rate of one every four or five minutes may be more effective in stimulating the progestational response than the control rate. One intromission delivered every half hour provided a density of stimulation of only 1 part per 7,200 (one intromission—250 msec—per half hour). This potency points to an exquisitely adapted form of neuroendocrine integration by which species-specific stimuli (the multiple intromissions) are stored by an adaptively specialized neural mechanism.

The operation of this entire pregnancy system can be conceptualized as a biological amplifier in which each stage lengthens the temporal characteristics of the previous one. Stimulation from the brief penile intromissions is stored and accumulated. The stimulation leads to a central nervous system event, the duration of which is undetermined but which may run for several hours (Barraclough and Sawyer, 1959). Pituitary involvement may last 12 days (Pencharz and Long, 1933); the ovary secretes large amounts of progesterone for 19 days (Morishige, Pepe, and Rothchild, 1973). The final stage, uterine pregnancy, continues for more than 20 days. In this sequence, the intromissions trigger the tonic secretion of progesterone.

The storage of the initial copulatory stimulation in the female rat resembles the other examples of reproductive mnemonic devices that were discussed earlier in the chapter. Adaptively specialized storage systems are, in fact, frequently occurring phenomena in reproductive physiology. The phenomenon of "delayed pseudopregnancy" represents a classic example (Everett, 1968); if proper parameters are used, electrical stimulation of the brain results in the induction of a progestational state in female rats, but only after a delay of hours or days.

Another example of reproductive storage occurs in the hamster, in which copulatory stimulation facilitates the subsequent parturition, more than 20 days after the stimulus (Diamond, 1972). Although exogenous progesterone injections can trigger the progestational response and permit a pregnancy to follow artificial insemination, parturition is not normal unless copulatory stimulation from a male hamster is provided at the time of insemination. The mechanisms by which the stimulus is stored in the female's neuroendocrine system is not yet known precisely in any of these examples, but phenomenologically, they all represent the storage and amplification of a triggering stimulus.

BEHAVIORAL INDUCTION OF SPERM TRANSPORT IN FEMALES. When first studying the copulatory influences on pregnancy in rats, we concentrated on the function of multiple intromissions in stimulating the neuroendocrine reflex that resulted in progesterone secretion and subsequent gestation. Since all of the female rats in our experiment, in both the high- and the low-intromission groups, had sperm and plug deposited in their vaginas, it was an easy assumption that sperm transport and fertilization were normal (Adler, 1969). In one experiment, however, we checked the condition of ova in the Fallopian tubes of the female rats three days after copulation.

Females that had received many preejaculatory intromissions all had developing ova in the blastocyst stage, whereas females that had received an ejaculation preceded by only one intromission had unfertilized and degenerating ova (Adler, 1968, 1969). From subsequent studies (Adler, 1969; Adler and Zoloth, 1970), we discovered that a number of preejaculatory intromissions were necessary to induce the normal transport of sperm from the vagina into the uterus of female rats that had just received an ejaculation.

Besides requiring the preejaculatory intromissions, the postejaculatory transport of sperm in female rats has two other behavioral prerequisites. First, a prolonged ejaculatory response is required. (In one experiment, males that dismounted in less than two seconds following ejaculation produced uterine sperm counts that were significantly lower than those produced by males that stayed on the female for two or more seconds; Matthews and Adler, 1977.)

It was also discovered that a period of behavioral quiescence by the male following ejaculation is necessary for the process of sperm transport in the female to be completed. Maximal numbers of sperm do not reach the uterus until six to eight minutes following ejaculation (Adler and Zoloth, 1970; Matthews and Adler, 1977). If, during this time, a female rat receives copulatory intromissions, the number of sperm in the uterus are reduced, and the size of her litter is diminished (Adler, 1974).

The potential disruption of sperm transport by postejaculatory copulatory stimulation may have functional significance for the organization of reproduction in this species. Theoretically, one male could "cancel" the effects of another male's copulation. If the second male begins copulating too soon after the previous male has completed an ejaculatory series, his multiple intromissons may prevent the first male's sperm from reaching the uterus, presumably by dislodging the plug. The second male's sperm would then be deposited upon his ejaculation and could fertilize the ova. To test this possibility, we arranged a series of mating tests involving albino female rats (Adler and Zoloth, 1970). An albino female was allowed to mate first with an albino male and was then mated with a pigmented male for a second ejaculatory series. Paternity could be established soon after the pups are born, since pups sired by albino fathers are light-colored and have clear eyes, whereas pups of pigmented fathers have dark skins and pigmented eyes. If the substitution of a pigmented for an albino male is made within the first few minutes after the initial ejaculation, approximately 60% of the offsprings are pigmented. If, however, 45–60 minutes elapse between copulations, only 23% of the offsprings are pigmented. Therefore, a male rat can, if he begins copulating soon enough, prevent the insemination of a given female by another male that had copulated previously (Adler and Zoloth, 1970). Thus, for effective sperm transport, the female rat must have no cervical stimulation for several minutes after receiving an ejaculation.

What, then, prevents a male that has just ejaculated from resuming his intromission during this critical time? We suggest that it is the male's postejaculatory refractory period that prevents him from resuming copulation too soon (Adler and Zoloth, 1970). The male rats in our laboratory require an average of 4.5 minutes after ejaculating before they deliver the first intromission of their next ejaculatory series. Since three intromissions on the average are required to dislodge the vaginal plug totally (Lisk, 1969), and since sperm transport is relatively complete within six to eight minutes, the postejaculatory refractory period is of the correct magnitude to permit effective sperm transport into the uterine lumen.

The hypothesized function of the postejaculatory refractory period may have ecological significance for rodent population dynamics. Under conditions of crowding, laboratory rats show persistent social pathology (Calhoun, 1962a). One type of behavioral abnormality is a kind of pansexual behavior in which males mount at a much higher rate than usual. In these crowded colonies, reproduction decreases, partly because of the pathological increase in mounting. Even where crowding is not a problem, colonies of rats with a higher percentage of males produce fewer pups than colonies with fewer males (Calhoun, 1962a). One of the reasons for reduced reproductive performance in such colonies may be copulatory interference with sperm transport.

Reproductive processes are also blocked in other species; the odor of strange males inhibits implantation in female mice (Parkes and Bruce 1961). Sperm are rejected by the bursa copulatrix of *Drosophila* females during interspecific mating (Dobzhansky, Ehrman, and Kastritsis, 1968); and prolonged auditory stimulation can reduce fertility in rats (Zondek and Tamari, 1967). All of these examples of disruptions in reproductive processing may be "pharmacological" in the sense that normally, behavioral processes—like the postejaculatory interval in male rats—protect the organism from reproductive dysfunction.

MECHANISMS RESPONSIBLE FOR ADAPTIVE COPULATORY PATTERNS IN RATS. If the postejaculatory refractory period of the male rat is an integral part of the copulatory process leading to sperm transport and successful pregnancy, its occurrence may be the result of an active physiological process of a type that normally ensures an adaptive behavioral inhibition. Several experiments now point to the operation of just such an active inhibitory process during the postejaculatory interval, when the male rat displays a pattern of "tonic immobility" (Dewsbury, 1967). Along with this behavior pattern, the hippocampal and cortical electroencephalograph (EEG) display the kind of spindling and slow-wave electrical activity (Kurtz and Adler, 1973) that often signals physiological inhibition (Gellhorn, 1967). Another feature of the postejaculatory interval that indicates its active nature is the 22 kHz vocalization emitted by the male during his "absolute refractory period" (Barfield and Geyer, 1975). When the EEG and vocalizations were recorded simultaneously, a correlation of approximately .95 was found between the inhibitory EEG spindling and the emission of the 22 kHz vocalizations.

On the basis of behavioral and physiological indices like those presented in the preceding paragraph, Kurtz was able to develop an opponent-process model to describe the male rat's copulatory pattern (Kurtz and Adler, 1973). The performance of the successive intromissions culminating in ejaculation is induced by a positive appetitive system. The function of this system is to produce the series of copulatory events necessary for ejaculation in the male and the induction of pregnancy in the female. The behavioral refractoriness of the male during his postejaculatory interval (necessary to permit sperm transport in the female) is under an inhibitory system, reflected by the EEG spindling.

A pattern of multiple control is also found in the sexual behavior of the female rat. There is an active (proceptive) phase in which she solicits and elicits male mounts (McClintock and Adler, 1978). During the male's mount with intromission, the penile contact with the cervix induces a momentary behavioral inhibition of the female (Diakow, 1974). Since cervical stimulation from intromission is necessary to induce pregnancy, it seems adaptive that the female rat should be inhibited from moving and should be less responsive to certain classes of stimuli while receiving an intromission. Komisaruk (1974) suggested that lordosis is an extensor reflex, which is the classical approach reflex and which would stabilize the female in her position on the substrate.

Finally, there is evidence that prolonged copulatory stimulation can, over the long run, inhibit or reduce female receptivity. The kind of cortical spindling that was described in male rats has also been found in female rats as they approach sexual satiety (Kurtz, 1975). Furthermore, the diminution of receptivity following copulation is a phenomenon not restricted to rats; it has been found in females of a wide variety of species, including hamsters, guinea pigs, turkeys, lizards, fruit flies, and some cockroaches (Barth, 1968; Carter and Schein, 1971; Crews, 1973; Goldfoot and Goy, 1970; Hardy and DeBold, 1972; Manning, 1967; Schein and Hale, 1965). It is by the precise integration of positive and inhibitory behavioral mechanisms that behavior is adaptively organized in sexually reproducing organisms.

Although there are many variations in the specific form of sexual behavior, and the physiological mechanisms controlling it, every sexually reproducing species must "solve" some basic problems of sexual synchronization: (1) the selection by an organism of a reproductively appropriate mate within the species; (2) the tying of reproductive activities to a spatially and temporally adequate set of environmental conditions; and (3) the coordination of the reproductive moods and copulatory movements of the mating pair, as well as the setting up of conditions compatible with the next stages of reproduction, pregnancy and parenthood. The purpose of this section has been to outline some of the ways that the physiological mechanisms controlling sexual behavior contribute to this synchronization.

SOME GENERAL PROPERTIES OF SOCIAL BEHAVIOR AND ITS MECHANISMS

Before discussing the second topic of this essay, the physiological basis of aggression, it is appropriate to make a few comments on the mechanisms controlling social behavior in general.

First of all, the emphasis here has been on *behavior*. This statement is not really a tautology, for the word *behavior* in this context denotes large-scale motor movement, often involving the entire organism. Psychology has always had at least two realms of discourse, and sometimes there are difficulties in translating from one to the other. The first realm is that of behavior, as defined above, while the second deals with subjective experience. Students of sexual behavior, for example, have the choice of defining their topic in terms of sexual responses and reflexes or in terms of sexual experience, love, affiliative tendencies, etc.

To be sure, analyses of emotion or bonding in animals are usually pinned to some overtly observable response (either behavior or physiological—especially autonomic—events). Nonetheless, the distinction between response-oriented and experience-oriented research is strategically, if not epistemologically, real.

Given an initial commitment to the "behavioral" tradition, there is a second set of choices. Behavior can be studied from a more molecular perspective, in which elementary units of response are analyzed, or higher-order units—molar behavior—can be analyzed. One of the major tasks of future research in physiological psychology and ethology will be to move from the analysis of overt motor patterns, and their sensory and neural control systems, to higher-order units of behavior. In this chapter, physiological mechanisms have been related to the first category: particular, discrete responses, such as hormonal facilitation of the lordosis reflex in female rats or courtship bowing and cooing in male ring doves. If we apply the hierarchical organization (discussed in some detail on pages 54-56) these smaller, motor movements are seen to be organized into larger categories of behavior (e.g., courtship). Many of the analyses in this volume deal with questions of *social organization*, *mating systems*, and *foraging patterns*. Concepts such as these are higher-order units that integrate (or at least summarize) the lower-level units of responsiveness. For example, in ring doves the pattern of sequentially shared *incubation duties* is a part of the *monogamous mating system*. To the extent that a particular hormone or neural system influences a more molecular response, it will influence the more molar behavioral unit. In the future, one of the major tasks in the analysis of physiological mechanisms is to determine the relationship between the proximal physiological causes and the larger units of social organization.

This kind of research will be especially important because it will fill in the intermediate links on the other axis of our analysis, that is, the temporal–causal dimension. Modern sociobiology has concentrated on relating genetic–evolutionary pressures and strategies (distal causes) to the larger units of social organization. Theories of parental investment, for example, relate reproductive–genetic strategies to concepts like monogamy. The more molecular behavioral constructs are given names like *cuckoldry, sequestering,* and *rape.* These terms are not really specific behavior patterns, as would be defined by physiological psychologists, but are molar categories. One rather unnecessarily extreme view would have it that we can dispense with lower-level units of behavioral analysis altogether. In the first chapter of his *Sociobiology* (1975), Wilson stated that the really important aspects of behavioral analysis are the linking of distal (genetic and ecological) factors directly to the larger units of social behavior. His view of what the field might (or should) include by the year 2000 consequently defines a large area for genes and consigns developmental and organismic factors to an "empty set."

A cautionary comment on the most extreme version of the sociobiological program is that there are too many degrees of freedom and that precise analyses of behavior and of proximal mechanisms are neglected. The careful study of the details of behavior characteristic of classical ethology and experimental psychology would be consciously neglected in this approach, if it were carried to extremes. Behaviorists are storytellers, and part of the tale is certainly the nature of the proximal mechanisms producing the responses.

Another reason for promoting the analysis of behavior and its physiological mechanisms is that this kind of research has the potential of enriching the evolutionary and ecological analyses of behavior, for by providing the intermediate links in the causal chain leading from gene to behavior, such analyses can both constrain and elaborate the causal nexus. Sociobiology would in turn be enriched and complemented.

This chapter is therefore written in an integrative spirit. The behavioral systems are defined, as often as possible, in terms of their functions (preparing for pregnancy, care of the young, warding off predation). The job of connecting the details of particular behavioral responses to larger behavioral categories is both a goal and a framework.

Part of the reason for the split between studies of the proximal and the distal causes of behavior may have been that different units of analyses proved useful in different fields. In the early days of the experimental analysis of behavior, for example, investigators concentrated on the causal factors controlling large categories of behavior, like sex and aggression. Instincts, with all the ambiguity of the term, were central concepts. When scientists began analyzing the role of specific physiological events, like the actions of a specific hormone, it became more useful to study changes in correspondingly specific responses. For example, intromission frequency in male rats became a standard measure, and often replaced more molar units like sexual arousal. With increasing experimental and technical sophistication during the past few decades, and with the infusion of an evolutionary–genetic concept, it may now be possible to build toward the higher units again.

A second general point concerning the physiological bases of social behavior is that by definition, at least two organisms are involved. Unlike the more molecular aspects of feeding and drinking, even sexual reflexes are performed with respect to, and in conjunction with, another organism. No matter how molecular the response, the proximal goal of each behavior has been social (for example, sexual union with a conspecific, or tissue damage of another animal as in some forms of aggression).

MOTIVATION

The variables discussed in this chapter are *behavioral* and *social*. A third characteristic of these responses is that they are *motivated*. There are obviously many ways to define and understand the concept of motivation (see discussions by Deutsch, 1960; Gallistel, 1979; Manning, 1972; Teitelbaum, 1967). It might be profitable to discuss some of these in the present context.

One criterion of motivation, popular among students of vertebrates, is that the animal will perform an arbitrary operant response if that response is followed (reinforced) by the opportunity to engage in the motivated behavior (Teitelbaum, 1967). A hungry animal, for example, learns to press a bar in a Skinner box if it is offered food reinforcement. Similarly, a female rat will press a bar if she is subsequently presented with a male rat (Bermant and Davidson, 1974). A male rat will learn a maze if it is permitted to intromit into a female at the end of the maze. This kind of operant test of motivation can be quite sensitive. For example, the latency between successive bar presses is a function of the *kind* of copulatory contacts. The latency after a mount is less than after an intromission, which in turn is less than after an ejaculation (Bermant & Davidson, 1974). Analogously, Thompson (1963, 1964) has shown that both game fowl and Siamese fighting fish will perform an arbitrary operant (passing through a plastic ring in the case of the Siamese fighting fish) if, following the operant, the animal is provided an opportunity to perform an aggressive display.

In demonstrating the existence of motivation, the "arbitrary" nature of the operant response has been stressed. In recent years, the notion of an "arbitrary" response has, however, been modified. It seems that a response may not be all that arbitrary for any given learning task; because of recent work on the biological boundaries of learning (Seligman and Hager, 1972), or pre-adaptation (Rozin and Kalat, 1971), the view has emerged that certain motor acts are easier to associate with a contingency if these responses are "naturally" related to the contingency. The classic example is the Garcia effect (see Seligman and Hager, 1972, for a review).

Despite the restriction on the class of the "arbitrary" behavior, it is generally conceded that an experimenter can increase the frequency of a response if the opportunity to engage in some motivated act is offered as a reinforcer.

The dependence of an experimentally defined operant response upon a specific reinforcer that follows it may have an analogue in the natural world. According to Craig (1918), the responses of animals may be divided into two broad categories, appetitive and consummatory. While such global terms may not be useful for modern, detailed analyses of behavior, they do highlight several properties of motivated sequences of behavior. Craig postulated that there are four stages in the performance of a response sequence. First, there is a state of deprivation (or *drive*). This leads the animal into an *appetitive* phase, in which it exhibits variable, searching behavior directed toward the attainment of the appetite stimulus. This is followed by the third stage, the performance of the often stereotyped consummatory response. The consummatory response then leads to a state of *satiety,* in which the postulated drive state is reduced.

In terms of this ethological analysis, the performance of the experimentally defined operant may represent a laboratory analog of Craig's appetitive behavior.

Hierarchical Organization

The sequence, in nature, of variable, goal-oriented "appetitive" response followed by performance of the fixed, stereotyped, species-general consummatory response, as well as the emission of an instrumental response followed by reinforcement in laboratory preparations may both indicate a motivationally dependent temporal organization. They both illustrate a general characteristic of motivated behavior: functionally related acts becoming temporally grouped (Manning, 1972). One of the ways of describing this grouping is by reference to a hierarchical organization (Gallistel, 1979; Tinbergen, 1952).

According to this hierarchical analysis, the simple units of motor behavior represent the output of the lowest level of the organismic hierarchy (Tinbergen, 1952). Motivational variables represent higher units of the hierarchy, and these higher units selectively facilitate or suppress the lower units. Gallistel (1979) has carried this analysis to the organization of motor behavior in general and in so doing has pointed out that this hierarchy is a "lattice hierarchy." In a lattice hierarchy, there are many different elemental motor patterns at the bottom of the hierarchy, with overlapping lines of control from higher centers. The result is that in a particular sequence, responses can be called into play by a number of different higher (motivational) systems.

To illustrate a lattice hierarchy, consider the lordosis reflex already discussed. This reflex occurs in receptive female rats as part of their sexual response system. The lordosis reflex is, however, simply a reflex that is defined by a curvature of the back and a correlated elevation of the perineal region. While adult *female* rodents display lordosis as part of their copulatory pattern only under sexual stimulation, both male and female guinea pigs display it in the absence of hormonal priming (see Adler, 1974, for a review of this work). In this context, neonatal lordosis is normally elicited by the mother's licking the rump of the pup. During the first month of life, the frequency of this elicited reflex declines, and the decline is, in fact, paralleled by an increase in the occurrence of the adult pattern of micturition. The functional significance of the neonatal lordosis is that it probably represents an exogenously stimulated release of urine and feces. Anyone who has tried to rear young rodents knows that one of the major problems is that micturition and elimination are not automatic (endogenously triggered) and must be stimulated (with a camel's hair brush or some other appropriate stimulus). As the brain matures, micturition comes under internal control, exogenously stimulated elimination reflexes are no longer needed, and consequently there is an increase in spontaneous elimination during the time that the elicitability of lordosis decreases. The basic spinal mechanisms for lordosis are presumably present during adulthood, but they are inhibited by higher centers and appear only in females when the proper hormonal milieu (e.g., ovarian estrogen and progesterone) and exogenous stimulation (a male's mounting) are present.

It can be concluded that the lordosis reflex is a low-level motor response that can be tapped into by a higher "elimination" system during infancy and, in the adult female, by the "sexual" system. (The general nature of sexual reflexes was presented earlier in this chapter).

Similarly, a courting male Japanese quail will mount a female, grab her head feathers in his beak, and pull her over on her side. This motor pattern is quite similar to the response of a male to another male during a fight. In the former case, it is part of the copulatory sequence and in the latter a component of aggression. (It may be significant that in the Orient, this species has undergone artificial selection for aggression and that the males have been used for sport, as fighting cocks are in the West.)

The general conclusion from this kind of work is that a given unit can occur in dissimilar social–motivational contexts. There is a large literature on the question of different drive states and especially the problem of unitary drive states. (That is, are there many individual drive states or fewer—perhaps one drive state—that can influence a range of behavior?) This literature has been discussed by Deutsch (1960), Gallistel (1979), Hinde (1959), and Valenstein (1970, 1971a,b).

Another characteristic of motivated behavior, which applies to the kinds of social responses discussed in this chapter, is that under increased levels of motivational stimulation, the threshold for eliciting units lower in the hierarchy is decreased.

The discussion of sexual reflexes showed how even relatively simple responses are potentiated under appropriate hormonal control. Genital flicks in the male rat and lordosis in the female were potentiated (either in magnitude or in frequency) under appropriate hormonal priming. In the next section, on aggression, it is noted that laboratory cats do not often spontaneously attack rats. Yet, under appropriate brain stimulation (Flynn, Vanegas, Foote, and Edwards, 1970), attack does occur. Analogously, in one study (Zemlan and Adler, 1977), female rats were given injections of estrogen at various doses. At the lower doses (6 mg), the lordosis to a male was weak and displayed no afterdischarge. At higher doses, the lordosis occurred more frequently (up to 100% of the time), was maintained for a time after the male dismounted (afterdischarge), and was quite strong (extreme curvature of the back). Finally, at the highest doses, the female spontaneously displayed "darting and hopping" before a male mounted. This darting and hopping may be part of the normal soliciting behavior that female rats are capable of displaying (Beach, 1976; McClintock and Adler, 1978).

AGGRESSION

GENERAL PROPERTIES

In the first part of this chapter, the physiological basis of sexual behavior was discussed. In the second section, some commonalities between the mechanisms controlling various kinds of social behavior were sketched. In the final sections of this chapter, aggression and the responses to aggression are treated.

Since some general properties of social behavior have already been considered, it might be useful at this point to present some of the *differences* between sex and aggression, especially as they relate to the biological mechanisms responsible for their production.

Both sex and aggression are molar behavior patterns, both are motivated, and both are social. Moreover, both classes are defined, or at least labeled, according to their function. There is a difference, however, in terms of the precise nature of the function. According to the distinction between proximal and distal functions, aggression refers to a more proximal end point, that is, tissue damage, threat of tissue damage, or the symbolic representation of such threat. Tissue damage is, conceptually, closer to the immediate result of the behavior than is, say, reproduction (sex), the gaining of nutritional resources (feeding), or the maintenance of body fluid equilibria (drinking). In fact, aggression often influences the survival of the behaving organism by virtue of its increasing the chance that the responding organism will have access to sex, food, or water. Tissue damage inflicted upon another organism is itself usually a part of a larger functional organization and has led some theorists to differentiate predatory aggression from intraspecific aggression and to further differentiation within the latter category, for example, sexual aggression, maternal aggression, and territorial aggression.

One thoughtful and influential taxonomy of aggression has been put forth by Moyer (1976). His categories are predatory aggression, intermale aggression, fear-induced aggression, maternal aggression, irritable aggression, and sex-related aggression.

These patterns are differentiated partly by the stimulus conditions eliciting them, partly by the object of the attack, partly by the motor patterns involved in the attack, and partly by the neural and hormonal systems controlling the behavior. It is interesting that territorial aggression, sometimes put forth as a separate class, is rejected as a distinct class by Moyer because this category seems to be explicable on the basis of the more fundamental forms of aggression listed above. Because it is possible to increase the occurrence of any aggressive response, no matter what its initial motivational source, if that response is followed by a positive reinforcement, Moyer has suggested that instrumental aggression should be added as a class.

The study of aggression is a vast one. The endocrine bases of this set class of responses have been admirably reviewed by Leshner (1978), and the work of Moyer (1976), already cited, gives a comprehensive overview. In this section, I concentrate on a limited case study to illustrate some points in the physiological control of aggression. A second intention is to show how physiological analyses can help behaviorists understand the organization of the behavior in general. Indeed, one of the bases of classifying the various forms of aggression is the analysis of their physiological mechanisms.

Neural Organization and the Kinds of Aggression

Much of our knowledge of the fundamental neural organization underlying aggression has been elaborated during the past decades by John Flynn and his collaborators. This work is a model of how the study of neural mechanisms can unravel complex behavior into elementary units.

First, let us attend to the problem of making distinctions among different patterns of aggression and how studies of physiology can help highlight the distinctions. It has been known for a number of years that stimulation of the hypothalamus can lead to aggressive behavior (Hess and Akert, 1955). Two qualitatively different patterns of attack behavior can be elicited by hypothalamic stimulation (Flynn *et al.*, 1970). These patterns have been termed (1) *affective attack* and (2) *quiet, biting attack*. The elicitation of each of these patterns does not seem attributable to individual differences between animals, since both patterns can be seen within a single animal upon stimulation of the brain at different sites.

In a typical study of affective attack in cats, the stimulus object is a rat.

Although the behavior pattern is sometimes called *affective defense,* the rat's behavior is not necessarily provocative (in fact, an anesthetized rat can be used effectively). The pattern of attack is characterized by a pattern of pronounced sympathetic arousal (Flynn *et al.,* 1970). The initial stages consist of behavioral alerting and dilation of the pupils. At lower stimulus intensities, the sequence goes no further than the alerting. As the stimulus intensity increases past threshold, piloerection develops, the tail becomes bushy and fluffed out, and hissing occurs. The animal leaps to its feet, begins to move with its head low to the ground, back arched, and claws unsheathed, salivating and breathing deeply. The cat comes up to the rat and stands poised. After a second or two, the cat raises a paw, with claws unsheathed, and then strikes with its paw, in a series of directed blows. Sometimes, the cat springs at the rat with a high-pitched scream and pounces, tearing at the rat. If the stimulus is continued, the cat will bite the rat, although the initial part of the attack is almost invariably with its claws.

The second form of attack (quiet, biting attack) resembles the stalking of prey. At lower intensities of brain stimulation, the alerting response, accompanied by pupillary dilation, appears quite suddenly. If stimulation continues, the cat walks about the cage but ignores the rat. Finally, the cat moves swiftly, with its nose low to the ground, approaches the rat, and bites at its head and neck. Unlike the affective attack, the paws are used primarily to knock the rat on its back in order to get at the throat. The paws are not used to strike the rat. In this form of attack, the animals do not growl, emit the high-pitched screams, or salivate.

Although mixtures of patterns are sometimes seen (Flynn *et al.,* 1970), the two patterns of aggression described above represent the classic forms of affective and quiet attack.

RELATION OF AGGRESSION TO OTHER MOTIVATIONAL SYSTEMS

FLIGHT. As already stated, aggression can be considered a more proximal effect that leads to a more distal function. Consequently, attention has been paid to the relationship of attack to flight and escape. Flynn *et al.* (1970) have noted that aggression-inducing stimulation of the brain *can* culminate in flight. (To simplify the experimental preparations, however, the investigators typically avoided CNS sites from which both effects are elicited.) Although noxious stimulation (presumably leading to flight) can produce rage (Bard and Rioch, 1937), and although some forms of affective attack were associated with noxious stimulation (Adams and Flynn, 1966), under other conditions, affective attack was not invariably associated with noxious stimulation. Nakao (1958) also found that flight and aggression could be dissociated: although both flight and aggressive reactions were accompanied by marked displays, cats exhibiting the *flight* reactions made obvious attempts to escape and did not attack the experimenter, while the aggressive cats did not attempt to escape but did attack the experimenter when the stimulation was sufficiently intense.

EATING. According to Hutchinson and Renfrew (1966), attacking rats is a component of food acquisition for cats. These investigators showed that eating could be elicited by stimulating the brain at the same site from which attack was evoked, although they noted that usually, the threshold for eating was lower than that for attack. Similarly, although Flynn *et al.* (1970) found brain sites that yielded similar results, they also found areas from which quiet attack was easily elicited—but from which eating could not be evoked at any stimulus intensity.

NEURALLY DEFINED COMPONENTS OF THE AGGRESSIVE RESPONSE

Flynn (1967) and Flynn *et al.* (1970) postulated three sets of neural mechanisms that control aggressive behavior. There are, at the most elementary level, *sensory and motor mechanisms* by which attack is carried out. Second, there are brain sites from which integrated patterns of attack can be elicited. These are termed *patterning mechanisms,* and they organize and integrate the units of aggressive responses. Finally, there are sites within the brain from which attack cannot normally be *elicited* by electrical stimulation but that can *modulate* the activity of the patterning mechanism.

PATTERNING MECHANISMS. Attack can be elicited from areas of the hypothalamus, the thalamus, the midbrain, and the stria terminalis (Bandler, 1977; Flynn, 1969; Flynn *et al.,* 1970; Nakao, 1958; Roberts, 1970). In summarizing this literature, Flynn *et al.* (1970) have concluded that while both affective attack and quiet, biting attack can be elicited from different sites within both the hypothalamus and the midbrain, only affective attack has been elicited from the stria terminalis and only quiet attack from the thalamus.

While the hypothalamus has been implicated in a wide variety of motivated behaviors, its role in patterning aggression may be less than the effect of midbrain areas (Bandler, 1977; Flynn *et al.,* 1970). To document this statement, Ellison and Flynn (1968) isolated the hypothalamus from the rest of the brain of cats by knife section. The animals were somewhat lethargic, but they would attack following the sight of a mouse or a pinch of the tail. In a careful parametric study, Bandler (1977) found that predatory-like attack could be elicited from both hypothalamic and midbrain stimulation—but that the threshold for the midbrain-elicited attack was three to four times less than for hypothalamic stimulation. These data on aggression seem to reinforce the notion, becoming increasingly popular, that midbrain structures are of critical importance in integrating information from both higher and lower areas in the central nervous system.

SENSORIMOTOR MECHANISMS. When stimulation of the hypothalamus or the midbrain elicits the integrated pattern of attack, there are also effects of the stimulation on both sensory and motor subsystems. If the patterning mechanism is thought to control the elicitability and the molar organization of the response, the sensorimotor components influence the specific form that the attack takes. For example, in aggression induced by stimulation of the central gray, only the paw contralateral to the side of stimulation strikes the rat (Flynn *et al.,* 1970). Also, in a remarkable series of experiments, MacDonnell and Flynn (1966a,b) demonstrated a direct effect of hypothalamic stimulation upon sensorimotor mechanisms in aggression.

First, they showed that when a tactile stimulus is applied to the cat's muzzle, the cat tends to move its head away from the stick to close its lips. In contrast to this case, if hypothalamic stimulation is delivered to a site that normally elicits aggression, then concurrent application of the tactile stimulus to the muzzle gives rise to two responses. First, the cat brings the midline of its mouth to the stick, and then the mouth opens when the lip is touched. Moreover, the *size* of the sensori-motor field is a function of the *intensity* of the stimulation. That is, the more intense the stimulation, the larger the area of the face from which the response can be evoked.

Responses to Aggression

One of the major activities of scientists engaged in the study of aggression has been the time-honored biological practice of creating a taxonomy of behavior. The discovery that different aggressive motor patterns can appear under different environmental conditions (or can be elicited by physiological stimulation of different neural systems within the organism) has led to at least a preliminary dissection of the concept of aggression into distinct subcategories. As was reviewed in the previous sections, it is quite common now to differentiate between *predatory attack* and *defensive aggression.* This latter category consists of two words, and logically it is possible to categorize the class of responses to which it refers as *either* aggression *or* defense.

Although there is a great deal of information on the physiological substrates of aggression in mammals, there is also a significant body of literature dealing with defense *against* aggression, especially in nonmammalian forms. Prey–predator relationships represent an important topic in ethology and are receiving increasing attention within physiological psychology.

In considering the defensive behavior of vertebrates, Ratner (1967) stated that there are four stages of antipredator devices: (1) freezing; (2) flight; (3) fight; and (4) immobility. The progression from one of these stages to another is, in his analysis, controlled by the distance of the predator. At great distances, freezing would render detection less likely. At the other extreme, at zero distance, to the extent that movement of the prey is a major stimulus for attack, immobility could serve to minimize additional stimulation. (Gallup, 1974; Gallup *et al.,* 1971). This general formulation has been supported in a number of species. For example, Gallup (1974) found that stronger immobility reactions were elicited if, prior to the induction of this immobility, there had been attempts to escape, suggesting a sequentially dependent relationship between earlier defensive reactions and subsequent immobility.

Ratner's scheme can provide an overall analysis of the patterns of response to aggression across many species. Like all large-scale summaries, it may not specifically describe the responses of every species examined, but it does highlight the extreme range of behavior that can be considered defensive.

For the purposes of the present discussion, one could adapt Ratner's scheme and treat the various classes of defensive behavior as lying along a continuum, the positions along the continuum being defined by the degree of activity of the defensive organism. At one end are included patterns of *active defense* (e.g., defensive aggression in mammals, mobbing in birds, and injection of poisons by stinging insects). At the other end are the classes of freezing, which includes the pattern of tonic immobility. This classification might be diagrammed as follows:

I.   Active defense
    A.   Attack predator
    B.   Symbolic attack (aposematic coloration and behavior)
II. Avoidance
    A.   Active escape and flight
    B.   Passive avoidance
        1.   Cryptic behavior and coloration
        2.   Freezing and tonic immobility

Although Ratner used his classification to describe sequential changes in behavior within the behavioral repertoire of a single animal, some species restrict their antipredator devices to only one behavior.

ACTIVE DEFENSE. In the discussion of aggression, we have already seen how students of mammalian neurophysiology have discovered neural sites that, when stimulated, produced affective defense. This general strategy of active defense is also seen in insects, some of which can inject lethal doses of poison into the predator.

Eisner (1970) distinguished insects that contain the poisons in specialized glands (either injectable or noninjectable) from those that employ poisons of non-glandular origin (toxins present in blood, gut, or elsewhere in the body).

The glandular poisons can be released in several different ways. Some organisms—like the swallowtail caterpillar—evert a gland when attacked. Others, like the millipede *Narceus gordanus,* contain a series of glands along the body that "ooze" poisons. The secretion lasts only for the duration of the attack and can be reabsorbed.

There can be quite intricate behavioral mechanisms that facilitate dispersal of the poison. In the carabid beetle *Galerita janus,* formic acid is sprayed from the rear. This spray is localized; it is produced from one of the two laterally placed glands, the direction of injection depending on the side from which the attack comes.

Often, the substance is stored in glands that are adapted for actively *shooting* the poison. In the millipede *Apheloria corrugata,* there are 22 glands arranged in pairs on most of the body segments. Each gland has two compartments, one containing mandelonitrile, the other containing an enzyme that promotes the dissociation of mandelonitrile into benzaldehyde and hydrogen cyanide. The products are liberated as vapors that enshroud the animal and that can serve as a protective screen. As much as 3.0 mg of mandelonitrile may be stored by a single *Apheloria,* producing about 0.6 mg hydrogen cyanide—which is several times the lethal dose for a mouse.

Eisner (1970) cited the *Apheloria* system as an example of "reactor glands." These glands are so constructed that the precursors of the defensive compound are stored separately and mixed at the moment of discharge, with the result that the active principles of the secretion are generated in the ejected fluid. One of the most spectacular examples of the reactor gland strategy is the hot secretion of the bombardier beetles, species of the genus *Brachinus*. Each gland is a two-compartment apparatus. The inner compartment reservoir contains an aqueous solution of hydroquinones and hydrogen peroxide, while the outer compartment contains a mixture of catalases and peroxidases (Schildknecht and Holoubek, 1961; Schildknecht, Maschwitz, and Maschwitz, 1968).

Discharge involves a series of closely timed events: some of the inner-chamber fluid is squeezed into the outer, the catalases promote the decomposition of hydrogen peroxide, and the peroxidases force the oxidation of the hydroquinones to their respective quinones. Under pressure of free oxygen, the mixture is explosively "popped" out (Eisner, 1970). Given the thermodynamic properties of the reaction, it was predicted that the secretion would be ejected with a high enough heat to bring the spray to the boiling point and to vaporize a portion of it. This prediction was confirmed (Aneshansley, Eisner, Widom, and Widom, 1969).

One of the most effective forms of chemical defense is the use of poisons of delayed effect, like the emetics and desiccants of arthropods (Ford, 1975; Eisner, 1970). These are active in relatively low concentrations and have primary actions that involve more-or-less delayed and usually systemic effects, rather than a topical effect of immediate onset. Another feature of these substances (one that raises interesting questions of evolutionary origin) is that they are frequently tolerated systemically by the organisms that produce them and may therefore be present in more-or-less general distribution through the blood and tissue, rather than being restricted to integumental glands (Eisner, 1970).

Some of these poisons are chemically similar to drugs long known from medicinal plants. One of the best-studied forms of chemical defense of this kind is that of the monarch butterfly, *Danaus plexippus,* which produces four glycosides (calotropagenin, calotoxin, calotropin, and calactin) (Eisner, 1970). Birds are principal enemies of the monarch, and both starlings and jays have vomited, within several minutes after the ingestion of monarchs or their extracts (see Alcock, 1975, for review).

Structurally, these glycosides are steroids (i.e., they contain a cyclopentanophenanthrene ring). Sometimes, the specific defensive compounds are identical to mammalian steroids. Aquatic beetles of the family Disticidae, for example, produce C21 corticosteroids (similar to adrenal mammalian adrenal products). (Schildknecht and Hotz, 1967; Schildknecht, Siewerdt, and Maschwitz, 1966, 1967). The amount of steroid may be extraordinarily high (0.4 mg of deoxycorticosterone) in *Dytiscus marginalis* (Schildknecht *et al.,* 1966). Commenting on the identity of these *arthropod* defensive substances with *vertebrate* steroid hormones, Eisner (1970) has drawn attention to the relation between *arthropods* and *plants*. He commented that there may be a

> . . . similar, although not strictly comparable case of the use of insect hormones by plants. Both ecdysonelike and juvenile hormonelike substances are known to be produced by a diversity of plants, which presumably employ them as a means for interfering with the development of their insect enemies. (p. 195)

SOME EVOLUTIONARY NOTES ON ANTIAGGRESSION MECHANISMS. This interesting analogy between arthropod and botanic chemical defense has other dimensions: there is some reasoned speculation that the insect defense substances, in some cases, *originate* in plants. Eisner (1970) compared the lists of arthropod defensive substances compiled by Weatherston (1967) with a similar list of "secondary substances" of plants (Karrer, 1958). He found that virtually all the major categories of compounds produced by the former group are also represented among the latter. Even the method of release is similar in certain cases. In plants, for example, hydrogen cyanide is usually generated by the hydrolysis of cyanohydrin glycosides, while a similar mechanism probably operates in the larvae of certain chrysomelid beetles.

While *some* arthropods do synthesize their antipredator toxins, there is now evidence that many organisms seem to acquire their chemical defenses from extrinsic sources, usually from plants (Eisner, 1970; Ford, 1975). While the evidence for such incorporation is only indirect, it is strongly suggestive.

Brower and Brower (1967) deduced that the unpleasant qualities of adult monarch butterflies were derived from the plants on which the larvae had fed. Part of their evidence was the fact that there was a strong correlation between the occurrence of noxious properties in a series of butterfly species and their larval food plants. This theory is made more plausible by the fact that many of these substances are steroids, since insects have only limited ability to synthesize steroids from nonsteroidal sources (Clayton, 1964).

The matter has been carried further. In 1967, Rothschild and Euw demonstrated that tissues of the monarch butterfly contain two powerful cardiac glycosides, (calotropin and calactin) derived from the larval food (Asclepiadaceae) and that it is these substances that protect the insects from predators (Euw, Fishelson, Parsons, Reichstein, and Rothschild, 1967; Rothschild, 1967).

Finally, Brower, Brower, and Corvino (1967) performed a difficult but compelling experiment to verify the hypothesis of the plant origin of glycosides. These investigators selected a strain of *D. plexippus* that would feed on cabbage (although the mortality was high). The resulting adults were nonpoisonous and fully acceptable to jays that had not learned from previous experience to avoid the insect.

The self-defense of insects, using systemic substances originally produced by plants, represents a striking example of the essential opportunism of the evolutionary process.

This example of active defense has many variations. In the examples just discussed, the toxin is present throughout the tissues of the insect. In some cases, it may suffice for the insect to take these chemicals into the gut, from which they may then be regurgitated and employed defensively. The regurgitate of the grasshopper *Romalea microptera* varies in repellency, depending on what was eaten. When given two of its natural food plants (*Eupatorium capillifolium* and *Salix nigra*), the regurgitate was strongly repellent to ants. An unnatural diet of *Myrica cerifera*, on the other hand, produced defensively ineffective regurgitates, although this plant has high intrinsic repellency itself. This finding suggested to Eisner (1970) that the repellent principles of *Myrica* are inactivated enterically by the grasshopper. He speculated that the enteric preservation of an ingested plant poison may be more adaptive than its detoxification, even in the evolutionary stage where a species has not yet developed the capacity to absorb the chemical and transmit it from one stage of the life cycle to the next. This provides a plausible sequence of evolutionary stages by which certain organisms, in this case exemplified by the arthropods, come to mobilize active defenses against predators.

In all these examples of active defense in arthropods (as well as the forms of affective defense in the mammalian case discussed in the sections on aggression), the attacker (e.g., the predator) faces the possibility of physical damage by the attacked. The behavioral and physiological adaptations serving the attacked organism can therefore be classified as *defensive aggression,* since the attacker generally "starts the fight," so to speak.

To focus on the the case of predation, since the proximal adaptation is to avoid being eaten (and the potential harm to the predator is only a means to this end), it would seem that the fundamental organization of the behavior involves avoiding being consumed rather than actually destroying the attacker. (In fact, the evolution of general toxins as defense substances, as in the monarch case, has presented a classic problem, that is, how the death of a predator—e.g., a blue jay—can be of any selective advantage to the butterfly that has already been consumed. R. A. Fisher (1958) was one of those that devoted attention to the genetic problems posed by this system and suggested something like kin selection as an explanation.)

Because the organisms that have been discussed in this section possess physiological adaptations that make them dangerous and/or repellent, it is not surprising that there are correlated behavioral adaptations that make the organisms conspicuous:

> Thus, the stink beetle *Eleodes* stops moving when touched and stands on its head; caterpillars with stinging hairs undulate conspicuously as they move over their food plant; wasps, bees, and rattlesnakes often engage in warning buzzes before they attack. (Alcock, 1975, pp. 380–381)

One familiar visual device making an organism conspicuous is the use of "eye spots." Although there has been criticism of the notion that eye spots have evolved and function to frighten potential predators, this phenomenon is remarkably widespread (Wickler, 1968). Besides the butterflies and caterpillars among insects, avoid markings have been described as eye spots in the American sparrowhawk *Falco sparverius,* in the pygmy owl *Glaucidiu,* and on the backs of the big cats (e.g., the serval) (Wickler, 1968).

To summarize the material in this last section—or in the entire chapter, for that matter—does not really require a restatement of the fact that physiological mechanisms influence behavior. That is almost a truism. What is important, I feel, is that the behaving organism is in a dynamic equilibrium between its evolutionary–genetic past and its potential for survival. The biological mechanisms that "produce" the behavior represent the final common path for all of the more distal causes of behavior. Therefore, these physiological mechanisms are, hopefully, of interest to students of behavior—no matter what their specific discipline.

References

Adams, D., and Flynn, J. P. Transfer of an escape response from tail shock to brain-stimulated attack behavior. *J. Exp. Anal. Behav.,* 1966, *8,* 401–408.

Adler, N. T. Effects of the male's copulatory behavior in the initiation of pregnancy in the female rat. *Anat. Rec.*, 1968, *160*, 304.

Adler, N. T. Effects of the male's copulatory behavior in successful pregnancy of the female rat. *J. Comp. Physiol. Psychol.*, 1969, *69*, 613–622.

Adler, N. T. The behavioral control of reproductive physiology. In W. Montagna and W. A. Sadler (eds.), *Reproductive Behavior*. Plenum Press, New York, 1974.

Adler, N. T., and Bell, D. Constant estrous: Vaginal, reflexive and behavioral changes. *Physiol. Behav.*, 1969, *4*, 151–153.

Adler, N. T., and Zoloth, S. R. Copulatory behavior can inhibit pregnancy in female rats. *Science*, 1970, *168*, 1480–1482.

Adler, N. T., Davis, P. G., and Komisaruk, B. K. Variation in the size and sensitivity of a genital sensory field in relation to the estrous cycle in rats. *Horm. Behav.*, 1977, *9*, 334–344.

Adler, N. T., Komisaruk, B. R., and Davis, P. Sensory field of the pudendal nerve in rats: Changes over the estrous cycle (abs.). *Proceedings*, 4th Ann. Meeting of the Society for Neuroscience, 1974, p. 113.

Adler, N. T., Resko, J. A., and Goy, R. W. The effect of copulatory behavior on hormonal change in the female rat prior to implantation. *Physiol. Behav.*, 1970, *5*, 1003–1007.

Alcock, J. *Animal Behavior: An Evolutionary Approach*. Sinauer, Sunderland, Mass., 1975.

Alexander, R. D. Arthorpods. In T. Seboek (ed.), *Animal Communication*. Indiana University Press, Bloomington, 1968.

Alleva, J. J., Waleski, M. V., and Alleva, F. R. A biological clock controlling the estrous cycle of the hamster. *Endocrinology*, 1971, *88*, 1368–1379.

Aneshansley, D., Eisner, T., Widom, J. M., and Widom, B. Biochemistry at 100 degrees centigrade: The explosive discharge of bombardier beetles (Brachinus). *Science*, 1969, *165*, 61–63.

Aron, C., Asch, G., and Roos, J. Triggering of ovulation by coitus in the rat. *Int. Rev. Cytol.*, 1966, *20*, 139–172.

Bandler, J. Predatory behavior in the cat elicited by lower brain stem and hypothalamic stimulation: A comparison. *Brain Behav. Evol.*, 1977, *14*, 440–460.

Bard, P., and Rioch, D. McK. A study of four cats deprived of neocortex and additional portions of the forebrain. *Bull. Johns Hopkins Hosp.*, 1937, *60*, 73–147.

Barfield, R. J., and Sachs, B. D. Sexual behavior: Stimulation by painful electrical shock to skin in male rats. *Science*, 1968, *161*, 392–396.

Barfield, T. J., and Geyer, L. A. The ultrasonic post-ejaculatory vocalization and the post-ejaculatory refractory period of the male rat. *J. Comp. Physiol. Psychol.*, 1975, *88*, 723–734.

Barraclough, C. A., and Sawyer, C. H. Induction of pseudopregnancy in the rat by reserpine and chlorpromazine. *Endocrinology*, 1959, *65*, 563–571.

Barth, R. H., Jr. The comparative physiology of reproductive processes in cockroaches: I. Mating behaviour and its endocrine control. *Adv. Reprod. Physiol.*, 1968, *3*, 167–207.

Beach, F. A. *Hormones and Behavior*. Hoeber, New York, 1948.

Beach, F. A. Sexual attractivity, proceptivity, and receptivity in female mammals. *Horm. Behav.*, 1976, *7*, 105–138.

Beamer, W., Bermant, G., and Clegg, M. Copulatory behavior of the ram, *Ovis aries:* II. Factors affecting copulatory satiation. *Anim. Behav.*, 1969, *17*, 706–711.

Bennet-Clark, H. C., and Ewing, A. W. The wing mechanism involved in the courtship of *Drosophila. J. Exp. Biol.*, 1968, *49*, 117–128.

Bennet-Clark, H. C., Ewing, A. W., and Manning, A. The persistence of courtship stimulation in *Drosophila melanogaster. Behav. Biol.*, 1973, *8*, 763–769.

Bermant, G. Sexual behavior of male rats: Photographic analysis of the intromission response. *Psychon. Sci.*, 1965, *2*, 65–66.

Bermant, G., and Davidson, J. M. *Biological Basis of Sexual Behavior*. Harper and Row, New York, 1974.

Blandau, R. J. On the factors involved in sperm transport through the cervix uteri of the albino rat. *Am. J. Anat.*, 1945, *77*, 253–272.

Brander, R. B. Movements of the female ruffed grouse during the mating season. *Wilson Bulletin*, 1967, *79*, 28.

Breland, K., and Breland, M. The misbehavior of organisms. *Am. Psychol.*, 1961, *16*, 681–684.

Brower, L. P., and Brower, J. Van Zandt. Birds, butterflies, and plant poisons: A study in ecological chemistry. *Zoologica*, 1964, *49*, 137–159.

Brower, L. P., Brower, J. van Z., and Corvino, J. M. Plant poisons in a terrestrial food chain. *Proceedings of the National Academy of Sciences*, 1964, *57*, 893–898.

Brower, L. P., Ryerson, W. N., Coppinger, L. L., and Glazier, S. C. Ecological chemistry and the palatability spectrum. *Science*, 1968, *161*, 1349–1351.

Brown-Grant, K., Davidson, J., and Grieg, F. Induced ovulation in albino rats exposed to constant light. *Journal of Endocrinology,* 1973, *57*, 7.

Bunning, E. *The Physiological Clock* (Rev. 3rd ed.). Springer-Verlag, New York, 1973.

Caggiula, A. R., & Eibergen, R. Copulation of virgin male rats evoked by painful peripheral stimulation. *Journal of Comparative and Physiological Psychology,* 1969, *69*, 414.

Caggiula, A. R., and Vlahoulis, M. Modifications in the copulatory performance of male rats produced by repeated peripheral shock. *Behav. Biol.,* 1974, *11*, 269–274.

Calhoun, J. B. *The Ecology and Sociology of the Norway Rat* (U.S. Public Health Service Pub. No. 1008). U.S. Government Printing Office, Bethesda, Md., 1962a.

Calhoun, J. B. Population and social pathology. *Sci. Am.,* 1962b, *206*, 139–48.

Campbell, B. *Sexual Selection and the Descent of Man.* Aldine, Chicago, 1972.

Capranica, R. R. *The Evoked Vocal Response of the Bullfrog.* MIT Press, Cambridge, Mass., 1965.

Carlsson, R. R., and De Feo, V. J. Role of the pelvic nerve vs. the abdominal sympathetic nerves in the reproductive function of the female rat. *Endocrinology,* 1965, *77*, 1014–1022.

Carr, W. J., Krames, L., and Costanzo, J. Previous sexual experience and olfactory preference for novel versus original sex partners in rats. *J. Comp. Physiol. Psychol.,* 1970, *71*, 216–222.

Carr, W. J., Krames, L., and Wylie, N. R. Responses to feminine odors in normal and castrated male rats. *J. Comp. Physiol. Psychol.,* 1966, *62*, 336–338.

Carter, C. S., and Schein, M. W. Sexual receptivity and exhaustion in the female golden hamster. *Horm. Behav.,* 1971, *2*, 191–200.

Clayton, R. B. The utilization of sterols by insects. *Journal of Lipid Research,* 1964, *5*, 3.

Collias, N. E., and Collias, E. C. Size of breeding colony related to attraction of mates in a tropical passerine bird. *Ecology,* 1969, *50*, 481–488.

Craig, W. Appetites and aversions as constituents of instincts. *Biol. Bull.,* 1918, *34*, 91.

Crews, D. Coition-induced inhibition of sexual receptivity in female lizards *(Anolis carolinensis). Physiol. Behav.,* 1973, *11*, 463–468.

Crow, J. F., and Kimura, M. *An Introduction to Population Genetics Theory.* Harper & Row, New York, 1970.

Crowley, W. R., Popolow, H. B., and Ward, B. O., Jr. From dud to stud: Copulatory behavior elicited through conditioned arousal in sexually inactive male rats. *Physiol. Behav.,* 1973, *10*, 391–394.

Darling, F. F. *Bird Flocks and the Breeding Cycle.* University Press, Cambridge, 1938.

Darling, F. F. *A Herd of Red Deer.* Doubleday, Garden City, N.Y., 1964.

Darwin, C. *On the Origin of Species.* Murray, London, 1859.

Darwin, C. *The Descent of Man and Selection in Relation to Sex.* Random House, New York, 1871.

Deutsch, J. A. *The Structural Basis of Behavior.* University of Chicago Press, Chicago, 1960.

Dewsbury, D. A. A quantitative description of the behavior of rats during copulation. *Behavior,* 1967, *29*, 154.

Dewsbury, D. A. Diversity and adaptation in rodent copulatory behavior. *Science,* 1975, *190*, 949–954.

Diakow, C. Male–female interactions and the organization of mammalian mating patterns. In D. S. Lehrman, J. S. Rosenblatt, R. A. Hinde, and E. Shaw (eds.), *Advances in the Study of Behavior,* Vol. 4. Academic, New York, 1974.

Diakow, C. Motion picture analysis of rat mating behavior. *J. Comp. Physiol. Psychol.,* 1975, *88*, 704–712.

Diamond, M. Intromission pattern and species vaginal code in relation to induction of pseudopregnancy. *Science,* 1970, *169*, 995–997.

Diamond, M. Vaginal stimulation and progesterone in relation to pregnancy and parturition. *Biol. Reprod.,* 1972, *6*, 281–287.

Diamond, M., and Yanagimachi, R. Induction of pseudopregnancy in the golden hamster. *J. Reprod. Fertil.,* 1968, *17*, 165–168.

Dobzhansky, T. *Evolution, Genetics, and Man.* Wiley, New York, 1955.

Dobzhansky, Th., Ehrman, L., and Kastritsis, P. A. Ethological isolation between sympatric and allopatric species of the *Obscura* group of *Drosophila. Anim. Behav.,* 1968, *16*, 79–87.

Doty, R. L. A cry for the liberation of the female rodent: Courtship and copulation in Rodentia. *Psychol. Bull.,* 1974, *81*, 159–172.

Edmonds, S., Zoloth, S. R., and Adler, N. T. Storage of copulatory stimulation in the female rat. *Physiol. Behav.,* 1972, *8*, 161–164.

Ehrman, L. Mating success and genotype frequency in *Drosophila. Anim. Behav.,* 1966, *14*, 332–339.

Ehrman, L. A genetic constitution frustrating the sexual drive in *Drosophila paulistorum. Science,* 1968, *131*, 1381–1382.

Ehrman, L. The mating advantage of rare males in *Drosophila. Proc. Nat. Acad. Sci.,* 1970, *65*, 345–348.

Ehrman, L., and Parsons, P. A. *The Genetics of Behavior.* Sinauer, Sunderland, Mass., 1976.

Eisner, T. Chemical defense against predation in arthropods. In E. Sondheimer and J. B. Simeone (eds.), *Chemical Ecology.* Academic, New York, 1970. Pp. 157–218.

Ellison, G. D., & Flynn, J. P. Organized aggressive behavior in cats after surgical isolation of the hypothalamus. *Archives Italiennes de Biologie,* 1968, *106*, 1.

Elliott, J. A., Stetson, M. H., and Menaker, M. Regulation of testis function in golden hamsters: A circadian clock measures photoperiodic time. *Science,* 1972, *178*, 771–773.

Euw, J. von., Fishelson, L., Parsons, J. A., Reichstein, T., & Rothschild, M. Cardenolides (heart poisons) in a grasshopper feeding on milkweeds. *Nature,* 1967, *214*, 25.

Everett, J. W. Central neural control of reproductive functions of the adenohypophysis. *Physiol. Rev.,* 1964, *44*, 373–431.

Everett, J. W. "Delayed pseudopregnancy" in the rat, a tool for the study of central neural mechanisms in reproduction. In M. Diamond (ed.), *Perspectives in Reproduction and Sexual Behavior.* Indiana University Press, Bloomington and London, 1968.

Everett, J. W., and Sawyer, C. H. A 24-hour periodicity in the "LH-release apparatus" of female rats, disclosed by barbiturate sedation. *Endocrinology,* 1950, *47*, 198–218.

Ewing, A. W. Body size and courtship behavior in *Drosophila melanogaster. Anim. Behav.,* 1961, *11*, 93–99.

Ewing, A. W. The genetic basis of sound production in *Drosophila Pseudoobscura* and *D. Persimilis. Anim. Behav.,* 1969, *17*, 555–560.

Ewing, A. W. The evolution of courtship songs in *Drosophila. Rev. Comp. Anim.,* 1970, *4*, 3–8.

Feder, H. H., Resko, A., and Goy, R. W. Progesterone levels in the arterial plasma of pre-ovulatory and ovariectomized rats. *J. Endocrinol.,* 1968, *41*, 563–569.

Fisher, A. Effects of stimulus variation on sexual satiation in the male rat. *J. Comp. Physiol. Psychol.,* 1962, *55*, 614–620.

Fisher, R. A. *The Genetical Theory of Natural Selection* (2nd rev. ed.). Dover, New York, 1958.

Flynn, J. P. The neural basis of aggression in cats. In D. C. Glass (ed.), *Neurophysiology and Emotion.* Rockefeller University Press, New York, 1967, pp. 40–59.

Flynn, J. P. Neural aspects of attack behavior in cats. *Ann. NY Acad. Sci.,* 1969, *159*, 1008–1012.

Flynn, J. P. Neural basis of threat and attack. In R. G. Grenell and S. Gabau (eds.), *Biological Foundations of Psychiatry.* Raven, New York, 1976.

Flynn, J. P., Edwards, S. B., and Bandler, R. J. Changes in sensory and motor systems during centrally elicited attack. *Behav. Sci.,* 1971, *16*, 1–19.

Flynn, J. P., Vanegas, H., Foote, W., and Edwards, S. Neural mechanisms involved in a cat's attack on a rat. In R. E. Whalen, R. F. Thompson, M. Verzeano, and N. W. Weinberger (eds.), *The Neural Control of Behavior.* Academic, New York, 1970.

Ford, E. B. *Ecological Genetics.* Wiley, New York, 1975.

Fowler, H., and Whalen, R. Variation in incentive stimulus and sexual behavior in the male rat. *J. Comp. Physiol. Psychol.,* 1961, *54*, 68–71.

Gallistel, C. R. *The Organization of Action: A New Synthesis.* LEA Press, Hillsdale, N.J., 1979.

Gallup, G. G., Jr. Animal hypnosis: Factual status of a fictional concept. *Psychol. Bull.,* 1974, *81*, 836–853.

Gallup, G. G., Jr., Nash, R. F., and Ellison, A. L., Jr. Tonic immobility as a reaction to predation: Artificial eyes as a fear stimulus for chickens. *Psychonom. Sci.,* 1971, *23*, 79–80.

Gaston, S., and Menaker, M. Photoperiodic control of hamster testis. *Science,* 1967, *158*, 925–928.

Gellhorn, E. *Principles of Autonomic-Somatic Integration: Physiological Basis and Psychological and Clinical Implications.* University of Minnesota Press, Minneapolis, 1967.

Goldfoot, D. A., and Goy, R. W. Abbreviation of behavioral estrus in guinea pigs by coital and vagino-cervical stimulation. *J. Comp. Physiol. Psychol.,* 1970, *72*, 426–434.

Grunt, J., and Young, W. C. Psychological modification of fatigue following orgasm (ejaculation) in the male guinea pig. *J. Comp. Physiol. Psychol.,* 1952, *45*, 508–510.

Hardy, D. F., and DeBold, J. F. Effects of coital stimulation upon behavior of the female rat. *J. Comp. Physiol. Psychol.,* 1972, *78*, 400–408.

Hart, B. L. Sexual responses and mating behavior in the male rat. *J. Comp. Physiol. Psychol.,* 1968, *65*, 453–460.

Hemmingsen, A. M., and Krarup, N. B. Rhythmic diurnal variations in the oestrous phenomena of the rat and their susceptibility to light and dark. *K. Dan. Vidensk. Selsk. Biol. Meddelelson,* 1937, *13*, 1–61.

Hess, W. R. & Akert, K. Experimental data on the role of hypothalamus in mechanisms of emotional behavior. *AMA Archives of Neurology and Psychiatry,* 1955, *73*, 127.

Hinde, R. A. Unitary drives. *Anim. Behav.,* 1959, *7*, 130–141.

Hjorth, I. Reproductive behavior in Tetraonidae, with special reference to males. *Viltrevy,* 1970, *7*, 271–328.

Hoffman, J. C. Effects of light deprivation on the rat estrous cycle. *Neuroendocrinology,* 1967, *2*, 1–10.

Hoffman, J. C. An effect of early lighting history on later response to light deprivation in the rat. *Fed. Proc.,* 1969, *28*, 382.

Hoffman, J. C. Light and reproduction in the rat: Effects of photoperiod length on albino rats from two different breeders. *Biol. Reprod.,* 1970, *2*, 255–261.

Hoffman, J. C. Influence of photoperiod on reproductive functions of female mammals. In S. R. Geiger (ed.), *Handbook of Physiological Endocrinology,* Vol. 2. American Physiology Society, Washington, D.C., 1973. Part 1, Ch. 3.

Hoy, R. R., and Paul, R. L. Genetic control of song specificity in crickets. *Science,* 1973, *180*, 82–83.

Hsiao, S. The effect of female variation on sexual satiation in the male rat. *J. Comp. Physiol. Psychol.,* 1965, *60*, 467–469.

Hutchinson, R. R., and Renfrew, J. W. Stalking attack and eating behaviors elicited from the same sites in the hypothalamus. *J. Comp. Physiol. Psychol.,* 1966, *61*, 360–367.

Jolly, A. Breeding synchrony in wild *Lemur catta.* In S. Altman (ed.), *Social Communication among Primates.* University of Chicago Press, Chicago, 1967. Pp. 3–14.

Karrer, W. *Konstitution und Vorkommen der organischen Pflanzenstoffe (exclusive Alkaloide).* Birkhauser, Basel, 1958.

Kollar, E. J. Reproduction in the female rat after pelvic nerve neurectomy. *Anat. Rec.,* 1953, *115*, 641–658.

Komisaruk, B. R. Neural and hormonal interactions in the reproductive behavior of female rats. In W. Montagna and W. A. Sadler (eds), *Reproductive Behavior,* Plenum, New York, 1974.

Komisaruk, B. R., Adler, N. T., and Hutchison, J. B. Genital sensory field: Enlargement by estrogen treatment in female rats. *Science,* 1972, *178*, 1295–1298.

Kow, L. M., and Pfaff, D. W. Effects of estrogen treatment on the size of receptive field and response threshold of pudendal nerve in the female rat. *Neuroendocrinology,* 1973–1974, *13*, 299–313.

Kruijt, J. P., and Hogan, J. A. Social behavior on the lek in black grouse, *Lyrurus tetrix tetrix (L.).* Ardea, 1967, *55*, 203–240.

Kuehn, R. E., and Beach, F. A. Quantitative measurement of sexual receptivity in female rats. *Behavior,* 1963, *21*, 282–299.

Kurtz, R. G. Hippocampal and cortical activity during sexual behavior in the female rat. *J. Comp. Physiol. Psychol.,* 1975, *89*, 158–169.

Kurtz, R., and Adler, N. T. Electrophysiological correlates of sexual behavior in the male rat. *J. Comp. Physiol. Psychol.,* 1973, *84*, 225–239.

Lack, D. 1968. *Ecological Adaptations for Breeding in Birds.* Methuen, London, 1968.

Larsson, K. *Conditioning and Sexual Behavior.* Almquist and Wiksell, Stockholm, 1956.

Larsson, L., and Sodersten, P. Mating in male rats after section of the dorsal penile nerve. *Physiological Behavior,* 1973, *10*, 567–571.

Leshner, A. I. *An Introduction to Behavioral Endocrinology.* Oxford University Press, New York, 1978.

Lincoln, G. A. The role of antlers in the behaviour of red deer. *J. Exp. Zool.,* 1972, *182*, 233–250.

Lisk, R. D. Cyclic fluctuations in sexual responsiveness in the male rat. *J. Exp. Zool.,* 1969, *171*, 313–326.

Lockard, R. B. Reflections on the fall of comparative psychology: Is there a message for us all? *Am. Psychol.,* 1971, *26*, 168–179.

Long, J. A., and Evans, H. Mc. The oestrous cycle in the rat and its associated phenomena. *Memoirs Univ. Calif.,* 1922, *6*, 1–148.

MacDonnell, M. F., and Flynn, J. P. Control of sensory fields by stimulation of hypothalamus. *Science,* 1966a, *152*, 1406–1408.

MacDonnell, M., and Flynn, J. P. Sensory control of hypothalamic attack. *Anim. Behav.,* 1966b, *14*, 399–405.

Manning, A. The effects of artificial selection for mating speed in *Drosophila melanogaster. Anim. Behav.,* 1961, *9*, 82–92.

Manning, A. Evolutionary changes in behaviour genetics. *Genetics Today, Proceedings* of the XI International Congress of Genetics, Pergamon, The Hague, Netherlands, 1963.

Manning, A. Drosophila and the evolution of behavior. *Viewpoints Biol.,* 1965, *4*, 125–169 (Butterworth, London).

Manning, A. The control of sexual receptivity in female *Drosophila. Anim. Behav.,* 1967, *15*, 239–250.

Manning, A. *An Introduction to Animal Behavior.* Addison-Wesley, Reading, Mass., 1972.

Matthews, M., and Adler, N. T. Facilitative and inhibitory influences of reproductive behavior on sperm transport in rats. *J. Comp. Physiol. Psychol.,* 1977, *91*, 727–741.

Mayr, E. *Animal Species and Evolution.* Belknap, Cambridge, Mass., 1963.

Mayr, E. *Principles of Systematic Zoology.* McGraw-Hill, New York, 1969.

McClintock, M. K., and Adler, N. T. The role of the female during copulation in wild and domestic Norway rats. *Behaviour,* 1978, *67*, 67–96.

McGill, T. E., and Coughlin, R. C. Ejaculatory reflex and luteal activity induction in *Mus musculus. J. Reprod. Fertil.,* 1970, *21*, 215–220.

Morishige, W. K., Pepe, G., and Rothchild, I. Serum luteinizing hormone, prolactin, and progesterone levels during pregnancy in the rat. *Endocrinology,* 1973, *92*, 1527–1530.

Moyer, K. E. *The Psychobiology of Aggression.* Harper & Row, New York, 1976.

Muller, H. J. Isolating mechanisms, evolution, and temperature. *Biol. Symp.,* 1942, *6*, 71–125.

Nakao, H. Emotional behavior produced by hypothalamic stimulation. *Am. J. Physiol.,* 1958, *194*, 411–418.

Nelson, J. B. The relationship between behavior and ecology in the Sulidae with reference to other sea birds. *Oceanogr. Mar. Biol. Ann. Rev.,* 1970, *8*, 501.

Parkes, A. S., and Bruce, H. M. Olfactory stimuli in mammalian reproduction. *Science,* 1961, *134*, 1049–1054.

Patterson, I. J. Timing and spacing of broods in the black headed gull *Larus ridibundus. Ibis,* 1965, *107*, 433.

Pencharz, R. I., and Long, J. A. Hypophysectomy in the pregnant rat. *Am. J. Anat.,* 1933, *53*, 117–135.

Petit, C. Le rôle de l'isolement sexuel dans l'évolution des populations de *Drosophila melanogaster. Bull. Biol. Fr. Belg.,* 1951, *85*, 392–418.

Pfaff, D. W., and Lewis, C. Film analyses of lordosis in female rats. *Horm. Behav.,* 1974, *5*, 317–335.

Ratner, S. C. Comparative aspects of hypnosis. In J. E. Gordon (ed.), *Handbook of Clinical and Experimental Hypnosis.* Macmillan, New York, 1967.

Richter, C. P. *Biological Clocks in Medicine and Psychiatry.* Springfield, Charles C Thomas, Ill., 1965.

Richter, C. P. Dependence of successful mating in rats on functioning of the 24-hour clocks of the male and female. *Commun. Behav. Biol* A, 1970, *5*, 1–5.

Ricklefs, R. E. *Ecology.* Chiron, Newton, Mass., 1973.

Robel, R. J. Booming territory size and mating success of the greater prairie chicken. *Anim. Behav.,* 1966, *14*, 328–331.

Roberts, W. W. Hypothalamic mechanisms for motivational and species-typical behavior. In R. L. Whalen, R. F. Thompson, M. Verzeano, and N. W. Weinberger (eds.), *The Neural Control of Behavior.* Academic, New York, 1970.

Rodgers, C. H. Influence of copulation on ovulation in the cycling rat. *Endocrinology,* 1971, *88*, 433–436.

Rodgers, C. H., and Schwartz, W. B. Diencephalic regulation of plasma LH, ovulation, and sexual behavior in the rat. *Endocrinology,* 1972, *90*, 461–465.

Rodgers, C. H., and Schwartz, N. B. Serum LH and FSH levels in mated and unmated proestrous female rats. *Endocrinology,* 1973, *92*, 1475.

Rodriguez-Sierra, J. F., Crowley, W. R., and Komisaruk, B. R. Vaginal stimulation in rats induces prolonged lordosis responsiveness and sexual receptivity. *J. Comp. Physiol. Psychol.,* 1975, *89*, 79–85.

Rowlands, I. W. (Ed.). *Comparative Biology of Reproduction in Mammals.* Zoological Society of London Symposia, Number 15, 1966.

Rothschild, M. Mimicry, the deceptive way of life. *Natural History,* 1967, *76*, 44.

Rozin, P., and Kalat, J. W. Specific hungers and poison avoidance as adaptive specializations of learning. *Psychol. Rev.,* 1971, *78*, 459–487.

Rusak, B., and Zucker, I. Biological rhythms and animal behavior. *Ann. Rev. Psychol.,* 1975, *26*, 137–171.

Sachs, B. D., and Barfield, R. J. Temporal patterning of sexual behavior in the male rat. *J. Comp. Physiol. Psychol.,* 1970, *73*, 359–364.

Sachs, B. D., and Barfield, R. J. Copulatory behavior of male rats given intermittent electric shocks: Theoretical implications. *J. Comp. Physiol. Psychol.,* 1974, *86*, 607–615.

Sachs, B. D., Macaione, R., and Fegy, L. Pacing of copulatory behavior in the male rat: Effects of receptive females and intermittent shocks. *J. Comp. Physiol. Psychol.,* 1974, *87*, 326–331.

Sade, D. S. Seasonal cycle in size of testes of freeranging *Macaca. mulatta. Folia Primatol.,* 1964, *2*, 171–180.

Sadleir, R. M. *The Ecology of Reproduction in Wild and Domestic Animals.* Methuen, London, 1969.

Schein, M. W., and Hale, E. B. Stimuli eliciting sexual behavior. In F. A. Beach (ed.), *Sex and Behavior.* Wiley, New York, 1965.

Schildknecht, H., and Holoubek, K. Die Bombardierkäfer und ihre Explosionschemie. V. Über Insekten-Abwehrstoffe. *Angew. Chem.,* 1961, *73*, 1–7.

Schildknecht, H., and Hotz, D. Identification of the subsidiary steroids from the prothoracic protective gland system of *Dytiscus marginalis. Angew. Chem. Intern. Ed. English,* 1967, *6*, 881.

Schildknecht, H., Maschwitz, E., and Maschwitz, U. Die Explosionschemie der Bombardierkäfer (Coleoptera, Carabidae). III. Isolierung und Charakterisierung der Explosionskatalysatoren. *Z. Naturforsch.,* 1968, *23b*, 1213–1218.

Schildknecht, H., Siewerdt, R., and Maschwitz, U. A vertebrate hormone as defensive substance of the water beetle *(Dytiscus marginalis). Angew. Chem. Intern. Ed. English,* 1966, *5*, 421.

Schinkel, P. G. The effect of the ram on the incidence and occurrence of oestrus in ewes. *Aust. Vet. J.,* 1954, *30*, 189–195.

Selander, R. K. On mating systems and sexual selection. *Amer. Nature,* 1965, *99*, 129–140.

Seligman, M. E. P., and Hager, J. L. *Biological Boundaries of Learning.* Meredith, New York, 1972.

Sinclair, A. N. A note on the effect of the presence of rams on the incidence of oestrus in maiden Merino ewes during spring mating. *Aust. Vet. J.,* 1950, *26*, 37–39.

Smith, M. S., Freeman, M. E., & Neill, J. D., The control of progesterone secretion during the estrous cycle and early pseudopregnancy in the rat: Prolactin gonadotropin and steroid levels associated with rescue of the corpus luteum of pseudopregnancy. *Endocrinology,* 1975, *96*, 219.

Smith, M. S. McLean, B. K., and Neill, J. D. Prolactin: The initial luteotrophic stimulus of pseudopregnancy in the rat. *Endocrinology,* 1976, *98*, 1370–1377.

Snow, D. W. Courtship ritual: The dance of the manakins. *Anim. Kingdom,* 1956, *59*, 86–91.

Snow, D. W. The display of the blue-backed manakin, *Chiroxiphia pareola*, in Tobago, W.I. *Zoologica,* 1963, *48*, 167–176.

Spies, H. G., and Niswender, G. D. Levels of prolactin, LH and FSH in the serum of intact and pelvic-neurectomized rats. *Endocrinology,* 1971, *88*, 937–943.

Tan, C. C. Genetics of sexual isolation between *Drosophila pseudoobscura* and *Drosophila persimilis. Genetics,* 1946, *31*, 558–563.

Teitelbaum, P. The biology of drive. In G. Quarton, T. Melnechuk, and F. D. Schmitt (eds.), *The Neurosciences: A Study Program.* Rockefeller, New York, 1967.

Thibault, C., Courit, M., Martinet, L., Mauleon, P., DuMesnil Du Buisson, F., Ortavant, P., Pelletier, J., and Signoret, J. P. Regulation of breeding season and oestrous cycles by light and external stimuli in some mammals. *J. Anim. Sci.,* 1966, *25*, Suppl., 119–142.

Thompson, T. Visual reinforcement in Siamese fighting fish. *Science,* 1963, *141*, 55–57.

Thompson, T. Visual reinforcement in fighting cocks. *J. Exp. Behav.,* 1964, 7, 45–49.

Tinbergen, N. *The Study of Instinct.* Oxford University Press, London, 1952.

Tinbergen, N. Some recent studies of the evolution of sexual behavior. In F. A. Beach (ed.), *Sex and Behavior.* Wiley, New York, 1965.

Trivers, R. L. Parental investment and sexual selection. In B. Campbell (ed.), *Sexual Selection and the Descent of Man.* Aldine, Chicago, 1972.

Valenstein, E. S. Stability and plasticity of motivation systems. In F. O. Schmitt (ed.), *The Neurosciences, Second Study Program.* Rockefeller University Press, New York, 1970.

Valenstein, E. S. Behavior elicited by hypothalamic stimulation: A prepotency hypothesis. *Brain Behav. Evol.,* 1971a, *2*, 295–316.

Valenstein, E. S. Channeling of responses elicited by hypothalamic stimulation. *J. Psychiat. Res.,* 1971b, *8*, 335–344.

Vandenbergh, J. G. Endocrine coordination in monkeys: Male sexual responses to females. *Physiol. Behav.,* 1969, *4*, 261–264.

Weatherston, J. The chemistry of arthropod defensive substances. *Quart. Rev.* (London), 1967, *21*, 297–313.

Wickler, W. *Mimicry in Plants and Animals.* World University Library, London, 1968.

Williams, G. C. *Adaptation and Natural Selection.* Princeton University Press, Princeton, N.J., 1966.

Wilson, E. O. *Sociobiology: The New Synthesis.* Belknap, Cambridge, Mass., 1975.

Wilson, J. R., Adler, N., and LeBoeuf, B. The effects of intromission frequency on successful pregnancy in the female rat. *Proc. Nat. Acad. Sci.,* 1965, *53*, 1392–1395.

Wilson, J., Kuehn, R., and Beach, F. A. Modification in the sexual behavior of male rats produced by changing the stimulus female. *J. Comp. Physiol. Psychol.,* 1963, *56*, 636–644.

Young, W. C. The hormones and mating behavior. In W. C. Young (ed.), *Sex and Internal Secretions* (Vol. 1). Williams & Wilkins, Baltimore, 1961, Pp. 1173–1239.

Young, W. C., Boling, J. L., and Blandau, R. J. The vaginal smear picture, sexual receptivity, and time of ovulation in the albino rat. *Anat. Rec.,* 1941, *80*, 37–45.

Zemlan, F. P., and Adler, N. T. Hormonal control of female sexual behavior in the rat. *Horm. Behav.,* 1977, *9*, 345–357.

Zimmerman, J. L. Polygyny in the dickcissel. *Auk,* 1966, *83*, 534–546.

Zimmerman, J. L. The territory and its density-dependent effect in *Spiza americana. Auk,* 1971, *88*, 591–612.

Zondek, B., and Tamari, I. The effects of auditory stimuli on reproduction. In G. E. W. Wolstenholme (ed.), *The Effects of External Stimuli on Reproduction.* Little, Brown, Boston, 1967.

3

The Analysis of Animal Communication

STEVEN GREEN AND PETER MARLER

INTRODUCTION

Communication consists of the transmission of information from one animal to another. Information is encoded by one individual into a signal. When received by another animal, this information undergoes decoding, while still retaining a specifiable relationship to the encoded information. The relationship is sometimes deterministic, sometimes only probabilistic. During such encoding and decoding, the carrier of the information and the format of the information undergo many transformations. Starting with the original designatum or referent, information passes through a series of steps internal to the signaling animal before effecting a change of state of the signaling organ. A signal is then propagated in a medium. Further steps follow, from transmitted signal to receptor organs of a recipient, from sensory to central processing, and eventually to a recipient's overt or covert response.

Viewed in this light, communication systems engage many scientific disciplines. Phenomena of memory and cognition are included as well as the physiology of transduction in receptor organs. Alterations in mechanisms can occur over many generations, with their fundamental regulation by natural selection, or by inter- and intragenerational learning, so that the study of animal communication impinges on the domains of sociobiology and evolutionary biology as well as ethology. We will not attempt to cover all of these areas but rather to highlight

STEVEN GREEN   Department of Biology, University of Miami, Coral Gables, Florida 33124.   PETER MARLER   Rockefeller University, Field Research Center, Millbrook, New York 12545. Partial support for this work derives from research grants MH 24269 (USPHS) to Steven Green, MH 14651 (USPHS) and BNS 77-16894 (NSF) to Peter Marler.

STEVEN GREEN AND
PETER MARLER

themes of current interest to students of animal behavior and psychology, in the context of a general scheme for examining animal communication. For our present purposes, the topic of animal communication includes only phenomena that satisfy the following three conditions:

1. *Nonconstancy of signals.* The signal itself is a discernible event, with its beginning and end marking a period much shorter than any phase of an individual's life cycle. Signal production is manifested by an observable change of state. Its detection by an observer is in some way contingent upon an external attribute that contrasts with the immediately preceding state. By use of this condition as a criterion, we intend for the most part to exclude from our consideration of signaling those attributes or signs that are constant within an individual's lifetime or that are strictly age-dependent.

Pelage color, for example, often mediates recognition of species, sex, age, or individual identity. With some special exceptions, such as fish (Baerends, Brouwer and Waterbolk, 1955; Leong, 1969; Heiligenberg, Kramer, and Schulz, 1972) and cephalopods (Moynihan, 1975), most body coloration changes occur over too long a period to qualify as signals by our definition. While the evolution of pelage color and pattern may well have incorporated selection for visibility or invisibility, these signs—and specialized structures that enhance visibility, such as the lamellae on butterfly wings—are not considered signals in and of themselves, although they may be used in signaling.

Some such features , involved as they are in recognition and discrimination of sex, age-classes, strangers, and kin, will fall within our purview, since any consideration of communication must clearly acknowledge that such basic information is often available to the communicant. However, we are inclined to treat them as contextual or ancillary components in the communicative process rather than as signals.

2. *Specialization.* Structural or behavioral adaptation for signal production and/or transmission and/or reception is a prerequisite for the phenomena we are considering, thus implying some specialization for communication. The energy transfer mediated by signal reception must serve as a response *trigger,* in the sense of Bullock (1961), rather than as a precipitant in its own right. To command someone to jump off a bridge is an act of communication; to push him is not (Cherry, 1966).

We shall be dealing primarily with intraspecific communication. There are, of course, cases of adaptive interspecific communication as in the signals of commensal beetles that live in ant colonies (Hölldobler, 1967, 1970). Interspecific communication may also be nonadaptive, as when an owl orients its strike to the squeal of a mouse. In such adventitious communication, one organism benefits from receiving another's signals without any benefit to the signaler. Such events may well be necessary precursors to natural selection for improved capabilities of receivers or for less readily detected signaling by transmitters, especially in communication between species. We will largely disregard adventitious communication, however, and concentrate instead on adaptations for mutually beneficial flows of information. For social communication, in the sense that we will use the term, potential two-way symmetry of communicating pairs is required, with both members subject to natural selection for better information transfer, yielding co-evolved, bidirectional signal production and signal perception (Otte, 1974; Marler, 1977b).

3. *Internal processing.* Signaling and receiving animals behave as if they internalize the encoding and decoding of signals. Communicative responses to the same signals in the same context may vary at different times. The variation in internal processing that is implied engages more than just receptor states. Although verbal reports on introspection are the best way to approach this issue, they are available only for analyzing our own communicative behavior. There are other criteria, however, which provide a basis for logical inference about similar processes in animals (Griffin, 1976).

Responses are defined as any change in the probability of subsequent behavior compared to expectations in the absence of signaling. Although a change may occur immediately or in the indefinite future (Heiligenberg, 1977), the practicalities of research generally restrict us to short-term changes of large magnitude. The nature of responses serves to inform us indirectly about the internal processes of encoding and decoding.

Note that conscious intention is not included as a criterion. While *intention*, defined operationally as goal-directed behavior (MacKay, 1972), is widespread in animal communication, rigorous criteria for intention are currently applicable only in man, although the possibility of extension to other species should not be excluded (Griffin, 1979). Communication characterized by the three criteria we have given can occur without any consciously determinable intention. For example, body and facial language often contradicts purposeful lying (e.g., Ekman, Friesen, and Ellsworth, 1972; Ekman and Friesen, 1974), yet it satisfies our criteria and is also congruent with our commonsense notions of communicative phenomena. Communication can also be mediated by physiological processes with little or no nervous component, such as the odors or swellings associated with mammalian estrus. Although these would not usually be considered intentional, we accept them as communicative, as long as other criteria, especially brevity and the existence of discernible end points, are met.

Our requirements for nonconstancy of signals and for specialized adaptations for communication cover common ground with more restrictive formulations of animal communication. A communicative interaction is a social event. It represents the essence of sociality. Our internalization requirement indicates that the state of one animal, a signal emitter, alters the state of another animal, a receiver. The vehicle for this alteration is the signal. Determination of the change of state of the receiver is based on its behavioral changes, as compared with probabilities for a different signal or for no signal at all. This "state" of the emitter is an internal process, contingent on its perception of certain past or present external events, referents, or designata.

The overall characteristics of a communication system are the result of chaining together the individual transformation steps in signaling transmission and reception, to yield a mapping function that describes the transfer of information from organism to organism. Each step can be affected by noise, error, and inherent biological variability.

STEVEN GREEN AND
PETER MARLER

The usual subjects of descriptive studies of the communicative behavior of animals are the signals. Sometimes, the relationships between referents and signals are studied, though usually without examining the chain of transformations within the emitter resulting in signal generation. Correlations between a receiver's behavior and an emitter's prior or parallel signal action are also frequency examined (Wiepkema, 1961; Stokes, 1962a,b; Nelson, 1964; Altmann, 1965; Hazlett and Bossert, 1965; Dunham, 1966; Dingle, 1969; Andersson, 1976; Baylis, 1976; Rand and Rand, 1976). Nonexperimental studies often lump all modes of signaling other than the one being examined together with other aspects of the behavioral context. Experimental studies tend to manipulate only the signals and to separate the effects of other components of the situation by employing balanced controls. Each method emphasizes only a few of the many information transformations that occur in the complete communication process. Depending on one's perspective, some aspects of communication are inherently more interesting than others. Whether we are concerned more with the stochastics of behavior or with information theory, receptor physiology or signal detection theory, competition or reproduction, or the evolution or maintenance of animal societies, our preoccupations will determine the most appropriate strategy.

There are, however, many other major but as yet relatively unstudied questions about the physiological and evolutionary processes that dictate relations among referents, signals, and responses. Some issues have received more attention than others, in part because they are accessible for study but perhaps also because of the lack of a coherent theoretical framework for identifying central issues in animal communication. This paper introduces some hypothetical constructs that, although they do not necessarily bear a one-to-one relationship with identifiable anatomical structures or physiological processes, can be used to describe phenomena of communication and may aid in their analysis.

SIGNAL PRODUCTION, TRANSMISSION, AND RECEPTION

THE SENDER

From a sender's vantage point, a signal must be producible at an intensity or concentration adequate for transmission over a required distance so that it can be received and acted upon in a way advantageous, on the average, to the sender's inclusive fitness. Some degree of matching inevitably arises between the form signals take and the nature and mode of operation of the special organs and motor equipment available for their production. Zoologists, linguists, and anthropologists have described a vast array of specialization for the production of signals, whether electric, photic, acoustic, chemical, or tactile (Sebeok, 1977). Thus, the constraints on sound production by cricket stridulation are quite different from those on bird vocalization, and the sounds produced differ accordingly. At a more subtle level, both birds and man use respiratory air flow to produce communicative sounds, but songbird and human vocal tracts operate differently. Laryngeal and syringeal mechanisms must be understood before differences in the acoustic structure of bird song and of speech become intelligible (Lieberman, 1967; Greenewalt, 1968).

By contrast with the diversity of studies on signal production, comparative information on the anatomical and physiological specializations for the encoding phases of signal production is virtually nonexistent. Only the comparison between man and nonhuman primates has yet been studied fruitfully. In this case, it is known that different parts of the brain relate to so-called affective and symbolic aspects of signal production (Robinson, 1975; Jurgens and Ploog, 1976; Lamandella, 1977).

Little is known about the direct consequences of signaling actions for the signaler, a potentially important issue, especially perhaps in cases where signal production is repeated continuously for some time (Haldane, 1953). Nelson (1965) has clear evidence that courtship actions of a male stickleback change the prospects of his future behavior. Eisenberg and Kleiman (1972, p. 26) have suggested that self-stimulation may be important to an olfactory signaler in some circumstances, in that production of a scent changes the odor field and arouses the individual in various ways, depending upon the nature of the change.

The hypothesis has been offered that adoption of the appropriate facial expression by human subjects facilitates a transition to the corresponding mood. Recent studies have supplied some supporting evidence (Izard, 1974; Schwartz, 1975; Schwartz, Fair, Salt, Mandel, and Klerman, 1976). Method-acting schools have expounded similar views for many years. If people gain some self-assurance by singing, whistling, talking, or shouting to themselves, why not animals? Such consequences for the signaler might involve not only positive but also negative feedback. In one of the few animal studies on this subject, Wilz (1970) has presented evidence that some of the courtship actions of the male three-spined stickleback function at least in part to change the state not of the female but of the male himself, in this case to reduce aggressiveness. Signaling actions that involve occlusion of sense organs, such as hiding the face, serving to "cut off" sources of stimulation may also have negative feedback consequences for the signaler (Chance, 1962).

The Receiver

From a receiver's viewpoint, selective pressures operate on its ability to detect and react to signals so as to enhance its inclusive fitness. Signals are thus part of an evolutionary feedback system that also reflects features of the receiver's own anatomy and physiology. Aside from the obvious need for possession of receptor systems in the appropriate sensory modality, the existence of particular predispositions within a modality—such as zones of high sensitivity or acuity, for example, or qualitative quantization of stimulus continua, as occurs in color vision (Kolers and von Grunau, 1975; Bornstein, Kessen, and Weiskopf, 1976; Ratliff, 1976)— will exert obvious influences on signal evolution. The details of such relationships are virtually unexplored (see Hailman, 1977) except for those between perception and production of human speech (page 99).

The range of frequencies best heard by animals as different as fish and orthoptera varies in parallel with the frequencies most strongly emphasized in their sounds (e.g., Nocke, 1972; Paton, Capranica, Dragsten, and Webb, 1977; Myrberg, 1978). Among birds, audiometric studies reveal species variations in frequency sensitivity, even though the overall range of audible frequencies may be similar across species. There is a general tendency for the emphasized frequencies of birdsong to be clustered around a species' own best frequency for hearing (Konishi, 1970, 1974; Dooling, Mulligan, and Miller, 1971).

Although there is necessarily coupling between signal structure and sensory systems, this is often very loose. Thus, one cannot predict that species with color vision will necessarily exploit colors in the design of their visual signals, although, if they do, a knowledge of the details of color perception should permit one to predict some of the rules governing how colors are used (cf. Hailman, 1977). Correspondingly, responsiveness to a wide range of sound frequencies is not necessarily predictive of an equivalent range in the vocal output.

Only when receptor systems are expressly and narrowly specialized for communication can knowledge of them permit precise predictions about properties of signals of the species. With social signal detection as the prime function, it may drive the structure and physiology of receptor design to the exclusion of other concerns. More versatile receptor systems, responsive to wider ranges of stimuli, are subject to many other selective influences, and the match with features of conspecific signals is correspondingly loosened.

Chemoreceptors of moths and hearing organs of frogs illustrate the close relationship that *can* evolve between signal structure and highly specialized receptors. Species differences in the chemical structure of female moth sex pheromones are sometimes, though not always, matched by the responsiveness of male antennal chemoreceptors (Schneider, 1962; Payne, 1974). In frogs, species differences in the frequency structure of male calling songs are beautifully matched to the best frequencies of the audiogram originating in the two primary hearing organs, the amphibian and the basillar papillae (Capranica, 1976). However, there is an obvious price to be paid for such specialization in that a species cannot maximize specificity to conspecific signals while retaining sufficient generality of responsiveness to be sensitive and efficient in detecting other stimuli.

SIGNAL DIRECTION

The ease with which a receiver can determine the direction of a distant signal varies with the sensory modality and the design of the receptor system that is used. Except for species with the most primitive light receptors, an animal can hardly detect a visual signal without at the same time getting a fair idea of where it comes from. Still, the accuracy of localization varies according to such structural features of the visual organ as retinal cell density, accommodation abilities, or, for compound eyes, whether ommatidia are of the apposition or superposition type (Horridge, 1975).

Unlike light rays, a diffusing chemical has minimal inherent directional qualities, so an animal sensing a pheromone from a distant source must localize it indirectly, by reference either to the differences in concentration at different locations or to the direction of movement of the medium carrying the scent, such as a breeze or a current, or both (Wright, 1958; Farkas and Shorey, 1974). Thus, for organisms relying heavily on chemical communication, sensitivity to small variations in stimulus concentration is a great advantage. This is, in fact, a general characteristic of both vertebrate and invertebrate olfactory systems (Adrian, 1928). Equally important is an ability to register the direction of air or water movements, an issue studied in some invertebrates (e.g., Camhi, 1969) and in fish, but virtually unexplored in mammals, whose vibrissae would seem prime candidates for such a function. The ease of locating the source of a chemical signal also varies according to its volatility and rate of diffusion as well as durability and the rate of production at the source (Bossert and Wilson, 1963; Wilson and Bossert, 1963; Wilson, 1968; Regnier and Goodwin, 1977).

Perhaps the most elaborate adaptations for easing or hindering the localizability of a signal source occur in the auditory capabilities of birds and mammals. Unlike insects, many of which possess receptors that are directly responsive to the vectorial properties of a sound wave, the ears of terrestrial vertebrates typically employ pressure receptors and must therefore rely mainly on binaural detection of differences of intensity, time of arrival of a sound, and phase relations. In certain circumstances, they can use all three methods, and localizations are most accurate in such cases. The available cues vary with the type of sound. Localization by means of intensity differences can be most accurate with high-frequency sounds, since wavelengths shorter than head dimensions permit the sound-shadowing effect to be greatest. Conversely, localization by means of phase differences is most accurate with frequencies low enough that their wavelength is longer than the distance between the ears (Konishi, 1977). Accurate localization by sensing the difference in time of arrival of the same sound at each ear depends on the presence of discontinuities and transient frequencies in the acoustic stimulus. All three types of cue are provided by sounds that are varying with time, broken, and repetitive, with a wide range of frequencies. These properties are shared by many animal sounds, but especially those where quick, accurate localization is at a premium (Marler, 1955).

However, a readily localizable signal is disadvantageous in some situations, as with small-bird alarm calls used in the presence of a hunting hawk or carnivore. If a sound is a relatively narrow-band pure tone, if its amplitude envelope begins and ends gradually, and if it has few transients or discontinuities, it is more difficult to locate, as Brown, Beecher, Moody, and Stebbins (1978) have shown with monkeys in the laboratory. Moreover, a high pitched sound, with its rapid attenuation with distance in air, can reduce the range of possible detection by predators while still effectively communicating danger to nearby companions (Konishi, 1973). Many birds and mammals have converged on the use of this type of ventriloquial sound as a signal for extreme danger (e.g., Collias, 1952; Orians and Christman, 1968; Melchior, 1971; Latimer, 1977; Vencl, 1977; Owings and Virginia, 1978), still localizable (Shalter and Schleidt, 1977; Shalter, 1978), but with greater difficulty (Konishi, 1973).

With signals originating close to the receiver or even directly touching its own body surface, as with the somesthetic and chemotactic senses, and with close-range olfaction, localization is direct and immediate. Odor-trail laying, exploited by many vertebrate and invertebrate animals, is a special case of this kind of contact or close-range signal orientation, elaborated with considerable refinement by ants and used by many other animals (Wilson, 1962, 1971a; Mykytowycz, 1974; Shorey, 1976). In some such cases, the location itself may be part of the signal rather than ancillary information. Touch patterns, whether gradual or sudden, weak or strong, localized or stroking across a surface, provide one of the elementary and widespread means available for communicants to exchange varied information of profound social significance (Geldard, 1977). Just where on the body surface one organism touches another, as well as the nature of the contact, can transform its communicative significance.

Spatial characteristics also affect encoding possibilities with other sensory modalities. Their relevance is most obvious with visual signals. The directionality of light and the discriminability of separate light sources permit the use of spatial patterns in encoding to a degree that is inconceivable for signals mediated by the other distance receptor systems. Even when communicating primarily by some other means, animals often exploit the visual channel as well for the particular directional advantages that visual signaling possesses.

NOISE

The background against which a given signal must be discriminated if it is to mediate effective communication, including other similar stimuli, may be viewed as noise. In almost all habitats, there is a background of environmental noise of nonbiological origin. A wind creates various kinds of acoustic noise that interfere with the processes of auditory communication. One of the factors favoring dawn and dusk as times of day for acoustic communication is the likelihood that convectional air movements will be at a minimum. The frequency properties of wind noise vary with the type of vegetation, with as yet unexplored consequences for the best frequencies for communicative use. Noise of biological origin may be even more significant than physical noise in some circumstances, as with the din of insect sounds through which vertebrate sounds must be detected and identified in a tropical rain forest (Waser and Waser, 1977) or the ubiquitous background noise of marine environments (Myrberg, 1978).

Signals of other organisms constitute a source of noise that can generate strong selective forces for specific distinctiveness of signals. One solution is to avoid simultaneous signaling (see Cody and Brown, 1969; Smith, 1977), manifest in patterns of pheromone production of closely related insects (Shorey, 1976) and perhaps an explanation for the specifically distinctive timing of participation of different bird species in the dawn chorus. Short-term avoidance of song overlap has been demonstrated between a flycatcher and a vireo (Ficken, Ficken, and Hartman, 1974). The nocturnal production of long-range calls by certain populations of orangutan has been interpreted as avoidance of intense competition with other primates and birds for use of acoustic channels at dawn. In geographic areas where some of the competitors are absent, calling at dawn is more typical than at night (MacKinnon, 1974). The contrapuntal singing of rival males of certain birds may also be viewed as a form of delivery that avoids temporal overlap.

Background noise of physical origin impinges even on electric communication in fish. A major source of electrical noise in tropical environments in South America and Africa, where electric fish are found, is lightning. Frequent thunderstorms produce interference in the same frequency range as those used by these fish for communication (Hopkins, 1973). Electromagnetic waves from lightning propagate with little attenuation, so that the pulses are detectable at great distances from storms. In the rivers in Guyana where the fish were studied, there was a steady but randomly organized background of electrical noise of this kind, against which the fish had to perceive each other's signals. Their tendencies to use continuous and regular trains of pulses is interpreted as an adaptation to favor contrast with this background (Hopkins, 1974), an interpretation also applied to the acoustic pulse trains of fish, amphibians, and birds in noisy environments (Myrberg, Espanier, and Há, 1978).

Presumably, chemical noise has a significant influence on the evolution of olfactory signaling, although it has been little studied. The chemical senses illustrate one means of dealing with the noise problem, namely, employing receptor systems narrowly tuned to a limited range of stimuli, thus eliminating masking that might result from the perception of stimuli outside that range (e.g., Roth, 1948; Tischner and Schief, 1954). The antennal olfactory receptors of some moths respond only to the sexual pheromone of females of the species and a few other closely related compounds (Schneider, 1962, 1970). With more versatile receptor systems that are responsive to broader ranges of stimuli, masking can be a serious problem, even when receptor subsets are narrowly tuned, as in audition (Scharf, 1970).

Adaptation to maximize contrast between signals and background is perhaps better known for the visual modality than for any other, though there has admittedly been little systematic effort to explore general relationships between variations in light quality in different environments and the visual signals used in them (Hailman, 1977; but see Burtt, 1977). There are many examples in animal coloration of patterns of color and shading that serve to emphasize the outlines of the shape of the body or some part of it (Cott, 1957). These are often focused on parts of the body exposed or moved in the course of signaling behavior, particularly those with significance to others, such as weapons or reproductive organs. Shading can emphasize three-dimensionality and hence, visibility. Black and white patterns or vivid coloration against a contrasting color of background also serve to increase discriminability from immediate surroundings (Hingston, 1933; Cott, 1957; Hamilton, 1973).

On the other hand, there is a rich literature concerning the opposite adaptation: animals subject to intense predation frequently blend with their visual background rather than contrasting with it. Similarly, some predators have visual aspects which make them difficult to detect, the tiger usually being offered as an example. Extreme cases are often exquisitely refined, involving resemblance not just to a general background but to a particular object or organism, gaining highly specific protection thereby (Tinbergen, 1951, 1953; Wickler, 1968).

STEVEN GREEN AND
PETER MARLER

Even more basic to communication than the directionality of signals is the distance from the signaler at which they can be detected and discriminated. This is of particular concern in exploring the nature of signals that mediate the differing organizations of social groups in animals. Species vary widely in their patterns of spatial distribution and therefore also in the optimal distances at which signals should be perceptible to competitors and companions, kin and strangers, predators and prey.

What determines the distance a signal travels and the degradation and distortion it suffers in the course of transmission? Much depends on how the signal spreads from the source—whether it is beamed, deposited, or transmitted omnidirectionally so that its intensity rapidly decreases in any given direction. Obstacles in the signal's path may absorb, reflect, refract, or distort it. These issues are obviously different for visual, acoustic, electrical, and chemical signals, the former most impeded by obstacles, the latter least. There are also variations within a modality depending on the particular physical properties of the signal and the environmental conditions of transmission. The alternatives have been most thoroughly explored with sound, as reviewed by Waser and Wiley (this volume), who describe frequency "windows" in relation to sound transmission under certain conditions (Morton, 1975; Marten and Marler, 1977; Marten, Quine, and Marler, 1977).

An analogous situation can occur in the ocean with a steep gradient at the thermocline near the water surface and another near the ocean floor resulting from compression. Payne and McVay (1971) have indicated that the "sofar channel" thus created can refract sounds away from energy-absorbing contact with the water surface and the ocean floor, and it may well be exploited by humpbacked whales. This species produces its very loud and elaborate songs at the range of intermediate depths where this sound channel occurs, and Payne and McVay speculate that under these conditions, the whales may be audible to one another at distances of hundreds of miles. Their suggestion appears to be plausible in light of the use by submarines of the special properties of the sofar channel for long-distance acoustic detection and communication.

Although whale sounds are audible over great distances, they are subject to considerable distortion in the process. The sound received at any one place is a sum of components that have different frequency-dependent histories of reflection and refraction. Parts of sounds with origins a few milliseconds apart may arrive simultaneously. An early part may be retarded by a longer transmission time if it has undergone more bends and bounces and hence travels a longer distance. Conversely, signals originating in a very short interval may arrive over a substantial spread of time. This raises an important but little studied issue. Signals detected at a distance may not only be faint but also degraded (Wiley and Richards, 1978; Richards and Wiley, in press). On both counts, they will be less easily detected against the background and less readily discriminated from each other, reducing the ease of selective identification. As we have mentioned earlier, selectivity and sensitivity cannot be simultaneously maximized, as the receptor requirements differ. However, a signal may include features that allow adaptations for both detection at a distance, when specific details of the signal may be minimal, and also selectivity when at closer range.

By no means all signals are adapted to maximize transmission distance. The amplitudes of different sounds in primate repertoires vary extensively, in some degree of harmony with their apparent function, sometimes favoring close-range, within-group transmission, and sometimes allowing longer-distance transmission, perhaps favoring audibility to neighboring troops (Marler, 1973; Waser and Waser, 1977). Similarly, frequency adjustments may serve to limit the range of detectability. The very high pitch of some of the "ventriloquial" alarm calls of birds not only diminishes the cues available to predators for localizing the origin but also, perhaps more importantly, diminishes the transmission range because of the greater attenuation of high frequencies (Konishi, 1973). The acoustic signals of aquatic animals may be adapted to contrast with the ambient noise in their environment (Winn, 1967; Myrberg, 1978). Furthermore, certain components of complex acoustic signals may be more closely adapted for long-range transmission than others (Morris, Kerr, and Gwynne, 1975; Gerhardt, 1974a, 1975, 1976).

In the chemical domain, calculations of the "active space" of pheromones—such as an alarm signal of ants, on the one hand, and a sexual pheromone of a moth, on the other—show that they differ strikingly in accord with their function, the former being much larger than the latter (Bossert and Wilson, 1963; Regnier and Goodwin, 1977). Simple economy dictates some adjustment of the energy expended in production of a signal to the socially appropriate transmission distance. But it is also likely that long-range transmission of some signals is not just uneconomical but positively disadvantageous, as would be so if a local alarm pheromone spread to all corners of an ant colony, or a hen's tidbitting call for its chicks was as far carrying as a cock's crowing.

Internal Transformations in Signal Processing

Transformation Rules

Communication can be characterized as a sequence of procedures yielding a transfer of information. If one set of data is processed to yield a second set, the two are related to each other by the rules or instructions that dictate the procedure, plus any errors or noise introduced. Whether we examine large or small segments of a communication sequence, the same scheme can be used for depicting the information transfer that takes place.

If we look at a single organism, the first set might contain referents external to a signaling animal, and the second set the signals it produces. At the level of a social dyad or a social group, the second set might be responses by signal recipients. Even at the physiological level within a single organism, we can imagine viewing the internal procedures as arrayed in tandem. Referents, the first set, would be processed by the sensory apparatus and the brain to yield perceptions as the second set. These in turn would comprise the input set for generating a second set of internal states, which we will call *assessments* of the referent data. Each assessment may or may not be processed to generate a signal, selected from the set of possible signaling outputs. Regardless of the scale we invoke, each link in the chain of information transfers in a communication system is logically and conceptually equivalent, although the physiological and psychological processes themselves may be quite different.

At each level, the result may be characterized by a process of mapping a body of input data onto output, which can in turn be part of the input for the next stage. The rules or instructions that describe how each member of the input is assigned to one of the possible outputs constitutes a mapping function.

The simplest kind of idealized mapping function is a listing of unique assignments: every member of the input set is linked to one and only one member of the output set, and vice versa. In such a case, as long as each of the specific links is given, knowing the identity of any member of either set implies knowledge of the identity of the corresponding member of the other set. In certain conditions, such a system can be very efficient. In the absence of noise and error, information transfer occurs without loss or degradation or the introduction of uncertainties.

In any natural process, particularly a biological one, these conditions are rarely satisfied. Noise (i.e., unpredictable variation in the linking process), misadventure (regularly mistaken connections at either the input or the output set), and dropouts (a lapse in the processing) are all apt to cause loss or spurious augmentation. The effects of such errors may be far from trivial, with a strong influence on survival and reproduction.

We can examine the ways in which natural selection should favor mapping functions to minimize the likelihood and severity of such hazards. As illustrations, we will present hypothetical rules that differ in the effectiveness with which they serve to transfer information. Some rules appear to be well represented by animal communication processes. Others seem to have major potential disadvantages and are not known to occur.

GENERALITY OF TRANSFORMATIONS

The rules governing signal selection are our first concern. When sensory input is combined with internalized information, either genetically determined or acquired, a signaling organism may assign the result to one of a number of assessment states. Assessments in turn become the input data linked to signal production. The links from input to output can be expressed as two parallel lists of assessments and signals, with each connection between them separately indicated.

For simple organisms, with few sensory inputs and small signal repertoires, a mapping function of this kind is readily envisaged (Figure 1). Even for complex organisms, well-endowed with sensory capacities, such a simple listing may suffice to describe the transformation of assessments into signals if, in the circumstances under study, the potential output set is limited. Consider, for example, a human infant in a state of discomfort. Although infants are complex organisms with multimodal sensory perceptions, each sensation and degree of discomfort may yield only a simple comfort assessment of "yes" or "no." These two assessments can

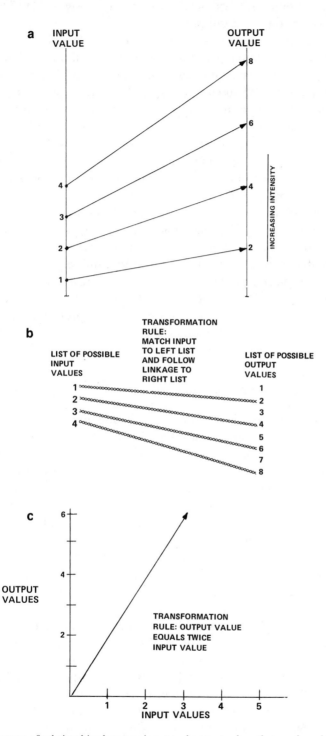

Fig. 1. (a) A diagram of relationships between input and output values that can be achieved either by (b) a set of linkages between parallel lists or (c) a general rule that can be applied to determine the output given any input. The same mapping function that describes (a) can be produced by the separate transformation rules shown in (b) or the general rule pictured in (c).

easily be mapped onto the vocal output set by a rule assigning "no" to crying and "yes" to silence or contented gurgling.

In more complex situations, however, it becomes less plausible to postulate a separate individual rule linking each and every pair of inputs and outputs. If, for example, an infant's assessments range over many intensities, reflecting different kinds and magnitudes of discomfort, and the output set varies from silence through minimal whimperings and thence louder and longer to full-blown screaming, then the list of rules linking each assessment to one of the vocal outputs would be extremely large. To internalize a list of rules embodying all such possible contingencies would require a staggering amount of information. An equivalent and more economical solution is achieved by applying one or more rules separately to each circumstance as it arises. A simple example would be a general rule specifying that the intensity value of the output data can be achieved by matching the intensity of the input. The greater the infant's hunger, for example, the louder its cry. Thus, one simple transformation function serves when needed to generate a relationship that maps input to output data and is fully equivalent to the separate determination of each output by matching the input against a list of input–output links. The result of transforming an assessment to a signal would be similar (Figure 1). Even with this type of more economical procedure, higher animals must have an enormous number of such rules, some as simple as this example, others much more abstract and complex.

Specificity of the Transformation

If each possible input is transformed into one and only one output, we say every input value *specifies* an output value. The resulting specific links from input to output are all deterministic, whether produced by a list of links or by application of a general rule. Examples can be found in production of those signals that have been described as "released" or "triggered." The input data set for a newly hatched herring gull, for example, includes one member that is a particular configuration of adult bill length, coloration, and movement. The output corresponding to this sensory input, specified by the process of internal transformation, is vigorous pecking at the bill tip (Tinbergen and Perdeck, 1950; Hailman, 1967; Tinbergen, 1973). The output in this example serves the direct function of obtaining food, which the adult carries to the chick, as well as an indirect one by signaling a need to the adult.

More than one input may specify the same output. Systematic experimental manipulation of the input can then determine the boundaries of the portion of the possible input set specifying a given output. In gulls, various hues, degrees of color contrast, shapes, and sizes can yield the pecking response in addition to the optimal set. Without access to further information at the physiological level, it is not possible to evaluate whether different effective stimuli yield different assessments, all specifying the same response, or whether all the effective stimuli result in the same assessment, one that is specifically linked to that response (see Figure 2).

To the extent that a transformation rule connects more than one member of the possible output set to an input, the mapping function is not specific. Such unspecific links may be parallel or alternate. The parallel case implies that two or more output items are simultaneously determined, a situation we will examine later. In the alternate case, there may be (1) an equiprobable random selection among outputs; (2) a fixed sequence of outputs, in which case the link is specified by the prior history of outputs as well as by the assessment; or (3) a nonuniform probabilistic determination of a range of outputs, or any mixture (Figure 3).

Unique Determination by the Transformation

If each possible output results from a transform of one and only one input, then we say that every output is uniquely determined by an input. Uniqueness is then the mirror image of specificity (p. 86).

A unique transformation implies that we can examine the output and ascertain which member of the input set is linked to it, thus permitting us to make inferences about the signaling animal's assessment of its own inputs. Adoption by a

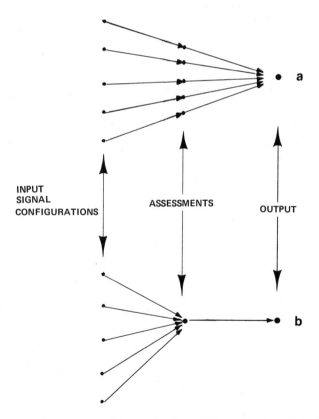

Fig. 2. Alternate routes for an array of input stimuli to yield specification of the identical output response. (a) Inputs are transformed into different assessments, each specifying the same output. (b) Each input is transformed into the same assessment, which specifies a single output.

STEVEN GREEN AND
PETER MARLER

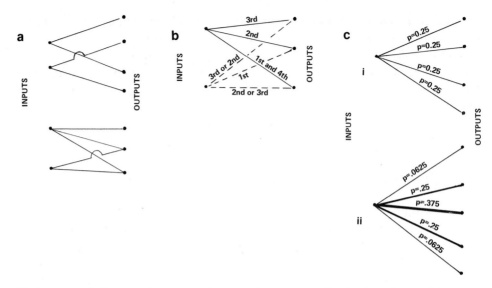

Fig. 3. Schematic diagram of transformation rules that are unspecific; that is, each input is linked to more than one kind of output. (a) More than one output is determined in parallel or simultaneous fashion. (b) Each input specifies an output that is not selected again until all other alternate outputs for that input have been specified. The sequence may be fixed or indeterminate. (c) Each input specifies an output with a fixed probability, but each such selection is independent of prior selections, so that (i) with equal probabilities of each output occurring, the transformations will be uniformly random, or (ii) with unequal probabilities, only the distribution of outputs can be predicted.

female bird of a typical precopulatory crouch would imply, if this posture is never otherwise elicited, that her assessment of the situation includes appropriateness for mating. Many sexual signals, however, appear in both mating and agonistic contexts. For these signals, which are not uniquely determined, no single inference is warranted. Examining additional signal components or knowing the broad context of signal production might provide further opportunities to refine our inferences (Figure 4).

UNIQUENESS AND SPECIFICITY

If each input is linked to exactly one output, and vice versa, the mapping is both specific and unique. Knowing the state of either input or output implies that we can infer the other. It must be remembered, however, that specificity and uniqueness are independent attributes of linkage relationships. Mapping functions may be fully asymmetrical relationships or only partly symmetrical.

Lack of symmetry presents an important practical problem when one attempts to examine the "assessment" of inputs by measuring responses. There is no *a priori* reason to expect exactly parallel mapping functions to link a single set of assessments to each of the separate possible output systems (Figure 5). The range of assessments that specify one output item might be much broader than those specifying another. If the outputs are used to gauge the richness of the assessments, it is easy to be misled by looking only at a single output system.

There are often arguments about whether animal signals and communication systems lack such attributes as digital coding, discreteness, arbitrariness, and openness. These terms are useful shorthand designations of extreme or limiting forms of transformation rules and the sets of signals or referent data on which they operate. Considering them as particular kinds of mapping functions provides a convenient, comparative framework for discussing human language and other animal communication systems.

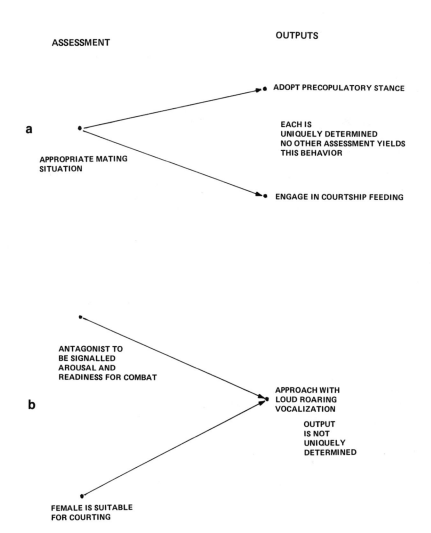

Fig. 4. (a) Precopulatory posturing and courtship feeding might each be uniquely determined by a bird's assessment that the situation is appropriate for mating. (b) A loud roaring vocalization by a male Japanese macaque is not uniquely determined; it may occur as part of a threat or during an agonistic chase or as part of a courtship sequence when approaching a female. An observer's inference after hearing the sound as to the male's assessment of the situation would be narrowed by knowledge of the context.

STEVEN GREEN AND
PETER MARLER

In signalers, we will take the input set as being the information available to the signaler and the output set as being the repertoire of possible signals. Thus, at the level of this discussion, two transformations are involved: input to assessment, and assessment to signal. For receivers, we will consider the next links in the chain of communication system transformations and reexamine signal transmission (the transformation from produced to received signal) and signal perception (reception through processing). For these receiver-oriented cases, the input set then consists of signals received, and the output set is an array of receiver's perceptions on which responses are based.

STEREOTYPY AND VARIABILITY

Lorenz (1935, reprinted 1970) originally focused attention on the existence of discrete, recurring, species-specific patterns of behavior in animals, epitomized in

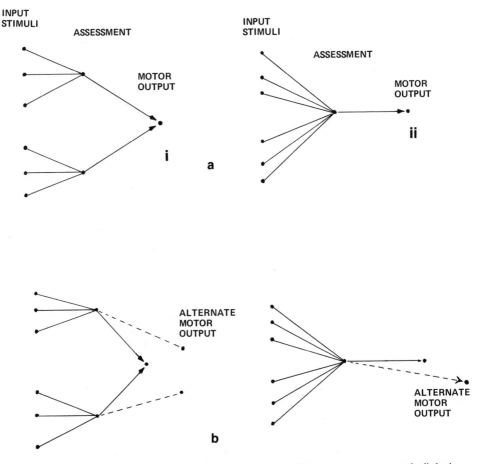

Fig. 5. (a) Alternate ways in which stimuli yielding the same or different assessments can be linked to a single motor output. Examination of the output does not allow one to distinguish whether the stimuli are perceived as the same or different: (i) stimuli are perceived to be of two kinds, but the same response occurs if (ii) they are perceived to be of the same kind. (b) The same stimuli may be shown to be perceived as different if a different response is measured as the output. Heart rate is frequently used, as it is often more sensitive than other measures.

his concept of the "fixed action pattern." Recently, ethologists have become concerned anew with the significance of signal variability. Substitution of the term *modal action pattern* is a significant step forward (Barlow, 1968, 1977), but there is still confusion about how to handle the problem of variation in the context of animal communication.

Stereotypy and *variability* are terms implying judgments about the degree of variation of behavior. In most ethograms, such judgments are usually made without explicit indication of their basis, but there is usually some implicit assumption of a criterion of acceptable physical variation. No signal is absolutely stereotyped, with no discernible variation. Given a small enough unit as a criterion for stereotypy, all nonsingular samples of any signal could be judged as variable, that is, with variation exceeding the criterion. When *stereotypy* is invoked as a descriptor, it usually implies that an animal produces the same signal in a recognizably similar or identical pattern, upon successive occasions. Another use is at the population or species level, namely, that all individuals produce the signal in a basically similar fashion.

We propose here that a logical and quantitative basis for determining which among a repertoire of patterns are the "same" signals (i.e., those appropriate for measuring within-signal variation) is to be found in the transformation rules operating in sending animals. We also suggest that selection of the most appropriate criteria for judging stereotypy is best accomplished by reference to the transformation rules operating in receiving animals. These are the two sides of the coin usually tendered under the rubric "natural units of behavior" (cf. Altmann, 1962).

CATEGORIES OF SIGNALER OUTPUT

Consider a signal repertoire comprising three readily characterized patterns, say, click trains of one, two, and three identical click elements. Two divergent approaches are available to describe signal variation in this repertoire. The first is to ignore all information not inherent in the signal itself. In this case, we derive appropriate descriptive statistics from counting the kinds of signal patterns produced. The statistical parameters estimated from our sampling can be used to compare degree of variation with another sampling of a different individual or population.

The second approach takes account of other kinds of information that permit inferences about the use of this repertoire. Each of the three elements might appear to be predominantly associated with a different intensity of threat. We can gauge the probability of agonistic behavior by observing events other than the kind of click signal given. Then, rather than measuring every signal in a sample, we could elect to measure variation only in signals putatively associated with one level of intensity. If, for example, single clicks predominate at the lowest intensity and triple clicks at the highest, these subsets will yield different estimates of variation than those based on all observed signals.

According to this procedure, we examine the social data available as input to the signaling animal, infer its assessments, and sample the signals according to the kind of assessment with which they seem to be associated. The measures of variation, although performed exclusively on the physical attributes of observed signals, reflect judgments about the mapping functions linking signals and assessments (see Figure 6).

Signals vary along many dimensions. One of the principal difficulties is to decide which parameters to ignore. The example of the click-train repertoire was phrased as if only the number of click elements was important in describing variation. Clicks may vary, however, in amplitude, rise time, frequency spectrum, beaming, phase relations, click duration, repetition rate, interclick interval, temporal modulation, and so on. Every signal can vary along the dimensions that physically describe it. Variation in some, however, may fail to be perceived. Thus,

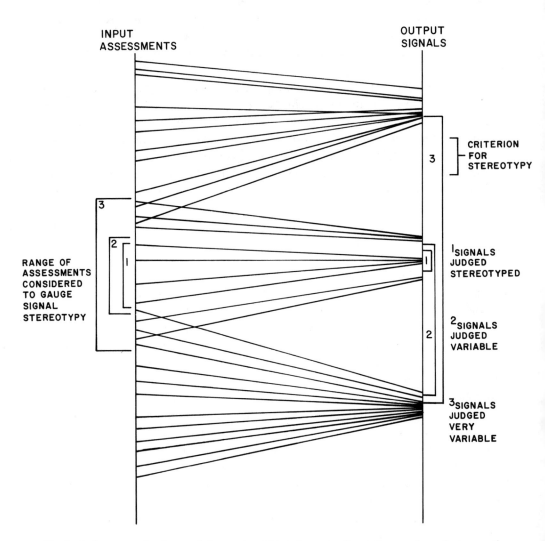

Fig. 6. A diagrammatic scheme of the way in which judgments of variation are dependent upon the breadth of the range of assessments transformed into signals. The signals linked to the smallest of the three ranges of input assessments, those within the #1 brackets, vary less than the indicated criterion for stereotypy. The variation of those linked to the assessments within the other two brackets exceed it.

not every bit of the signal-pattern information theoretically available is necessarily assessed or utilized by a receiver.

To decide whether physical variability is potentially meaningful to others, we must select a criterion and employ it systematically. The choice of subjects must be specified. The sample of signals for measurement may be obtained by repeating observations on one individual in the same circumstances, or it may be gathered in a naturally varied range of circumstances. The choice depends on the nature of the signal variation we seek to quantify. If we are examining population variability, the sample will be obtained from different individuals, either in the natural range of signaling circumstances or in some subset.

If any member of a sample set of signals differs by more than our criterion from some normative value, such as an arithmetic mean, we may say these signals are not stereotyped. We could equally well require a probabilistic rather than a threshold judgment of stereotypy, such as that no more than a certain fraction differ from the normative value by our criterion. If our measurements of the variable are taken along one dimension, the criterion will be a simple unidimensional constant. Analogous arguments apply for multidimensional signal variation. The major question is which criterion to use. Although any arbitrary value could be chosen for systematic comparisons, the particular selection predetermines whether signals are judged to be stereotyped or not. Procedures for sampling signals and for establishing criteria clearly determine whether our studies of stereotypy are biologically interesting or merely exercises in quantitative description.

Suppose that with our repertoire of three kinds of clicks, we try to characterize stereotypy looking at only the number of clicks. If we select one click as a threshold criterion for range of allowable variation, then any sample containing all three kinds of signals will clearly be considered variable; only samples that represent a single kind or just two kinds, including the double click, will be judged as stereotyped. With a criterion that variation should not exceed the mean or median number of clicks plus or minus one, then equal numbers of each kind of pattern will suggest a stereotyped repertoire. A different judgment of stereotypy could result if the same criterion is applied to a different sample taken from the same repertoire, one in which the single- and triple-click signals are not found in exactly equal numbers. Just as important as the magnitude of the criterion is how it is used and selection of the sample to which it is applied.

Another important consideration is the external-stimulus situation. By experimentally manipulating sensory input, we could probably find a narrow range of stimulation over which only one signal type would be elicited. The output would thus be deemed stereotyped. It might also be possible for a stimulus range of the same magnitude to cross a boundary between inputs linked to two different assessments, and to different signal types. We would then characterize the signals as variable (Figure 7). It is thus quite possible that the same restricted repertoire, produced from the same system and using the same criteria, would be characterized as stereotyped in some cases and variable in others.

In nonexperimental situations, such as is commonplace in field studies of communication, study of the combination of signals emitted in a given behavioral

STEVEN GREEN AND
PETER MARLER

situation and of the surrounding context can facilitate the formation of hypotheses about which input data are processed to achieve the same assessment. These can be tested by formal analysis, just as they are by the much-vaunted "intuition" of ethologists. The latter, although rarely explicitly recognized, is usually an internalized procedure for testing different ways of associating members of the signal set with external referents or presumptive internal states. Whether tested formally or intuitively, the basic procedure is the same. Variation of signals associated with one assemblage of input data is compared with variation under other schemes for classifying the signaler's input data and its inferred assessments. By a trial-and-error process, the assemblage that corresponds to the set of signals showing least variation is presented as the best estimate of the situation yielding that set of signals (Green, 1975a).

This method employs hidden assumptions about the relative importance of both signal variables and input variables. For senses that we ourselves possess, and for vertebrates, with which we have some empathy founded on familiarity and a

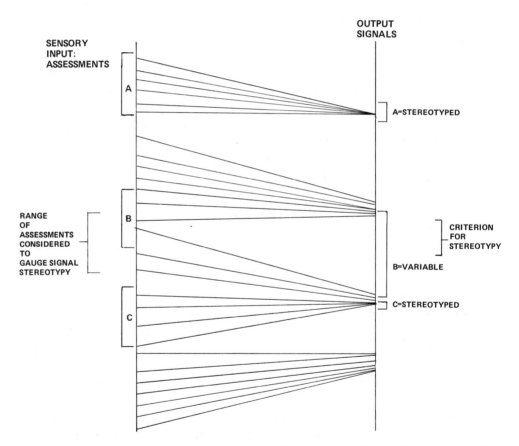

Fig. 7. A diagrammatic scheme of the way in which judgments of variation are dependent upon the nature of input assessments (represented by location) transformed into signals. Each of the three regions of input assessments covers a range of the same magnitude, but they are linked to signals with differing variation. Although the signals linked to ranges A and C would be judged stereotyped, those linked to B would be judged variable. The input range at location B includes a boundary between inputs mapped onto two different signal clusters.

shared evolutionary history, we rarely attack the issues of signal classification and stimulus-parameter salience from first principles. Instead, we usually rely, often quite appropriately, on a reasonable guess. Variation is measured on what we infer, using our own sense organs, to be the biologically relevant signal properties. Thus, for vertebrate vocalizations, we generally measure temporal changes of frequency and amplitude but ignore phase, unless we are concerned with localization problems. In the final analysis, only experimental manipulation can establish unequivocally which parts of a signal are relevant and therefore suitable for measurements of biologically meaningful variability, although this becomes glaringly obvious only when dealing with signals that activate sensory apparatus of other taxa quite different from our own (cf. Griffin, 1978). Lacking the ultrasonic sensitivity of bats or rodents, we are liable to lump all of their sounds as "squeaks," if we hear them at all.

Receiving Animals: Input

Signal stereotypy implies not so much a lack of variation as a judgment of "sameness." If we assess the receiving animal's ability to distinguish one signal from another, the JND (just noticeable difference) so derived is one useful starting point for establishing criteria for stereotypy. Clearly, if the "sameness" criterion is set at much less than a JND, we will be labeling signals as variable that the recipients perceive as identical. Conversely, if it is set at more than one JND, then it is possible that two signals judged to be the same (i.e., stereotyped) could actually produce two different assessments by a recipient. A criterion roughly equal to the JND for a given dimension is a good starting point.

Most signals are complex patterns that vary simultaneously along several dimensions. Although sensory JNDs may be useful for examining biologically relevant similarities and differences among signal patterns that vary along a single dimension, we lack sufficient psychophysical expertise to combine them with confidence when considering more complex signals. Perceptual tests are required to inform us about the presence and magnitude of interactions that affect minimal discriminable differences between complex signals not readily predicted from separate JNDs. The interactions between hue, saturation, and intensity in color-vision tests are examples of such complex effects. If we are to use the responders' assessments of input data as guidelines for constructing signal measurement and classification schemes appropriate to each species and sensory modality, more such perceptual tests are essential.

Use of any criterion level for judgments of stereotypy must take full account of what is known about sensory psychophysics. Detectable differences might be of dissimilar perceptual magnitudes in different zones of the overall range of variation. A familiar example is the operation of the Weber–Fechner law, which describes ratio relationships for difference limens; we thus describe JNDs in logarithmic terms, as with decibels for acoustic intensity. In general, there is no *a priori* reason to expect JNDs to be uniform. The size of regions in which test pairs of stimuli are all labeled similarly by a receiver may vary, depending upon their absolute location on a stimulus continuum.

Given multidimensional signal variation, the interaction of JNDs on different dimensions could yield perceptual categories of markedly different sizes. Small variations in one variable could lead to a judgment of difference between two test stimuli at one setting of the other parameters, while being judged similar at other settings (Gautier and Gautier-Hion, 1977; Beecher, Petersen, Zoloth, Moody, and Stebbins, in press; Zoloth and Green, in press).

It follows that judgments of variability or stereotypy are not generally made with sufficient information in hand to be taken at face value. As they appear in the literature, many such judgments are nevertheless informative because they are given in a comparative framework. When one species is judged as producing *more* or *less* stereotyped signals than another, this implies application of the same criterion to both species. Even though the criterion may not have been explicitly given, or perhaps even determined, such comparisons are valuable when considering the adaptiveness of signal morphology and evolutionary trends in signal usage.

Digital versus Analog Coding in Signals

These terms apply to signal structures with only two stereotyped signals or states possible *(digital)* and to those in which continuous variation is possible along a given dimension *(analog)*. The terms are often confused with *arbitrary* and *iconic*, which apply to mapping functions and not to signal patterns themselves (see below). Analog signals can reflect assessments along a range of continuous judgments, for example, more–less. Digital signals are capable of reflecting two classes of input assessments, for example, yes–no. If a recipient perceives the two elements of a digital signaling system as different, the signals can form the basis for digital coding. A special case of digital signaling is presence versus absence of a single stereotyped element.

If the set of signal patterns in a repertoire, or the range of signal variants of a given type, is such that a receiver can detect an intermediate form between any two of them, then these signals form an analog array. They can thus form the basis for analogic coding.

Clearly, it is possible to have a repertoire in which some signal types are digital and others analog. Similarly, it is possible to have a repertoire in which some signals are stereotyped, each physically discontinuous from all others, and others are variable, with neighbors abutting or overlapping so as to form an analog continuum.

The recipients of such signals may assess them either by digital or by analog means, regardless of the digital or analogic nature of the signals themselves. Analogic signals may be assessed as present or absent regardless of which variant is received. In the case of a visual signal, for example, there is an intergraded set of variable threatening facial expressions common to many anthropoids (van Hoof, 1962, 1967). Regardless of which variant a dominant male gives, a youthful subordinate perceiving it is likely to respond by fleeing. An older respondent, more nearly a social equal, may, however, adjust its response to the "more intense" or "less intense" information coded analogically, rather than acting purely on the digital presence or absence of threat.

We can view every signal as conveying digital information in terms of its presence or absence. Thus, there is always some hierarchical duality of signal structure. Similarly, digital signals may be assessed by summing them over time, so that an analogic rate is derived from digital occurrences. These two kinds of mapping functions from signal input to assessment may even operate on the same signal (e.g., Konishi, 1963; Wilson and Bossert, 1963; Ramsay, 1969).

The signal and response ends of communication systems can then be described as employing digital and analog processes simultaneously at different levels. We may conclude that although digital and analog modes are clear logical alternatives, the terms by themselves are of limited usefulness without specifying which properties of the signal are being considered and which aspects of a respondent's mapping of the signal onto its assessment are under discussion.

ARBITRARINESS VERSUS ICONICITY

Signals are said to be arbitrary if the mapping function generating them cannot be described by a generalized transformation rule. In this case, each member of the signal set is linked to input information by specific assignments that can be characterized only by listing them separately. The spoken names of primary colors are arbitrary signals in this sense, each linked to a somewhat different sensory input range in different languages and cultures (Rosch-Heider, 1971, 1972).

Signals are said to be iconic if variations in the physical configuration of the referent are transformed into parallel variations along dimensions of the signal. Ordering relationships are preserved by iconic mapping functions, a change in the referent being mirrored by a corresponding change in some signal variable. For the signal to be completely iconic, all perceived properties of the referent need to be reflected in the signal; the signal would be in some literal sense an image. The hand signals of American Sign Language are rich in iconic imagery (Stokoe, 1975; Bellugi and Klima, 1976), and onomatopoeic sounds recur in our speech. A predator alarm signal in which duration or amplitude increases with the increased size of the predator could be said to represent predator size iconically.

Although a similar ordered relationship can occur between a signaler sensing the presence of a predator and its assessment of the degree of danger present, the resulting signals are not necessarily iconic if this danger assessment is transformed into alarm-signal variation. *Iconicity* refers directly to physical attributes and thus to external referents, not to internal assessments, even though the transformation process might be analogous.

The relationship between the perceived predator and the signal form that it elicits may be noniconic and yet by no means arbitrary. Although an arbitrary relationship between signal morphology and referent cannot, by definition, be an iconic one, and although an iconic one is never arbitrary, many regular relationships between signals and physical properties of their referents are neither iconic nor arbitrary.

A low-intensity call might be given with a certain predator seen at a great distance and become louder or longer at shorter distances. Such a series would not usually be considered to iconically reflect distance, as ordering relationships are not preserved but reversed. They perhaps reflect the retinal image size and the visual perception of the predator by the signaler, but the signals then follow rules similar to iconic mapping of the assessment, not a measurable attribute of the referent. The referent has not changed its physical dimensions in the same way as the signal. Such a signal would usually be deemed analogic but not iconic. Note, however, that some situations can be difficult to classify. If there were an increase in signal repetition rate as the predator came closer, the time between signals *would* be iconically diminishing with decreased distance, but the average signal intensity over time would not. We therefore suggest that iconic be applied to situations where either positive or negative ordering relationships exist.

Perhaps the most celebrated of all animal communication systems, the dance language of honeybees, illustrates iconicity in the relationship between the direction of a resource in relation to the sun's observed or inferred position and the orientation of the waggle run. This is direct on a horizontal surface and angled to gravity when translated to a vertical surface (von Frisch, 1923, 1967; Lindauer, 1961; Gould, 1976). Other waggle-dance features bear an iconic relationship to resource distance. These include tempo, rates and numbers of waggles, and the duration of the bursts of sound produced in the waggle dance (Esch, 1961; Wenner, 1962), though it is still not certain which convey distance to other workers.

Dance meaning is further enriched both by olfactory and other cues brought back from the resource and by the context provided by the audience. The general excitedness of the dance corresponds with the relative "quality" of the food. However, "quality" relates in turn to current needs of the hive, conveyed to the dancer by how long it takes to share the incoming load with with other bees. If this takes more than about a minute, dancing will rarely occur:

> For example, water—which is used to air-condition the hive—is normally not well received by the colony. If the day gets hot, however, foragers returning with very sweet nectar will no longer be able to distribute their loads quickly. Bees gathering dilute nectar or water, on the other hand, will be relieved of their loads very rapidly. The nectar foragers will stop dancing while the water collectors will begin to dance vigorously. (Gould, 1976, pp. 215–216)

Only analog signals such as sound-pulse number or waggle-run duration in the dance language can be used for iconic representations of physical attributes that are themselves continuous, such as food distance (Gould, 1975). However, it is also logically possible for analogic signals to be linked in some *arbitrary* fashion to a continuum of intergraded referent data or assessments, although the likelihood of communication errors in such a system would restrict its evolution to very special situations (cf. Altmann, 1967).

Digital signals can also be used iconically, but only to represent physical attributes with just two states. Signaling systems that are neither analog nor digital can have some attributes of both. Repertoires may be formed, for example, of an array of discretely distinctive stereotyped patterns drawn from a continuum but without intermediates. If the range of variation within each pattern is much less than the distance between them, such signals are often called discrete. Signals of this kind could be used as iconic representations of attributes that are similarly discrete, as if stepped levels of signal intensity represented the number of predators in an attacking group. They are also available as the output set from arbitrary transformations of either continuous or discontinuous assessments, or from a nonarbitrary mapping function that, although noniconic, is very regular, such as stepped intensities of signal representing degrees of threat. Such discrete signals cannot be used for iconic representation of any physically continuous attribute, such as predator size (Figure 8).

CATEGORICAL AND CONTINUOUS PERCEPTION

It is an obvious but often neglected point that what an animal makes of a signal it receives cannot be determined by analyzing the signal. The information transfer from sense organ to assessment is governed by rules that we are unable to discern no matter how closely we examine signal morphology. This point is exemplified by tests performed on humans listening to sounds of speech. Presented with neighboring pairs of stimuli from an array of speech sounds spaced equidistantly along a single acoustic dimension, listeners assign only one label to both members of some pairs, yet classify others as representing two different stimulus categories (Liberman, Cooper, Shankweiler, and Studdert-Kennedy, 1967). The dimensions tested include such features as voice–onset–time and formant slope. If we examine other aspects of performance during the listening task, however, it is apparent that information on within-category discrimination is available, although this is not evident if listeners employ the usual labeling procedure (Cooper, Delattre, Liberman, Borst, and Gerstman, 1952; Pisoni and Tash, 1974) (Figures 9 and 10).

As viewed spectrographically through time, normal speech is a continuously changing pattern of frequency and amplitude modulations. To the listener,

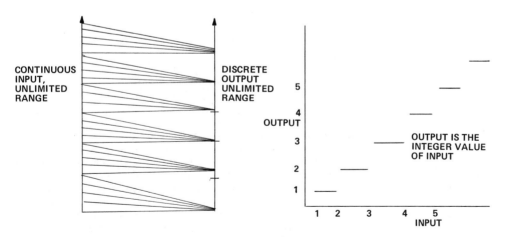

Fig. 8. To the left is a schematic diagram of a mapping function which transforms the continuous input at the left margin into the discrete outputs on the right. The graph on the right side illustrates the kind of orderly and non-arbitrary transformation rule which can generate such a regular and systematic, but non-iconic, mapping.

STEVEN GREEN AND
PETER MARLER

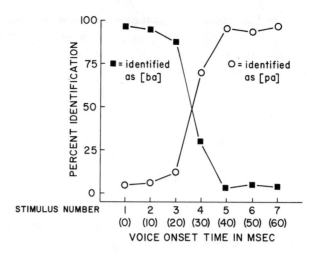

Fig. 9. Average identification scores of nine subjects listening to seven steps in a synthetic speech, voice-onset–time continuum (cf. Pisoni and Tash, 1974). There is a consistent partitioning of the stimulus continuum into the two categories [ba] and [pa]. Stimuli in which laryngeal voicing starts early in the sound are heard as the voiced consonant *b*. Sounds with a later voicing onset are heard as the unvoiced consonant *p*.

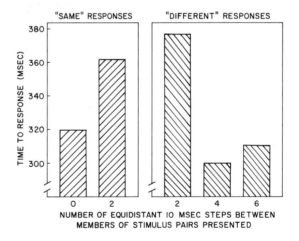

Fig. 10. Mean time for nine subjects listening to paired stimuli and judging them as "same" or "different" to respond correctly. The number of 10 msec steps between members of a pair is the difference between their assigned stimulus numbers, each (as listed below) representing a stimulus with a specific timing of voice onset as given in Figure 9. Within category (= same) pairs with zero difference are 1–1 (stimulus number one paired with itself) and 3–3 for [ba], 5–5 and 7–7 for [pa]; those with a two-step difference are 1–3 [ba], and 5–7 [pa]. Across category (= different) pairs are 3–5 (two-step [ba]–[pa]), 2–6 (four-step [ba]–[pa]), and 1–7 (six-step [ba]—[pa]). Note the across-category responses to stimuli near the category boundary (located between 3 and 5 in Figure 9) are slower than to those pairs whose members have a greater degree of acoustic disparity in the timing of voice onset. The within-category responses to the acoustically two-step different stimuli are slower than to pairs with identical members although in both cases the stimuli are each given the same phonetic label [ba] or [pa] by subjects. Thus, differences in processing are revealed which would be obscured if only the question of same or different identification or of phonetic labeling were addressed. (See Pisoni and Tash (1974) for a full account.)

however, it appears to be a stream of closely spaced discrete elements (Liberman *et al.*, 1967). The mapping function of speech perception is then of the kind shown in Figure 11, a set of discrete labels, or assessments, each linked to a small portion of the total range of intergraded signal morphologies. In the speech literature, this kind of transformation is called categorical processing of a continuous signal.

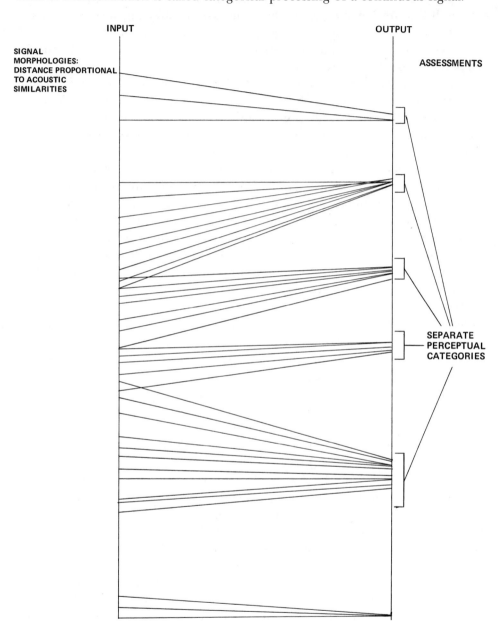

Fig. 11. Diagram of a mapping function describing categorical assessment of signals with continuous variation as revealed by listening tests using speech signals. Samples taken from acoustically continuous speech variation are labeled as belonging to separate perceptual phonetic categories. Variants within some ranges are all labeled similarly. Variants which differ by lesser amounts, however, may be labeled as belonging to two different categories. There are small boundary zones where variants are sometimes identified as belonging to one category and at other times another. Listeners do not identify sounds from these zones as belonging to an intermediate category.

We are as yet unable to define which of the physical attributes of the vocal signal are invovled in most kinds of assessments made in speech processing. The labeling process leads us to infer that the processing normalizes for differences in the speaker's age, sex, systematic distortion (e.g., regional accent), and idiosyncracies, all of which change the values of the parameters describing spoken phonemes. It appears that our only reliable method for establishing the salient units of speech is to employ human listeners, a situation with important implications for students of animal vocal signals (Marler, 1976c, 1977a; Green, 1977; Beecher *et al.*, in press; Zoloth and Green, in press).

The phenomena of categorical perception and the attendant normalization for cues that are irrelevant to phonemic identity dramatize the difficulty of deriving biologically relevant signal classifications. In some important intuitive sense, a variable sampling of the same spoken phoneme from a single speaker or a selection of different speakers contains signals more similar to each other than they are to other phonemes. To establish an analytic procedure yielding this same result, we would first have to determine the important dimensions used in speech-pattern recognition and then establish the appropriate criterion for stereotypy for different parts of the range of natural variation. This is somewhat of a paradox, since categorical perception implies that any criterion may be vanishingly small across boundaries between perceived categories, although the signals are clearly physically continuous. In fact, the differences between phonemes can be *less* than the variation within a sample of the same phoneme. Not only do extreme signal forms that abut a boundary differ little, but even central or median patterns of different kinds can differ less than the difference across the range of one of them. This perceptual phenomenon of auditory categorization is probably more general than is acknowledged (Cutting and Rosner, 1974; Kuhl and Miller, 1975; Pastore, 1976) and is likely to play an increasingly important role in analyzing animal communicative systems, especially as ethologists become more familiar with speech research.

The human propensity to perceive sounds categorically probably inclines us to label animal signal repertoires as stereotyped or discrete even when a physical analysis does not fully support this judgment (contrast Winter, Ploog, and Latta, 1966, with Schott, 1975). This may be a more serious problem in forming differences of opinion on vocal repertoire size and degrees of vocal variability than the lack of uniform criteria or the undersampling of repertoires. Similar processes occur in sensory modalities other than audition. Here, too, repertoire characterizations that rely on human pattern-recognition may be informing us more about the number of categories that we can comfortably erect than about the signals themselves (e.g., Miller, 1956; Moynihan, 1966, 1970; Bertrand, 1969; Wilson, 1972; Eisenberg, 1974, 1976).

Of course, continuously variable signals are not necessarily perceived categorically and may also be assessed in a continuous fashion. It appears that the crest display of Stellar's jay, for example, yields a continuously variable assessment of the agonistic intent of the signaler (Brown, 1964, and Figure 12), as does the extension of median fins in fish (Rasa, 1969). Furthermore, continuous and categorical perception of the same continuum may occur together, but at different

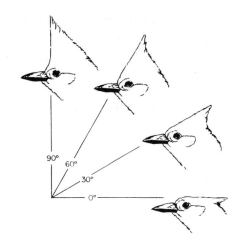

Fig. 12. Continuous gradation in the degree of
crest elevation in Steller's jay in various behavioral
contexts. After Brown (1964).

levels, just as there may be concurrent digital and analog processing. The best
example, again, comes from human speech. While the linguistic content may be
assessed by categorizing the speech signals into phonetic elements, intonation
patterns can yield continuous assessments of mood.

Lastly, discontinuous or discrete signals may be perceived in a continuous or
noncategorical fashion (Figure 13). Although rarely considered explicitly, the
mapping function describing this kind of transformation may play an important
role in many communication systems, as discussed next.

DISCRETE AND GRADED COMMUNICATION SYSTEMS

Consider an organism that produces signals in conjunction with a number of
different assessments, each derived from differing combinations of current and
previously internalized data. If we picture an animal using a regular, nonarbitrary
mapping function, its signals will bear some readily specifiable relationships to the
assessments. In this simple, hypothetical situation, assessments that are similar will
be linked to similar signals. Those with distinctly different assessments will be
linked to signals with very different parameters. The repertoire would then
consist of some signals closely spaced along a dimension of physical similarity and
others that are distant from their neighbors, the degree of separation reflecting
relationships among their underlying assessments. There would be a complementary set of signal–assessment relationships in a receiving animal. By engaging the
converse receptive mapping function, similar signals would yield neighboring
assessments, while perceptions of distinctly different signals would yield very
different assessments (assuming that the other inputs into the assessment, such as
context and prior experience, remain constant).

Signal patterns necessarily change somewhat during transmission. If the
effects of noise and degradation are equivalent for all elements of a signal
repertoire, we can predict that certain relationships will be preserved. For a signal
that is originally different enough from neighboring signals, transmission degradation will result in a received signal that still matches its own original form more

closely than any other. With lesser differences, two signals may be indistinguishable after transmission.

Given such a simple, generalized communication system, any input assessment by the signaler will produce a signal that elicits an assessment in the receiver
within a defined range of probabilities. The size of the range and the sharpness of
the probability peaks will be functions of such factors as the noise, error, and

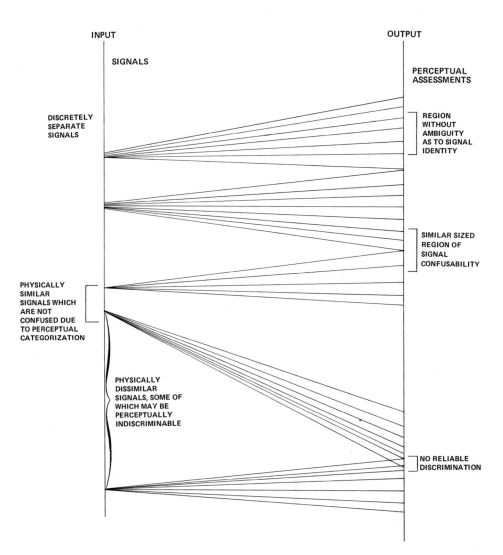

Fig. 13. Diagram of a mapping function by which discretely separate signals may not be perceived as
such. The perceptual assessments represented by the upper bracket on the right all derive from one
discrete set of signals. Those from the bracket below it can be generated from signals of two sets which
are discretely separate. The signals embraced by the square bracket at the left generate widely different
perceptions. Those more discontinuous embraced by the curved brackets generate a continuous range
of similar perceptions including a range of overlapping perceptual assessments. Signal discontinuity of
greater or lesser degree may or may not be transformed into continuous, discontinuous, or overlapping
perceptions, depending upon the mapping function rather than exclusively upon the degree of signal
similarity.

variability in sender and receiver processing; the continuous or categorical nature
of signal perception in the receiver; the degrees of dissimilarity among closely
spaced signals; and, particularly, for distinctively different signals, the effects of
transmission.

If all the signal varieties in a repertoire that reflect different input assessments
are so widely spaced that even after taking account of variation and allowing for
the maximum signal degradation that occurs during normal transmission, differences between them larger than a JND are still preserved at the receiver, the result
is a *discrete* communication system. Such a system is composed of stereotyped
signals (regardless of the degree of physical variation), is digitally coded (each
assessment is signaled in a yes–no fashion), and comprises signals that are perceived as distinct categories. With the categorical processing (i.e., there are very
small JNDs at some boundary points between signals), discriminable signals can
be relatively more similar to each other than with continuous processing. When
transmission losses are negligible, as in operation over short distances, discriminability can be retained without increasing dissimilarity. Such a system permits
completely arbitrary mapping functions to be used without diminished effectiveness or increased likelihood of error compared with nonarbitrary ones. It pro-
hibits analogical communication, although with continuous processing of these
discrete signals, some of the subtlety of analogic communication of ordered series
can be preserved.

A *graded* communication system would be the opposite, one in which signals
are both so closely similar to each other and also variable enough that a pair deriving from neighboring assessments will on occasion be judged to be identical. In
this system, signals originally different by more than a JND may become indistinguishable after transmission. Analogic signaling would be possible and continuous
perception likely. Although some of the advantages of discrete systems could be
preserved by imposing categorical perception on the receiver, the disadvantages
in terms of error would be enormous unless very regular nonarbitrary mapping
functions for production and perception or some other error-reducing procedure
were employed, such as a high degree of redundancy.

Probably only the very simplest organisms communicating in a single sensory
modality can be characterized as having fully discrete or completely graded
communication signals. Most animals are likely to employ a mixture of discrete
and graded signal ranges within any sensory modality, although one can imagine a
multimodal system that approximates a graded one by multiplexing signals of
different modality, each of which operates discretely. No animal system is well
enough known to determine whether the potential of such multimodal communication is realized.

The evolution of systems with discrete and graded properties has been
treated by Moynihan (1964), Marler (1965, 1975), Gautier (1974, 1978; Gautier
and Gautier-Hion, 1977), and others, although initially applied to signals and their
transmission rather than entire systems. Briefly, they conclude that discretely
organized primate vocal repertoires are favored when auditory signals must
operate without complementation by other sensory modalities, as in signaling at
night or in intergroup calling in the day over long distances in the forest.

Conversely, graded sound signals are more common in close-range signaling, often within-group, where rich supplementation by visual and tactile signals is the rule.

Open and Closed Systems

If we define an open communication system as always having the potential for production of new signals, and a closed system as having a preordained signal set, the graded portion of any system is clearly open in the sense that intermediate signals can always be added to reflect intermediate assessments. With a shared regular, nonarbitrary mapping function and continuous perception, intermediate assessments by recipients would follow. Apart from transmission problems, the limits on such systems will derive from the receiver's capabilities for refined discriminations and from the signaler's capacity for fine control of signal output, so that intermediate signals are likely to reflect intermediate assessments rather than effects of noise or variation. Expansion can occur within these physiological limits until additional intermediates can no longer be reliably produced and accurately transmitted, received, and assessed. Such systems are not open, however, with respect to expansion of the range of input data to which signals are linked, since this is preordained by the original mapping function.

The discrete portion of any system is always open to expansion of the range of referents. This can be done by adding new discrete signals or by embroidering variations on existing signals. They can thus be transformed into a new graded portion of the repertoire, assuming that parallel changes in receiver processing and the other criteria are met.

Characterization as graded or discrete is least useful with systems in which signals and perceptions may differ, as, for example, if signals vary continuously and perceptions are categorical, and with a mapping function that is arbitrary or listlike. Such systems are always open in the sense that a lexicon is open: new signals can be assigned new links both for the emitter (to additional referent data configurations) and the receiver (yielding new labels or output assessments). Human language is our best-known case for this kind of openness, but the specification of new, arbitrary links may also occur in animal communication systems.

There are then two independent substrates on which evolution can act to provide for the openness of communication systems. On the one hand, there can be selection for the capacity to generate new arbitrary individual links. On the other hand, there can be selection of processing and producing systems that allow a precise refinement of signal variability and its perception. We usually think of the former as a capacity to learn and of the latter as refinement of neuromuscular and sensory skills, each known to occur to some degree in all animals.

While this is not the place to pursue an argument on the origins of social communication, we can suggest a few premises. First, *all* systems are open. The traditional distinction between open and closed systems is a matter of timetable, that is, whether new communicative usages occur within a single life span as opposed to more leisurely, evolutionary changes. If heritable augmentation of signaling behavior occurs without the parallel or preexisting development of receiver capabilities, natural selection is unlikely to favor it. Thus, either perceptual capabilities develop earlier in phylogeny than the signaling behaviors that utilize them, *or* they emerge simultaneously. In the latter case, it is most likely that simultaneity would occur in progeny or siblings that have inherited part of the same parental genotype associated with the new signals. Regardless of which animal produces signals—parent, offspring, or sibling—corresponding perceptions and assessments are more likely to occur when common transformation rules govern both processes and are associated with the same genetic material, a point we return to in the next section.

In the case of new linkages, those that are relearned within each individual's development, social usage is likely to spread first among relatives, both because of kinship-related physical proximity in many animals and also as a result of their sharing whatever component of this learning capability that is heritable. To the extent that such new linkages enable greater individual success and inclusive reproductive fitness, the propensity for such learning will spread. Once the traits associated with such capabilities become widespread, the stage is set for the cultural transmission of these linkages, that is, of learned and shared agreement on the rules specifying signal usages, both in perception and in production. Perhaps bird and monkey vocal dialects are expressions of this process (Marler and Mundinger, 1971; Green, 1975b).

The Heredity and Ontogeny of Communication

In the course of communication, signal senders and receivers can benefit most from the use of closely matched procedures. Errors will be reduced, and information loss will be kept to a minimum. Given the advantages of sharing basic procedures for signaling and reception, variations of lesser or greater effectiveness among individuals are subject to natural selection to the extent that the apparatus, rules, and procedures are heritable. The social organization of most animals requires that uniform rules extend far beyond a simple communicative dyad of mother and offspring or mated pair to include families, larger kin groupings, local clusters or aggregates, social networks, demes, all species members, and, to a degree, even broader phyletic units. A variety of means can be employed to ensure that the necessary degree of rule sharing is achieved.

Neither biologists nor psychologists have yet accumulated a sufficient body of empirical information to encourage formulation of theories about rule transmission in animals. Even in our own species, though language is a target of much current research, rules for linguistic, syntactic, and speech processing are still largely a matter of speculation. The deficiencies in studies of human communication are somewhat complementary to those in other species.

In animals, there is an extensive literature on the phylogeny of signaling actions, a major theme in ethological research since Lorenz's (1941) classical analysis of display behaviors in ducks. Ethologists have properly emphasized that genetic mechanisms must play a dominant role, though some have argued that the importance of learning has been underplayed.

By comparison, there is almost no ethological information on the phylogeny or ontogeny of encoding and decoding procedures. While the development of many signal actions is largely innate, it seems probable that, at least in higher animals, learning plays an important role in the acquisition and development of functionally appropriate "assessments" of situations or signals. Thus, one may argue that the focus on the morphology of signaling behaviors in past animal research has led to overemphasis on the inherited component of the communicative performance.

If we compare the current state of understanding of the development of human behavior, a different bias emerges. Few hesitate to acknowledge the dominant or even exclusive role of individual experience in the ontogeny of language. This is perhaps in part because we are aware of the great diversity of human languages and dialects, and are introspectively conscious of the processes of encoding and decoding speech signals. In the minds of many, this environmental viewpoint extends to the development of all other human signaling behavior. However, this extension is probably less appropriate than is often supposed. Innate, species-specific components in human signaling behavior are in fact widespread in human facial expressions (e.g., Eibl-Eibesfeldt, 1972) and even in human speech behavior (Eimas, 1975; Eimas and Tartter, in press), although we are rarely conscious of them. In recent years, the revival of interest in nativistic interpretations of human communicative behavior has given promise of a more sensible balance, acknowledging both the essential role of hereditary influences in human communication and also the greater importance in animals of environmental influences, including some that may be properly viewed as cultural.

SIGNALING, SENSATION, AND PERCEPTION

Although we have indicated examples of extensive mutual evolutionary interactions between mechanisms of signal production and of sensation, such interactions are most evident in species with nonversatile receptor systems. When service for other functions is required in addition to communication, mechanisms of signal perception become more deeply embedded in the basic perceptual operations performed on sensory stimuli in general. Studies of perceptual development thus come to bear directly on the ontogeny of communication. We can hardly do justice here to a theme on which there is an extensive literature in both philosophy and psychology (e.g., Boring, 1942; Gibson, 1966; Uhr, 1966; Warnock, 1967; Gibson, 1969; Sutherland, 1973; Rosinski, 1977).

Perception involves not just the ability to sense changes in the environment but also the ability to organize and interpret what is sensed and to act on the basis of those interpretations. It is evident from this definition that the construct we have called *assessment* has much in common with perception in the broad sense. Indeed, it is probably best viewed as a special case of the more general phenomenon.

There is evidence that perceptual development includes something equivalent to building up structural representation of the external world (Craik, 1943; Sutherland, 1973; Gregory, 1974). In ways that are still mysterious, objects and events become classified into categories, with definite boundaries between them. The process of assessment that we have invoked is closely allied to this classificatory process.

Aside from the purely sensory aspects of interaction with the external world that contribute to the ontogeny of internalized representations of external phenomena, there is a growing appreciation of the importance of motor involvement (Turvey, 1977; Weimer, 1977). In addition to the importance of actions that directly aid the gathering of sensations, such as searching movements with the distance receptors and their supporting body parts (e.g., Hebb, 1949 ; Yarbus, 1967), there is also evidence that functional involvement with the environment plays a role in the emergence of perceptual categories (Rosch, 1973, 1975; Nelson, 1974). Given the intimate association between human perception and action, it is but a small step to the invocation of sensorimotor interactions as a factor in the development of animal communication. In fact, such interaction is implied by the construct of *sensory templates* (reviewed in Marler, 1976b), invoked by students of auditory communication in animals as varied as crickets, frogs, and birds.

SHARED PROCEDURES FOR PRODUCTION AND PERCEPTION

We want to develop the notion that the perception and production of both human and animal signals requires only one kind of algorithm linking external signal to internal state. There is a sense of economy in designing communicative physiology so that common mechanisms serve this role in both signal senders and signal receivers. One line of argument favoring common physiological mechanisms underlying both signal production and perception derives from studies of effects of temperature on the behavior of cold-blooded animals. In a pioneering study, Walker (1957) demonstrated that a critical species-specific difference between the calling songs of males of different species of tree crickets lies in the rate of pulsation of the stridulatory sounds. Within groups of sympatric cricket species, he found that females respond selectively to conspecific male pulse rates by approaching the loudspeaker. It is well known that song pulse rates are temperature-dependent in a regular fashion, and Walker was able to show the responsiveness of females to pulse-rate changes in parallel, so maintaining specific discrimination over a range of temperatures that would otherwise completely confuse the discrimination process. It is economical to postulate that the temperature dependence of both male song production and female song responsiveness is mediated by a common mechanism. In another study of this type, Gerhardt's (1978) work with tree frogs has shown that species-specific pulse-repetition rates and pulse durations in male calling are highly dependent on temperature, and that female responsiveness for each species studied marches in parallel.

Study of the behavior of hybrid crickets leads to a similar interpretation. Having demonstrated that the calling songs of hybrids are uniquely different from those of either parental species, Bentley and Hoy went on to show that hybrid females prefer hybrid male songs to either of the two parental male songs (Bentley and Hoy, 1972; Hoy and Paul, 1973; Hoy, 1974; Hoy, Hahn, and Paul, 1977). Common genetic control of signal production and reception is indicated, and Hoy *et al.* (1977) went on to speculate that

> the existence of neurones common to both central pattern generators (male) and to hypothetical feature detectors or templates (female) would help explain the coupling of male and female auditory behavior. Genetic control could be achieved by identical sets of genes acting on the same neurone types in both male and female. Thus behavioral and genetic coupling would have a common basis.

BIRDSONG: PRODUCTION AND PERCEPTION

Studies of vocal communication in birds have provided another type of evidence in favor of sensorimotor neural templates as shared mechanisms for perceiving, producing, and responding to birdsongs. Since many songs are learned, it is possible to extend interpretations beyond what is appropriate for the cricket and frog findings, where the innate patterns of sound production are under more-or-less strict genetic control.

It is clear that learning plays a dominant role in the development of the perceptions that birds have of their own vocal signals. This is true even in cases where the patterns of production are not only innate but develop in the absence of auditory feedback, as in the domestic chicken (Konishi, 1963). In spite of this apparent lack of plasticity in the motor coordinations of sound production, there are strong hints that chickens derive much of their mature perception of conspecific sounds through learning (Evans, 1972; Evans and Mattson, 1972; Guyomarc'h, 1972, 1974a,b). Similarly, in birds with more plastic vocal behavior, a variety of evidence indicates that songbirds engage in extensive perceptual learning. While there is an innate basis for song recognition (e.g., Marler and Peters, 1977), songbirds also acquire responsiveness to many details of the male territorial song, such as local dialects, individual differences, and variations associated with changing motivation (e.g., Falls, 1969; Falls and Brooks, 1975; Milligan and Verner, 1971; Brooks and Falls, 1975a,b; Wiley and Wiley, 1977; Kroodsma, 1978).

Auditory learning plays a role in motor aspects of vocal development in many songbirds, so that their vocal behavior is abnormal if reared in social isolation (Marler and Mundinger, 1971). The accuracy with which sounds can be imitated indicates that vocal learning can proceed by reference to auditory information (Konishi and Nottebohm, 1969). The extreme abnormality of the singing behavior of males of some songbirds deafened in youth, before singing, is further evidence of the crucial role of auditory learning in vocal development (Konishi, 1963, 1964, 1965, 1966; Marler, Konishi, Lutjen, and Waser, 1973; Marler and Waser, 1977). In one closely related group of sparrows, deafening has been found almost to eliminate species song differences, again indicating the major role of audition in guiding species-specific signal production.

Sensorimotor interplay is also indicated by the tendency for singing to develop later than song learning. The initiation of the perceptual phase of song learning tends to precede production in many birds, sometimes overlapping in time and sometimes not. When singing begins, there is a gradual transition from subsong to full song that often proceeds without further access to models. Sequences of vocal transformations occur such as might be expected if the bird were improving its skill at controlling operations of the complex syringeal apparatus, thereby achieving a better and better match with the memory of sounds heard earlier in life. We can conceive of the acoustic information used in this matching process as embodied in a sensory template that is modifiable through auditory experience (e.g., Marler, 1970).

A further role for perceptual mechanisms in avian vocal development is implied by evidence of selectivity in initial stages of the learning process. Whereas some birds are interspecific mimics, either by nature or in artificial circumstances of captivity, some species that develop a highly abnormal song when reared in social isolation are then nevertheless quite selective in what sound patterns they accept for imitation (Thorpe, 1958, 1961; Marler, 1970; Marler and Peters, 1977; Konishi, 1978). Evidently, some birds exhibit an innate auditory predisposition to learn certain classes of sounds more readily than others.

If recent studies are any guide, the initial specifications may be quite simple and incomplete (Marler, 1978). Although lacking in many details, the specifications are sufficient to endow the singing of a naive young male with more normal traits than is the case if he is deafened. Given auditory experience with normal species-specific songs, additional features are memorized, with delayed effects on learned song patterns when the male begins singing later. The learned song is obviously a closer match to the wild type than that of a bird without this experience. Thus, we may confidently postulate an engram or schema of the learned song, then used template fashion during the process of learning to sing. In the brain of an adult bird, equivalent processes are presumably used in song recognition as well as in song production (Marler, 1976b).

That mechanisms with some similar properties exist in the brains of nonsinging females is indicated by the elicitation of female song by treatment with male sex hormones. In the white-crowned sparrow, a species with well-marked song dialects, the normal male song is learned (Marler and Tamura, 1964; Marler, 1970). A female who hears a local dialect in her youth not only will sing under the influence of testosterone but will render that particular dialect (Konishi, 1965). This acquired information is presumably normally used in the process of mate selection by female sparrows (Milligan and Verner, 1971; Baker and Mewaldt, 1978). Thus, a common mechanism is indicated for perceptual and motor development, shared by males and females, though normally put to different uses by the two sexes.

Learning plays a major role in the development of this shared mechanism. The neuroanatomical nature of the mechanism is unexplored. Although it is conceptualized as having unity of operation, it may comprise few or many physiological components, with separate elements selecting different acoustic features from external sounds and from the animal's own vocal performance. Components exhibiting developmental plasticity may be distinct from or identical with those that underlie the innate selective perception of an untrained bird. Mechanisms might operate in series or in parallel, with control shifting from one to another as learning takes place.

While the particular structures involved are yet to be identified, together they achieve the template-matching function we have outlined. It also seems conceivable that they operate in analogous fashion to the developing internalizations of past experiences involved in the control of other kinds of perception and movement that physiologists are beginning to infer, however dimly, from interactions between operations in different parts of the brain (Evarts, Bizzi, Burke, DeLong, and Thach, 1971; Mountcastle, 1976).

The Motor Theory of Speech Perception

There is a remarkable parallel here with the motor theory of speech perception as developed by Liberman *et al.* (1967; Studdert-Kennedy, Liberman, Harris, and Cooper, 1970). Noting that some anomalies of speech-sound recognition disappear if one thinks of them in terms not of acoustic features but of the vocal gestures producing them, it was proposed that a common mechanism underlies both perception and production. They suggest that we

> think in terms of overlapping activity of several neural networks—those that supply control signals to the articulators and those that process incoming neural patterns from the ear—and to suppose that information can be correlated by these networks and passed through them in either direction.

In its original form, there was no commitment to any particular kind of ontogenetic history. In the seminal and widely used taxonomy of "distinctive features" of speech patterns, acoustic criteria mingle with production operations (Jakobson, Fant, and Halle, 1952). There has been some tendency to adduce primacy for mechanisms of sound production in view of our tendency to make use of gestures of tongue and palate that exhibit a degree of acoustic stability, with little variation in the sounds produced with errors of placement (Stevens, 1972; Lieberman, 1977). In other accounts, the metaphor is used of an internalized dynamic representation of the vocal tract and its operation, terms immediately reminiscent of the "schemata" used by psychologists to conceptualize other kinds of internalized perceptual phenomena (Bartlett, 1932; Oldfield and Zangwill, 1942–1943).

With the discovery that pre-speech infants are responsive to some of the same distinctions between phonemes that adults make (Eimas, Siqueland, Jusczyk, and Vigorito, 1971), it now seems reasonable to think of auditory rather than motor predispositions as taking the initiative in the development of the very complex task of analyzing speech sounds. According to this line of interpretation, perceptions of speech would first be elaborated in infancy. Then, speaking would begin, guided by memories of what has been learned, much as has been postulated in the learning of birdsong. There will follow a period of overlap between the ability to learn new speech perceptions and new productions, as mature speech behavior emerges.

A common mechanism is postulated, developing during infancy through the conjoint operations of speaking and listening to speech, which then takes part in the control of both kinds of operation in the mature organism. Processes of encoding and decoding would thus employ some of the same brain mechanisms, an illustration of the kind of economy we may expect to be widespread.

Sensory Templates and Schemata

Using examples from auditory communication, we have developed a case for overlap or even correspondence between the biologist's *sensory template* and the psychologist's *schema*. At least partly because we are conscious of the operation of our own external auditory feedback channel, the argument seems intuitively plausible in this case. Even with audition, however, it is likely that the bulk of sensorimotor matching occurs unconsciously. It is worth remembering that the neurologist Henry Head emphasized the frequency of unconscious processing in his original conception of brain "schemata" for bodily movements (Oldfield and Zangwill, 1942–1943; Mason, this volume).

Adult humans and chimpanzees, for example, are remarkably clever at imitating what they see others doing (e.g., Hayes and Hayes, 1952). This imitation extends to facial expressions. Recent studies have shown that 2-week-old human infants can imitate both facial and manual gestures, a result that implies a remarkable ability on the baby's part. It must first perceive the configuration of the stimulus face and then generate a matching motor output. This could only be achieved by reference to some internalized representation of patterns of previous proprioceptive experience from his own unseen facial movements or by direct mapping onto an appropriate motor output (Meltzoff and Moore, 1977). At least, as adults, we are not conscious of either kind of operation. During ontogeny, such sensorimotor brain mechanisms as are nevertheless implied for the infant must surely become enormously elaborated and also enriched by developing visual experience and growing skill in operation of the visual signaling apparatus. Again, we postulate the likelihood that shared mechanisms are involved in both perception and production.

In several of the examples we have discussed, much of the adult communicative behavior of higher organisms is heavily influenced by learning. There is nevertheless repeated evidence of perceptual constraints emerging early in life. In some cases, these are known to be innate. We view these indications as most important in understanding how perceptual abilities develop. The importance of shared rules for encoding and decoding of signals is obvious if communication is to operate efficiently. To the extent that signaling behaviors are modified and elaborated through learning, it becomes more difficult to ensure that an adequate degree of rule sharing for production and perception will persist among all communicants, especially with signals as complex as speech or human facial expressions. However, with both processes performed by common mechanisms that develop with some close degree of genetic control, we can visualize how this might be accomplished.

Innate instructions to the young organism as to how to embark on the process of perceptual analysis would be valuable both in ensuring a choice of efficient procedures and in encouraging all species members to tackle the problem in the same basic fashion. It may be that some classical ethological illustrations of innate responsiveness are actually better interpreted as innate instructions for embarking on a certain trajectory of perceptual learning, rather than for designing animals as behavioral automata (Marler, 1978). To the extent that this strategy of innately guided perceptual development is successful, it will ensure a degree of rule sharing, while still allowing freedom for learned variability in both signal perception and production.

Signal Structure and Function

Although recent reviews have analyzed many aspects of animal signals and their contributions to patterns of social organization (e.g., Brown, 1975; Hailman, 1977; Sebeok, 1977; Smith, 1977), no comprehensive system is yet available for the study of animal semantics. More progress has been made in interrogating animals on questions of semantic meaning using human languagelike systems (e.g., Gardner and Gardner, 1971, 1975; Premack, 1971, 1976; Rumbaugh, 1976; Fouts and Rigby, 1977) than by studying communication in nature. Clearly new approaches are needed.

The Importance of Context and Past Experiences

We sometimes think of a signal receiver as though it were in a passive, neutral condition, waiting for external instruction as to what to do next. It is obvious, however, that in all but the simplest animals, a potential recipient already has a great deal of foreknowledge it can call upon in planning future action. A bird that has just passed through a section of woodland has gathered information about who else is there and what they are doing. Probability judgments have been possible about the likelihood of a neighboring rival's encroaching, or whether he is too preoccupied with newly hatched young. Memories of unduly anxious behavior by recently encountered neighbors may hint at the possibility that a hawk has changed its hunting beat and could soon pass over again. Awareness of the changing seasons may rekindle older memories of annual migrations of other species, preparing expectations of encounters with unaccustomed signals, some perhaps similar enough to its own to have been confusing in the past and thus the object of refined discriminative learning.

An exhaustive list of internalized contextual information would be enormous, requiring much deeper empathy with the perceptual world of animals than we now possess. Yet, it is clear that when an animal receives a signal, various kinds of information stored in memory can influence its assessment of what a given signal means (Wiley, 1976). The communication of animals, like that of people, must involve a great deal of guesswork. The more information from the past that can be brought to bear on a given situation, the better the chance of guessing correctly. For this reason, if no other, it would be surprising if animals were not constantly consulting their memories in deciding what signals mean (cf. Griffin, 1976).

It must often happen that an animal receives a faint sound, an odor, or a glimpse of a display, sufficient to ascertain receipt of a signal but not enough to determine its precise nature. Memories of past events often suffice, however, to form a reliable judgment as to the signal's probable nature and meaning—that a neighboring rival has chosen this moment to make its customary evening transit for water or has discovered the predator that has been sleeping for the past few days in a boundary tree. Above all, such an unidentified signal specifies a moment in time at which a receiver might well choose to pause in ongoing maintenance activities for attentive surveillance. By consulting past knowledge and present perceptions of the organization of natural events in familiar habitats, it is often possible to make a reasonable guess at the nature of the unknown signal and to plan accordingly. It is hard for the laboratory scientist to appreciate the extent of this kind of ordering, which prevails in both time and space in the natural flow of events. There is every reason to suppose that many animals can become aware of such patterns, but few serious attempts have yet been made to incorporate this possibility in the interpretation of communicative behavior.

Suppose that an animal receives an unidentified signal, which may or may not be repeated. What might be inferred from variations in the timing of delivery alone? Schleidt (1973, 1977) has drawn a useful distinction between phasic and tonic signals, many of the latter being invariant and thus excluded from consideration here. While some signals are given singly, or in relatively brief bursts at irregular intervals, others are given at a regular rate over periods of time. These two delivery patterns relate to phenomena with different time courses, and a receiver might draw some inferences about them even in the absence of any other input from the signaler. A phasic characteristic correlates with a rapid change in a signaler state, as might ensue upon perception of a discrete event. A tonic pattern of delivery is more likely to designate an ongoing, or only slowly changing, state of the signaler. Examples of the former might be discovery of a predator or food. The latter might include the onset of physiological readiness for mating or parental care, though only general temporal features would be specifiable without further information.

Depending on its own circumstances and its physiological condition, a receiver may respond either phasically or tonically to a tonic signal. A continuously reiterated male birdsong may elicit slow physiological changes culminating in the ovulation of a mated female, while also evoking the rapid, phasic response of fleeing by a casually intruding male neighbor.

A different issue is raised by a receiver's past experience with the rate of signal reception in general. The significance of perceiving a single unidentified signal would be very different to an animal living in a group, surrounded night and day by a host of signaling companions, than to a solitary one with rare social contacts. In the latter case, the "stimulus contrast" would be high (Andrew, 1964), and the likelihood and nature of reactions would differ accordingly. The receiver accustomed to common signal reception is less likely to investigate an unidentified signal further than one for whom reception is rare.

Thus, even if a receiver has failed to identify an unknown signal, it can gain a great deal by interpreting the location, circumstances, and timing of the event in light of prior experiences of the probabilities of contextual events. Such information is equally relevant to a recipient's assessment of the meaning of accurately identified and highly differentiated signals. Thus, we fully concur with the emphasis placed by Smith (1965, 1968, 1977) upon the importance of context in understanding the meanings of animal signals.

IDENTIFYING SIGNALER SPECIES

What kind of assessment can a receiver derive when, irrespective of other aspects of signal meaning, the species of a signaler becomes known? Most ethological research on species recognition focuses on discrimination between the receiver's own species and others. Typically, little attention is given to the value of discrimination among "others." Cross-species identification can nevertheless make a valuable contribution to the context in which a species' own signals are assessed.

As migrating birds strive to locate appropriate summering or wintering habitats, a history of experience with the resident fauna in these habitats contributes to selection of opportune geographical locations for settling. On a more local scale, movements and foraging patterns of some species are closely correlated with those of others. Fish (Barlow, 1974a,b; Itzkowitz, 1977), monkeys (Gautier and Gautier-Hion, 1969; Struhsaker and Gartlan, 1972; Marler, 1973; Gautier-Hion and Gautier, 1974), and birds, especially in the tropical rain forest, habitually form mixed-species groups (Moynihan, 1962; Morse, 1970; Wiley, 1971; Buskirk, Powell, Wittenberger, Buskirk, and Powell, 1972). The gain from identifying another species can be substantial and immediate, such as locating a newly fruiting tree or a swarm of army ants which disturbs thousands of otherwise cryptic insects in the vanguard of its columns (Willis, 1966). There are equivalent illustrations of cross-species recognition in food location in temperate woodland birds (Krebs, 1973), predator communities on the African savanna (Kruuk, 1972; Schaller, 1972), and territorial defense in the coral reef (Myrberg and Thresher, 1974), all contributing to the contextual background for intraspecific communication.

Cross-species signal recognition can be equally important in the assessment of potential hazards, alarm calls being an obvious case, undoubtedly helping to sharpen assessments of the meaning of conspecific alarm signals. Interspecies dominance relations among food competitors is a significant source of selection pressure in some communities (e.g., Morse, 1970), and is probably sufficient to encourage the discrimination of other species' signals. An animal with food might well decide to behave cryptically upon detecting signals of another belonging to a dominant and competing species, again with implications for intraspecific signaling as well. It seems safe to assume that animals living in complex communities and with appropriate perceptual abilities rarely classify signals of other species into a single category. Rather, they tend to develop abilities to discriminate among them insofar as they constitute a sensitive and dynamic component in the contextual background for conspecific signal assessments.

There can be no doubt, however, that the discrimination of own from other species is the most critical of all. The functions served are legion. Some are relatively simple, as in aiding the location of suitable microhabitats for reproduction or overwintering or the choice of migration routes. Selection of a habitat by some lizard species is favored if they see other species members there, made more conspicuous by their frequent visual signaling (Kiester and Slatkin, 1974). A similar function has been suggested for male song in crickets (Ulagaraj and Walker, 1973) and for bird sounds (Falls, 1978).

SIGNAL SPECIES-SPECIFICITY

How are conspecific signals discriminated from others? Aspects other than signal structure sometimes play a critical role, as is illustrated by insect sex pheromones. While some species have pheromones with a unique molecular structure, others do not. Experiments show that sympatric moths may be equally responsive to one another's sex pheromones (e.g., Schneider, Kafka, Beroza, and Bierl, 1977). However, in nature there are different annual and circadian rhythms both of female sex pheromone production and of male responsiveness, resulting in a form of contextual species-specificity that does not rely on chemical individuality (Roelofs and Cardé, 1974; Shorey, 1976). In some beetles with the potential of cross-species chemical attraction, odors from other sources, such as the different trees on which they live, provide a species-specific context or act synergistically with pheromones that are inactive without them (Borden, 1974; Lanier and Burkholder, 1974).

Given the noisiness of most natural environments, the multitude of animal signals broadcast into them, and the frequent advantages of providing receivers with clear, unequivocal evidence of species identity, there is often strong selection pressure for signal distinctiveness within given animal communities. Species-specificity of signal structure can be achieved in many ways. In pheromones, as Wilson (1968) indicated, "organic odorants provide an immense array of potential signals. With an increase in molecular weight in any given homologous series, molecular diversity increases exponentially." Verifiable predictions have been made of the range of molecular weights that insect pheromones should have, with strong selection pressure for species-specificity (Wilson and Bossert, 1963). Signal specificity is sometimes matched by receptor specificity, so that pheromone receptors are highly tuned to respond only to the sex pheromone of the species and a few closely related compounds (e.g., Schneider, 1962, 1970).

The temporal patterning of damselfish chirps conveys precise information used in species recognition as well as for more subtle social functions (Myrberg *et al.*, 1978). In electric fish communities, both species-specific waveforms and the rates of repetition of electrical discharges differ distinctively among species members. The fish themselves prove to be clearly responsive to these features (Hopkins, 1974), and there is evidence that entire electroreceptor systems are attuned to waveforms of conspecific signals (Hopkins, 1974, 1976; Hopkins and Heiligenberg, 1978).

Species-specificity often accrues in a signal repertoire as a consequence of morphological adaptations that are primarily ecological rather than social in nature. When a number of similar species from a single taxonomic family are sympatric, they often form a series of distinct size classes, each with different niche specifications. In general, the pitch of acoustic signals bears an inverse relationship to the size of the sound-producing apparatus. Thus, the frequency contrasts that exist among sounds of species of frogs, birds, or primates that live together may be in a large part attributable to their ecological differentiation which results in species size differences (Blair, 1956, 1958; McAlister, 1959, 1961; Schneider, 1967, 1974, 1977; Martin, 1972a,b; Lorcher and Schneider, 1973; Bergmann, 1976; Eisenberg, 1976), although in some cases we also find divergent properties of structures involved in phonation, such as extralaryngeal vocal sacs and special neuromuscular control mechanisms (e.g., Negus, 1949; Gautier, 1971; Gautier and Gautier-Hion, 1977).

In crickets and grasshoppers, the sound spectrum of calling songs seems less dependent on body size or wing loading than on the way in which the file and scraper are employed (Dumortier, 1963; Morris, 1970)—that is, on patterns of neuromuscular activity, with or without afferent feedback interaction (e.g., Elsner and Hirth , 1978; review in Huber, 1975). While many orthopteran songs are relatively simple pulse trains, some require elaborate central motor programs for their production (e.g., Otte, 1972). In Uhler's katydid, with the most complex orthopteran song yet described, there is nothing unusual about the structure of the file of this species, implying that the complexities must be centrally generated (Walker and Dew, 1972). In frogs, a species-specific temporal pattern can be as important as size-related spectral structure in species recognition (Capranica, 1965, 1966; Loftus-Hills and Littlejohn, 1971; Capranica, Frishkopf, and Nevo, 1973; Gerhardt, 1974b), and again, central nervous pattern generators are implicated (Schmidt, 1974).

In European warblers, a survey of song revealed that some other features than song pitch also correlated with body weight. The tempo tends to be slower in heavier species, and song syllables tend to be longer (Bergmann, 1976). Moreover, some birds have special resonant structures that affect the pitch of their song (Stresemann, 1928). In general, however, syringeal structure is highly conservative among close relatives (Ames, 1971; Warner, 1972), and species-specific bird-song features must often be attributed to variations in the temporal pattern of neuromuscular activation of the syringeal musculature and respiratory patterns (Nottebohm, 1975).

Many such properties prove significant in the discrimination of conspecific song from others. Pitch differences are often relevant, as in the spotted sandpiper (Heidemann and Oring, 1976), the golden-winged warbler (Ficken and Ficken, 1973), and in song discrimination by the sympatric goldcrest and firecrest (Becker, 1976). In the latter case, temporal features seem less important in species recognition, whereas in others such as the white-throated sparrow (Falls, 1969) and the brown thrasher (Boughey and Thompson, 1976), timing and sequential organization are more important than frequency. Descriptive analyses of song specificity often emphasize temporal differences (e.g., Guttinger, 1978). There is much redundancy, however, in the species-specific information contained in male bird-songs, and the most common finding is that several acoustic features play a role in species recognition (e.g., Tretzel, 1965; Bremond, 1968a,b, 1972, 1976; Thompson, 1969; Schubert, 1971; Emlen, 1972; Shiovitz, 1975).

While there is a tendency for species to rely especially on features that are most stable throughout all members (Emlen, 1971, 1972), this is not necessarily the case (e.g., Bonelli's warbler, Bremond, 1976). By far the most attention has been focused on species-specificity of male birdsong, where selection pressures relating to reproductive and ecological isolation must place an especially high premium on rapid, reliable recognition. There are already indications that issues of species-specificity in calls, rather than song, may be just as important, even more subtle, and ultimately of even greater interest (e.g., Thielcke, 1971, 1976; Stephanski and Falls, 1972a,b).

Species recognition can be viewed as a special case of the more general phenomenon of discrimination of a signal from noise (p. 80). It follows that variations in signal environment will affect the kind of adaptations that optimize specific discrimination. The occurrence of "character displacement" is circumstantial evidence of such effects. Signals of related species presumed to be subject to selection for specific distinctiveness sometimes show more divergence in zones of sympatry than where they are allopatric (e.g., Brown and Wilson, 1956; Blair, 1968; Little-john, 1971; reviews in Straughan, 1973, and Brown, 1975). There are opposite cases in which signals seem to converge in zones of sympatry. When this occurs with birdsong, it appears that cross-species competition is especially intense, with evidence of interspecific territoriality (Marler, 1960; Cody, 1969, 1974), so that song assumes a rather different function than usual.

It should be emphasized that extreme signal species-specificity is by no means a universal advantage. While the benefits are obvious with signals that play a pivotal role in reproductive and competitive isolation, such as sex pheromones, typical birdsongs, and the "loud calls" of adult male forest monkeys, the advantages are much reduced with other signal functions. Some signals are very similar across species and are effective interspecifically. This seems to be true of some alarm signals, whether pheromones, calls, or displays, and also of some aggressive signals (Marler, 1957, 1973; Wilson and Bossert, 1963; Struhsaker, 1970; Zann, 1975; Gautier and Gautier-Hion, 1977; Morton, 1977), although this is not a universal rule (e.g., S. M. Evans, 1972).

A receiver's assessment of a signal identified as from a member of its own species depends on context (Prushka and Maurus, 1976). The song of a territorial male bird such as a chaffinch is assessed differently by reproductive and nonreproductive female chaffinches, by settled male neighbors, and by males seeking space for a territory (Marler, 1956). Such differences in the assessment of the same signal perceived in different contexts may be radical. Consequences may be cooperative in one case and competitive in another.

Consider, for example, an adult reproductive male rhesus monkey, recently emigrated from his natal group. While solitary, he will be seeking another group into which he can gain entry for reproduction. As he searches, any call identified as from a rhesus macaque, irrespective of other connotations, will lead to approach, further investigation, and, if circumstances are propitious, attempts to become a group member. A few weeks later, that same signal experienced in a changed context would be assessed quite differently, as evidence of a competing group. Instead of advancing to solicit social acceptance, the same male, now a resident member of his group, may instead take part in an attack.

We are reminded that of all possible communicants, members of the same species offer by far the widest range of alternative assessments. While their signals are potential markers for social companionship, cooperation, and reproduction, they also signify the most potent and general class of competitors, with maximally overlapping needs and similar methods for satisfying them. Again, the major burden in assessing how to respond to conspecific signals in general must be carried by knowledge from other sources, both current and past. In this sense, meaning is again as much a function of context as of particular signal structure (cf. Prushka and Maurus, 1976).

This portion of our review emphasizes auditory signals, which have been the subject of a majority of signaling studies. Similar principles pertain to the visual domain, as exemplified by such systems as the flashing patterns of fireflies and other manifestations of visual communication in insects (Soucek and Carlson, 1975; Lloyd, 1966, 1977; Markl, 1974; Carlson and Copeland, 1978), the displays and colorations of lizards (e.g., Carpenter, 1962; Hunsaker, 1962; Kiester, 1977), and the displays, plumage patterns, and other morphological signaling characters in birds (Sibley, 1957; Hamilton and Barth, 1962; Moynihan, 1968; Brown, 1975; Smith, 1977). There is also an enormous literature on visual signals with a false species-specificity, mimicking other sympatric organisms and serving a wide variety of functions, with a multitude of complex and intricate adaptations brought into service (reviews in Cott, 1957; Wickler, 1968; Hailman, 1977).

Further Recognition of Signaler Identity

When a signal is perceived, there is a wide range of precision over which the signaler's identity may be ascertained. At one extreme is the basic discrimination between social signals and inanimate stimuli. At the other extreme is personal recognition of individual signalers. While individual recognition is virtually absent from insect societies apart from certain special exceptions such as bumblebees and *Polistes* wasps (Wilson, 1971b, 1975b), it is widespread among vertebrates.

Individual Recognition

Wilson (1971b) offers the generalization that

> the members of an insect colony employ signals that are for the most part uniform throughout the species. The one known exception is the colony odor, which is acquired at least in part from food and nesting material and is used to distinguish nest mates, all of them together, from members of other colonies. (p. 402)

Among vertebrates, however, individual signaler recognition probably extends through all sensory modalities, certainly olfaction, audition, and vision.

Olfaction mediates individual recognition in fish (e.g., Fricke, 1973) and is involved in species and group recognition as well, along with vision (Myrberg, in press). Canids can discriminate individually among group members by smell, probably on the basis of proportions of salient compounds in urine and glandular secretions (Mech, 1970). In the vocal domain, wolf howling is individually distinctive (Theberge and Falls, 1967). Some nonhuman primate sounds are known to be individually distinctive, such as the pant-hooting of chimpanzees (Marler and Hobbet, 1975). Yet, while it may be widespread, only in a few cases has individual recognition of calls been confirmed by experiment or playback of recordings (Waser, 1975a, 1976; Hansen, 1976; Pereira and Bauer, in press). Nowhere is the personal individuality of signals more evident than in vocalizations of birds, and playback studies have repeatedly demonstrated that individuals are indeed discriminated by voice (e.g., Brooks and Falls, 1975a,b; Falls and Brooks, 1975; Kroodsma, 1976; Wiley and Wiley, 1977; Falls, 1978). Similarly, with visual signals, at least for social birds, there is evidence of individual recognition, which seems to involve especially features of the face (Guhl and Ortman, 1953; Candland, 1969).

Young Canada geese can reliably select group members from birds of similar age but from strange groups (Radesäter, 1976). However, it is not clear in this case whether this is a class discrimination of familiar versus unfamiliar age-mates or whether each group member is recognized personally. Parallel problems of interpretation arise in other studies of individual recognition. In much bird research, behavior related to hierarchical status is used as a criterion for individual recognition. But it is not always clear whether the data exclude the possibility that the discrimination involves not multiple individuals but two classes, one higher in rank and one lower (Wiley and Hartnett, in press).

The problem is confounded by the involvement of some of the visual characters, known by experiment to play a role in individual recognition, in the actual establishment of dominance rank. For example, both Guhl and Ortman (1953) and Candland (1969) found that of all disguises, modification of the comb of hens and cocks caused the maximum disruption of dominance relations. There is evidence that relative comb size is a good predictor of future dominance relations as birds become acquainted (Collias, 1943; Guhl and Ortman, 1953; Marks, Siegel, and Kramer, 1960), no doubt because it tends to reflect androgen levels. As an equivalent illustration from a nondomesticated bird, comb size in the willow ptarmigan also correlates well with dominance rank (Gjesdal, 1977). The antler size of deer covaries with social dominance and may help to establish rank (Espmark, 1964). Similarly, behavioral signals that correlated with dominance rank, such as tail position in baboons (Hausfater, 1977), might play a role in identifying hierarchies, without the *necessity* of individual recognition. Thus, care is needed to demonstrate personal recognition of group members unequivocally, even though general observation repeatedly confirms that it is indeed widespread.

DISCRIMINATION OF A FAMILIAR FROM OTHERS

More robust evidence is available that signals from particular individuals may be discriminated from those of all others as a class, as in the relationships between mates or between parent and young (e.g., Mills and Melhuish, 1974; Petrinovich,

1974). Miller and Emlen (1975), for example, changed the appearance and modified the sound production of ring-billed gull chicks, thus showing that they are discriminated from other young by parents after about seven to nine days posthatching. Visual cues were the more important of the two. The adequacy of vocal signals when they alone are available has been demonstrated with a variety of seabirds (e.g., Tschanz, 1968; reviews in Beer 1970, 1975). Similarly, in the relationship between a mated monogamous pair, as in gannets, experiments reveal that the discrimination of mate versus nonmate vocalizations can often readily be made (White, 1971).

Many species appear to rely on chance or growth-related differences in morphology or behavior as a basis for such discriminations, although the unusually high variability of such signal features as aspects of the face and the plumage patterns of chicks has been noted (Marler, 1961; Buckley and Buckley, 1970, 1972). In other cases, signal learning is clearly involved. Thus, in goldfinches, twites, and other cardueline finches, details of the flight call are modified so that mated pairs are matched. Playback demonstrates that they do indeed respond more strongly to the mate's call than to the calls of others (Mundinger, 1970; Marler and Mundinger, 1975). A more extreme case is provided by the elaborate, highly coordinated, and pair-specific duets that mates of some bird species produce (Todt, 1970, 1975; Helversen and Wickler, 1971; Payne, 1971; Thorpe, 1972; Wickler, 1972a,b, 1973, 1976; Kunkel, 1974; Seibt and Wickler, 1977; Wiley and Wiley, 1977).

Such behavior sometimes incorporates neighbors in addition to the mated pair, though their kinship relations are not known. Certainly, in species with close-knit and durable family bonds, one can readily see how signal-learning processes could encompass all members. Call modification of finches can occur in such circumstances (Marler and Mundinger, 1971), serving, along with other signals, to foster discrimination between members of other groups and members of the family, whether immediate or extended.

STRANGENESS, FAMILIARITY AND KIN RECOGNITION

For social birds and mammals, especially colony dwellers and herding species, animals are reared in a close-knit group in which everyone probably knows everyone else. The discrimination of strangers' signals from those of the familiar group is likely to be a component in the recognition process by which kin may be distinguished from nonkin. It is surely more than coincidental that strange conspecific individuals provide the strongest stimuli for hostility in a variety of species (see Bernstein, 1964; Southwick, 1967; Southwick, Siddiqi, Farooqui, and Pal, 1974; Rosenblum, Levy, and Kaufman, 1968; Scruton and Herbert, 1972; Wade, 1976, for primate examples; Balph, 1977, for an avian example; review in Marler, 1976a). If we are to improve our understanding of the mechanisms of communication between animals, it is essential that we learn more about the distribution of familiarity in natural animal communities and about the rules governing its generation and decay. Not only is an understanding of this distribution basic to the analysis of how animals assess signals in their daily lives, but it is also important from a theoretical viewpoint.

With our growing appreciation of the theoretical importance of kinship relationships in understanding the evolution of social structure, it is important to learn more about how kin networks are distributed in nature and about what means, if any—whether spatial, morphological, or behavioral—are employed for discriminating close kin from others and with what accuracy. One possibility would be communication by cues that directly reflect genetic constitution, perhaps most likely to be chemical in nature. Demonstrations of mating preferences among mouse strains bred for divergent immunological traits may hint of such a possibility (Yamazaki, Boyse, Mike, Thaler, Mathieson, Abbot, Boyse, Zayas, and Thomas, 1976; Yamaguchi, Yamazaki, and Boyse, 1978). Another candidate is surely intimate communicative familiarity. There is no better way to appreciate the importance of this factor than to observe social reactions to complete strangers. As we have indicated, strangeness constitutes one of the most potent accentuators of aggression in many species. It has profound consequences for dispersing species members and groups (Waser and Wiley, this volume), acting as a powerful modifier of the effects of distance-increasing and -decreasing signals, as well as of those signals that maintain dispersal or proximity (Tinbergen, 1959; Marler, 1968, 1976a; Kummer, 1971). Xenophobia in man lends itself to the perpetration of a group structure in which spatial companions tend to remain together. These are likely to be kin in both man and many other species. Indeed most of the conditions we have listed as favoring intimacy of communication in a group tend to increase the likelihood that communicants will be more closely related than randomly selected individuals from a deme, a virtual precondition for the evolution of shared, compatible mechanisms for signal generation and perception.

Communicative familiarity thus becomes a fundamental issue. Much signaling may be designed to permit companions to expose themselves to each other in many different circumstances, with ample opportunity for each to know how the others smell and sound, as well as how they look and how they are likely to behave in a variety of situations. The dynamics of marginal acquaintanceship, of forgetting what companions are like and what they do, may prove fundamental in separating the in-group from the out.

We know of examples of animals' forgetting one another. Something like this must occur, for example, when a troop of primates divides, severing long-established bonds and gradually turning familiar companions into strangers (e.g., Angst, 1973). Species differences in social organization may derive in part from variations in the rates at which strangers can become familiar and differences in what they must do to achieve this familiarity. Equally important may be the rates at which previously familiar individuals become strangers, the divergence perhaps hastened by their failure to perform particular activities, such as mutual grooming or greeting behaviors, that might otherwise delay the schism (e.g., Barash, 1974a). The delicate balance between strangeness and familiarity may be the ultimate function of much highly redundant and time-consuming signal behavior (Marler, 1976a), perhaps also involved in within-group discrimination of immediate from more distant kin (e.g., Massey, 1977).

STEVEN GREEN AND
PETER MARLER

A more complex signal vehicle for discriminating kinship groupings from others is provided by learned dialects in some bird songs (Marler and Mundinger, 1971). Several attempts have been made to explain their functional significance by perhaps providing reproductive advantages for individuals bound in kin groups or regional demes. One possibility is that if the dialects serve as population markers and encourage birds to settle and mate with members of the birthplace population, they perhaps act to perpetuate local physiological adaptations or races (e.g., Marler and Tamura, 1962; Nottebohm, 1969, 1975, 1976; Nottebohm and Selander, 1972). Both male and female white-crowned sparrows are most sensitive to the dialect learned in youth. In addition, there is direct evidence that a dialect boundary blocks gene flow by diverting the settling patterns of the young of both sexes back into the natal dialect area (Marler, 1970; Milligan and Verner, 1971; Baker, 1974; Baker and Mewaldt, 1978).

Dialects may be a special case of a more general propensity for birds to vary their behavior according to the unfamiliarity of a stranger's song. Playback of recorded bird songs has revealed a widespread tendency for stranger's signals to evoke more intense attack and repulsion than the familiar songs of immediate neighbors (e.g., Falls, 1969; Kroodsma, 1976; Wiley, 1976). Given that young birds are prone to settle near their birthplace, repulsion of birds with strange songs may also encourage the formation of local kinship groupings. A significant amount of signaling behavior may in fact be directly or indirectly concerned with the genetic structuring of local populations, serving by one means or another to aid the discrimination of close kin from nonrelatives.

SEX AND AGE

Another significant contribution to social organization derives from signal features that permit a receiver to identify a signaler's sex and age class. Static properties of the organism are often involved, such as coloration or size of the body or external structures. The issue of sexual dimorphism in signals would merit independent treatment. There are many cases of signals that are present in the repertoire of one sex and absent from the other, as, for example, in bird vocalizations (Nottebohm, 1975). The extent of such discrepancies varies in relation to many considerations, one being the intensity of sexual selection (Selander, 1972). It is especially acute in polygamous species, which tend to exhibit the most extreme sexual differences in signal repertoires, as in grouse (Wiley, 1974).

Size differences may contribute to age-specific signal structure, as in anuran songs. In the bullfrog, sounds of intermediate pitch, such as are offered by subadult males, actually inhibit the responsiveness of fully adult males to them (Capranica, 1966). Gautier and Gautier-Hion (1977) have plotted the changes of pitch with age in *Cercopithecus* monkeys, proving a ready basis for determining the age of the signaler. More subtle are the increases in the song-repertoire size of canaries with age, described by Nottebohm and Nottebohm (1978). Age-related song features may recur in other songbirds, providing possible cues by which females can compare the ages of potential mates. Even more elaborate in this regard are the temporal castes of social insects (Wilson, 1976).

The Signal Address

Some signals point to an addressee, and some point to an external referent. We need to distinguish clearly between these two alternatives. Hailman (1977) has adopted Charles Pierce's term *index* and has used it for both functions, although he indicated that the original application was for signs that point out their referent objects. We propose that the term *indexical* be kept for signals that indicate referents and that the term *deictic* be used for signals that point out addressees.

Deictic Signals

The response given to a signal may vary, depending on whether a receiver perceives itself or someone else as the addressee. The possibilities of addressing vary with the sensory modality used. It is most direct and unambiguous with tactile and chemotactic signals (by touching the addressee) and with visual signals (looking toward or otherwise orienting to the addressee). As Hailman (1977) illustrated, there are abundant animal examples of deictic addressing in the orientation of threat or courtship displays by fish, birds, and mammals, often clarified by special structures and markings.

Students of human nonverbal communication have found multitudes of examples of the use of looking, either unilateral or mutual, in deictic specification of signal addressees. The mode and temporal patterning of looking also serves as a mediator for meanings of other signals, such as speech, for which it provides an important accompaniment (Kendon, 1967; von Cranach, 1971; Exline, 1971; Argyle and Cook, 1976; Duncan and Fiske, 1977). Primatologists are becoming aware of the importance of recording the directed gazes within groups of monkeys and apes in the process of establishing patterns of social interaction (Chance, 1967; Chance and Jolly, 1970). There can be little doubt that the study of social looking behavior would be revealing in other mammals and in birds.

In speech we use what may be defined as *nominal addressing* in the form of personal or group names. There is a sense in which the distinctive contributions that each pair member makes to duets in many birds and certain primates could be thought of as names, eliciting as they do a response from only one particular individual.

Selective Addressing

Independent of the existence of deictic and nominal signal components, there is another sense in which one may think of signals as being addressed. Many signals appear to select a particular subset from the audience as respondents. We call this *selective addressing*. Consider, for example, an impala giving an alarm snort on seeing a leopard, a male bird singing on its territory, and an infant monkey

STEVEN GREEN AND
PETER MARLER

screaming after being left unattended by its mother. Even though there need be no deictic component in any of these, the implicit or selected addressees can be inferred in each case from the potential range of responding animals, varying from broad to narrow.

The range of potential responders to the impala call is large, including not only its own neighbors and kin but all other herd members and other species, including baboons, as well (Washburn and DeVore, 1961). The birdsong is also broadcast, but it is addressed to a narrower audience—a mate and several rival males—and normally evokes responses only from these two classes of receivers. The infant monkey, although not necessarily directing or beaming its screams, is nevertheless calling its mother and will probably evoke no response from any other group member unless eventually a sibling or its mother's sister responds.

Thus, one may think of the range of selected addressees for even a broadcast signal as broad in some cases and narrow in others. For each signal, the size of the class of respondent animals is a different proportion of all animals receiving it. This interpretation can be extended further. A sexual signal might be thought of not so much as commanding sexual behavior in respondents as selecting or "addressing" respondents already predisposed to sexual interaction.

When a receiver perceives a signal originating some distance away, often the first detectable response is no more than a change in its orientation or spatial relationship to the signaler. Indeed, the dynamics of social spacing are important in building the distinctive attributes of societies (Kummer, 1974; McBride, 1978; Waser and Wiley, this volume). Both aggressive and alarm signals may elicit the withdrawal of a receiver. Signals that eventually elicit very different responses—attack or copulation—may first elicit an identical response, namely, signaler approach. Response patterns diverge later in the interaction, only after further signals have been received or more contextual information is available.

Approach to a signaler may be followed by many types of interaction. While it is implicit in much of our thinking that the eventual response selected in the signal receiver is specified by the same signal that elicited approach, we must remember that not all who receive a given signal approach in the first place. This is obvious in the case of the infant monkey screaming for its mother or an adult female soliciting for copulation. A female monkey who has recently given birth has a different set of response predispositions than an adult male engaged in consort-ship behavior.

One may think of an infant distress call and a female copulation signal as being, in this sense, directed to different selected addressees, rather than simply as triggering sexual or parental behavior. The specification of selected addressees might comprise a supraspecies grouping, an individual or group of conspecific animals, or a subgroup of a particular age, sex, rank, or kin class. It might also be made according to transitory physiological states, as when a food signal evokes responses from hungry animals but not from satiated ones. Finally, the specification might also be made indirectly by selectively addressing respondents finding themselves in a particular context, as when alarm calls elicit a response from animals out in the open but not from others deep in cover. We are reminded that the receiver's context is just as important as that of the signaler in determining whether and what kind of response a signal evokes (Prushka and Maurus, 1976).

A signaler can indicate an external referent to a receiver indirectly, by iconic or noniconic means, or directly, by indexing. We have surely underestimated the power of indexing in animals by orienting the gaze, the body, or external structures such as a pinna toward the referent (Hailman, 1977). Indexing becomes especially informative in combination with affective expressions of arousal. The point is best illustrated with a quotation from Norbert Wiener (1948):

> Suppose I find myself in the woods with an intelligent savage who cannot speak my language and whose language I cannot speak. Even without any code of sign language common to the two of us, I can learn a great deal from him. All I need to do is to be alert to those moments when he shows the signs of emotion or interest. I then cast my eyes around, perhaps paying special attention to the direction of his glance, and fix in my memory what I see or hear. It will not be long before I discover the things which seem important to him, not because he has communicated them to me by language, but because I myself have observed them. (p. 157)

Affect plus Indexing

As long as the receiver is aware of the context of a signal production, the cooperation of indexical and affective signal properties has an enormously rich communicative potential. In a discussion of the origins of language, Premack (1975) developed further this theme that it is easy to underestimate the communicative potential of a combination of indexical and affective signaling:

> Consider two main ways in which you could benefit from my knowledge of the conditions next door. I could return and tell you, "The apples next door are ripe." Alternatively, I could come back from next door, chipper and smiling. On still another occasion I could return and tell you, "A tiger is next door." Alternatively, I could return mute with fright, disclosing an ashen face and quaking limbs. The same dichotomy could be arranged on numerous occasions. I could say, "The peaches next door are ripe," or say nothing and manifest an intermediate amount of positive affect since I am only moderately fond of peaches. Likewise, I might report, "A snake is next door," or show an intermediate amount of negative affect since I am less shaken by snakes than by tigers.(p. 591)

Premack thus indicated the further increment in information about external referents that can accrue if a receiver not only perceives affective signal components but also identifies the signaler. Given foreknowledge of, for example, individual idiosyncrasies in feeding preferences or in fearfulness of different types of predator, a receiver may be able to guess at the nature of a particular signaler's external referent quite accurately, even without indexical signal elements. With these added, the precision is even greater. It seems probable that animals, like children (Goldin-Meadows and Feldman, 1977), do a great deal of communicating about external phenomena by this combination of relatively simple signal elements and a comprehensive knowledge of signaler predispositions based on intimate social familiarity.

Enemy Specifications

Data are difficult to gather, but there are promising leads. Careful study of the external referents of alarm signals, for example, is yielding new insights. Even with the alarm pheromones of ants, a high degree of enemy specification is sometimes achieved (Wilson, 1975a). The same is true of ground squirrels' alarm calls, although here there is also the possibility of supplementary information from the signaler's identity. There are striking sex- and age-class differences in the frequency with which different ground squirrels' alarm calls are uttered (Sherman, 1977). It would be most interesting to know whether the effective predator situations for alarm calling differ consistently between these classes and whether receivers can sex or age a caller and modulate their responses accordingly.

There is a potential for using signal indexing in enemy specification. Sherman (1977, p. 1251) described how alarm callers usually sit upright, often on prominent rocks, and look directly toward the advancing predator, thereby seemingly directing the attention of conspecifics toward it. He noted that "I could often locate the predator by following the gaze of several alerted animals, whether or not they were calling. I do not know whether ground squirrels also use this cue." He added, "In eleven instances a ground squirrel probably could not see an advancing predator because of the ground squirrel's position in a swale: on eight of the occasions (73%), the ground squirrel sat up and oriented itself in the same direction as a conspicuous, calling conspecific, thus towards the apparently unseen predator."

Melchior's (1971) study of Arctic ground squirrels adds a further component. Noting that an observer could follow the course of a ground predator through a squirrel population by orienting to the squirrel sounds, he added that if the predator moves directly toward a squirrel, the squirrel typically runs down its burrow, calling as it does so. The result is a series of fading chat calls that locate the predator's position more precisely, even if it is invisible to a human receiver. Whether the squirrels can also locate the position using this cue has to be determined.

Signal features that correlate with varying degrees of arousal elicited by the referent are important in locating an unseen predator by the calling of others. Leger and Owings (1978) studied alarm calls in California ground squirrels, which, like many squirrels, have two classes of alarm calls: "chatter-chats," especially for ground predators, and "whistles." The latter are given mainly for aerial predators, though occasionally in social chases. Leger and Owings went on to comment on whistles as follows:

> It is also possible that the multitude of dimensions along which these calls vary provide sufficient diversity to permit division of the signal spectrum into a graded subset referring to predators and a second lower alarm level graded subset referring to social interactions. Our anecdotal observations are compatible with this latter hypothesis.

For example, whistles elicited by social chases seem to have lower sound intensities than those evoked by flying raptors. Similarly, predators such as bobcats (*Lynx rufus*) and coyotes (*Canis latrans*) elicit highly frequency-modulated chatters with about seven notes, whereas one- or two-note noisy calls signal agonistic interactions (Leger and Owings, 1978). Equivalent data are reported for the round-tailed ground squirrel (Dunford, 1977).

There are, of course, many examples from animals of correlations between such measures of signal intensity as concentration, amplitude, rate, and morphology, and the intensity of stimulation that the signaler receives. However, the ground squirrel data hint at the possibility that, assuming receivers to be responsive to such signal properties, they may infer more from such signal variations than just an intensity judgment, given access to enough additional information in natural contexts.

Arousal, Emotion, and External Referents

While signals that are mainly a reflection of degrees of arousal can in some circumstances convey a great deal of information about external referents, there are obvious limits to what such a system can achieve. It would be advantageous if the signaler could add even a general indication of the class of referents being signaled about. Otherwise, a hungry youngster, for example, might approach a referent indicated by its mother as worthy of positive arousal, only to discover that it denotes not a choice morsel but a desirable mate. If only on the basis of time and effort saved, we would expect natural selection to favor means by which a signaler could indicate whether the referent is environmental or social in nature. Environmental referents might include hazards, such as predators or bad weather, or resources, such as food, drink, or a safe resting place. Social referents might include a favored companion or an infant in need of care, both worthy of approach. An enraged male or a protective mother would be social referents to be avoided.

If we consult the literature on the complexities of human emotional states and their classification, it is clear that much more than a single arousal dimension is involved. There is some concurrence that four dimensions go a long way toward a comprehensive classification of the various human emotions. As an illustration, we present here a diagram from Plutchik (1970), with the major categories in the center and some equivalent ethological categories of ongoing behavior about which signals might be emitted in the outer ring (see Figure 14). It will be noted that two of these, C and D can be matched with classes of social referents and environmental referents, respectively. The other two may be viewed as an arousal dimension (A) and an approach–withdrawal dimension (B). Such a hypothetical system for human emotions can reasonably be generalized to animals, at least to birds and mammals. Looking at the patterns of behavior indicated in the outer ring, one could readily assign different signals, both visual and auditory, to each of them and reasonably infer that a receiver's assessment would include the external referents so indicated.

Such a hypothetical emotion-based signaling system would provide an economical explanation for much of the signaling behavior of animals, especially if one allows for some degree of mingling of emotional states and for variations in the intensity of each. Both Eisenberg (1976) and Green (1975a) have described socially complex primate signaling-systems that can be viewed in this light. A system of this type would suffice for receivers to assess that a signaler has perceived quite specific referents.

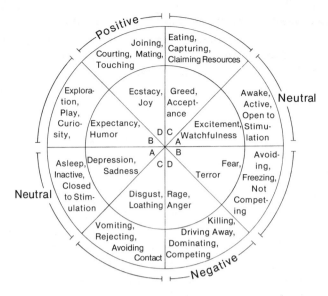

Fig. 14. Human emotional states (inner ring) with some equivalent ethological activities (outer ring) arranged according to whether their connotations are positive, negative, or neutral. A–A = a possible arousal-depression dimension. B–B = a locomotor approach–withdrawal dimension. C–C = an object acceptance–rejection dimension. D–D = a social engagement–disengagement dimension. Modified after Plutchik (1970).

FOOD SPECIFICATION

There are reliable descriptions of food calls in such birds as quail, jungle fowl, and other gallinaceous birds (Collias and Joos, 1953; Kruijt, 1964; Williams, Stokes, and Wallen, 1968; Stokes, 1971; Stokes and Williams, 1972; Anderson, 1978). The calls are used by males as a component of courtship feeding to attract females and by both sexes to attract young to food, often in conjunction with a visual "tidbitting" display. The melding of feeding and sexual behaviors perhaps illustrates the possibility of mixed emotional states already alluded to above and as is described in much of the ethological literature on display analysis (Tinbergen, 1940, 1952; Moynihan, 1955; Morris, 1956). Leaving on one side those species in which the behavior has become more ritualized and involves nonfood objects, such food calls clearly denote an external referent. Moreover, they are used not for just any edible item but for highly preferred foods, such as live insects (Williams *et al.*, 1968). That an intensity component is involved is indicated by the increased likelihood of quails' food-calling to nonpreferred food if they have been deprived (Williams *et al.*, 1968). Similarly, among primates, the rough grunting of the chimpanzee that this species uses as a food call (Marler, 1976c; Marler and Tenaza, 1977) attracting others to come and share is given only to highly preferred foods, such as palm fruits or bananas.

SYMBOLIC SIGNALING: ALARM CALLS

There are cases of more narrowly specified external referents, however, that seem to call for still further-refined internal representations. We have already commented on the recurrence of two types of alarm calls in ground squirrels, one for terrestrial predators and the other for aerial ones. Owings and Virginia (1978) found that the great majority of California ground squirrels' whistles were given to flying raptors, usually when they were less than 15 meters above the ground. In the few cases of whistling in a social chase, there were indications that the calls were softer, as already mentioned. In separate tests with dogs as predators, whistles were heard as the dog rushed to the squirrel, which retreated into a burrow, but the great majority of trials elicited the chatter-chat alarm call instead. Owings and Virginia noted a further intensity dimension in that the number of notes per chatter-chat call increased when a dog abruptly changed its speed or direction of movement, and calling rates were higher at the beginning of an encounter with a dog than at the end. Note-duration and the number of calls containing an ascending frequency-modulation component also decrease in the course of a bout. Although there appeared to be several referent-related intensity dimensions to these calls, it does not follow that the most significant aspect of whistle and chatter-chat calls is stimulus intensity, as opposed to stimulus quality.

Leger and Owings (1978), in fact, made a special point of emphasizing the specificity of the external referents for these two kinds of calls. Their description of the responses to the playback of the two calls notes that a basic qualitative difference is exhibited even though there is always a quantitative element as well. Both kinds evoke immediate running, but whereas whistles then typically evoke walking and any upright posturing is considerably delayed, the upright position follows chatter-chat immediately, facilitating search for a terrestrial predator. Adopting the upright posture immediately after perceiving a call that signifies a nearby raptor would be an invitation to attack, a significant point since predators are known to pursue and strike at squirrels giving alarm calls (Sherman, 1977). Thus, the squirrels behave as though the two alarm calls have qualitatively different meanings for them, even though a change in the number of separate components in a chatter-chat also modifies the intensity of receiver responses.

Many birds have two equivalent classes of alarm calls for the same two types of predator (e.g., Marler, 1955, 1957). Again, there are referential intensity components, as when a male chaffinch that typically gives a whistle call to a flying raptor also utters it to a person approaching his nest with young. Yet, intensity variations alone do not suffice to explain the very different responses to the two calls: flight to cover, stationary crouching, and upward visual scanning in response to whistles, and conspicuous approach and mobbing behavior, in the case of the "chink" alarm call, the functional equivalent of the ground squirrel's chatter-chat.

Struhsaker (1967) discovered a remarkable array of alarm calls in the vervet monkey (Table 1). Two have rather generalized external referents and seem to function primarily to alert others. One, the "chutter," is associated with either a man or a snake, especially the latter, possibly with a difference in structure for these two referents. The "threat-alarm-bark" is given on sighting a major predator, typically a carnivore. It evokes not approach and mobbing, as is the case with the chutter, but precipitant flight to cover and ascent into trees. The "chirp" call of females has similar external referents, and receivers respond similarly. Finally there is a sixth call, the "rraup," for which the most typical referent is the initial sighting of an eagle, generally in flight. Here, the response is almost the opposite

STEVEN GREEN AND
PETER MARLER

TABLE I. VERVET MONKEY ALARM CALLS[a]

	Uh!	Nyow!	Chutter	Rraup	Threat alarm-bark	Chirp
Typical stimulus	Minor mammal predator near	Sudden movement of minor predator	Man or venomous snake—but the chutter is structurally different for man and snake	Initial sighting of eagle	Initially and after sighting major predator (leopard, lion, serval, eagle)	After initial sighting of major predator (leopard, eagle)
Typical response of troop members	Become alert, look to predator	Look to predator, sometimes flee	Approach snake and escort at safe distance	Flee from tree-tops and open areas into thickets	Attention and then flight to appropriate cover	Flee from thickets and open areas to branches and canopy

[a]All calls are given by adults of both sexes, except the female "chirp." After Struhsaker (1967) and Cheney and Seyfarth (personal communication).

of that for the threat-alarm-bark and the chirp, namely, sudden dropping out of the treetops, as well as fleeing from open areas into thickets. Signal reactions are somewhat context-dependent, differing according to whether the receiver is in the treetops or out in the open. In each case, one can see the adaptiveness of the particular mode of response. Again, there are obvious intensity components, but variations in arousal level alone are inadequate to explain this remarkable array of signals and receiver responses.

The conclusion seems inescapable that these calls serve as labels or symbols for the different classes of external referent that they represent. This function is supplemented in many and perhaps all cases by varying degrees of arousal or affect that indicates to receivers the degree of priority they should give in assessing signal meaning.

ARTIFICIAL COMMUNICATION SYSTEMS

That there is a rich *capacity* for use of signaling behaviors as symbols for objects , attributes, operations, and even concepts is indicated by the performance of apes trained to use artificial communication systems based on human language and used between animals (Savage-Rumbaugh, Rumbaugh, and Boysen, 1978) as well as between animal and experimenter. Aware of the extent to which chimpanzees use their hands in natural communication, Gardner and Gardner (1971, 1975) used the hand sign language of the deaf, American Sign Language (Fouts and Rigby, 1977). With various training techniques, including shaping, guidance, and observational learning, as well as imitation, they were able to teach the young female chimpanzee Washoe to perform 85 signs, each equivalent to a word, in a three-year period. Included were many nouns, such as *flower, dog,* and *toothbrush,* adjectives such as *red* and *white,* prepositions such as *up* and *down,* and verbs such as *help, hug,* and *go.* Many words were used in appropriate combinations, such as the invitation for a walk, *You me go out hurry,* or the request *Please gimme sweet drink.* The appropriateness of combinations of actions and objects indicates a grammar not very different from that of young children in early two-word sentences (Brown, 1970; Gardner and Gardner, 1974). Another young chimpanzee, Lana, has demonstrated her prowess with a languagelike system based on keyboard signals to a computer, which talks back to her in a similar fashion (Rumbaugh, 1976).

The chimpanzee Sarah was trained by Premack (1971) to use colored plastic shapes instead of words, these shapes serving as symbols for objects and actions. A blue plastic triangle served as the symbol for *apple.* The one for *banana* was a red square, and so on. The relation between symbol and referent was noniconic, the shape lacking any physical resemblance to the object to which it referred. After Sarah was trained to present the appropriate shapes when she wanted a piece of fruit, other nouns and then verbs were introduced, such as *give, wash,* and *insert,* each performed by the experimenter when Sarah presented the appropriate symbol.

Within her repertoire of about 130 words were not only many nouns, verbs, and adjectives but also more complex constructions, such as *same,* and *different,* questions, and the conditional *if–then.* A particular word order was required of

Sarah in arranging the symbols on a board. Premack aimed more to test the conceptual abilities of Sarah than to see whether she could use language, reasoning that in our own species, the one is closely mirrored in the other.

Can one infer that Sarah thinks in the language of these plastic shapes? Premack says yes. One test, he feels, is the ability "to generate the meaning of words in the absence of their internal representation." Premack asked Sarah to perform a feature analysis of an apple, using the plastic words to name its color and shape, the presence or absence of a stalk, and so on. Asked to perform a similar analysis of the plastic word for apple, the blue triangle, she answered by describing an apple once more and not the blue shape. This test bears on a further point, Sarah's ability to consider something that is not there at the moment— implying internalization and illustrating the critical language requirement of displacement in time.

The importance of appreciating the natural motives of a subject in trying to understand its use of language is well illustrated by errors that Sarah made in the use of shapes for different fruits. Required to present the appropriate shape for a fruit before she was allowed to eat it, she chose the wrong word surprisingly often. In a moment of inspiration, Premack wondered whether Sarah was asking for what she preferred rather than for what was before her. An independent series of tests of her fruit preferences provided the explanation. The word for banana offered when confronted with an apple was not an error but an attempt to get the experimenter to give her something else, suggesting again that she truly understood the symbolic significance of the shapes.

The accomplishments of chimpanzees using languagelike systems of signaling to converse with an experimenter are surely the highest animal attainments demonstrated so far. Yet, they also raise a curious dilemma. If a chimpanzee can indeed achieve some elementary competence with language when provided with an appropriate vehicle, why is the evidence for symbolic usage in nature so limited? It may well be that the paucity of our knowledge of natural communication in animals is such that we can hardly judge whether such abilities are demonstrated in nature or not. However, it is also possible that in most social interactions, animals have little use for languagelike patterns of communication but that occasions do arise where those individuals and families possessing better cognitive capacities and signaling competence are more likely to survive, thus favoring the evolution of languagelike capabilities. The circumstances may be infrequent but the selection pressures strong.

From a biological viewpoint, symbolic communication is highly specialized, working most efficiently with particular kinds of problems. For many of the uses to which animals can put their signals—largely social in nature and taking place within groups in which members have become familiar with one another over a long history of acquaintanceship—other kinds of signal usage can probably do the job better.

SIGNALS AND INTERNAL REFERENTS

Our treatment of communication emphasizes the pivotal roles of internalization in both signal production and signal reception. Production depends on a prior assessment of the situation made by the signaler. The instigation of an assessment is often triggered by an encounter with an external referent in a given context. However, we have noted that there are variations in the uniqueness of connections between a signal and its input data. One major source of multiplicity of inputs to a given signal arises from contributions to the assessment by both external and internal referents.

Thus we use the word *food* both in response to food placed before us and in association with memories of food, as when we become hungry. A nestling bird gives begging calls spontaneously when it is hungry, although calling can also be triggered by the sudden appearance of food or of a food provider, or even of a stimulus that is an adventitious but regular accompaniment of the arrival of the provider, such as jogging of the nest.

Similarly, an ovulating female finch may break into the sexual solicitation display spontaneously or upon confrontation by her courting mate. The situation is somewhat different here, however, than in the case of a begging nestling. While the external referent for the latter is clearly food or something associated with it, the appropriate external referent for a copulation call is not so easy to identify. It seems inappropriate to name the male mate as the external referent and more pertinent to name as an internal referent for the call the current, transient internal state of the female, namely, her readiness to copulate.

At this point, the importance of internalized assessments again becomes evident. The assessment incorporates not only external referents but the entire context, both external and internal. Thus, for a female finch at the time of ovulation, the arrival of her courting mate has a similar signification to that of her own current physiological state, namely, that this is an appropriate moment for copulation and for the production of a signal that will ensure this response from her mate. Similarly, in the case of begging calls, despite their potential linkage to both internal and external referents, the underlying assessment for spontaneous begging and for begging triggered by food is similar, namely, that this is an appropriate moment for feeding solication.

INTERNAL AND EXTERNAL TRIGGERING

It should be the rule rather than the exception that many signals can be both externally and internally triggered, since the same fundamental assessment can often be precipitated by different trains of events. As functional alternatives, internal and external triggering are, of course, vitally important. While internal triggering is frequent in the case of food signaling, it is rare or even absent for alarm calling in most ordinary situations. Alternatively, in the case of a male birdsong with largely tonic communicative functions (Schleidt, 1973, 1977; Heiligenberg, 1977), triggering is primarily internal, although again external triggering is possible on, say, hearing the song of a neighbor.

Giving internalized assessments a central role makes it easier to incorporate the contribution of affective or emotional factors to signal production. Say that a male signaler is in the mood for reproductive behavior. This might arise because of some long-term physiological trend that reflects such changes in the physical environment as day length, or because of an endogenous reproductive trend (e.g., Gwinner, 1975), or because of a carryover from recent sexual encounters, or because of entry into an environmental situation in which sexual encounters have occurred in the past. These factors may all influence the assessment of, say, copulation calls from the female of a neighboring pair and may increase the likelihood that he will then invade their territory and direct aggressive signals at the neighboring male, perhaps then stealing a copulation from his mate. On another occasion, perhaps at a different season, when the male is preoccupied with feeding his own young, there might be no visible response to a female's copulation signals at all.

In no case can one ignore the role of internal factors in determining the nature of a signal-generating assessment. Indeed, this is true not only of signal production but of all stimulus–response situations. Even in the most reflexive behavioral mechanisms, internal factors play a major role in determining which sensations evoke responses and which properties of a response are stimulus-locked, rather than being internally programmed (Marler and Hamilton, 1966; Bullock, 1961).

Consider as another example a male black-and-white colobus monkey giving a threat display and roaring at an intruding group. The signals are clearly provoked by the intrusion, and members of a neighboring troop might be able to infer the presence of the invading group from the signals perceived. The assessment by members of the intruding group would include the fact of having been detected by the resident male. Although the referent is intrusion, the most significant aspect of the signaling male's assessment is that this is an occasion for expressing rage and, ultimately, physical assault. The linkage between signal form and underlying assessment makes it easier for us to understand the similarities, from the signaler's viewpoint, between these circumstances of colobus roaring and another situation in which it is given, namely, overflight by a monkey-preying eagle (Marler, 1972; Oates, 1977). There is no specific and unique external triggering that might be thought of as a referent for all roaring, but the signaler's underlying assessment might well be similar—that this is an occasion for a state of aroused hostility and alertness. Thus, members of a neighboring troop might not be able to distinguish on the basis of the roaring signal alone whether the referent is an eagle flying over or a colobus intrusion. The task would be made easier if males in other troops in the area began roaring, as often happens during eagle flights.

COMMUNICATIVE FAMILIARITY AND SOCIAL ORGANIZATION

Communication is both an instrument for organizing societies and a mirror for social organization. Just as processes of communication serve to establish and operate networks of social interaction among animals (Hinde, 1976; Hinde and Stevenson-Hinde, 1976), so the details of the social matrix within each society establish the contexts on which communication depends. When an animal makes an assessment of a signal with social import, it takes account of the current situation and of relevant past social experiences. The details of social networks vary from species to species and population to population. The chain of logical steps linking communication systems to diverse patterns of social organization is long and difficult to analyze, requiring a finer appreciation of social structure than we now possess. While no comprehensive analysis of relationships between semantics and social organization is yet feasible, one general principle is likely to pertain.

In certain circumstances, such as when communicants are completely familiar with one another and with the events precipitating signaling, prior experience makes a maximal contribution to the process of signal assessment. Such circumstances are especially likely to arise with long-term pair bonds and in species that are long-lived, with overlapping and cohabiting generations residing in assemblages of relatively stable membership. Another factor favoring complete familiarity is a social structure in which, at one time or another, members play a variety of social roles, such as dominant and subordinate, mother and daughter, young and adult. Adding further to familiarity are individual life histories in which animals pass through phases more than once in a lifetime—as with recurring reproductive cycles as opposed to a single period in a lifetime. Thus, lengthy, multipurpose, mixed assemblages are more predisposing to general communicative familiarity than those formed for a special behavioral function, such as a reproductive lek or a transient feeding group. The physical environment intrudes considerably into social organization, and intimacy with particulars of geography is another predisposing circumstance, as arises in philopatric species that are either permanently resident in an area or return to it repeatedly in the course of a life span.

There are, of course, many difficulties with such a prediction, such as defining the extent of "familiar groupings." It is obvious that a lion pride qualifies, but perhaps more solitary carnivores have a range of familiar acquaintances almost as wide, as Leyhausen (1975) has suggested for the domestic cat. The same may be true of other so-called solitary species (Eisenberg and McKay, 1974; Waser, 1975b). Both Brown (1964) and Barash (1974b) have shown in different ways that the range of acquaintanceship of solitary mammals and a pair-living bird extends into the neighboring community. In social circumstances that fulfill all of these conditions, many communicative interactions have been repeatedly rehearsed. As a result, participants are often able to anticipate the prospective features of evolving interactions. We may therefore expect to see effective communication achieved by experienced interactants with signals that are uncompleted and undramatized, including subtly changing points along graded signal continua. The social organization of most nonhuman primates satisfies these conditions remarkably well (Crook, 1970; Eisenberg, Muckenhirn, and Rudran, 1972; Struhsaker, 1975), and there is in fact evidence of very subtle acoustic discriminations used in their vocal communication (Gautier, 1974, 1978; Green, 1975a; Eisenberg, 1976; Gautier and Gautier-Hion, 1977). Other animals that might well qualify are wolves and lions, porpoises and whales, bats, elephants, some ungulates, and perhaps some birds such as the long-lived social species of corvids, larids, galliformes, anseriformes, and psittaciformes. In all of these, there is reason to suspect that within-group signaling is subtle and that contextual cues play a major role in determining how signal receivers respond.

NEW DIRECTIONS

While the framework we have suggested for viewing animal communication is, at best, a tentative formulation, it serves to reveal significant gaps in current knowledge. Filling these gaps will be important for developing alternative frameworks. Progress will depend in a fundamental way on advances in understanding the evolution of sociality and the physiology of behavior. In addition, we suggest that attention to the following topics may be profitable.

SIGNALING: SPECIFICATION OF CONDITIONS FOR SIGNAL PRODUCTION

There is an urgent need for progress in understanding the rules, and perhaps the mechanisms, by which a signaling animal forms an "assessment" of a situation. In addition to defining the range of external situations in which signals occur, it is equally important to specify the internal conditions for the production of different elements of a signal repertoire. Means are not currently at hand to investigate much of the physiology of signaling behavior. For example, to determine just one small but crucial component of an animal's internal state, we need techniques for rapid tracking of circulating levels of hormones.

As a more indirect route to specifying the internal state of a signaler, one can describe its prior history and immediate context. If field studies reveal developmental histories that differ consistently among individuals producing different signals in the same situations, the variables identified can be systematically manipulated in experimental studies. As demonstrated by studies of the ontogeny of birdsong, control of experiential factors can illuminate sources of individual variability. Experiments ranging in complexity from habituation studies to investigations of the internalization processes that underlie imprinting, for example, are appropriate but all too infrequent in animal communication research. We are just beginning to see serious attention paid to the effects on signaling of the presence of strange as opposed to familiar recipients. Closer attention to the effects of proximity of a signaler's close relatives on its signaling can only help in solving some of the puzzles emerging in the study of the evolution of communication behavior.

SIGNAL FORM: SELECTIVE PRESSURES AND DESCRIPTION

When a study suggests that the structure of a few signals, or even an entire species repertoire, can be best understood as the product of selection for such characteristics as localizability or maximizing transmission distance, it seems likely that there is often more to it than that. If hypotheses about signal form and function are to have predictive value, descriptions of signal morphology are required that are sufficiently precise to facilitate a comparative review of variation of the appropriate signal parameters and experimental manipulation of them. Perhaps one reason that questions about the adaptive features of signals are so frequently suggested but so rarely pursued is that signal patterns are difficult to define empirically and thus are elusive as a basis for theorizing.

The apparent simplicity of the process of physically describing a signal is deceptive. With some sensory modalities, such as taste or odor, molecular characterization is conceptually straightforward although technically difficult. With other kinds of signals, such as visual and auditory, questions of classification immediately thrust one into the complex arena of multivariate pattern analysis.

Signals can be described parametrically, by the use of many variables. The initial task facing a classifier is to reduce the number of items while retaining those that are biologically relevant to the species under study. Sometimes, an explicit statement of the grounds for selecting variables and strategies for subsequent signal classification is presented, but all too frequently it is lacking. Many investigators have understandably relied on the availability of instrumental methods to select the dimensions for analysis. Thus, temporal patterning, frequency modulation, and amplitude modulation of acoustic signals may be emphasized but phase rarely mentioned. By the time a scheme for classifying repertoires is presented, the rationale for categorizing some elements as together and others as apart is often obscure. The lack of uniformity among researchers, even when examining closely related species, can only hinder the advance of animal communication studies.

With these difficulties in mind, we offer a few suggested guidelines about information to include in signal descriptions. Often, the effort involved in establishing signal repertoire categories also generates the data needed for interpreting them. For example, an explicit discussion of the rationale behind the choice of the stimulus dimensions used would enhance the usefulness of many studies by serving as a basis for testing alternative descriptive schemes, as well as facilitating comparative work. If technically feasible, electing to describe and classify signals along variables known to be perceptually salient for a species is often illuminating. Sometimes, patterns of signal usage provide clues to the likely relevance and importance of variation in different dimensions. Similarly, if the choice of boundaries between signal categories and the criteria for gauging variability within categories can be related to what is known of the sensory psychophysiology of the species, the usefulness of the classification is increased.

The presentation of data can both encourage and impede their use for further comparisons. Scatter diagrams describing simultaneous variation in two dimensions reveal more about the animals' natural signal units than statistical digests of the same information given separately. In like fashion, a histogram of the incidence of signal elements arrayed against the parameters used to erect repertoire categories is more revealing than a listing of boundary demarcations and a simple judgment as to whether the repertoire is organized in discrete or graded fashion.

While it may seem pedantic to enumerate such basic concerns about the presentation of quantitative data, literature surveys have convinced us that a recitation that may be self-evident to most readers is not so to all. Trying to relate signal form to social, environmental, and phylogenetic determinants is difficult enough without the handicap of insufficient and unsuitable empirical evidence.

CORRELATIONS BETWEEN SIGNAL PERCEPTION AND PRODUCTION

One fundamental goal of studies of animal communication is to identify the distinguishing features of signals that receivers use to classify them into socially significant categories. A related objective is to characterize the relations between the structure of a signal repertoire and the nature of the perceptual processing brought to bear on it (e.g., Zoloth *et al.,* in press). It would be surprising if a species' signaling did not take advantage of the general sensitivity and acuity of its sensory capabilities. We must also consider the possibility of perceptual specializations, mutually adapted for the processing of communication signals. As epitomized in the concept of "innate release mechanisms," such specializations have long played a cardinal role in ethological theorizing about the mechanisms underlying social communication (Lorenz, 1970; Tinbergen, 1951). However, the interpretation of any degree of matching between signal and perceptual categories necessitates developmental studies as well (Marler, 1978).

The most extensive developmental studies, those examining birdsong, are concentrated on production aspects. Only recently has attention shifted to the effects of experience on perceptual performance (but see Peters, Searcy, and Marler, in press; Marler, 1978). Hybridization studies, chiefly on orthopterans and anurans, suggest a common genetic basis for production and perception. Much more work is needed on species that depend heavily on experiential factors (our own species included) if we are to determine whether a common neural substrate is involved (Liberman *et al.*, 1967). In addition to deprivation experiments, cross-fostering and hybridization studies are also needed, using avian genera that require auditory feedback for song development. The fact that in some bird species females can be hormonally induced to sing provides another avenue of approach to the relation between signal perception and production.

Progress in characterizing any commonality of rules dictating signal production and their perception is probably limited more by the paucity of perception studies than by any other factor. While there is a long and distinguished tradition of studies of sensation, relatively few of these have explored the areas critical to communication. Even with audition, the most extensively examined modality, we have little information on JNDs for the discrimination of complex acoustic signals and virtually none on changes in JNDs over the range of the acoustic signal parameters pertinent to the perceptual processing of a species' signals. Except for a few investigators now probing categorical perception in animals, the nature of multidimensional stimulus categories is unexplored (see Bullock, 1977, for reports of a recent conference on these issues).

Perception of socially significant signals in animals, if it parallels perception in man, involves more than simply sensory processing. Context-dependence and attention sets are involved, as well as other phenomena that call upon memory and collateral information. Is it meaningful to ask, for example, whether an animal detecting a stimulus can process it either as a communicative signal or not, depending on its character, as some think man can do, after deciding whether a sound is speech or nonspeech (Lane, 1965)?

A related area of inquiry, also rarely addressed, is the degree to which there are cross-modal perceptual interactions such as masking, facilitation, or more complex possibilities, yielding different percepts entirely for multimodal signals than expected on the basis of simple additivity.

RESPONSES: EFFECTS OF SIGNAL PERCEPTION ON BEHAVIOR

Looking at what an organism does after receiving a signal would seem the most straightforward route for studying communication. The approach has been put to fruitful use in many studies, attacking the issue of temporal or sequential correlations, as the principal way to establish putative cause-and-effect relationships.

In most descriptive studies, contingencies of acts in a behavioral sequence or social interaction are reported qualitatively; for example, "The male usually does cartwheels after the female nods her head and rolls over." Wiepkema's (1961) studies of bitterling reproductive behavior were influential in developing quantitative analyses of intraindividual sequences of actions. Stokes's (1962a) study of blue tits employed similar quantitative techniques but emphasized interindividual sequence pairs. The preceding action by one animal was considered part of a signal to the other, whose response was measured. By comparing the degree to which response frequencies were contingent upon the presence or absence of antecedent acts, a quantitative foundation for inferring effectiveness of communication was constructed. Dunham (1966) elaborated on these methods in studying grosbeaks. He also measured proportions of different response categories contingent upon preceding actions but then used different combinations of single elements as the initial action.

Altmann (1965) elaborated stochastic analysis further in rhesus monkeys by examining the preceding actions further antecedent than the immediately prior event and calculating the additional reductions in uncertainty obtained by taking these into consideration. Actions were classified as gross patterns of behavior, apparently occurring as "natural units" (Altmann, 1962).

With today's easy access to computation facilities far more sophisticated than those available when these pioneering studies were performed, it is surprising how little advancement there has been on this front. In spite of severe methodological constraints on combining data gathered on different individuals and different dyads for sequence and interaction analyses (Chatfield and Lemon, 1970), this approach should be used more often, with inferences presented in ways that are interpretable to readers who do not wish to wade through enormous transition matrices. The major weakness in many applications of stochastic methods appears to be the neglect of a temporal dimension. Often, sequential action pairs are scored identically regardless of the time interval between components.

Applying somewhat different analytic methods to hermit crabs, Hazlett and Bossert (1965) emphasized the difference between the the number of actions (responses) of each kind observed after each category of prior action (signal) and the number otherwise predicted. Expanding on these methods, Dingle (1969) compared such differences at different stages of interindividual agonistic bouts in mantis shrimp. By contrasting the figures from early, middle, and final periods of these encounters, he could determine how responses to signal-category actions are influenced by the contextual factor of elapsed time. Baylis (1976) also employed a transition matrix of preceding and following acts and used it to compare divergences between observed and expected value but added the novel twist of using the observed values of one species of cichlids to calculate the expected values for a different species against which the observed for this latter species were compared. He was thus able to perform interspecific analyses that provide a quantitative basis for judging similarities and differences in patterns of social communication.

The analyses mentioned above, comparing observed and expected numbers of responses, all concentrate on responses that occur much more often than expected (facilitated) and less frequently than expected (inhibited). Many responses, however, appear to follow particular signals about as frequently as one would predict in the absence of that signal. The preceding actions are therefore anomalous as signals when examined by these response-oriented techniques. The methods, however, do not purport to look at the possibility of signal effects other than those reflected in the very next actions of the respondent.

Nelson (1964) addressed this issue in a study of courtship in glandulocaudine fish by methods that deserve further application. Employing the comparison of observed and expected frequencies of responses, he also added the cumulative effect of prior actions by combining them into categories of preceding behavior in a fashion similar to Altmann's (1962) calculations of higher-order stochastic transitions. Nelson's analysis also examined the responses at intervals of varying duration after the signal actions. His study thus combines many of the best features of the other methods, permitting the sorting of signal actions according to the time for which they influence subsequent actions of a partner.

Rand and Rand (1976) extended the stochastic analysis methods by not only looking at transitions from signal patterns to subsequent behavior but also examining the joint effect of sequences of signal exchanges between individuals. Feedback of information on the nature of responses to the signaler, though little studied, must be important in many social species.

These latter two studies begin to address the issue of internalization of signal information by social interactions, only later manifest in behavior. Studies of sensitive periods, as in imprinting or song learning, illustrate other cases in which adult responses are influenced by information internalized early in life. Effects of signals on responses over interim periods that are neither very recent nor during a sensitive period early in life embody the majority of an animal's experience. Yet, studies that explore effects of communication on an animal's behavior beyond the immediate future are virtually unknown. This neglected area is undoubtedly procedurally difficult, but the rewards could be substantial.

With Smith (1977), we have tried to emphasize that responses to signals vary as a function of context. In the above studies, only encounter duration was explicitly considered as a contextual factor, although some of the antecedent signal categories, as defined, included contextual variables. The significance of context is rarely examined in its own right, although for some considerations it may be of fundamental importance. Knowledge of the dependence of responses on the genetic relatedness of signaler and respondent, for example, will surely generate new hypotheses about the evolution of social communication. Studying the variability of responses to the same signal in different stimulus contexts will help to refine our understanding of signal perception much as figure–ground contrast experiments in visual perception led to a better understanding of the physiological mechanisms underlying vision (Ratliff, 1976). Similar methods can enable us to explore which signal dimensions become salient as a result of contrast with their long-term context, as in the classic examples of a hawk silhouette becoming salient to turkeys (Schleidt, 1961), and search images which are modified by the experience.

A special case of context-dependence in communication is the possibility of intermodal interactions of signals. Do signals received through different channels interact in semantic-like fashion or should we consider information in one modality a part of the context that influences responses to signals arriving in another modality?

Similarly, the effects of varying the temporal order of signal elements can be gauged best only by studies of conspecific responses. Are sequential signals combined syntactically, or are early ones incorporated by a respondent as contextual information that tempers responsiveness to later ones (Beer, 1976; Wiley, 1975)? Regardless of evidence gathered by studying signaling, only by directing attention to responses can such issues be resolved.

In all such research, we must guard against narrowing our attention too early. If an alien being were to study human speech as a nonparticipant observer, how impoverished our communication might seem if tiny details of phonology were ignored in favor of the major features of mood-conveying intonation. And how confused the observer might be by the change of responses to an utterance with the same phonemes but different intonations. Inability to participate fully in social interactions would be a serious obstacle, to be overcome only by learning about the social structure and the relationships and prior histories of individuals and by gaining an appreciation of the factors that lead to the stereotypy and variability of responses. Discovery of which features of signal variability are disregarded by respondents and in which circumstances would help a great deal. And at some stage, the experimental introduction of appropriate signals and signaler models would be essential to make a final choice between alternative hypotheses about the nature of communicative operations, the underlying physiological mechanisms, and the associated cognitive processes.

Acknowledgments

Our thanks to Dorothy Cheney, Donald R. Griffin, Arthur Myrburg, Keith Nelson, Robert Seyfarth, and R. Haven Wiley, whose constructive criticisms greatly improved earlier drafts. The formulations, interpretations, and conclusions are our own responsibility, however, for we have rejected some substantive suggestions.

REFERENCES

Adrian, E. D. *The Basis of Sensation.* Christophers (Publishers), London, 1928.
Altmann, S. A. A field study of the sociobiology of rhesus monkeys, *Macaca mulatta. Ann. N.Y. Acad. Sci.,* 1962, *102*, 338–435.
Altmann, S. A. Sociobiology of rhesus monkeys. II. Stochastics of social communication. *J. Theoret. Biol.,* 1965, *8*, 490–522.
Altmann, S. A. The structure of primate social communication. In S. A. Altmann (ed.), *Social Communication Among Primates.* University of Chicago Press, Chicago, 1967.
Ames, P. L. The morphology of the syrinx in passerine birds. *Peabody Mus. Nat. Hist. Bull.,* 1971, *37*, 1–194.
Anderson, W. L. Vocalizations of scaled quail. *Condor,* 1978, *80*, 49–63.
Andersson, M. Social behavior and communication in the great skua. *Behaviour,* 1976, *58*, 40–77.

Andrew, R. J. Vocalization in chicks, and the concept of "stimulus contrast." *Anim. Behav.,* 1964, *12*, 64–76.

Angst, W. Pilot experiments to test group tolerance to a stranger in wild *Macaca fascicularis. Amer. J. Phys. Anthropol.,* 1973, *38*, 625–630.

Argyle, M., and Cook, M. *Gaze and Mutual Gaze.* Cambridge University Press, Cambridge, England, 1976.

Baerends, G. P., Brouwer, R., and Waterbolk, H. T. Ethological analyses of *Lebistes reticulatus* (Peters). I. An analysis of the male courtship pattern. *Behaviour,* 1955, *8*, 249–334.

Baker, M. C. Genetic structure of two populations of white-crowned sparrows with different song dialects. *Condor,* 1974, *76*, 351–356.

Baker, M. C., and Mewaldt, L. R. Gene flow and song dialects in white-crowned sparrows, *Zonotrichia leucophrys nuttalli. Evolution,* 1978, *32*, 712–722.

Balph, M. H. Winter social behaviour of dark-eyed juncos: Communication, social organization and ecological implications. *Anim. Behav.,* 1977, *25*, 859–884.

Barash, D. P. The evolution of marmot societies: A general theory. *Science,* 1974a, *185*, 415–420.

Barash, D. P. Neighbor recognition in two "solitary" carnivores: The raccoon (*Procyon lotor*) and the red fox (*Vulpes fulva*). *Science,* 1974b, *185*, 794–796.

Barlow, G. W. Ethological units of behavior. In D. Ingle (ed.), *The Central Nervous System and Fish Behavior.* University of Chicago Press, Chicago, 1968.

Barlow, G. W. Contrasts in social behavior between Central American cichlid fishes and coral reef surgeon fishes. *Amer. Zool.,* 1974a, *14*, 9–34.

Barlow, G. W. Extraspecific imposition of social grouping among surgeon fishes (Acanthuridae, Pisces). *J. Zool. Lond.,* 1974b, *174*, 333–340.

Barlow, G. W. Modal action patterns. In T. A. Sebeok (ed.), *How Animals Communicate.* Indiana University Press, Bloomington, 1977.

Bartlett, F. C. *Remembering: A Study in Experimental and Social Psychology.* Cambridge University Press, London and New York, 1932.

Baylis, J. R. A quantitative study of long-term courtship. II. A comparative study of the dynamics of courtship in two New World cichlid fishes. *Behaviour,* 1976, *59*, 117–161.

Becker, P. H. Artkennzeichnende Gesangsmerkmale bei Winter- und Sommergoldhähnchen (*Regulus regulus, R. ignicapillus*). *Z. Tierpsychol.,* 1976, *42*, 411–437.

Beecher, M., Petersen, M., Zoloth, S., Moody, D., and Stebbins, W. Perception of conspecific vocalizations by Japanese macaques: Evidence for selective attention and neural lateralization. *Brain, Behavior and Evolution,* in press.

Beer, C. Individual recognition of voice in the social behavior of birds. In D. S. Lehrman, R. A. Hinde, and E. Shaw (eds.), *Advances in the Study of Behavior,* Vol. 3. Academic Press, New York, 1970.

Beer, C. G. Multiple functions and gull displays. In G. Baerends, C. Beer, and A. Manning (eds.), *Function and Evolution in Behaviour.* Clarendon Press, Oxford, 1975.

Beer, C. G. Some complexities in the communication behavior of gulls. In S. R. Harnad, H. D. Steklis, and J. Lancaster (eds.), *Origins and Evolution of Language and Speech.* New York Academy of Science, New York, 1976.

Bellugi, U., and Klima, E. S. Two faces of sign: Iconic and abstract. In S. R. Harnad, H. D. Steklis, and J. Lancaster (eds.), *Origins and Evolution of Language and Speech.* New York Academy of Science, New York, 1976.

Bentley, D. R., and Hoy, R. R. Genetic control of cricket song patterns. *Anim. Behav.,* 1972, *20*, 478–492.

Bergmann, H.-H. Konstitutionsbedingte Merkmale in Gesängen und Rufen europäischer Grasmücken (Gattung *Sylvia*). *Z. Tierpsychol.,* 1976, *42*, 315–329.

Bernstein, I. S. The integration of rhesus monkeys introduced to a group. *Folia Primatol.,* 1964, *2*, 50–63.

Bertrand, M. The behavioral repertoire of the stumptail macaque. *Biblio. Primatol.,* 1969, *11*, Karger, Basel.

Blair, W. F. Call difference as an isolating mechanism in south western toads. *Texas J. Sci.,* 1956, *8*(1), 87–106.

Blair, W. F. Mating call in the speciation of anuran amphibians. *Amer. Nat.,* 1958, *92*, 27–51.

Blair, W. F. Amphibians and reptiles. In T. A. Sebeok (ed.), *Animal Communication.* Indiana University Press, Bloomington, 1968.

Borden, J. H. Aggregation pheromones in the Scolytidae. In M. C. Birch (ed.), *Pheromones.* Elsevier, New York, 1974.

Boring, E. G. *Sensation and Perception in the History of Experimental Psychology.* Appleton-Century-Crofts, New York, 1942.

Bornstein, M. H., Kessen, W., and Weiskopf, S. Color vision and hue categorization in young human infants. *J. Exp. Psychol., Human Perception and Performance,* 1976, *2,* 115–129.

Bossert, W. H., and Wilson, E. O. The analysis of olfactory communication among animals. *J. Theoret. Biol.,* 1963, *5,* 443–469.

Boughey, M. J., and Thompson, N. S. Species specificity and individual variation in the songs of the brown thrasher *(Toxostoma rufum)* and catbird *(Dumetela carolinensis). Behaviour,* 1976, *57,* 64–90.

Bremond, J. C. Recherches sur la sémantique et les éléments vecteurs d'information dans les signaux acoustiques du Rouge-Gorge *(Erithacus rubecula). La Terre et Vie,* 1968a, *2,* 109–220.

Bremond, J. C. Valeur spécifique de la syntaxe dans le signal de défense territoriale du Troglodyte *(Troglodytes troglodytes). Behaviour,* 1968b, *30,* 66–75.

Bremond, J. C. Recherche sur les paramètres acoustiques assurant la reconnaissance spécifique dans les chants de *Phylloscopus sibilatrix, Phylloscopus bonelli* et d'un hybride. *Gerfaut,* 1972, *62,* 313–323.

Bremond, J. C. Specific recognition in the song of Bonelli's warbler *(Phylloscopus bonelli). Behaviour,* 1976, *58,* 99–116.

Brooks, R. J., and Falls, J. B. Individual recognition by song in white-throated sparrows. I. Discrimination of songs of neighbors and strangers. *Canad. J. Zool.,* 1975a, *53,* 879–888.

Brooks, R. J., and Falls, J. B. Individual recognition by song in white-throated sparrows. III. Song features used in individual recognition. *Canad. J. Zool.,* 1975b, *53,* 1749–1761.

Brown, C. H., Beecher, M. D., Moody, D. B., and Stebbins, W. C. Localization of primate calls by old world monkeys. *Science,* 1978, *201,* 753–754.

Brown, J. L. The integration of agonistic behavior in the Steller's jay *Cyanocitta stelleri* (Gmelin). *U. Cal. Publ. Zool.,* 1964, *60,* 223–328.

Brown, J. L. *The Evolution of Behavior.* W. W. Norton, New York, 1975.

Brown, R. The first sentences of child and chimpanzee. In R. Brown (ed.), *Psycholinguistics.* The Free Press, New York, 1970.

Brown, W. L., and Wilson, E. O. Character displacement. *Syst. Zool.,* 1956, *5,* 49–64.

Buckley, P. A., and Buckley, F. G. Color variation in the down and soft parts of royal tern chicks. *Auk,* 1970, *87,* 1–13.

Buckley, P. A., and Buckley, F. G. Individual egg and chick recognition by adult royal terns *(Sterna maxima maxima). Anim. Behav.,* 1972, *20,* 457–462.

Bullock, T. H. The origins of patterned nervous discharge. *Behaviour,* 1961, *17,* 48–59.

Bullock, T. H. (ed.). *Recognition of Complex Acoustic Signals.* Dahlem Konferenzen, Berlin, 1977.

Burtt, E. H., Jr. The coloration of wood warblers (Parulidae), Ph.D. thesis, University of Wisconsin, Madison, 1977.

Buskirk, W. H., Powell, G. V. N., Wittenberger, J. F., Buskirk, R. E., and Powell, T. U. Interspecific bird flocks in tropical highland Panama. *Auk,* 1972, *89,* 612–624.

Camhi, J. M. Locust wind receptors. *J. Exp. Biol.,* 1969, *50,* 335–348, 349–362, 363–373.

Candland, D. K. Discriminability of facial regions used by the domestic chicken in maintaining the social dominance order. *J. Comp. Physiol. Psychol.,* 1969, *69,* 281–285.

Capranica, R. R. The evoked vocal response of the bullfrog: A study of communication by sound. *M.I.T. Research Monog.,* 1965, *33.*

Capranica, R. R. Vocal response of the bullfrog to natural and synthetic mating calls. *J. Acoust. Soc. Am.,* 1966, *40,* 1131–1139.

Capranica, R. R. Morphology and physiology of the auditory system. In R. Llinas and W. Precht (eds.), *Frog Neurobiology.* Springer-Verlag, Berlin, 1976.

Capranica, R. R., Frishkopf, L., and Nevo, E. Encoding of geographic dialects in the auditory system of the cricket frog. *Science,* 1973, *182,* 1272–1275.

Carlson, A. D., and Copeland, J. Behavioral plasticity in the flash communication systems of fireflies. *Amer. Sci.,* 1978, *66,* 340–346.

Carpenter, C. C. A comparison of patterns of display of *Ursosaurus* and *Streptosaurus. Herpetologica,* 1962, *18,* 145–152.

Chance, M. R. A. An interpretation of some agonistic postures: The role of "cut-off" acts and postures. *Symp. Zool. Soc. Lond.,* 1962, *8,* 71–89.

Chance, M. R. A. Attention structure as the basis of primate rank orders. *Man,* 1967, *2,* 503–518.

Chance, M. R. A., and Jolly, C. J. *Social Groups of Monkeys, Apes and Men.* Dutton, New York, 1970.

Chatfield, C., and Lemon, R. E. Analyzing sequences of behavioral events. *J. Theoret. Biol.,* 1970, *29,* 427–445.

Cherry, C. *On Human Communication,* 2nd Ed. M.I.T. Press, Cambridge, Mass., 1966.

Cody, M. L. Convergent characteristics in sympatric populations: A possible relation to interspecific territoriality. *Condor,* 1969, *71,* 222–239.

Cody, M. L. *Competition and Structure of Bird Communities.* Princeton University Press, Princeton, N.J., 1974.

Cody, M. L., and Brown, J. H. Song asynchrony in neighboring bird species. *Nature,* 1969, *222,* 778–780.

Collias, N. E. Statistical analysis of factors which make for success in initial encounters between hens. *Amer. Nat.,* 1943, *77,* 519–538.

Collias, N. E. The development of social behavior in birds. *Auk,* 1952, *69,* 127–159.

Collias, N. E., and Joos, M. The spectrographic analysis of sound signals of the domestic fowl. *Behaviour,* 1953, *5,* 175–188.

Cooper, F. S., Delattre, P. C., Liberman, A. M., Borst, J., and Gerstman, L. F. Some experiments on the perception of synthetic speech sounds. *J. Acoust. Soc. Amer.,* 1952, *24,* 597–606.

Cott, H. B. *Adaptive Coloration in Animals.* Methuen, London, 1957.

Craik, K. J. W. *The Nature of Explanation.* Cambridge University Press, Cambridge, England, 1943.

Cranach, M. von. The role of orienting behavior in human interaction. In A. Esser (ed.), *Behavior and Environment.* Plenum Press, New York, 1971.

Crook, J. H. *Social Behavior in Birds and Mammals.* Academic Press, New York, 1970.

Cutting, J. E., and Rosner, B. Categories and boundaries in speech and music. *Perception and Psychophysics,* 1974, *16,* 564–570.

Dingle, H. A statistical and information analysis of aggressive communication in the mantis shrimp *Gonodactylus bredini* Manning. *Anim. Behav.,* 1969, *17,* 561–575.

Dooling, R., Mulligan, J., and Miller, J. Auditory sensitivity and song spectrum of the common canary *Serinus canarius. J. Acoust. Soc. Amer.,* 1971, *50,* 700–709.

Dumortier, B. Morphology of sound emission apparatus in Arthropoda. In R. G. Busnel (ed.), *Acoustic Behaviour of Animals.* Elsevier, Amsterdam, 1963.

Duncan, S., Jr., and Fiske, D. W. *Face to Face Interaction.* Lawrence Erlbaum, Hillsdale, N.J., 1977.

Dunford, C. Kin selection for ground squirrel alarm calls. *Amer. Nat.,* 1977, *111,* 782–785.

Dunham, D. W. Agonistic behavior in captive rose-breasted grosbeaks, *Pheucticus ludovicianus* (L.). *Behaviour,* 1966, *27,* 160–173.

Eibl-Eibesfeldt, I. Similarities and differences between cultures in expressive movements. In R. A. Hinde (ed.), *Non-verbal Communication.* Cambridge University Press, Cambridge, England, 1972.

Eimas, P. D. Speech perception in early infancy. In L. B. Cohen and P. Salapatek (eds.), *Infant Perception: From Sensation to Cognition,* Vol. 2. Academic Press, New York, 1975.

Eimas, P. D., Siqueland, E. R., Jusczyk, P., and Vigorito, J. Speech perception in infants. *Science,* 1971, *171,* 303–306.

Eimas, P. D., and Tartter, V. C. On the development of speech perception: Mechanisms and analogies. In H. W. Reese and L. P. Lipsitt (eds.), *Advances in Child Development and Behavior,* Vol. 13. Academic Press, New York, in press.

Eisenberg, J. F. The function and motivational basis of hystricomorph vocalizations. *Symp. Zool. Soc. Lond.,* 1974, *34,* 211–247.

Eisenberg, J. F. Communication mechanisms and social integration in the black spider monkey, *Ateles fusciceps robustus,* and related species. *Smithson. Contr. Zool.,* 1976, *213,* 1–108.

Eisenberg, J., and Kleiman, D. Olfactory communication in mammals. *Ann. Rev. Ecol. Syst.,* 1972, *3,* 1–32.

Eisenberg, J. F., and McKay, G. M. Comparison of ungulate adaptations in the New World and Old World tropical forests with special reference to Ceylon and the rainforests of Central America. In V. Geist and F. Walther (eds.), *The Behaviour of Ungulates and Its Relation to Management.* International Union for Conservation of Nature and Natural Resources, Morges, Switzerland, 1974.

Eisenberg, J. F., Muckenhirn, N. A., and Rudran, R. The relation between ecology and social structure in primates. *Science,* 1972, *176,* 863–874.

Ekman, P., and Friesen, W. V. Detecting deception from the body or face. *J. Personality and Social Psychol.,* 1974, *29,* 288–298.

Ekman, P., Friesen, W. V., and Ellsworth, P. *Emotion in the Human Face.* Pergamon Press, New York, 1972.

Elsner, N., and Hirth, C. Short- and long-term control of motor coordination in a stridulating grasshopper. *Naturwiss.,* 1978, *65,* 160.

Emlen, S. T. The role of song in individual recognition in the Indigo Bunting. *Z. Tierpsychol.,* 1971, *28,* 241–246.

Emlen, S. T. An experimental analysis of the parameters of bird song eliciting species recognition. *Behaviour,* 1972, *41,* 130–171.

Esch, H. Ueber die Schallerzeugung beim Werbetanz der Honigbiene. *Z. vergl. Physiol.,* 1961, *45,* 1–11.

Espmark, Y. Studies in dominance subordination relationships in a group of semi-domesticated reindeer (*Rangifer tarandus* L.). *Anim. Behav.*, 1964, *12*, 420–426.

Evans, R. M. Development of an auditory discrimination in domestic chicks (*Gallus gallus*). *Anim. Behav.*, 1972, *20*, 77–87.

Evans, R. M., and Mattson, M. E. Development of selective responses to individual maternal vocalizations in young *Gallus gallus*. *Can. J. Zool.*, 1972, *50*, 777–780.

Evans, S. M. Specific distinctiveness in the calls of cordon bleus (*Uraeginthus spp.*: Estrildidae). *Anim. Behav.*, 1972, *20*, 571–579.

Evarts, V., Bizzi, E., Burke, R. E., DeLong, M., and Thach, W. T. Jr., Central control of movement. *Neurosci. Res. Program Bull.*, 1971, *9*(1).

Exline, R. V. Visual interaction: The glances of power and preference. In J. K. Cole (ed.), *Nebraska Symposium on Motivation*, Vol. 19. University of Nebraska Press, Lincoln, 1971.

Falls, J. B. Function of territorial song in the white-throated sparrow. In R. A. Hinde (ed.), *Bird Vocalizations*. Cambridge University Press, Cambridge, 1969.

Falls, J. B. Bird song and territorial behavior. In L. Krames, P. Pliner, and T. Alloway (eds.), *Aggression, Dominance, and Individual Spacing*. Plenum Press, New York, 1978.

Falls, J. B., and Brooks, R. J. Individual recognition by song in white-throated sparrows. II. Effects of location. *Canad. J. Zool.*, 1975, *53*, 1412–1420.

Farkas, S. R., and Shorey, H. H. Mechanisms of orientation to a distant pheromone source. In M. C. Birch (ed.), *Pheromones*. Elsevier, New York, 1974.

Ficken, M. S., and Ficken, R. W. Effect of number, kind and order of song elements on playback responses of the golden-winged warbler. *Behaviour*, 1973, *46*, 114–128.

Ficken, R. W., Ficken, M. S., and Hartman, J. P. Temporal pattern shifts to avoid acoustic interference in singing birds. *Science*, 1974, *183*, 762–763.

Fouts, R. S., and Rigby, R. L. Man–chimpanzee communication. In T. A. Sebeok (ed.), *How Animals Communicate*. Indiana University Press, Bloomington, 1977.

Fricke, H. W. Individual partner recognition in fish—Field studies on *Amphiprion bicinctus. Naturwiss.*, 1973, *4*, 204–205.

Frisch, K. von. Über die Sprache der Bienen, ein tierpsychologische Untersuchungen. *Zool. Jahrb. Abt. Allg. Zool. Physiol. Tiere*, 1923, *40*, 1–186.

Frisch, K. von. *The Dance Language and Orientation of Bees*. Belknap Press, Harvard University Press, Cambridge, Mass., 1967.

Gardner, B. T., and Gardner, R. A. Two-way communication with an infant chimpanzee. In A. M. Schrier and F. Stollnitz (eds.), *Behavior of Nonhuman Primates* (Vol. 4).Academic Press, New York, 1971.

Gardner, B. T., and Gardner, R. A. Comparing the early utterances of child and chimpanzee. *Minn. Symp. on Child Psychol.*, 1974, *8*, 3–24.

Gardner, R. A., and Gardner, B. T. Early signs of language in child and chimpanzee. *Science*, 1975, *187*, 752–753.

Gautier, J.-P. Etude morphologique et fonctionelle des annexes extra-laryngées des cercopithecinae; Liaison avec les cris d'espacement. *Biologia Gabonica*, 1971, *7*,2, 229–267.

Gautier, J.-P. Field and laboratory studies of the vocalization of talapoin monkeys (*Miopithecus talapoin*). *Behaviour*, 1974, *51*, 209–273.

Gautier, J.-P. Répertoire sonore de *Cercopithecus cephus. Z. Tierpsychol.*, 1978, *46*, 113–169.

Gautier, J.-P., and Gautier-Hion, A. Les associations polyspécifiques chez les Cercopithecidae du Gabon. *La Terre et la Vie*, 1969, *2*, 164–201.

Gautier, J.-P., and Gautier-Hion, A. Communication in Old World Monkeys. In T. A. Sebeok (ed.), *How Animals Communicate*. Indiana University Press, Bloomington, 1977.

Gautier-Hion, A., and Gautier, J.-P. Les associations polyspécifiques de Cercopithèques du plateau de M'passa, Gabon. *Folia Primat.*, 1974, *22*, 134–177.

Geldard, F. A. Tactile communication. In T. A. Sebeok (ed.), *How Animals Communicate*. Indiana University Press, Bloomington, 1977.

Gerhardt, H. C. The significance of some spectral features in mating call recognition in the green treefrog (*Hyla cinerea*). *J. Exp. Biol.*, 1974a, *61*, 229–241.

Gerhardt, H. C. The vocalizations of some hybrid treefrogs: Acoustic and behavioral analyses. *Behaviour*, 1974b, *49*, 130–151.

Gerhardt, H. C. Sound pressure levels and radiation patterns of the vocalizations of some North American frogs and toads. *J. Comp. Physiol.*, 1975, *102*, 1–12.

Gerhardt, H. C. Significance of two frequency bands in long distance vocal communication in the green treefrog. *Nature*, 1976, *261*, 692–694.

Gerhardt, H. C. Temperature coupling in the vocal communication system of the gray tree frog, *Hyla versicolor*. *Science*, 1978, *199*, 992–994.

Gibson, E. J. *Principles of Perceptual Learning and Development*. Prentice-Hall, Englewood Cliffs, N.J., 1969.

Gibson, J. J. *The Senses Considered as Perceptual Systems*. Houghton Mifflin, Boston, 1966.

Gjesdal, A. External markers of social rank in willow ptarmigan. *Condor*, 1977, *79*, 279–281.

Goldin-Meadows, S., and Feldman, H. The development of language-like communication without a language model. *Science*, 1977, *197*, 401–403.

Gould, J. L. Communication of distance information by honey bees. *J. Comp. Physiol.*, 1975, *104*, 161–173.

Gould, J. L. The dance-language controversy. *Quart. Rev. Biol.*, 1976, *51*, 211–244.

Green, S. Communication by a graded vocal system in Japanese monkeys. In L. A. Rosenblum (ed.), *Primate Behavior*. Vol. 4. Academic Press, New York, 1975a.

Green, S. Dialects in Japanese monkeys, vocal learning and cultural transmission of locale-specific behavior. *Z. Tierpsychol.*, 1975b, *38*, 304–314.

Green, S. M. Comparative aspects of vocal signals including speech. Group report. In T. H. Bullock (ed.), *Recognition of Complex Acoustic Signals*. Dahlem Konferenzen, Berlin, 1977.

Greenewalt, C. H. *Bird Song: Acoustics and Physiology*. Smithsonian Institution, Washington, D.C., 1968.

Gregory, R. L. *Concepts and Mechanisms of Perception*. Scribner's, New York, 1974.

Griffin, D. R. *The Question of Animal Awareness*. Rockefeller University Press, New York, 1976.

Griffin, D. R. The sensory physiology of animal orientation. Harvey Lectures, Series, 1978, *71*, 133–172. Academic Press, New York.

Griffin, D. R. Prospects for a cognitive ethology. *Behavioral and Brain Sciences*, 1979, *1*.

Guhl, A. M., and Ortman, L. L. Visual patterns in the recognition of individuals among chickens. *Condor*, 1953, *15*, 287–298.

Guttinger, H. R. Verwandschafts bezeihungen und Gesangsaufbau bei Steiglitz (*Carduelis carduelis*) und Grunlings erwandten (*Chloris* spec.). *J. Ornithol.*, 1978, *119*, 172–190.

Guyomarc'h, J.-C. Les bases ontogénétiques de l'attractivité du gloussement maternel chez la poule domestique. *Rev. Comportement Anim.*, 1972, *6*, 79–94.

Guyomarc'h, J.-C. L'empreinte auditive prénatale chez le poussin domestique. *Rev. Comportement Anim.*, 1974a, *8*, 3–6.

Guyomarc'h, J.-C. Le rôle de l'expérience sur la sémantique du cri d'offrande alimentaire chez le poussin. *Rev. Comportement Anim.* 1974b, *9*, 219–236.

Gwinner, E. Circadian and circannual rhythms in birds. In D. S. Farner and J. A. King (eds.), *Avian Biology*, Vol. 5. Academic Press, New York, 1975.

Hailman, J. P. Ontogeny of an instinct. *Behaviour Suppl.*, 1967, *15*, 1–59.

Hailman, J. P. *Optical Signals: Animal Communication and Light*. Indiana University Press, Bloomington, 1977.

Haldane, J. B. S. Animal ritual and human language. *Diogenes*, 1953, *4*, 3–15.

Hamilton, T. H., and Barth, R. H. The biological significance of season change in male plumage appearance in some New World migratory bird species. *Am. Naturalist*, 1962, *96*, 129–144.

Hamilton, W. J., III. *Life's Color Code*. McGraw-Hill, New York, 1973.

Hansen, E. W. Selective responding by recently separated juvenile rhesus monkeys to the calls of their mothers. *Dev. Psychobiol.*, 1976, *9*, 83–88.

Hausfater, G. Tail carriage in baboons *(Papio cynocephalus)*: Relationship to dominance rank and age. *Folia Primatol.*, 1977, *27*, 41–59.

Hayes, K. J., and Hayes, C. Imitation in a home raised chimpanzee. *J. Comp. Physiol. Psychol.*, 1952, *45*, 450–459.

Hazlett, B. A., and Bossert, W. H. A statistical analysis of the aggressive communications systems of some hermit crabs. *Anim. Behav.*, 1965, *13*, 357–373.

Hebb, D. O. *The Organization of Behavior*. Wiley, New York, 1949.

Heidemann, M. K., and Oring, L. W. Functional analysis of spotted sandpiper (*Actitis macularia*) song. *Behaviour*, 1976, *56*, 181–193.

Heiligenberg, W. Releasing and motivating functions of stimulus patterns in animal behavior: The ends of a spectrum. *Ann. N.Y. Acad. Sci.*, 1977, *290*, 60–71.

Heiligenberg, W., Kramer, U., and Schulz, V. The angular orientation of the black eye-bar in *Haplochromis burtoni* (Cichlidae, Pisces) and its relevance to aggressivity. *Z. vergl. Physiol.*, 1972, *76*, 168–176.

Helversen, D. V., and Wickler, W. Über den Duettgesang des afrikanischen Drongo *Dicrurus adsimilis* Bechstein. *Z. Tierpsychol.*, 1971, *29*, 301–321.

Hinde, R. A. Interactions, relationships and social structure. *Man (N.S.)*, 1976, *11*, 1–17.

Hinde, R. A., and Stevenson-Hinde, J. Towards understanding relationships: Dynamic stability. In P. P. G. Bateson and R. A. Hinde (eds.), *Growing Points in Ethology*. Cambridge University Press, Cambridge, England, 1976.

Hingston, R. W. G. *The Meaning of Animal Colour and Adornment*. Edward Arnold, London, 1933.

Hölldobler, B. Zur Physiologie der Gast-Wirt-Beziehungen (Myrmecophilie) bei Ameisen. I. Das Gastverhältnis der *Atemeles-* und *Lomechusa*-Larven (Col. Staphylinidae) zu *Formica* (Hym. Formicidae). *Z. vergl. Physiol.*, 1967, *56*:1–21.

Hölldobler, B. Zur Physiologie der Gast-Wirt-Beziehungen (Myrmecophilie) bei Ameisen. II. Das Gastverhältnis des imaginalen *Atemeles pubicollis* Bris. (Col. Staphylinidae) zu *Myrmica* und *Formica* (Hym. Formicidae). *Z. vergl. Physiol.*, 1970, *66*, 215–250.

Hooff, J. A. R. A. M. van. Facial expressions in higher primates. *Symp. Zool. Soc. Lond.*, 1962, *8*, 97–125.

Hooff, J. A. R. A. M. van. The facial displays of the Catarrhine monkeys and apes. In D. Morris (ed.), *Primate Ethology*. Weidenfeld and Nicholson, London, 1967.

Hopkins, C. D. Lightning as background noise for communication among electric fish. *Nature*, 1973, *242*, 268–270.

Hopkins, C. D. Electric communication in fish. *Amer. Sci.*, 1974, *62*, 426–437.

Hopkins, C. D. Stimulus filtering and electroreception: Tuberous electroreceptors in three species of gymnotoid fish. *J. Comp. Physiol.*, 1976, *111*, 171–207.

Hopkins, C. D., and Heiligenberg, W. F. Evolutionary designs for electric signals and electroreceptors in gymnotoid fishes of Surinam. *Behav. Ecol. Sociobiol.*, 1978, *3*, 113–134.

Horridge, G. A. (ed.). *The Compound Eye and Vision of Insects*. Oxford University Press, Oxford, England, 1975.

Hoy, R. R. Genetic control of acoustic behavior in crickets. *Amer. Zool.*, 1974, *14*, 1067–1080.

Hoy, R. R., Hahn, J., and Paul, R. C. Hybrid cricket auditory behavior: Evidence for genetic coupling in animal communication. *Science*, 1977, *195*, 82–84.

Hoy, R. R., and Paul, R. C. Genetic control of song specificity in crickets. *Science*, 1973, *180*, 82–83.

Huber, F. Sensory and neuronal mechanisms underlying acoustic communication in orthopteran insects. In R. Galun, P. Hillman, I. Parnas, and R. Werman (eds.), *Sensory Physiology and Behavior*. Plenum Press, New York, 1975.

Hunsaker, D. Ethological isolating mechanisms in the *Sceloporus torquatus* group of lizards. *Evolution*, 1962, *16*, 62–74.

Itzkowitz, M. Social dynamics of mixed species groups of Jamaican reef fishes. *Behav. Ecol. Sociobiol.*, 1977, *2*, 361–384.

Izard, C. E. Patterns of emotions and emotion communication in "hostility" and aggression. In P. Pliner, L. Krames, and T. Alloway (eds.), *Advances in the Study of Communication and Affect*, Vol. 2. *Nonverbal Communication of Aggression*. Plenum Press, New York, 1975.

Jakobson, R., Fant, C. G. M., and Halle, M. *Preliminaries to Speech Analysis*. M.I.T. Press, Cambridge, Mass., 1952.

Jurgens, U., and Ploog, D. Zur Evolution der Stimme. *Arch. Psychiat. Nervenkr.*, 1976, *222*, 117–137.

Kendon, A. Some functions of gaze-direction in social interaction. *Acta Psychol.*, 1967, *26*, 22–63.

Kiester, A. R. Communication in amphibians and reptiles. In T. A. Sebeok (ed.), *How Animals Communicate*. Indiana University Press, Bloomington, 1977.

Kiester, A. R., and Slatkin, M. A strategy of movement and resource utilization. *Theoret. Pop. Biol.*, 1974, *6*, 1–20.

Kolers, P. A., and von Grunau, M. Visual construction of color is digital. *Science*, 1975, *187*, 757–759.

Konishi, M. The role of auditory feedback in the vocal behavior of the domestic fowl. *Z. Tierpsychol.*, 1963, *20*, 349–367.

Konishi, M. Effects of deafening on song development in two species of juncos. *Condor*, 1964, *66*, 85–102.

Konishi, M. The role of auditory feedback in the control of vocalization in the white-crowned sparrow. *Z. Tierpsychol.*, 1965, *22*, 770–783.

Konishi, M. Effects of deafening on song development in two species of juncos. *Condor*, 1966, *66*, 85–102.

Konishi, M. Comparative neurophysiological studies of hearing and vocalizations in songbirds. *Z. vergl. Physiol.*, 1970, *66*, 257–272.

Konishi, M. Locatable and nonlocatable acoustic signals for barn owls. *Amer. Nat.*, 1973, *107*, 775–785.

Konishi, M. Hearing and vocalization in songbirds. In I. J. Goodman and M. W. Schein (eds.), *Birds: Brain and Behavior*. Academic Press, New York, 1974.

Konishi, M. Spatial localization of sound. In T. H. Bullock (ed.), *Recognition of Complex Acoustic Signals*. Dahlem Konferenzen, Berlin, 1977.

Konishi, M. Auditory environment and vocal development in birds. In R. D. Walk and H. L. Pick (eds.), *Perception and Experience*. Plenum Press, New York, 1978.

Konishi, M., and Nottebohm, F. Experimental studies in the ontogeny of avian vocalizations. In R. A. Hinde (ed.), *Bird Vocalizations*. Cambridge University Press, London and New York, 1969.

Krebs, J. R. Social learning and the significance of mixed-species flocks of chickadees (*Parus* spp.). *Can. J. Zool.*, 1973, *51*, 1275–1288.

Kroodsma, D. E. The effect of large song repertoires on neighbor "recognition" in male song sparrows. *Condor,* 1976, *78*, 97–99.

Kroodsma, D. Aspects of learning in the ontogeny of bird song: Where, from whom, when, how many, which and how accurately? In M. Bekoff and G. Burghardt (eds.), *Development of Behavior*. Garland, New York, 1978.

Kruijt, J. P. Ontogeny of social behaviour in Burmese red jungle fowl *(Gallus gallus spadiceus)* Bonaterre. *Behav. Suppl.,* 1964, *12*.

Kruuk, H. *The Spotted Hyena. A Study of Predation and Social Behavior.* University of Chicago Press, Chicago, 1972.

Kuhl, P. A., and Miller, J. D. Speech perception by the chinchilla: Voiced-voiceless distinction in alveolar plosive consonants. *Science,* 1975, *190*, 69–72.

Kummer, H. Spacing mechanisms in social behavior. In J. Eisenberg and W. S. Dillon (eds.), *Man and Beast: Comparative Social Behavior*. Smithsonian Institution Press, Washington, D.C., 1971.

Kummer, H. Distribution of interindividual distances in patas monkeys and gelada baboons. *Folia Primatol.,* 1974, *21*, 153–160.

Kunkel, P. Mating systems of tropical birds: The effect of weakness or absence of external reproduction-timing factors, with special reference to prolonged pair bonds. *Z. Tierpsychol.,* 1974, *34*, 265–307.

Lamandella, J. T. The limbic system in human communication. *Studies in Neurolinguistics,* 1977, *3*, 157–222.

Lane, H. L. The motor theory of speech perception: A critical review. *Psychol. Rev.,* 1965, *72*, 275–309.

Lanier, G. N., and Burkholder, W. E. Pheromones in speciation of Coleoptera. In M. C. Birch (ed.), *Pheromones*. Elsevier, New York, 1974.

Latimer, W. A comparative study of the songs and alarm calls of some Parus species. *Z. Tierpsychol.,* 1977, *45*, 414–433.

Leger, D. W., and Owings, D. H. Responses to alarm calls by California ground squirrels: Effects of call structure and maternal status. *Behav. Ecol. Sociobiol.,* 1978, *3*, 177–186.

Leong, C. T. The quantitative effect of releasers on the attack readiness of the fish *Haplochromis burtoni* (Cichlidae, Pisces). *Z. vergl. Physiol.,* 1969, *65*, 29–50.

Leyhausen, P. *Verhaltensstudien an Katzen.* Paul Parey, Berlin, 1975.

Liberman, A. M., Cooper, F. S., Shankweiler, D., and Studdert-Kennedy, M. Perception of the speech code. *Psychol. Rev.,* 1967, *74*, 431–461.

Lieberman, P. *Intonation, Perception and Language.* M.I.T. Press, Cambridge, Mass., 1967.

Lieberman, P. *Speech Physiology and Acoustic Phonetics: An Introduction.* Macmillan, New York, 1977.

Lindauer, M. *Communication among Social Bees.* Harvard University Press, Cambridge, Mass., 1961.

Littlejohn, M. J. A reappraisal of mating call differentiation in *Hyla cadaverina* (=*Hyla californiae*) and *Hyla regilla*. *Evolution,* 1971, *25*, 98–112.

Lloyd, J. E. Studies on the flash communication system in Photinus fireflies. *Misc. Publ. Mus. Zool.,* 1966, University of Michigan No. 130, 1–95.

Lloyd, J. E. Bioluminescence and communication. In T. A. Sebeok (ed.), *How Animals Communicate*. Indiana University Press, Bloomington, 1977.

Loftus, Hills, J. J., and Littlejohn, M. J. Pulse repetition rate as the basis for mating call discrimination by two sympatric species of *Hyla. Copeia,* 1971, 154–156.

Lorcher, K., and Schneider, H. Vergleichende bio-akustiche Untersuchungen an der Kreuzkröte, *Bufo clamitans* (Laur.), und der Wechselkröte, *Bufo v. viridis* (Laur.). *Z. Tierpsychol.,* 1973, *32*, 506–521.

Lorenz, K. Vergleichende Bewegungstudien bei Anatiden. *J. Ornithol.,* 1941, *89*, 194–294.

Lorenz, K. *Studies in Animal Behavior,* Vol. 1. Harvard University Press, Cambridge, Mass., 1970.

MacKay, D. M. Formal analysis of communicative processes. In R. A. Hinde (ed.), *Non-verbal Communication*. Cambridge University Press, Cambridge, England, 1972.

MacKinnon, J. The behaviour and ecology of wild orang-utans (*Pongo pygmaeus*). *Anim. Behav.,* 1974, *22*, 3–74.

Markl, H. Insect behavior: Functions and mechanisms. In M. Rockstein (ed.), *The Physiology of Insecta*, Vol. 3. Academic Press, New York, 1974.

Marks, H. L., Siegel, P. B., and Kramer, C. Y. Effect of comb and wattle removal on the social organization of mixed flocks of chickens. *Anim. Behav.*, 1960, *8*, 192–196.

Marler, P. Characteristics of some animal calls. *Nature (London)*, 1955, *176*, 6–7.

Marler, P. The voice of the chaffinch and its function as a language. *Ibis*, 1956, *98*, 231–261.

Marler, P. Specific distinctiveness in the communication signals of birds. *Behaviour*, 1957, *11*, 13–39.

Marler P. Bird songs and mate selection. In W. E. Lanyon and W. N. Tavolga (eds.), *Animal Sounds and Communication. Amer. Inst. Biol. Sci. 7*, 1960.

Marler, P. The logical analysis of animal communication. *J. Theoret. Biol.*, 1961, *1*, 295–317.

Marler, P. Communication in monkeys and apes. In I. DeVore (ed.), *Primate Behavior*. Holt, Rinehart and Winston, New York, 1965.

Marler, P. Aggregation and dispersal: Two functions in primate communication. In P. Jay (ed.), *Primates: Studies in Adaptation and Variability*. Holt, Rinehart and Winston, New York, 1968.

Marler, P. A comparative approach to vocal learning: Song development in white-crowned sparrows. *J. J. Comp. Physiol. Psych.*, 1970, *71*, Suppl. 1–25.

Marler, P. Vocalizations of East African monkeys. II. Black and white colobus. *Behaviour*, 1972, *42*, 175–197.

Marler, P. A comparison of vocalizations of red-tailed monkeys and blue monkeys, *Cercopithecus ascanius* and *C. mitis*, in Uganda. *Z. Tierpsychol.*, 1973, *33*, 223–247.

Marler, P. On the origin of speech from animal sounds. In J. F. Kavanagh and J. E. Cutting (eds.), *The Role of Speech in Language*. M.I.T. Press, Cambridge, 1975.

Marler, P. On animal aggression: The roles of familiarity and strangeness. *Amer. Psychol.*, 1976a, *31*, 239–246.

Marler, P. Sensory templates in species-specific behavior. In J. Fentress (ed.), *Simpler Networks: An Approach to Patterned Behavior and Its Foundations*. Sinauer, New York, 1976b.

Marler, P. Social organization, communication and graded signals: The chimpanzee and the gorilla. In P. P. G. Bateson and R. A. Hinde (eds.), *Growing Points in Ethology*. Cambridge University Press, Cambridge, England, 1976c.

Marler, P. Development and learning of recognition systems. In T. H. Bullock (ed.), *Recognition of Complex Acoustic Signals*. Dahlem Konferenzen, Berlin, 1977a.

Marler, P. The evolution of communication. In T. A. Sebeok (ed.), *How Animals Communicate*. Indiana University Press, Bloomington, 1977b.

Marler, P. Perception and innate knowledge. In W. H. Heidcamp (ed.), *The Nature of Life*. University Park Press, Baltimore, 1978.

Marler, P., and Hamilton, W. J., III. *Mechanisms of Animal Behavior*. Wiley, New York, 1966.

Marler, P., and Hobbet, L. Individuality in a long-range vocalization of wild chimpanzees. *Z. Tierpsychol.*, 1975, *38*, 97–109.

Marler, P., Konishi, M., Lutjen, A., and Waser, M. S. Effects of continuous noise on avian hearing and vocal development. *Proc. Nat. Acad. Sci. (Washington)*, 1973, *70*, 1393–1396.

Marler, P., and Mundinger, P. Vocal learning in birds. In H. Moltz (ed.), *Ontogeny of Vertebrate Behavior*. Academic Press, New York, 1971.

Marler, P., and Mundinger, P. Vocalizations, social organization and breeding biology of the twite, *Acanthus flavirostris. Ibis*, 1975, *117*, 1–17.

Marler, P., and Peters, S. Selective vocal learning in a sparrow. *Science*, 1977, *198*, 519–521.

Marler, P., and Tamura, M. Song dialects in three populations of white-crowned sparrows. *Condor*, 1962, *64*, 368–377.

Marler, P., and Tamura, M. Culturally transmitted patterns of vocal behavior in sparrows. *Science*, 1964, *146*, 1483–1486.

Marler, P., and Tenaza, R. Signaling behavior of apes with special reference to vocalization. In T. A. Sebeok (ed.), *How Animals Communicate*. Indiana University Press, Bloomington, 1977.

Marler, P., and Waser, M. S. Role of auditory feedback in canary song development. *J. Comp. Physiol. Psychol.*, 1977, *91*, 8–16.

Marten, K., and Marler, P. Sound transmission and its significance for animal vocalization. I. Temperate habitats. *Behav. Ecol. Sociobiol.*, 1977, *2*, 271–290.

Marten, K., Quine, D., and Marler, P. Sound transmission and its significance for animal vocalization. II. Tropical forest habitats. *Behav. Ecol. Sociobiol.*, 1977, *2*, 291–302.

Martin, W. F. Evolution of vocalization in the toad genus *Bufo*. In W. F. Blair (ed.), *Evolution in the Genus Bufo*. University of Texas Press, Austin, 1972a.

Martin, W. F. Mechanics of sound production in toads of the genus *Bufo:* Passive elements. *J. Exp. Zool.,* 1972b, *176,* 273–294.

Massey, A. Agonistic aids and kinship in a group of pigtail macaques. *Behav. Ecol. Sociobiol.,* 1977, *2,* 31–40.

McAlister, W. H. The vocal structures and method of call production in the genus *Scaphiopus* Holbrook. *Texas J. Sci.,* 1959, *11,* 60–77.

McAlister, W. H. The mechanics of sound production in North American Bufo. *Copeia,* 1961, *1,* 86–95.

McBride, G. Society evolution. *Proc. Ecol. Soc. Aust.,* 1978, *1,* 1–13.

Mech, L. D. *The Wolf: The Ecology and Behavior of an Endangered Species.* Natural History Press, New York, 1970.

Melchior, H. R. Characteristics of Arctic ground squirrel alarm calls. *Oecologia,* 1971, *7,* 184–190.

Meltzoff, A., and Moore, M. K. Imitation of facial and manual gestures by human neonates. *Science,* 1977, *198,* 75–78.

Miller, D. E., and Emlen, J. T. Individual chick recognition and family integrity in the Ring-billed Gull. *Behaviour,* 1975, *52,* 124–144.

Miller, G. A. The magical number seven, plus or minus two: Some limits on our capacity for processing information. *Psychol. Rev.,* 1956, *63,* 81–97.

Milligan, M. M., and Verner, J. Inter-populational song dialect discrimination in the white-crowned sparrow. *Condor,* 1971, *73,* 208–213.

Mills, M., and Melhuish, E. Recognition of mother's voice in early infancy. *Nature,* 1974, *252,* 123–124.

Morris, D. The function and causation of courtship ceremonies. In *L'Instinct dans le comportement des animaux et de l'homme.* Fondation Singer-Polignac, Masson et Cie Editeurs, Paris, 1956.

Morris, G. K. Sound analysis of *Metrioptera sphagnorum* (Orthoptera: Tettigoniidae). *Canad. Entom.,* 1970, *102,* 363–368.

Morris, G. K., Kerr, G. E., and Gwynne, D. T. Calling song function in the bog katydid, *Metrioptera sphagnorum* (F. Walker) (Orthoptera, Tettigoniidae): Female phonotaxis to normal and altered song. *Z. Tierpsychol.,* 1975, *37,* 502–514.

Morse, D. H. Ecological aspects of some mixed-species foraging flocks of birds. *Ecol. Monog.,* 1970, *40,* 119–168.

Morton, E. S. Ecological sources of selection on avian sounds. *Amer. Nat.,* 1975, *109,* 17–34.

Morton, E. S. On the occurrence and significance of motivation/structural rules in some bird and mammal sounds. *Amer. Natur.,* 1977, *111,* 855–869.

Mountcastle, V. The world around us: Neural command functions for selective attention. *N.R.P. Bull. 14,* Suppl. April 1976.

Moynihan, M. Some aspects of reproductive behavior in the black-headed gull (*Larus ridibundus ridibundus* L.) and related species. *Behaviour Suppl,* 1955, *4,* 1–201.

Moynihan, M. The organization and probable evolution of some mixed-species flocks of neotropical birds. *Smithson. Misc. Collect.,* 1962, *143,* 1–140.

Moynihan, M. Some behavior patterns of platyrrhine monkeys. I. The night monkey (*Aotus trivirgatus*). *Smithson. Misc. Coll.,* 1964, *146,* 1–84.

Moynihan, M. Communication in *Callicebus. J. Zool. Lond.,* 1966, *150,* 77–127.

Moynihan, M. Social mimicry: Character convergence versus character displacement. *Evolution,* 1968, *22,* 315–331.

Moynihan, M. Control, suppression, decay, disappearance and replacement of displays. *J. Theoret. Biol.,* 1970, *29,* 85–112.

Moynihan, M. Conservatism of displays and comparable stereotyped patterns among cephalopods. In G. Baerends, C. Beer, and A. Manning (eds.), *Function and Evolution in Behavior.* Clarendon Press, Oxford, 1975.

Mundinger, P. C. Vocal imitation and individual recognition in finch calls. *Science,* 1970, *168,* 480–482.

Mykytowycz, R. Odor in the spacing of mammals. In M. C. Birch (ed.), *Pheromones.* Elsevier, New York, 1974.

Myrberg, A. A., Jr. Ocean noise and the behavior of marine animals: Relationships and implications. In J. L. Fletcher and R. G. Busnel (eds.), *Effects of Noise on Wildlife.* Academic Press, New York, 1978.

Myrberg, A. A. Sensory mediation of social recognition processes in fishes. In J. E. Bardach, J. J. Magnuson, R. C. May, and J. M. Reinhart (eds.), *Fish Behaviour and Its Use in the Capture and Culture of Fishes.* I.C.L.A.R.M., Manila, Phillipines, in press.

Myrberg, A. A., Espanier, E., and Há, S. J. Temporal patterning in acoustical communication. In E. S. Reese (ed.), *Contrasts in Behavior.* Wiley, New York, 1978.

Myrberg, A. A., Jr., and Thresher, R. E. Interspecific aggression and its relevance to the concept of territoriality in reef fishes. *Amer. Zool.*, 1974, *14*, 81–96.

Negus, V. E. *The Comparative Anatomy and Physiology of the Larynx.* Grune and Stratton, New York, 1949.

Nelson, K. The temporal patterning of courtship behaviour in the glandulocaudine fishes (ostariophysi, Characidae). *Behaviour*, 1964, *24*, 90–146.

Nelson, K. After effects of courtship in the male three-spined stickleback. *Z. vergl. Physiol.*, 1965, *50*, 569–597.

Nelson, K. Concept, word and sentence: Interrelations in acquisition and development. *Psych. Rev.*, 1974, *81*, 267–285.

Nocke, H. Physiological aspects of sound communication in crickets. (*Gryllus campestris* L.). *J. Comp. Physiol.*, 1972, *80*, 141–162.

Nottebohm, F. The song of the chingolo, *Zonotrichia capensis*, in Argentina: Description and evaluation of a system of dialects. *Condor*, 1969, *71*, 299–315.

Nottebohm, F. Vocal behavior in birds. In D. Farner (ed.), *Avian Biology*, Vol. 5. Academic Press, New York, 1975.

Nottebohm, F. Continental patterns of song variability in *Zonotrichia capensis*: Some possible ecological correlates. *Amer. Natur.*, 1976, *109*, 605–624.

Nottebohm, F., and Nottebohm, M. E. Relationship between song repertoire and age in the canary, *Serinus canarius. Z. Tierpsychol.*, 1978, *46*, 298–305.

Nottebohm, F., and Selander, R. K. Vocal dialects and gene frequencies in the chingolo sparrow (*Zonotrichia capensis*). Condor, 1972, *74*, 137–143.

Oates, J. F. The social life of a black-and-white colobus monkey, *Colobus guereza. Z. Tierpsychol.*, 1977, *45*, 1–60.

Oldfield, R. C., and Zangwill, O. L. Head's concept of the schema and its application in contemporary British psychology I–IV. *Br. J. Psychol.*, 1942–1943, *32*, 267–286; *33*, 58–64, 113–129, 143–147.

Orians, G. H., and Christman, G. M. A comparative study of the behavior of red-winged, tricolored, and yellow-headed blackbirds. *Univ. Calif. Publ. Zool.*, 1968, *84*, 1–81.

Otte, D. Simple versus elaborate behavior in grasshoppers. An analysis of communication in the genus *Syrbula. Behaviour*, 1972, *42*, 291–322.

Otte, D. Effects and functions in the evolution of signaling systems. *Ann. Rev. Ecol. Syst.*, 1974, *5*, 385–415.

Owings, D. H., and Virginia, R. A. Alarm calls of California ground squirrels. *Z. Tierpsychol.*, 1978, *46*, 58–70.

Pastore, R. E. Categorical perception: A critical re-evaluation. In S. K. Hirsh, D. H. Eldredge, I. J. Hirsch, and S. R. Silverman (eds.), *Hearing and Davis: Essays Honoring Hallowell Davis.* Washington University Press, St. Louis, 1976.

Paton, J. A., Capranica, R. R., Dragsten, P. R., and Webb, W. W. Physical basis for auditory frequency analysis in field crickets (Gryllidae). *J. Comp. Physiol.*, 1977, *119*, 221–240.

Payne, R. B. Duetting and chorus singing in African birds. *Ostrich Sup.*, 1971, *9*, 125–146.

Payne, R., and McVay, S. Songs of humpback whales. *Science*, 1971, *173*, 585–597.

Payne, T. L. Pheromone perception. In M. C. Birch (ed.), *Pheromones.* Elsevier, New York, 1974.

Pereira, M. E., and Bauer, H. R. Maternal recognition of individual juvenile offspring "coo" calls in Japanese macaques *(Macaca fuscata). Z. Tierpsychol.*, in press.

Peters, S., Searcy, W., and Marler, P. Species song discrimination in choice experiments with territorial male swamp and song sparrows. *Anim. Behav.*, in press.

Petrinovich, L. Individual recognition of pup vocalization by northern elephant seal mothers. *Z. Tierpsychol.*, 1974, *34*, 308–312.

Pisoni, D. B., and Tash, J. Reaction times to comparisons within and across categories. *Perception and Psychophysics*, 1974, *15*, 285–290.

Plutchik, R. Emotions, evolution and adaptive processes. In M. B. Arnold (ed.), *Feelings and Emotions.* Academic Press, New York, 1970.

Premack, D. On the assessment of language competence in a chimpanzee. In A. Schrier and F. Stollnitz (eds.), *Behavior of Nonhuman Primates* (Vol. 4). Academic Press, New York, 1971.

Premack, D. On the origins of language. In M. S. Gazzaniga and C. B. Blakemore (eds.), *Handbook of Psychobiology.* Academic Press, New York, 1975.

Premack, D. *Intelligence in Ape and Man.* Wiley, New York, 1976.

Prushka, H., and Maurus, M. The communicative function of some agonistic behavior patterns in squirrel monkeys: The relevance of social context. *Behav. Ecol. Sociobiol.*, 1976, *1*, 185–214.

Radesäter, T. Individual sibling recognition in juvenile Canada geese (*Branta canadensis*). Can. *J. Zool.*, 1976, *54*, 1069–1072.

Ramsay, A. Time, space and hierarchy in zoosemiotics. In T. A. Sebeok and A. Ramsay (eds.), *Approaches to Animal Communication*. Mouton, The Hague, 1969.

Rand, W. M., and Rand, A. S. Agonistic behavior in nesting iguanas: A stochastic analysis of dispute settlement dominated by the minimization of energy cost. *Z. Tierpsychol.*, 1976, *40*, 279–299.

Rasa, O. A. E. Territoriality and the establishment of dominance by means of visual cues in *Pomacentrus jenkinsi* (Pisces: Pomacentridae). *Z. Tierpsychol.*, 1969, *26*, 825–845.

Ratliff, F. On the psychophysiological bases of universal color terms. *Proc. Amer. Philosoph. Soc.*, 1976, *120*, 311–330.

Regnier, F. E., and Goodwin, M. On the chemical and environmental modulation of pheromone release from vertebrate scent marks. In D. Müller-Schwarze and M. M. Mozell (eds.), *Chemical Signals in Vertebrates*. Plenum Press, New York, 1977.

Richards, D. G., and Wiley, R. H. Reverberations and amplitude fluctuations in the propagation of sound in a forest: Implications for animal communication. *Am. Natur.*, in press.

Robinson, B. W. Limbic influences on human speech. *Ann. N.Y. Acad. Sci.*, 1975, *280*, 761–771.

Roelofs, W. L., and Cardé, R. T. Sex pheromones in the reproductive isolation of lepidopterous species. In M. C. Birch (ed.), *Pheromones*. Elsevier, New York, 1974.

Rosch, E. On the internal structure of perceptual and semantic categories. In T. E. Moore (ed.), *Cognitive Development and the Acquisition of Language*. Academic Press, New York, 1973.

Rosch, E. H. Universals and cultural specifics in human categorization. In R. Breslin, S. Bochner, and W. Lonner (eds.), *Cultural Perspectives on Learning*. Sage/Halsted, New York, 1975.

Rosch-Heider, E. "Focal" color areas and the development of color names. *Developmental Psych.*, 1971, *4*, 447–455.

Rosch-Heider, E. Universals in color naming and memory. *J. Exptl. Psych.*, 1972, *93*, 10–20.

Rosenblum, L. A., Levy, E. J., and Kaufman, I. C. Social behaviour of squirrel monkeys and the reaction to strangers. *Anim. Behav.*, 1968, *16*, 288–293.

Rosinski, R. R. *The Development of Visual Perception*. Goodyear, Santa Monica, California, 1977.

Roth, L. M. A study of mosquito behavior. *Amer. Midl. Nat.*, 1948, *40*, 265–352.

Rumbaugh, D. M. *Language Learning by a Chimpanzee: The Lana Project*. Academic Press, New York, 1976.

Savage-Rumbaugh, E. S., Rumbaugh, D. M., and Boysen, S. Symbolic communication between two chimpanzees *(Pan troglodytes)*. *Science*, 1978, *201*, 641–644.

Schaller, G. B. *The Serengeti Lion; A Study of Predator-Prey Relations*. University of Chicago Press, Chicago, 1972.

Scharf, B. Critical bands. In J. V. Tobias (ed.), *Foundations of Modern Auditory Theory*, Vol. 1. Academic Press, New York, 1970.

Schleidt, W. M. Reaktionen von Truthühnern auf fliegende Raubvögel und Versuche zur Analyse ihrer AAM's. *Z. Tierpsychol.*, 1961, *18*, 534–560.

Schleidt, W. M. Tonic communication: Continual effects of discrete signs in animal communication systems. *J. Theor. Biol.*, 1973, *42*, 359–386.

Schleidt, W. M. Tonic properties of animal communication systems. *Ann. N.Y. Acad. Sci.*, 1977, *290*, 43–50.

Schmidt, R. S. Neural correlates of frog calling. *J. Comp. Physiol.*, 1974, *88*, 321–333.

Schneider, D. Electrophysiological investigation on the olfactory specificity of sexual attracting substances in different species of moths. *J. Insect. Physiol.*, 1962, *8*, 15–30.

Schneider, D. Olfactory receptors for the sexual attractant (bombykol) of the silk moth. In F. O. Schmitt (ed.), *The Neurosciences: Second Study Program*. Rockefeller University Press, New York, 1970.

Schneider, D., Kafka, W. A., Beroza, M., and Bierl, B. A. Odor receptor responses of male gypsy and nun moths (Lepidoptera, Lymantriidae) to disparlure and its analogues. *J. Comp. Physiol.*, 1977, *113*, 1–15.

Schneider, H. Rufe und Rufverhalten des Laubfrosches, *Hyla arborea arborea* (L.). *Z. vergl. Physiol.*, 1967, *57*, 174–189.

Schneider, H. Structure of the mating calls and relationships of the European tree frogs (Hylidae, Anura). *Oekologia (Berl.)*, 1974, *14*, 99–110.

Schneider, H. The acoustic behavior and physiology of vocalization in the European tree frog, *Hyla arborea* (L.). In D. H. Taylor and S. I. Guttman (eds.), *The Reproductive Biology of Amphibians*. Plenum Press, New York, 1977.

Schott, D. Quantitative analysis of the vocal repertoire of squirrel monkeys (*Saimiri sciureus*). *Z. Tierpsychol.*, 1975, *38*, 225–250.

Schubert, G. Experimentelle Untersuchungen über die artkennzeichnenden Parameter im Gesang des Zilpzalps. *Behaviour*, 1971, *38*, 289–314.

Schwartz, G. E. Biofeedback, self-regulation and the patterning of physiological processes. *Am. Sci.,* 1975, *63*, 314–324.

Schwartz, G. E., Fair, P. L., Salt, P., Mandel, M. R., and Klerman, G. L. Facial muscle patterning to affective imagery in depressed and nondepressed subjects. *Science,* 1976, *192*, 489–491.

Scruton, D. M., and Herbert, J. The reaction of groups of captive talopoin monkeys to the introduction of male and female strangers of the same species. *Anim. Behav.,* 1972, *20*, 463–473.

Sebeok, T. A. (ed.). *How Animals Communicate.* Indiana University Press, Bloomington, 1977.

Seibt, U., and Wickler, W. Duettieren als Revier-Anzeige bei Vögeln. *Z. Tierpsychol.,* 1977, *43*, 180–187.

Selander, R. K. Sexual selection and dimorphism in birds. In B. Campbell (ed.), *Sexual Selection and the Descent of Man, 1871–1971.* Aldine, Chicago, 1972.

Shalter, M. D. Localization of passerine seet and mobbing calls by goshawks and pygmy owls. *Z. Tierpsychol.,* 1978, *46*, 260–267.

Shalter, M. D., and Schleidt, W. M. The ability of barn owls *Tyto alba* to discriminate and localize avian alarm calls. *Ibis,* 1977, *119*, 22–27.

Sherman, P. W. Nepotism and the evolution of alarm calls. *Science,* 1977, *197*, 1246–1253.

Shiovitz, K. A. The process of species-specific song recognition by the indigo bunting, *Passerina cyanea,* and its relationship to the organization of avian acoustical behavior. *Behaviour,* 1975, *55*, 128–179.

Shorey, H. H. *Animal Communication by Pheromones.* Academic Press, New York, 1976.

Sibley, C. G. The evolutionary taxonomic significance of sexual dimorphism and hybridization in birds. *Condor,* 1957, *59*, 166–191.

Smith, W. J. Message, meaning and context in ethology. *Amer. Natur.,* 1965, *99*, 405–409.

Smith, W. J. Message-meaning analyses. In T. A. Sebeok (ed.), *Animal Communication.* Indiana University Press, Bloomington, 1968.

Smith, W. J. *The Behavior of Communicating.* Harvard University Press, Cambridge, Mass., 1977.

Soucek, B., and Carlson, A. D. Flash pattern recognition in fireflies. *J. Theoret. Biol.,* 1975, *55*, 339–352.

Southwick, C. H. An experimental study of intragroup agonistic behavior in rhesus monkeys (*Macaca mulatta*). *Behaviour,* 1967, *28*, 183–209.

Southwick, C. H., Siddiqi, M. F., Farooqui, M. Y., and Pal, B. C. Xenophobia among free-ranging rhesus groups in India. In R. L. Holloway (ed.), *Primate Aggression, Territoriality and Xenophobia.* Academic Press, New York, 1974.

Stephanski, R. A., and Falls, J. B. A study of distress calls of song, swamp, and white-throated sparrows (Aves: Fringillidae). I. Intraspecific responses and functions. *Can. J. Zool.,* 1972a, *50*, 1501–1512.

Stephanski, R. A., and Falls, J. B. A study of distress calls of song, swamp, and white throated sparrows (Aves: Fringillidae). II. Interspecific responses and properties used in recognition. *Can. J. Zool.,* 1972b, *50*, 1513–1525.

Stevens, K. N. Quantal nature of speech. In E. E. David, Jr., and P. B. Denes (eds.), *Human Communication: A Unified View.* McGraw-Hill, New York, 1972.

Stokes, A. W. Agonistic behavior among blue tits at a winter feeding station. *Behaviour,* 1962a, *19*, 118–138.

Stokes, A. W. The comparative ethology of great blue marsh and coal tits at a winter feeding station. *Behaviour,* 1962b, *19*, 208–218.

Stokes, A. W. Parental and courtship feeding in red jungle fowl. *Auk,* 1971, *88*, 21–29.

Stokes, A. W., and Williams, H. W. Courtship feeding calls in gallinaceous birds. *Auk,* 1972, *89*, 177–180.

Stokoe, W. C., Jr. The shape of soundless language. In J. F. Kavanagh and J. E. Cutting (eds.), *The Role of Speech in Language.* M.I.T. Press, Cambridge, Mass., 1975.

Straughan, I. R. Evolution of anuran mating calls: Bioacoustical aspects. In J. L. Vial (ed.), *Evolutionary Biology of the Anurans.* University of Missouri Press, Columbia, 1973.

Stresemann, E. Aves. In W. Kükenthal and T. Krumbach (eds.), *Handbuch der Zoologie.* W. de Gruyter, Berlin, 1928.

Struhsaker, T. T. Auditory communication among vervet monkeys *(Cercopithecus aethiops).* In S. A. Altmann (ed.), *Social Communication among Primates.* University of Chicago Press, Chicago, 1967.

Struhsaker, T. T. Phylogenetic implications of some vocalizations of Cercopithecus monkeys. In J. R. Napier and P. H. Napier (eds.), *Old World Monkeys.* Academic Press, New York, 1970.

Struhsaker, T. T. *Behavior and Ecology of Red Colobus Monkeys.* University of Chicago Press, Chicago, 1975.

Struhsaker, T. T., and Gartlan, J. S. Polyspecific associations and niche separation of rain-forest anthropoids in Cameroon, West Africa. *J. Zool.,* 1972, *168*, 221–264.

Studdert-Kennedy, M., Liberman, A. M., Harris, K. S., and Cooper, F. S. The motor theory of speech perception: A reply to Lane's critical review. *Psych. Rev.*, 1970, *77*, 234–249.

Sutherland, N. S. Object recognition. In E. C. Carterette and M. P. Friedman (eds.), *Handbook of Perception*, Vol. 3. Academic Press, New York, 1973.

Theberge, J. B., and Falls, J. B. Howling as a means of communication in timber wolves. *Amer. Zool.*, 1967, *7*, 331–338.

Thielcke, G. Versuche zur Kommunikation und Evolution der Angst-, Alarm-, und Rivalenlaute des Waldbaumläufers *(Certhia familiaris). Z. Tierpsychol.*, 1971, *28*, 505–516.

Thielcke, G. *Bird Sounds.* University of Michigan Press, Ann Arbor, 1976.

Thompson, W. L. Song recognition by territorial male buntings (*Passerina*). *Anim. Behav.*, 1969, *17*, 658–663.

Thorpe, W. H. The learning of song patterns by birds, with especial reference to the song of the chaffinch, *Fringilla coelebs. Ibis*, 1958, *100*, 535–570.

Thorpe, W. H. *The Biology of Vocal Communication and Expression in Birds.* Cambridge University Press, London, 1961.

Thorpe, W. H. Duetting and antiphonal singing in birds. Its extent and significance. *Behaviour Suppl.*, 1972, *18*, 1–197.

Tinbergen, N. Die Übersprungbewegung. *Z. Tierpsychol.*, 1940, *4*, 1–40.

Tinbergen, N. *The Study of Instinct.* Oxford University Press, Oxford, 1951.

Tinbergen, N. "Derived" activities: The causation, biological significance, origin and emancipation during evolution. *Quart. Rev. Biol.*, 1952, *27*, 1–32.

Tinbergen, N. *The Herring Gull's World.* Collins, London, 1953.

Tinbergen, N. Comparative studies of the behaviour of gulls (Laridae): A progress report. *Behaviour*, 1959, *15*, 1–70.

Tinbergen, N. *The Animal in Its World*, Vols. 1 and 2. Harvard University Press, Cambridge, Mass., 1973.

Tinbergen, N., and Perdeck, A. C. On the stimulus situation releasing the begging response in the newly-hatched herring gull chick (*Larus a. argentatus* Pont.). *Behaviour*, 1950, *3*, 1–38.

Tischner, H., and Schief, A. Fluggeräusch und Schallwarnehmung bei *Aedes aegypti* L. (Culicidae). *Verh. Deutsche Zool. Gesell.*, 1954, *51*, 453–460.

Todt, D. Die antiphonen Paargesänge des ostafrikanischen Grassängers *Cisticola hunteri prinioides* Neumann. *J. Ornithol.*, 1970, *111*, 332–356.

Todt, D. Effect of territorial conditions on the maintenance of pair contact in duetting birds. *Experientia*, 1975, *31*, 648–649.

Tretzel, E. Imitation und Variation von Schäferpfiffen durch Haubenlerchen (*Galerida c. cristata* L.). Ein Beispiel für spezielle Spottmotiv-Prädisposition. *Z. Tierpsychol.*, 1965, *22*, 784–809.

Tschanz, B. Trottellummen. Die Entstehung der persönlichen Beziehungen zwischen Jungvogel und Eltern. *Z. Tierpsychol.*, 1968, *4*, 51–100.

Turvey, M. T. Preliminaries to a theory of action with reference to vision. In R. Shaw and J. Bransford (eds.), *Perceiving, Acting, and Knowing.* Wiley, New York, 1977.

Uhr, L. *Pattern Recognition.* Wiley, New York, 1966.

Ulagaraj, S. M., and Walker, T. J. Phonotaxis of crickets in flight: Attraction of male and female crickets to male calling songs. *Science*, 1973, *182*, 1278–1279.

Vencl, F. A case of convergence in vocal signals between marmosets and birds. *Amer. Natur.*, 1977, *111*, 777–816.

Wade, T. D. The effects of strangers on rhesus monkey groups. *Behaviour*, 1976, *56*, 194–214.

Walker, T. J. Specificity in the response of female tree crickets (Orthoptera, Gryllidae, Oecanthinae) to calling songs of the males. *Ann. Ent. Soc. Amer.*, 1957, *50*, 626–633.

Walker, T. J., and Dew, D. Wing movements of calling katydids: Fiddling finesse. *Science*, 1972, *178*, 174–176.

Warner, R. W. The anatomy of the syrinx in passerine birds. *J. Zool. Lond.*, 1972, *168*, 381–393.

Warnock, G. J. *The Philosophy of Perception.* Oxford University Press, Oxford, 1967.

Waser, P. M. Experimental playbacks show vocal mediation of intergroup avoidance in a forest monkey. *Nature*, 1975a, *255*, 56–58.

Waser, P. Spatial associations and social interactions in a "solitary" ungulate: The bushbuck *Tragelaphus scriptus* Pallas. *Z. Tierpsychol.*, 1975b, *37*, 24–36.

Waser, P. M. Individual recognition, intragroup cohesion and intergroup spacing: Evidence from sound playback to forest monkeys. *Behaviour,* 1976, *60*, 28–84.

Waser, P. M., and Waser, M. S. Experimental studies of primate vocalization: Specializations for long-distance propagation. *Z. Tierpsychol.*, 1977, *43*, 239–263.

Washburn, S. L., and DeVore, I. The social life of baboons. *Sci. Am.,* 1961, *204*(6), 62–71.

Weimer, W. B. A conceptual framework for cognitive psychology: Motor theories of the mind. In R. Shaw and J. Bransford (eds.), *Perceiving, Acting and Knowing.* Lawrence Erlbaum Assoc., Hillsdale, N.J., 1977.

Wenner, A. M. Sound production during the waggle dance of the honeybee. *Anim. Behav.,* 1962, *10*, 79–95.

White, S. J. Selective responsiveness by the Gannet (*Sula bassana*) to played-back calls. *Anim. Behav.,* 1971, *19*, 125–131.

Wickler, W. *Mimicry in Plants and Animals.* McGraw-Hill, New York, 1968.

Wickler, W. Aufbau und Paarspezifität des Gesangduettes von *Laniarius funebris* (Aves, Passeriformes, Laniidae). *Z. Tierpsychol.,* 1972a, *30*, 464–476.

Wickler, W. Duettieren zwischen artverschiedenen Vogeln im Freiland. *Z. Tierpsychol.,* 1972b, *31*, 98–103.

Wickler, W. Artunterschiede im Duettgesang zwischen *Trachyphonus d'arnaudii* usambiro und den anderen Unterarten von *T. d'arnaudii. J. Ornithol.,* 1973, *114*, 123–128.

Wickler, W. The ethological analysis of attachment. *Z. Tierpsychol.,* 1976, *42*, 12–28.

Wiener, N. *Cybernetics.* Wiley, New York, 1948.

Wiepkema, P. R. An ethological analysis of the reproductive behaviour of the bitterling (*Rhodeus arnarus* Block). *Arch. Neerl. Zool.,* 1961, *14*, 103–199.

Wiley, R. H. Cooperative roles in mixed flocks of ant wrens *(Formicariidae). Auk,* 1971, *88*, 881–892.

Wiley, R. H. Evolution of social organization and life history patterns among grouse. *Quart. Rev. Biol.,* 1974, *47*, 129–152.

Wiley, R. H. Multidimensional variation in an avian display: Implications for social communication. *Science,* 1975, *190*, 482–483.

Wiley, R. H. Communication and spatial relationships in a colony of common grackles. *Anim. Behav.,* 1976, *24*, 570–584.

Wiley, R. H., and Hartnett, S. A. Mechanisms of spacing in groups of juncos: Aggression, approach, and avoidance in relation to proximity of opponents. *Anim. Behav.,* in press.

Wiley, R. H., and Richards, D. G. Physical constraints on acoustic communication in the atmosphere: Implications for the evolution of animal vocalizations. *Behav. Ecol. Sociobiol.,* 1978, *3*, 69–94.

Wiley, R. H., and Wiley, M. S. Recognition of neighbors' duets by stripe-backed wrens, *Campylorhynchus nuchalis. Behaviour,* 1977, *62*, 10–34.

Williams, H. W., Stokes, A. W., and Wallen, J. C. The food call and display of the bobwhite quail *(Colinus virginianus). Auk,* 1968, *85*, 464–476.

Willis, E. O. The role of migrant birds at swarms of army ants. *Living Bird,* 1966, *5*, 187–231.

Wilson, E. O. Chemical communication among workers of the fire ant, *Solenopsis saevissima* (Fr. Smith). 1–3. *Anim. Behav.,* 1962, *10*, 134–164.

Wilson, E. O. Chemical systems. In T. A. Sebeok (ed.), *Animal Communication, Techniques of Study and Results of Research.* Indiana University Press, Bloomington, 1968.

Wilson, E. O. *The Insect Societies.* Belknap Press of Harvard University Press, Cambridge, Mass., 1971a.

Wilson, E. O. The prospects for a unified sociobiology. *Amer. Sci.,* 1971b, *59*, 400–403.

Wilson, E. O. Animal communication. *Sci. Amer.,* 1972, *227*(3), 52–60.

Wilson E. O. Enemy specification in the alarm-recruitment system of an ant. *Science,* 1975a, *190*, 798–800.

Wilson, E. O. *Sociobiology: The New Synthesis.* Harvard University Press, Cambridge, Mass., 1975b.

Wilson, E. O. Behavioral discretization and the number of castes in an ant species. *Behav. Ecol. Sociobiol.,* 1976, *1*, 141–154.

Wilson, E. O., and Bossert, W. H. Chemical communication among animals. *Rec. Prog. Hormone Res.,* 1963, *19*, 673–716.

Wilz, K. J. Causal and functional analysis of dorsal pricking and nest activity in the courtship of the three-spined stickleback *Gasterosteus aculatus. Anim. Behav.,* 1970, *18*, 115–124.

Winn, H. E. Vocal facilitation and the biological significance of toadfish sounds. In W. N. Tavolga (ed.), *Marine Bio-acoustics,* Vol. 2. Pergamon Press, New York, 1967.

Winter, P., Ploog, D., and Latta, J. Vocal repertoire of the squirrel monkey (*Saimiri sciureus*), its analysis and significance. *Exp. Brain Res. (Berlin),* 1966, *1*, 359–384.

Wright, R. H. The olfactory guidance of flying insects. *Can. Entomol.,* 1958, *90*, 81–89.

Yamaguchi, M., Yamazaki, K., and Boyse, E. A. Mating preference tests with recombinant congenic strain BALB.H.T.G. *Immunogenetics,* 1978, *6*, 261–264.

158

STEVEN GREEN AND
PETER MARLER

Yamazaki, K., Boyse, E. A., Mike, V., Thaler, H. T., Mathieson, B. J., Abbot, J., Boyse, J., Zayas, Z. A., and Thomas, L. Control of mating preferences in mice by genes in the major histocompatability complex. *J. Exp. Med.*, 1976, *144*, 1324–1335.

Yarbus, A. L. *Eye Movements and Vision.* Plenum Press, New York, 1967.

Zann, R. Inter- and intra-specific variation in calls of three species of grassfinches of the subgenus *Poephila* (Gould) (Estrildidae). *Z. Tierpsychol.*, 1975, *39*, 85–125.

Zoloth, S., and Green, S. Monkey vocalizations and human speech: Parallels in perception? *Brain, Behavior and Evolution,* in press.

Zoloth, S. R., Petersen, M. R., Beecher, M. D., Green, S., Marler, P., Moody, D., and Stebbins, W. Species specific perceptual processing of vocal sounds by monkeys. *Science,* in press.

Mechanisms and Evolution of Spacing in Animals

PETER M. WASER AND R. HAVEN WILEY

Animals of the same species are rarely distributed randomly. Each individual's movements are influenced by those of its neighbors, with the result that any population exhibits a characteristic pattern of individuals' locations and activities in space.[1] In this chapter, we discuss in turn three approaches to understanding individuals' spatial relationships: quantitative specification of patterns of spacing; analysis of the behavioral mechanisms that control spacing; and identification of the effects of natural selection on the evolution of spacing. This division separates discussion of the proximate controls of spacing, in our initial sections, from consideration of the ultimate controls, with which we conclude.

The literature on spacing relies heavily on two simple concepts: home range and territoriality, Recently, it has become apparent that important variation in spacing patterns and mechanisms is concealed by the application of these common terms. Consider "territorial" birds. In some species, like bicolored antbirds (*Gymnopithys bicolor*) (Willis, 1967), individuals overlap widely in their movements, although each manifests clear dominance over intruders within its territory. In other species with similar patterns of spatial variation in domanice, individuals

---

[1]Where individuals form cohesive groups, these groups often behave in a manner similar to that of individuals in more solitary species. Except in discussions of fitness or unless otherwise indicated, the term *individual* in this paper includes cohesive social groups.

PETER M. WASER Department of Biological Sciences, Purdue University, West Lafayette, Indiana 47906.   R. HAVEN WILEY Department of Zoology, University of North Carolina, Chapel Hill, North Carolina 27514. Our research on spatial relationships in vertebrate societies has been supported by the National Institute of Mental Health (MH22316 to Wiley), the National Science Foundation (DEB 77–23671 to Waser), and a National Institute of Health training grant to Rockefeller University (GM01789).

occupy largely exclusive areas. Tree sparrows *(Spizella arborea)* provide a well-documented example (Weeden, 1965). Tree sparrows and antbirds thus share "territorial" characteristics in spacing behavior, but they differ dramatically in the degree of isolation they maintain from neighbors. It is time to recognize that spatial variation in an individual's agonistic behavior, activities, and isolation from neighbors varies in complex ways from species to species.

In this chapter, rather than pursue unitary concepts, we attempt to address this variation in spacing by examining methods for measuring spatial patterns of individuals' activities, isolation, and aggression; by considering the behavioral mechanisms that can control these manifestations; and by proposing a framework for explaining their evolution.

In the first section, "Quantitative Description of Spacing Patterns," we review attempts to measure aspects of spacing. For clarity in describing variation in spacing patterns , we introduce the use of two "fields" (Wiley, 1973; Black and Wiley, 1977), which can be defined for any individual.

The distribution of an individual's time as a function of location defines an *activity field*. The word *field* is used here in the mathematical sense as "a function of . . . position in space measured in a rectangular coordinate system" (Feynman, Leighton, and Sands, 1964, II:2-2). The value of an individual's activity field at any point is the proportion of its time spent there in all activities. The boundaries of this field delimit the individual's home range or activity space (Burt, 1943; Weeden, 1965). Alternatively, such a field could include only particular activities of importance to resource use, for instance, time spent feeding. An activity field that pertains to an individual's use of a particular resource is sometimes called a "utilization distribution" (van Winkle, 1975).

The relative exclusiveness of an individual's use of space as a function of location further defines an *isolation field*. The value of an individual's isolation field at any location (x, y) is the ratio: time spent by the subject at location (x, y) divided by time spent by all individuals including the subject at (x, y). This ratio varies from 1, when the subject has exclusive use of the location, to 0, when the subject never uses the location but others do. A set of individuals' isolation fields thus both describe their pattern of spacing and, in combination with information on resource distribution, indicate the degree to which each individual monopolizes access to resources.

In the second section, "Behavioral Mechanisms of Spacing," we discuss the behavioral tendencies that are the proximate determinants of spacing patterns. As Marler (1976) has emphasized, the same spacing pattern can in principle arise through alternate behavioral strategies of individuals. Consider arboreal forest primates that maintain largely exclusive territories: in some, like titi monkeys *(Callicebus moloch)* (Mason, 1968; Robinson, in press), gibbons *(Hylobates lar)* (Ellefson, 1968), and red-tailed monkeys *(Cercopithecus ascanius)* (Struhsaker, 1975), close-range aggressive encounters at boundaries are a regular feature of neighboring groups' interactions; in others, like blue monkeys *(Cercopithecus mitis)* (Struhsaker, 1975), black-and-white colobus *(Colobus guereza)* (Marler, 1972; Struhsaker, 1975), and some howler monkeys *(Alouatta* species) (Chivers, 1969; Altmann, 1959; Neville, 1972), neighboring groups meet at close range much less frequently. In the latter species, loud calls seem to aid in maintaining distance between neighboring groups without frequent close-range encounters, while in titi monkeys and gibbons, loud calls at dawn seem, in contrast, to lead neighboring groups into close-range interactions at boundaries. Similar patterns of isolation are maintained by different balances between overt aggression and avoidance.

The behavioral "rules" that determine spacing in a population will, in general, be influenced by the previous histories of individuals, the identities and characteristics of opponents, the proximity of opponents, and especially the location of encounters. The last of these effects produces spatial variation in individuals' agonistic tendencies. Because this phenomenon has such crucial importance for spacing, we introduce a third field (Wiley, 1973), an *aggression field;* the value of an individual's aggression field at any location is defined by its probability there of attack or retreat. Determining the way in which aggression and activity fields interact to produce the pattern of isolation fields in a population is a basic goal for studies of spacing.

In the third section, "Communication of Advertisement and Threat," we take up the use of signals as substitutes for physical contact. Spacing signals greatly increase the area over which an individual influences its neighbors' movements; in this section, we discuss constraints on the evolution of such signals.

In the fourth section, "Evolution of Spacing Behavior," we turn to the evolution of the diversity in patterns of animal spacing. Most previous evolutionary explanations for spacing patterns have addressed the relative advantages and disadvantages of the defense of a resource. But defense is not a simple phenomenon, particularly when alternate behavioral mechanisms can lead to isolation. We develop theories that deduce the optimal spacing of resident individuals in a population from the spatial and temporal distribution of critical resources. This approach provides more comprehensive evolutionary explanations of relationships between movement patterns and isolation fields of individuals in a population.

QUANTITATIVE DESCRIPTION OF SPACING PATTERNS

ACTIVITY FIELDS AND MOVEMENT PATTERNS

The first challenge in a study of spacing is a choice of methods for recording and then measuring the movements of individuals and the consequent activity and isolation fields. The technique selected for recording animals' movements can constrain the range of answerable questions about spacing.

Methods for recording animal movements have ranged from direct observation of individuals (e.g., Altmann and Altmann, 1970; Gottfried and Franks, 1975; Struhsaker, 1975) to such imaginative indirect methods as positioning smoked kymograph paper in the pathways used by individually toe-clipped mice (Justice, 1961; Metzgar, 1973a) or mounting spools on the backs of turtles, which then leave their tracks in unwound thread (Stickel, 1950). Field methods usually require some trade between the time or effort required and the quality of data obtained (see Sanderson, 1966; Taber and Cowan, 1971). In addition, methods differ in suitability for measuring the spatial distribution of an individual's time, as opposed to the temporal sequence of its movements.

Direct observation of an individual yields the greatest information: the overall area used by the individual, the distribution of the individual's time within that area, and the spatial distributions of particular behavior patterns. Direct observation also gives information on location as a function of time, including rates of movement and rates of return to specific areas. Complete information is, however, acquired at the cost of considerable time and effort and requires an easily observable subject. Tagging individuals with visual, radioactive, sonic, or radio beacons can facilitate direct visual observation (Montgomery, Cochran, and Sunquist, 1973; Buchler, 1976), but in practice, information must often be sacrificed through the use of tracking or mark-recapture techniques.

Tracking methods can often be devised for animals not observable by direct means. These techniques preserve information on sequence of movement, but they often lose information on variation in rates of movement and are of limited use in measuring the form of activity fields. As a result, tracking methods are most useful where the details of neighbors' movements relative to each other are of interest (Peters and Mech, 1976) or where they generate data on the distribution of behavior patterns, such as site-specific defecation, which are relevant to interindividual spacing (Bearder and Randall, 1978).

Mark and recapture methods retain information on the form of activity fields but lose all information on movements within the intervals between captures. "Capture" need not disrupt the movements of the animals under study; repeated censusing of banded birds, radio fixes, detection of radioactive tags, and use of dyes to generate marked urine or feces (Frantz, 1972; Evans and Griffith, 1973) are all forms of mark-recapture methods. Recording of individually distinctive tracks on kymograph paper, photography of birds and mammals by activity-triggered remote cameras, and microphone arrays to record locations of loud vocalizations (Schleidt, in press; Watkins, 1976) are similar to mark-recapture methods in recording the locations of individuals at irregular intervals. Although such techniques are often simpler than direct observation or tracking, they can have the disadvantage of recording locations only during certain activities. In particular, locations at which individuals are live-trapped can misrepresent the overall use of space by those individuals (Brown, 1962; Metzgar, 1973a; Robinson and Falls, 1965). "Over a period of time the investigator accumulates a series of dots on a map or chart and is not certain what they mean, and rarely knows why the animals came near the traps when they were caught" (Sanderson, 1966, p. 222).

Despite this shortcoming, for many species mark-recapture techniques are the only feasible way to record movements. If captures or observations are repeated at time intervals that are reasonably short in relation to the animal's rate of movement, mark-recapture becomes a form of instantaneous sampling (J. Altmann, 1974) and can in principle be used to estimate both activity-field and sequence-of-movement data. Statistical techniques for assessing the reliability of such estimates are not, as yet, available.

The next decision in a study of spacing is a selection of procedures for the quantitative description of an individual's use of space. The traditional measure of an animal's use of space is home range size. Home range, "the area over which an animal normally travels in pursuit of its routine activities" (Jewell, 1966, p. 103), has been widely accepted as an indication of the amount of space (and, by extension, resources) used by an individual (McNab, 1963; Schoener, 1968a; Turner, Jennrich, and Weintraub, 1969). Home range area, or more precisely the area enclosed by a convex perimeter around an animal's locations, is attractively simple as a measure of the spatial distribution of its activities. Nevertheless, the concept has serious drawbacks.

Much disagreement has resulted from conflicting conventions in estimating home range size (Sanderson, 1966). The application of a variety of commonly used techniques to the same set of data obtained by continuous following of individuals can yield measures of range size that differ severalfold (Waser and Floody, 1974). Problems become especially severe when an individual's activities are concentrated in a relatively few scattered locations and the intervening areas are occupied briefly in passing, if at all. For instance, in feral cats the area utilized "consists of a varying number of more or less regularly visited localities connected by an elaborate network of pathways" (Leyhausen, 1965, p. 252). This situation seems to characterize many mammals (Ewer, 1968; see Adams and Davis, 1967; Bailey, 1974; and Eaton, 1970, for recent examples) as well as other animals, like butterflies, bees, and hummingbirds, which practice "trap-line" foraging (Janzen, 1971). In these cases, the size of an animal's home range has no clear relation to its ecology or behavior.

A more general problem in estimating the sizes of home ranges arises from effects of the length of study. Cumulative range size tends to approach an asymptote as length of sampling time increases. To reduce the effects of sampling time, Odum and Kuenzler (1955) have suggested that range size be defined at the point where each further observation increases the measured area by 1% or less. Other methods for estimating the asymptotic area of a home range, analogous to those for estimates of species number from nested quadrats in botanical communities (Preston, 1962) or repertoire size from samples of the frequencies of behavior categories (Fagen and Goldman, 1977), have not, to our knowledge, been applied to home range data. Any estimate of the asymptotic area of a home range encounters problems when animals focus their activities successively in different subsections of their ranges. Then, the cumulative home-range area passes several successive "asymptotes," like steps, as observations continue (Figure 1).

Temporary shifts in habitat use, occasional movements outside the usual area, unutilized "lacunae," and other manifestations of uneven use of space make it virtually impossible to propose universally satisfactory methods for measurement of home range size. Yet, just such complications may have critical consequences for spacing. This dilemma points up the major shortcomings of any single parameter, like area, as a measure of the distribution of an animal's activities in space. Intensity of use varies with location; an activity field is rarely specified by one parameter.

Probabilistic models of home ranges provide a limited analysis of differences

PETER M. WASER
AND R. HAVEN
WILEY

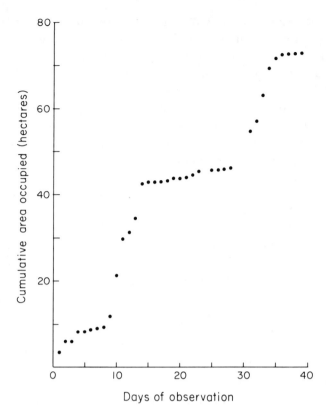

Fig. 1. Cumulative area occupied by one mangabey group. The group was followed continuously. From Waser and Floody, 1974.

in the intensity of an individual's use of locations. These models require stringent assumptions concerning the form of the activity field: probability of use must fall off from the center of the home range according to a specified probability distribution, either univariate (Dice and Clark, 1953; Hayne, 1949; Harrison, 1958; White, 1964) or bivariate (Calhoun and Casby, 1958; Jennrich and Turner, 1969; Metzgar, 1972; Mazurkiewicz, 1971). The use of two parameters to describe an activity field, in bivariate models, is potentially a modest advance over a single parameter, like asymptotic home-range size. These models require "that the actual utilization distribution conform to rather specific constraints . . . which are frequently not satisfied, even within rather homogeneous habitats" (van Winkle, 1975, p. 12). Worse, where spacing is at issue, the properties of the assumed probability distribution are most crucial at the edge of the home range, where data are often least adequate.

A more complete description results from the tabulation of intensity of use on a grid of quadrats superimposed over the home range. Continuous (or instantaneously sampled) data have been transformed into maps of intensity of use by molding and weighing clay "tracks" (Adams and Davis, 1967), by hand tabulation of observational data (Weeden, 1965; Chivers, Raemakers, and Aldrich-Blake, 1975; Struhsaker, 1975) and by digital computer (Siniff and Jessen, 1969; Nicholls and Warner, 1972; Archibald, 1975; Harding, 1976). Such maps (Fig. 2), which are called "activity spaces" by Weeden (1965), are more accurately termed *activity fields*.

The flexibility of machine computation permits rapid comparisons of activity fields with different quadrat sizes. While quadrat size could be selected for biological reasons (for instance, to approximate the area that might be scanned for resources from the position of a moving animal or to match the size of resource patches), it could also be chosen to allow direct comparisons between species or habitats.

Frequencies of quadrat use by radio-tracked red foxes *(Vulpes fulva)* and snowshoe hares *(Lepus americanus)* fit a zero-truncated negative binomial distribution (Siniff and Jessen, 1969). This distribution provides yet another method for

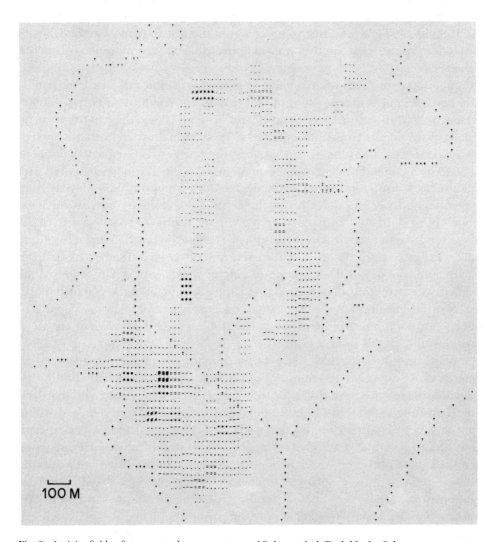

Fig. 2. Activity fields of one mangabey group over a 10-day period. Each block of characters represents a 50-m × 50-m quadrat, with optical density of characters proportional to the number of mangabeys sighted there during systematic half-hourly scan periods while the group was continuously followed. From Waser, 1976.

PETER M. WASER
AND R. HAVEN
WILEY

estimating the size of a home range, from the sum of expected quadrat frequencies, including the zero class, of the negative binomial distribution. More important, if a wide variety of species' activity fields are found to fit such a distribution, and if values of the distribution's parameters are (as Siniff and Jessen suggested) species-specific, its parameter k will provide a comparative index of clumping or nonrandomness of an activity field (Siniff and Jessen, 1969). Other candidates for such an index of nonuniformity of an activity field might include various statistics of environmental "grain" (Goodall, 1970; Pielou, 1969) or a simple statement of the fraction of total utilized area in which X percent of time is spent.

None of the analyses so far described preserves sequential information. Yet, among those parameters on which selection can act to increase efficiency of resource utilization, there are theoretical reasons to believe that movement sequence and rate are of particular importance (Cody, 1971, 1974; Schoener, 1971; Smith, 1974; Krebs, this volume). Given the distribution of an individual's locations in space, what are the "transition probabilities" for movements between these locations?

The simplest model of an animal's movements assumes that each movement to a new location is independent of all previous movements. Although animals seldom follow this assumption (Siniff and Jessen, 1969), the deviation of an animal's movements from those predicted by such first-order stochastic models can elucidate spacing patterns. For instance, the rate at which sequential locations of an individual tend to drift away from an initial position can be compared with that predicted for a random walk; the degree to which observations deviate from expectation provides an index of attachment to a home site (Waser, 1976). Some models of random walk incorporate changes in the probability of turns toward the home range center as distance from center increases ("centrally biased random walk"; Holgate, 1969; Rohlf and Davenport, 1969). More complex models can incorporate changes in the direction or rate of movement as a function of the animal's location. For instance, Beeler (1973) has investigated the potential movements of an imaginary worm crawling on a hexagonal lattice, whose choice of direction at each intersection of the lattice is dictated by rules depending on its previous "use" of the intersection.

Siniff and Jessen (1969) have taken a more pragmatic approach to the description of animal movements. Working with radio-tracked foxes and hares, the authors measured the distances traveled between sequential radio fixes and the relative angles between successive steps. Siniff and Jessen found these distributions to vary with species and habitat. Cody (1971) has tabulated similar distributions of step length and angle of turn for flocks of desert finches. He suggested that flocks both maximize coverage of areas within the home range and adjust the rates of return to given subareas to coincide with renewal rates of resources. Clutton-Brock (1975) has applied similar reasoning to the movements of red colobus *(Colobus badius)* feeding on growing shoots and leaves in East African forests. There are no precise measurements of rates of return for any animal.

In computer simulation of animal movements with either real or idealized distributions of step lengths and angles of turn, Siniff and Jessen concluded that these two parameters could produce activity fields statistically indistinguishable from real data. Considering that their initial simulations explicitly ignored both the possibility of attachment to familiar sites and interactions with neighbors, it is not surprising that their simulations tended to produce activity fields that were less clumped and larger in area than those from which the data were originally obtained; but these differences were statistically significant in only a few simulations. The degree to which these simulations resemble actual activity fields underscores the possibility that an individual's movements, without reference to interactions with its neighbors, might in some cases account for the major characteristics of its activity field.

SPATIAL RELATIONS BETWEEN INDIVIDUALS

How are an individual's activity field and movements related to those of its neighbors? There are two basic approaches in answering such a question. One focuses on the simultaneous positions or movements of individuals, the other on the spatial relationships of individuals' activity fields.

Methods for measuring the instantaneous dispersion of individuals, particularly those based on nearest-neighbor distances, are readily extended from plants, for which they were developed (Clark and Evans, 1954, 1955), to sedentary animals or such bases of activity as anthills (Brian, Hibble, and Kelly, 1966), bird nest sites (Krebs, 1971), and mammalian or crustacean burrows (Lighter, 1975), or to moving individuals whose positions can be simultaneously recorded. For instance, Miller and Stephen (1966) applied these techniques to aerial photographs of sandhill cranes *(Grus canadensis)*. By comparing the distribution of nearest-neighbor distances with that expected from a set of randomly positioned points, one can classify populations as *overdispersed* (when close spacing of individuals is less frequent than expected), *random,* or *aggregated* (when close spacing is more frequent than expected at random) (Hutchinson, 1953).

For most species, particularly when animals' movements are rapid and extensive or individuals are scattered or elusive, simultaneous location of numerous individuals is impractical. Groups of gray-cheeked mangabeys *(Cercocebus albigena)* in western Uganda, which occur at a density of less than 1 per km² in dense forest (Waser, 1976), provide an example. Yet, since large home ranges and poor visibility hinder not only an observer but also the animals' efforts to maintain exclusive use of a resource, data on spacing behavior in such species are of particular interest.

For gray-cheeked mangabeys, movements of two groups can in general be monitored only while groups are separated by less than 500 m. When groups are this close together (an unusual occurrence in this population), it is possible to record intergroup distances at regular time intervals.

From these data, the relative probabilities of approach or withdrawal can be calculated as a function of intergroup distance (Waser, 1976). A "radius of repulsion," if one exists, can be detected by statistical comparison of these probabilities with null probabilities of approach or withdrawal with respect to an arbitrarily chosen point or to a noninteracting neighboring group. For mangabeys, groups 2 km away and thus well beyond any possibility of interaction were used to generate "null" probabilities. If it is difficult to observe more than one individual simultaneously, as is the case for mangabey groups, this straightforward approach is limited by small sample sizes, which result from just those low probabilities of close approach that constitute the phenomenon of interest.

These same data can also be tested against hypotheses predicting frequencies of encounters or approaches to a specified separation. A simple null hypothesis is that movements are independent and random. In this case, frequency of approach (Z) to any specified distance (d) can be computed from simple considerations of statistical mechanics for a two-dimensional perfect gas with density ρ and velocity v. When all individuals but one are stationary, $Z = 2\rho v\sigma$, where $\sigma = d + s$ and s is the diameter of an individual (or group of individuals). If all individuals move at the same velocity v,

$$Z = \frac{8\rho v\sigma}{\pi}$$

Such models can be extended to incorporate probability distributions of velocities, rather than constant v, or cases in which velocities of two individuals differ; in fact, however, predicted encounter frequencies are relatively insensitive to such refinements in the model.

Comparison of observed and expected frequencies of approach at given distances can determine whether or not avoidance occurs, as well as the radius of avoidance, if such exists (Waser, 1975b, 1976). When applied to mangabeys, this approach indicates that groups avoid each other at distances of several hundred meters, a conclusion supported by experiments that mimic intergroup encounters through the playback of specialized intergroup vocalizations (see section on "Communication of Advertisement and Threat").

The literature on primates frequently states an impression that groups avoid each other, so that "actual contact between groups is even less than expected" (DeVore and Hall, 1965, p. 36). Nevertheless, the data necessary to evaluate this hypothesis (ρ, v, d, and the observed frequencies of approach) are rarely reported (Table I). In fact, when such data are presented (or reasonable values can be inferred), in only one case does such a statement appear to be clearly warranted. For titi monkeys *(Callicebus moloch)*, the null hypothesis predicts approach within 50 m approximately 6 times more frequently than intergroup confrontations actually occur (Mason, 1968). In contrast, according to the data presented by Schaller (1963), gorilla groups approach each other within 50 m 25 times *more* frequently than expected on the assumption that movements are independent. This result suggests a level of familiarity between groups that approaches the casual associations of chimpanzees.

Differences between observed and expected frequencies of approach might result either from a lack of independence or a lack of randomness of individuals' movements. In addition to tendencies to approach or avoid conspecifics, such factors as an avoidance of areas where previous encounters were lost or a concentration of activity in familiar areas could lead to such deviations. We return to these possibilities in the next section.

Only a few quantitative models are available for independent but nonrandom movements. Jorgenson (1968a,b) has calculated the joint probability of quadrat occupancy assuming circular home ranges and neglecting all locations of an individual farther than its 95% recapture radius from its home range center. A potentially more general method, though requiring the assumption that activity fields can be described by bivariate normal distributions, has recently been developed by Dunn and Gipson (1977). Simultaneous movements of neighboring individuals were used to measure both home range overlap and canonical correlation of movements between neighboring individuals. These methods also provide expected distributions of interanimal distance given observed parameters of movement.

The spatial relationships of activity fields are another major concern in studies of individual's spacing. The simplest measure of the spatial relationships of activity fields is the percentage of an individual's home range overlapped by those of neighbors. In the case of the mangabeys described above, overlap was 72% for one group observed for a year. Such a measure is relatively straightforward to obtain, and methods exist for evaluating the probability of its deviation from the overlap expected if similar home ranges were randomly distributed in space (Metzgar and Hill, 1971). But such an overlap figure (1) is highly dependent on the observer's criteria for home range boundaries and (2) completely neglects differences in intensity of use of overlap areas. In many animals, overlap includes only those areas used occasionally (DeVore and Hall, 1965, describe a classic example among the primates). Thus arises the common conclusion that "core areas" do not overlap. In other cases, however, boundaries pass through areas of heavy use (Klopfer and Jolly, 1970).

Indices of overlap that take intensity of use into account include measures of overlap in the use of a spectrum of resources. These indices can serve just as well

TABLE I. OBSERVED AND EXPECTED RATES OF INTERGROUP ENCOUNTERS IN SELECTED PRIMATE SPECIES

Species	ρ Groups/km²	v m/day	σ m	Encounters/day Expected	Encounters/day Observed
Cereocebus albigena (Waser, 1976)	.25	1,200	190	.15	.01
Colobus badius (Struhsaker, 1974)	5.92	649	100	.98	.59
Colobus guereza (Oates, 1974)	10.0	535	75	1.02	.73
Papio anubis (Harding, 1973)	.15	5,000	300[a]	.57	.30[b]
Gorilla gorilla (Schaller, 1963)	.14	532	100[a]	.02	.26[b]
Callicebus moloch (Mason, 1968)	131.00	635	75[a]	15.89	1.4

[a]These studies do not provide precise values of σ, but estimates of probable group spread and mean distance at which "encounters" occurred are possible from the data presented.

[b]Rates of encounter/day were calculated as total (encounters/total observation hours) × (10 hours observation/day).

for studies of spacing, with quadrats substituted for resources. A numerically simple index was suggested by Holmes and Pitelka (1968; see also Schoener, 1968a; Baker and Baker, 1973):

$$O_{ij} = 1 - 1/2 \sum_a |P_{ia} - P_{ja}| \qquad (1)$$

where O_{ij} is the index of overlap between individuals i and j, P_{ia} is the probability of use by i of quadrat a, and P_{ja} is the probability of use by j of quadrat a. Alternative measures of resource overlap include one derived from information theory (Horn, 1966; Morse, 1970) and several from competition coefficients (α), which are in fact measures of overlap in resource use (Colwell and Futuyma, 1971; May, 1975). May argues on mathematical grounds in favor of Pianka's (1975) measure:

$$O_{ij} = \frac{\sum_a P_{ia}P_{ja}}{\sqrt{\left(\sum_a P_{ia}^2\right)\left(\sum_a P_{ja}^2\right)}} \qquad (2)$$

However, the shortcomings of other formulations, as discussed by May, do not appear to apply to studies of overlap in space. The relative merits of the various indices as measures of spatial overlap remain to be worked out. The only index of overlap so far used for intensities of quadrat use is the product–moment correlation coefficient of the frequencies of use by animals i and j in all quadrats used by either animal (Adams and Davis, 1967); this correlation coefficient is identical in form mathematically to equation (2), with $(P_{ia} - \bar{P}_i)$ and $(P_{ia} - \bar{P}_j)$ substituted for P_{ia} and P_{ja}, respectively.

The degree to which any of these measures of spatial overlap estimate competition between individuals depends on the relationship between the renewal periods of resources in each quadrat and the time intervals between visits to those quadrats by different individuals. The latter can be estimated by repeated sampling of short-term overlap (see Schoener, 1970), but so far no attempts have been made to measure this parameter.

Just as information about an animal's movements is lost by reducing its activity field to a single parameter, such as area or k from the negative binomial distribution, information about spatial relationships is lost by reducing an individual's isolation field to an index of overlap. Determination of an individual's isolation field follows directly from determinations of all overlapping activity fields. Thus, all of the considerations discussed above for the measurements of activity fields apply equally to isolation fields. In particular, the observer must choose an appropriate quadrat size and decide whether continuous recording, instantaneous sampling at regular intervals, or trapping will optimize the balance between feasibility and accuracy in describing an individual's probability of occupying the specified quadrats. In addition, because an isolation field expresses a relationship between individuals, isolation fields with respect to different sets of opponents often differ (see the next section).

Although almost no measurements of isolation fields are now available, it is clear that isolation varies a great deal even among species with territorial behavior, in the sense that individuals attack or dominate intruders within a fixed area. Anecdotal observations suggest that many territorial species have isolation fields with pronounced convexity with respect to the center of the individual's range. The isolation fields of territorial dwarf cichlids *(Apistogramma ramirezi)* in a large aquarium illustrate this pattern (Black and Wiley, 1977). In cross-sections halfway through four individuals' isolation fields (Figure 3), the values of each individual's isolation ratio are a convex function of distance from the center of its range. Some territorial species lack such strong convexity in their isolation fields (see Wiley, 1973). For example, bicolored antbirds *(Gymnopithys bicolor)* (Willis, 1967), mentioned earlier, and Steller's jays *(Cyanocitta stelleri)* (Brown, 1963) seem not to occupy any areas with high isolation ratios. Even ovenbirds *(Seiurus aurocapillus)*, long thought to occupy exclusive areas, wander extensively within neighbors' areas (Zach and Falls, in press). This unobtrusive trespassing was detected only by carefully following marked individuals in early spring before foliage had grown enough to interfere with observations. Zach and Falls's data suggest that isolation ratios for a territorial ovenbird are high, but probably do not reach 1.0, near the center of its territory and decrease gradually away from the center (Figure 4). Thus, even though ethologists and ecologists have seldom measured isolation

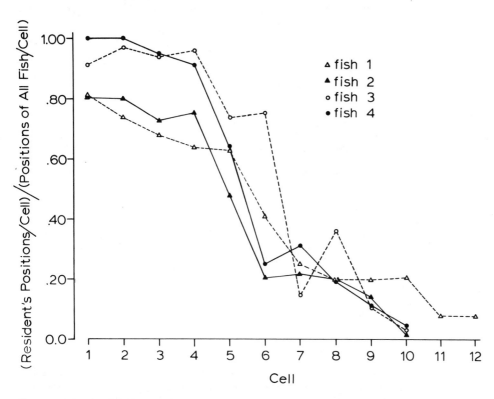

Fig. 3. Cross-sections halfway through four residents' isolation fields for the dwarf cichlid *Apistogramma ramirezi* in a large aquarium. Ordinate, isolation ratio (see text). Abscissa, 5-cm² quadrats along an unobstructed corridor from the center of an individual's territory to the periphery. From Black and Wiley, 1977.

PETER M. WASER
AND R. HAVEN
WILEY

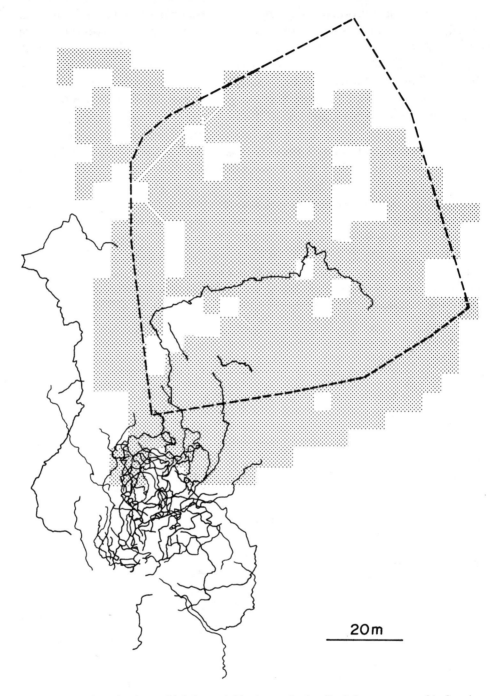

Fig. 4. Trespassing of male ovenbirds into neighboring territories. Shaded area: area used in foraging by Male 5. Dashed line: boundary of Male 5's "song territory" (minimum convex polygon surrounding all song perches). Solid lines: foraging paths of Male 6, Male 5's neighbor. From Zach and Falls, in press.

fields, it is clear that species differ considerably in this regard, even among species with at least superficially similar patterns of aggression.

In the past, ecologists and ethologists have debated whether the essence of territoriality was site-dependent dominance or exclusive occupation of an area, in other words, characteristics either of spatial variation in aggression or of isolation fields. We propose to abandon the search for a unitary definition of territoriality and any simple dichotomy between territorial and nonterritorial species. Instead, we shall address the variation among species in relationships of aggression, isolation, and activity fields, first by considering the behavioral mechanisms that control these relationships (in the next two sections), then by considering the selection pressures that can explain their evolution (in the fourth section).

BEHAVIORAL MECHANISMS OF SPACING

The behavioral mechanisms that control spacing have to explain the causal relations among an individual's activity field, isolation field, and agonistic tendencies (its tendencies to approach, avoid, threaten, and attack) for each category of opponents. There has never been a systematic review of the possible behavioral mechanisms of spacing or variation in these mechanisms among species. This section integrates evidence from laboratory and field in order to make a start in this direction. Many of the phenomena discussed here have clear implications for the evolution of spacing behavior, but we confine our discussion in this section to the proximate relationships between spacing behavior and pattern. This section treats mechanisms of spacing; subsequent sections consider evolutionary adaptations.

We emphasize that ethology has much yet to learn about the determinants of spatial variation in agonistic tendencies and its causal relationships with activity and isolation fields. Rather than attempt to reach definite conclusions, our discussion has two goals: (1) to systematize hypotheses about the behavioral mechanisms that can generate patterns of spacing, so that future studies might succeed more often in discriminating among the possibilities; and (2) to indicate the relevance of laboratory studies of aggression and dominance to the control of spacing behavior in natural populations.

Before proceeding, it is important to dispel two oversimplifications. First, agonistic tendencies in encounters do not completely determine individuals' isolation fields. One additional factor is the probability that individuals will detect each other's presence. This probability, like agonistic tendencies, might well vary with an opponent's location or proximity. As a consequence, *frequencies* of aggressive encounters are not necessarily good indices of aggressive *tendencies*. For instance, consider the inverse relation between the frequency of aggression between territorial neighbors and the sizes of their territories (van den Assem, 1967; Post, 1974). Individuals on smaller territories would presumably detect each other's presence near a boundary more frequently; thus, situations evoking agonistic behavior would occur more frequently. Two separate variables are involved: the frequency of encounters and behavioral tendencies during encounters. This

PETER M. WASER
AND R. HAVEN
WILEY

section will focus on agonistic tendencies after detection of an opponent; the third section will return to the problems of detection.

Second, similar patterns of spacing can result from different behavioral mechanisms. Although exclusively occupied areas are often interpreted as evidence for site-specific defense, different mechanisms can generate exclusive areas. To pick an extreme case, extensive isolation could simply result from wide separation of patches of resources or suitable habitat. Traveling to a distant patch on the chance of using some of it might not be energetically profitable even in the absence of defense by another individual. For instance, mangabeys occupy exclusive areas where unsuitable habitat partially delimits their home ranges (Chalmers, 1968a; Waser, 1976) but not, apparently, where suitable habitat is continuous (Cashner, 1972). Other possible examples of such constraints on spacing include certain marmots *(Marmota)* (Barash, 1973) and talapoin monkeys *(Miopithecus talapoin)* (Gautier-Hion, 1971). Thus, direct responses by individuals to the distribubution of resources might explain their spatial relationships.

Similar spacing patterns could also result from different balances between aggression and avoidance (Marler, 1976). Zoologists have focused on animals' tendencies to threaten and attack conspecifics rather than on their tendencies to avoid them. Yet, avoidance is clearly an important component of spacing behavior (see "Reactions to an Opponent's Proximity" below). Because the dominance relationship between two individuals at a particular location depends on their relative agonistic tendencies there, a change in dominance relationship could result from changes in either tendencies to approach and threaten or tendencies to withdraw. Largely exclusive territories could result not only from tendencies to attack and supplant other individuals in the center but not near the periphery, but also from each individual's tendencies to avoid others in the periphery but not in the center of its range.

REACTIONS TO AN OPPONENT'S PROXIMITY

The behavioral mechanisms that regulate the dispersion of activity fields and the nature of isolation fields often hinge on spatial variation in agonistic tendencies. Before addressing variation in aggression with location, however, we first consider reactions to the proximity of opponents. Our discussion will indicate that changes in agonistic tendencies with an opponent's proximity have important consequences for the likely simultaneous positions of individuals but cannot alone generate overdispersed activity fields.

Early ethologists noted that individuals of many species tended to maintain characteristic separations by means of threat and avoidance at closer distances (Hediger, 1950). These individual distances are particularly noticeable in animals that gather in flocks or herds (Emlen, 1952; Crook, 1961). Marler (1955a,b, 1956b, 1957) measured changes in the probability of agonistic interactions as a function of the separation between chaffinches *(Fringilla coelebs)* feeding from movable hoppers in aviaries. His experiments, conducted during the autumn and winter, when chaffinches normally forage in flocks, were the first to measure variation in agonistic behavior with proximity of opponents. He established that the frequency of aggression increased as separation decreased. At any separation, males were more aggressive toward other males or toward females disguised with male coloration than toward normal females.

Variation of agonistic tendencies with the separation between opponents is probably a general phenomenon. Male fiddler crabs *(Uca terpsichores)* increase their rate of claw-waving in response to a test stimulus (a tethered crab) as the stimulus distance decreases (Zucker, 1974). The response of groups of gray-cheeked mangabeys to the playback of a call used in intergroup spacing depends strongly on their distance from the playback speaker (Figure 5) (Waser, 1975a).

Does spacing in natural circumstances ever result from agonistic tendencies that vary solely with separation between opponents? Evidence that individuals avoid each other without relation to their locations is available for mangabeys and for cheetahs *(Acinonyx jubatus)*. The tendency of mangabey groups to move away from spacing calls of other groups within a few hundred meters does not depend on the group's location in the home range; groups showed no significant differences in responses at their home range center and periphery (Waser, 1975a). Moreover, there is no preference for retreat toward the center of the group's range. Observations and experiments also confirm that mutual long-distance avoidance occurs without respect to the relative sizes of interacting groups.

Groups of cheetahs also avoid each other at a distance, although persistent olfactory signals rather than long-range acoustic signals mediate the interactions (Eaton, 1970). Observations of cheetahs' natural movements suggest that the locality at which an individual contacts another's trail does not influence its immediate reaction. Adult males in small bisexual groups leave olfactory marks by directional urination every 30–100 m as the groups move. When a group detects another's mark, they tend to spread out until a second mark is located and then depart approximately at right angles to the predecessors' trail. The urine marks evoke reactions from later groups for about 24 hours after deposit. This study, however, could not eliminate the possibility that the locations of olfactory contacts might have some influence on the followers' subsequent direction of movement or that marking might differ in frequency in different parts of a group's range.

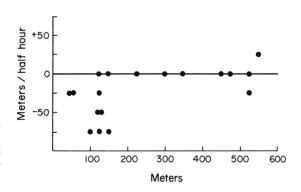

Fig. 5. Net change in rate of movement of mangabey groups as a function of the distance from site of spacing-call playbacks to nearest individual in the group. From Waser, 1976.

PETER M. WASER
AND R. HAVEN
WILEY

Mutual avoidance of other individuals or their signs, without regard to the location of encounters, generates "time-plan" dispersion (Leyhausen and Wolff, 1959), in which at any instant an individual is unlikely to have others nearby. If, in addition, individuals practiced long-term avoidance of areas in which contacts with others were too frequent, then site-independent avoidance could generate regularly spaced activity fields or even exclusive areas. The spacing of feral house cats, mangabeys, and cheetahs might indeed illustrate these conditions (Leyhausen and Wolff, 1959; Eaton, 1970), although the arrangement of activity fields and the nature of isolation fields need further study in these species.

Regular dispersion of activity fields in suitable habitat characterizes populations from diverse taxa, including pumas *(Felis concolor)* (Hornocker, 1969), antbirds *(Gymopithys bicolor)* (Willis, 1967), American robin *(Turdus migratorius)* (Young, 1951), and lizards *(Uta stansburiana)* (Tinkle, 1965). Overdispersion of activity fields may persist even when overlap is extensive, as in olive baboons *(Papio anubis)* in Nairobi National Park, Kenya (DeVore and Hall, 1965). Mutual avoidance without regard to location, in combination with long-term avoidance of areas in which other individuals or their signs are frequently encountered, could theoretically produce such patterns, but regular spacing usually results from some pattern of variation in agonistic tendencies with location.

Agonistic behavior that varies solely with the separation between opponents would be sufficient to generate overdispersed territories in one special case: small territories that residents can survey in their entirety from habitual locations. Nesting black-headed gulls *(Larus ridibundus)* exemplify this situation. Patterson (1965) has shown that the tendencies of a resident to attack or threaten a strange intruder depend entirely on the intruder's distance from the resident's current location rather than its distance from the resident's nest or habitual perch. Resident gulls maintain nearly exclusive territories because each usually perches at a "station" near the center of its small territory. Thus, an intruder near the center of the territory is also usually near the resident.

Effects of proximity and location on aggression can interact, as during the transition from winter flocks to spring territories in certain passerine birds. Often, an individual establishing a territory first localizes its activities around certain preferred singing sites, and then the distance at which opponents evoke aggression gradually increases (Conder, 1949, 1956; Marler, 1956a,c). Eventually, the resident's agonistic tendencies come to depend more on the location of an encounter with an intruder than on the intruder's proximity. There are, however, no quantitative studies of this interaction of location and proximity in determining a territorial resident's agonistic tendencies.

In conclusion, when individuals' activity fields are overdispersed, with less overlap than predicted for randomly positioned activity fields, the spacing of activity fields and the form of individuals' isolation fields often develop from some pattern of spatial variation in the individuals' agonistic tendencies. To generate such overdispersion, individuals both evoke withdrawal by others from specific areas, either by employing long-range or persistent signals or by directly challenging intruders, and avoid individuals or their signs in other areas.

In the earliest accounts, a territory was recognized as the locus of positions in which the resident won agonistic encounters. When territorial individuals met opponents beyond this locus, they either reliably "lost" or the outcome was less predictable, depending on whether the opponent was within its territory or not (Howard, 1920; Nice, 1941). Site-specific dominance has subsequently become an explicit criterion for territoriality (Emlen, 1957). Beginning with Huxley's (1934) analogy between a bird's territory and a rubber disc, permitting limited contraction under external pressure, ethologists have proposed that a territorial resident's aggressiveness decreases away from the center of its territory (Fitch, 1940: van Iersel, 1958; Tinbergen, 1960; Harris, 1964; van den Assem, 1967).

In documenting such spatial variation in agonistic tendencies, one must carefully distinguish between the *frequencies* of agonistic encounters and each individual's behavioral *tendencies* during encounters. Evidence for spatial variation in agonistic tendencies requires studies of an individual's responses to similar opponents in different locations. For example, laughing gulls *(Larus atricilla),* which defend nesting territories within a colony, react less frequently with threats and chases as the distance of an intruder from the subject's nest increases (Burger and Beer, 1975). In three-spined sticklebacks *(Gasterosteus aculeatus),* standard opponents evoke progressively less aggression from a territorial male the farther the opponent is from the resident's nest (van Iersel, 1958).

Experiments with playbacks of tape-recorded vocalizations have suggested that several species of territorial passerines respond more intensely to playbacks from the center of their territories than to playbacks of the same stimulus from the periphery (Dhondt, 1966; Ickes and Ficken, 1970; Brooks and Falls, 1975). However, a difference in average responses to playbacks in central and peripheral positions might also arise if subjects were less likely to detect a peripheral stimulus promptly. Definite confirmation of an effect of the location of playback on aggressive tendencies might involve examining the subjects' responses after approaching the speaker or, even better, locating the subject before each playback in order to control for the initial distance between the subject and the speaker.

Observations of site-dependent dominance in the field also suggest that individuals' agonistic tendencies vary with location. A number of these studies have focused on territorial passerines that reside year round near their breeding areas but range more widely during winter months than during the breeding season. Territorial Steller's jays *(Cyanocitta stelleri)* during the winter become progressively lower in rank at feeding stations as they move farther from the locations of their breeding territories (Brown, 1963). Other examples are birds specialized for feeding at swarms of army ants in tropical forests. Individuals frequently must travel considerable distances to find a swarm on any particular day. Among bicolored antbirds *(Gymnopithys bicolor),* each pair has an area within which it dominates all other conspecific individuals at ant swarms, and each individual's rank drops the farther it is from this territory (Willis, 1967, 1972). An example of a mammal with site-dependent dominance is the chipmunk *(Tamias striatus*) (Dunford, 1970). In this species, an individual's area of dominance corresponds to the central portion of its range.

Variation with location in an individual's aggression toward opponents suggests a third function of spatial coordinates, in addition to activity and isolation fields, with special relevance for the behavioral control of spacing: an *aggression field*. We can define this field as the value of some measure of an individual's agonistic tendencies in encounters with specified opponents at different locations. As we have seen, an individual's agonistic tendencies toward an opponent often vary with its proximity to the subject as well as its absolute location. The concept of an aggression field is best restricted to variation in a subject's agonistic tendencies with an opponent's absolute location, when proximity to the subject is controlled. In this sense, the concept serves to emphasize the special importance of this aspect of agonistic behavior for the behavioral mechanisms that regulate spacing.

No aggression field has ever been measured in any detail. Perhaps van Iersel (1958) came closest when he determined the decline in aggressiveness of male sticklebacks toward standard opponents as distance from the subject's nest increased. Van den Assem (1967) called this function an "aggression gradient." Patterson (1965) and Burger and Beer (1975) obtained similar measurements for nesting gulls.

Accurate measurement of an individual's aggression field might encounter a difficulty not met with activity and isolation fields. If an individual's tendencies to attack and avoid do not strongly covary across locations, no aggression field of a single variable can completely describe spatial variation in an individual's tendencies in encounters. Nevertheless, the available observations in natural situations suggest, as a good first hypothesis, that a single variable can often describe changes with location in an individual's agonistic tendencies toward specified opponents.

Variation in agonistic tendencies with location might result from any one, or a combination, of three influences on agonistic behavior, considered in turn below: effects of familiarity with the site of an encounter; effects of previous experience at the site of an encounter; and effects of external referents for aggression. These effects have received considerable attention in experimental studies, but their importance for spacing in natural populations has had no systematic appraisal.

LOCATION EFFECTS AS A RESULT OF DIFFERENTIAL FAMILIARITY WITH THE ENCOUNTER SITE. The predictable polarity in the interactions of intruders with residents in their territories was early attributed to the psychological advantage of the individual on familiar ground (Howard, 1920; Nice, 1941). Familiarity with the site of an encounter has such a strong effect on an encounter's outcome that it is standard practice to control this variable in experimental studies of aggression. Early experiments with fish, lizards, doves, and mice have established that prior residence in an enclosure confers an advantage, often insurmountable, in encounters with intruders (Evans, 1936: Ulrich, 1938; Diebschlag, 1941: Guhl and Allee, 1944; Braddock, 1949; Baerends and Baerends-van Roon, 1950; Ritchey, 1951). Recently, Zayan (1975, 1976) found for platyfish *(Xiphophorus)* hybrids that prior residence in an aquarium for three hours was sufficient to establish an individual's dominance over subsequently introduced individuals.

In natural circumstances as well, prior residence often confers dominance. For instance, among tits of several species of *Parus,* individuals gather in winter flocks in which the highest-ranking individual is the male whose previous breeding territory is included in the flock's range. Sometimes, this male's area of dominance is greater in winter than during the breeding season, so that he comes to dominate during the winter his former territorial neighbors (Dixon, 1963, 1965; Hartzler, 1970; Glase, 1973). In addition, chickadees transported to a new area become subordinate to the resident individuals (Odum, 1941), although this result does not separate effects of unfamiliar opponents from effects of an unfamiliar location.

It seems probable that this effect of familiarity with the site of an encounter on aggressive tendencies is related to the effects of novel environments on exploratory and "emotional" or " fearful" behavior. A recent experiment with territorial jewelfish *(Hemichromis bimaculatus)* (Heuts and Boer, 1973) suggests this connection. When transferred to a new aquarium, the fish tended to establish their new territories in close relationship to conspicuous objects that resembled those in their previous territories. These results, however, do not allow us to separate the individual's tendencies to remain near familiar objects from the effects of those familiar objects on their agonistic tendencies.

The connection between reactions to novel environments and aggressiveness has received only intermittent attention, in spite of some interesting results. Mice bred for lower defecation rates in novel environments (an indication of "fearful" or "emotional" behavior) are also more aggressive (Hall and Klein, 1942); conversely, mice bred for aggressiveness have lower defecation rates in a novel environment (Lagerspetz, 1961). For the fish *Trichogaster trichopterus,* prior residence in an aquarium, which predisposes an individual to dominance over others introduced later, reduces indications of fear but does not increase aggression (Frey and Miller, 1972). Tendencies to avoid strong stimuli, including threatening conspecifics, in novel circumstances would have clear relevance for spacing behavior.

The effects of prior residence on agonistic tendencies can result in territories of different sizes, depending on whether or not individuals establish themselves simultaneously. To obtain the maximum number of territorial individuals in experimental situations, usually small fish in large aquaria, the investigator must introduce all individuals into the enclosure simultaneously (see van den Assem, 1967). When individuals are introduced sequentially, those with precedence are able to exclude latecomers from much larger areas. Knapton and Krebs (1974) have documented a similar phenomenon in wild song sparrows *(Melospiza melodia).* Populations are denser when a habitat is settled synchronously rather than asynchronously. In this case, however, the latecomers are also younger individuals. Maynard Smith (1974a) presented a formal model of this effect of synchrony in territory establishment.

LOCATION EFFECTS AS A RESULT OF PREVIOUS ENCOUNTERS AT THE SITE. The value of an individual's aggression field might be expected to correlate point by point with the value of its activity field for two reasons: (1) as discussed above, an individual's familiarity with any location, as determined by the intensity of its use,

PETER M. WASER
AND R. HAVEN
WILEY

affects its dominance there; or (2) it might avoid locations where it had previously lost encounters. The two possibilities are not mutually exclusive. In the early stages of territory establishment, chance differences in the values of the activity field in the zone of overlap might influence the outcomes of encounters there; if neighbors tended to avoid locations where they had lost encounters, the centers of their activity fields might subsequently shift farther apart.

A lasting tendency to avoid sites of low dominance would also explain the persistence of boundaries during the replacement of a territorial resident by a newcomer. In such circumstances, the newcomer often comes to have nearly the same boundaries as its predecessor (for instance, Owen-Smith, 1975; Wiley, 1973), so that boundaries in a population of territorial individuals become traditional. There are no experimental studies of the mechanisms that maintain such traditions in the locations of boundaries.

EXTERNAL REFERENTS FOR AGONISTIC TENDENCIES. Proximity to external referents, such as mates, nests, or critical food sources, can also influence an individual's agonistic tendencies at a particular location. The importance of proximity to an external referent is especially clear when the referent moves. For parents of many species, their young serve as external referents for threat and attack when conspecifics approach too close. In many species, protection of young is the primary determinant of aggressive behavior by females.

In species that form pair affiliations, partners often direct aggression or threat to nearby individuals other than the partner. This phenomenon has been variously interpreted as defense of the mate, redirection of aggressive tendencies evoked by proximity to the mate, and coupling between the motivational systems of aggression and sexual behavior. Among wildebeest *(Connochaetus taurinus)*, as in many other ungulates, males in sedentary populations maintain exclusive mating rights within fixed areas to which they attempt to attract female herds, but in some migratory populations, wildebeest males attempt instead to set up temporary exclusive areas with respect to the locations of females rather than fixed spatial referents (Estes, 1969; Jarman, 1974). In many primates and ungulates, males form consort relations with estrous females and attack other males that approach too closely.

Tree squirrels of the genus *Tamiasciurus* demonstrate another possible relationship of agonistic tendencies to mates as an external referent (Smith, 1968). Both sexes maintain largely exclusive territories throughout the year. During the mating season, several males enter the territory of an estrous female on the one day that copulations occur. During this day, females relax their aggressive tendencies toward intruding males. One male quickly establishes its dominance over the others and then follows the female closely, except for forays to chase other approaching males.

Individuals of the opposite sex sometimes are external referents for agonistic tendencies even when individuals occupy stationary territories. A male yellow-hooded blackbird *(Agelaius icterocephalus)*, for instance, is more likely to attack or threaten a strange male near the periphery of its territory or even in neighbors' territories when the stranger has closely approached a female. Males of this neotropical species maintain territories in marshes and attract a succession of females to nest in their territories. During the three to four days immediately preceding egg laying by one of a male's mates, he becomes aggressive even toward other females within several meters of the mate (Wiley, personal observation).

The effects of females on agonistic interactions between males have received surprisingly little experimental investigation. In domestic mice, the presence of a female or odors from females reduce fighting between males (Fredericson, Story, Gurney, and Butterworth, 1955; Mugford, 1973). Prior sexual experience reduces a previously naive male's aggression in a subsequent encounter with another male four days later (Lagerspetz and Hautojarvi, 1967). In laboratory colonies of wild rats *(Rattus norvegicus),* males do not usually fight in the presence of an estrous or proestrous female, but males do begin to fight after a female leaves them (Barnett, 1963) or when two or more males visit a site marked by an estrous female (Calhoun, 1962).

In contrast, recent experiments with zebra finches *(Taeniopygia guttata)* have shown that a male's aggression toward a male partner increases dramatically in the presence of a female (Caryl, 1975). The effectiveness of the stimulus female declines sharply with her distance from the two males. In comparison with a strange female, a male's mate has a slightly greater effect on his aggression toward a male partner. These effects seem likely to increase the spacing of males near females.

A den, a nest, or localized food also often serves as an external referent for an individual's agonistic tendencies. For instance, aggression within a group of mangabeys increases tenfold when they exploit the basketball-sized fruits of *Treculia* (Chalmers, 1968b), an effect repeatedly noted in studies of artificially provisioned primates (Wrangham, 1974). This effect of concentrated food sources is taxonomically widespread; coconut crabs *Birgus latro* have an elaborate repertoire of agonistic behaviors displayed on encounters at opened coconuts (Hel, 1975). Aggressive behavior near concentrated food in some cases could result entirely from the proximity of individuals in these circumstances, but in mangabeys, coconut crabs, and other cases, the presence of concentrated food evokes aggression when similar proximity of individuals in other circumstances does not.

The converse of this situation is demonstrated by cases of low aggression in the absence of a referent. Oates (1976) found that the normally aggressive relationships between groups of black-and white colobus *(Colobus guereza)* can break down when these normally arboreal, leaf-eating monkeys visit small ponds to forage on aquatic vegetation; ranges of many otherwise territorial groups overlap at this location, and groups intermingle peacefully. In baboons and vervets, aggressive interactions are often suppressed at waterholes, which represent spatially limited but not ecologically limiting resources (S. Altmann, 1974; DeVore and Hall, 1965; Struhsaker, 1967).

In species that show little agonistic behavior of other sorts, individuals still frequently attack or threaten conspecifics at the nest or den. In one experiment to determine the influence of nests on an aggression field, the nests of female red-winged blackbirds *(Agelaius phoeniceus)* were moved to new locations near or across the original male's boundary (Nero and Emlen, 1951). Males did not expand their territories to include the new positions of their mates' nests, perhaps because red-winged blackbirds lack strong associations with their mates once the females begin incubation. In contrast, studies of a tropical congener, the yellow-hooded blackbird, suggest that changes in activity fields, and subsequent changes in aggression fields, follow shifts in the location of active nests in a male's territory (Wiley, personal observation). In this species, unlike red-winged blackbirds, the male constructs the nests in his territory.

The influences of external referents on individuals' agonistic tendencies probably include avoidance of other individuals' referents. For instance, male common grackles *(Quiscalus quiscula)* seldom closely approach females accompanied by other males (Wiley, 1976a). Male hamadryas baboons *(Papio hamadryas)* refrain from challenging one another for females associated with another male (Kummer, Götz, and Angst, 1974). Somewhat analogous is the "protected threat" of many primate species, which depends on avoidance by the threatened individual as a result of the presence of another, referent individual.

Proximity to an external referent, such as a particular female or nest, presumably both increases one individual's aggressive tendencies and reduces the other's. In the defense of a mate or young, the relevant distance that influences an individual's aggression is probably that between the referent and the opponent, while protected threat probably depends on the distance between an individual and the referent. However, no experimental studies have yet documented the variation in agonistic tendencies with changes in the pertinent separations between subject, referent, and opponent.

In conclusion, the proximate control of spatial variation in an individual's agonistic tendencies includes effects of (1) the individual's proximity to opponents; (2) its proximity to external referents for aggression; (3) its opponent's proximity to such referents; and (4) its familiarity with the location and previous experience in agonistic encounters there. The determinants of an individual's activity field and its aggression field are likely to have reciprocal effects on each other.

INDIVIDUAL AND POPULATION DIFFERENCES IN AGONISTIC TENDENCIES

The preceding sections have examined the interactions among an individual's agonistic tendencies, its spatial relationships with opponents and external referents, and its familiarity with different locations. The available literature, for the most part, documents these interactions only vaguely. Nevertheless, it is clear that both spacing and agonistic behavior vary with age and season for any one individual and among populations and species.

Physiological, genetic, and experiential determinants of these differences remain largely unexplored. Endocrine and genetic differences with sex, age, and season, which have extensively documented effects on dominance and aggressiveness in laboratory situations, are almost certainly associated with these same differences in agonistic behavior under natural circumstances. In one of the few attempts to administer steroid hormones to animals in natural circumstances (Emlen and Lorenz, 1942), results dramatically matched naturally occurring changes in agonistic behavior and interanimal spacing. In this case, implants of an androgen in male valley quail*(Lophortyx californicus)* during the winter resulted in prompt increases in aggressive behavior by the implanted birds in their covey and, within a few weeks, their separation from the covey, behavior that normally coincides with the start of breeding activity in the spring. Individual differences in agonistic tendencies depend in complex ways on differences in hormone levels and previous social experience. Androgen levels and success in territorial interactions can mutually reinforce each other (Bramley and Neaves, 1972).

EFFECTS OF PREVIOUS EXPERIENCE. One effect of social experience that might influence spacing behavior is a change in agonistic tendencies as a result of the frequency of interactions in a preceding period. In laboratory rodents, isolation induces increased aggression in tests with pairs of isolated males (Valzelli, 1969; Banerjee, 1971; Spencer, Gray, and Dalhouse, 1973). Incidence of aggression by such pairs increases with the duration of isolation. Conversely, aggression eventually decreases between isolated mice subjected to repeated tests at approximately weekly intervals (Banerjee, 1971). Isolation of hermit crabs *(Pagurus samuelis)* similarly increases an individual's dominance, its probability of initiating aggression, and its frequencies of high-intensity aggressive actions in tests with group-held opponents (Courchesne and Barlow, 1971). After a period of deprivation from any opportunity to see rivals, damselfish *(Microspathodon chrysurus)* spend more time in a small chamber with a view of a rival (Rasa, 1971). Since the subjects performed normal aggressive displays in the chamber when in sight of a rival, Rasa concluded that the amount of time spent in the small chamber was a measure of the subject's readiness to fight.

Other experiments have led to the opposite conclusion: isolation from opponents reduces aggressiveness. For example, when hermit crabs (*Clibanarius* species) are held at high or low densities (17 and 35 cm²/crab) for a week, those with experience of low densities retreat from opponents at nearly twice the distance as those from high densities. Consequently, crabs from low densities lose most of their encounters with opponents from high densities (Hazlett, 1974). In another example, the cichlid *Haplochromis burtoni* becomes less aggressive toward small, blinded stimulus fish after being deprived of normal opponents (Heiligenberg and Kramer, 1972).

Two basic parameters of these experiments have received little systematic attention: the specificity of the deprived stimulation and the specificity of the effects for different responses or stimulus preferences. For instance, "isolation" in most experiments involves deprivation from all stimulation except a bare cage. In these circumstances, mice become hyperreactive and hyperkinetic (Valzelli, 1969; Banerjee, 1971). Are changes in aggressiveness the primary effects of such deprivation? Does contact with partners of different sex or age have different tonic effects on aggressive tendencies? Is exposure to conspecifics without contact as effective as exposure with contact? Rasa (1971) explored these questions in a preliminary way. She determined, for instance, that a moving inanimate stimulus did not substitute for a rival fish in reducing the effects of deprivation and thereby ruled out a decrease of stimulation in general as an explanation for her results. In

PETER M. WASER
AND R. HAVEN
WILEY

addition, she concluded that the effects of deprivation were not entirely explained by an increase of activity in general, although changes in activities other than clear aggression occurred after deprivation. In these first attempts to determine the specificity of the stimulus and the effects of deprivation, Rasa included no investigation of nonaggressive interactions with conspecifics.

When the opponent's previous social experience is manipulated, in addition to the subject's, the behavior of isolated male mice and gerbils depends on the treatment of the opponent. Isolated animals tested with animals from groups often do not fight. Isolated male gerbils are more likely to investigate their partners during tests in a new environment, while males with continuous social experience investigate objects rather than their partner in the test (Spencer *et al.,* 1973). This difference in the orientation of exploratory behavior leads to more frequent fights when isolates are tested together than when isolates are tested with nonisolates or when nonisolates are tested together. The predominant orientation of isolated animals to their partners in tests perhaps explains why isolated mice are not more dominant or more likely to initiate aggression when tested in their own, as opposed to the partner's, home cage (Banerjee, 1971).

A related effect of previous experience might also influence spacing: a history of defeats or wins in dyadic encounters results in tonic suppression or facilitation of aggression toward strangers (Collias, 1943; Scott and Fredericson, 1951; Lagerspetz, 1961). This effect probably has little influence on spacing behavior in natural populations, where individuals usually withdraw from encounters before serious defeat and, by moving to new areas, can avoid long histories of defeat. Within cohesive groups, in contrast, suppressed aggression following repeated losses probably has important effects on the structure of agonistic behavior. Spacing is perhaps most directly affected by this mechanism when some individuals remain as subordinates associated with territorial individuals rather than establishing their own exclusive areas, as do male white rhinoceros *(Ceratotherium simum)* (Owen-Smith, 1972, 1975).

When rates of social interaction with opponents have tonic effects on an individual's agonistic tendencies, these effects tend to damp any changes in spacing in response to transient changes in population pressure. Morse (1976) found that the sizes of warblers' *(Parulidae)* territories changed less rapidly than did population density over a period of several years, an indication that such inertia in spacing behavior occurs in the field. Tonic increases in individuals' aggressive tendencies in sparse populations would counteract abrupt changes in spacing in response to changes in the numbers of individuals seeking to establish themselves.

Experiments on the effects of previous experience on aggression have generally not attempted to elucidate the control of spacing in natural circumstances. Studies should consider (1) a greater range of the subjects' responses, including avoidance; (2) different kinds of stimulation from social interactions; and (3) different rates of exposure to social stimulation. Conclusions about the effects of different rates and kinds of social interaction on aggressiveness would have direct relevance to an understanding of individual and population differences in spacing in natural circumstances.

EFFECTS OF FOOD AVAILABILITY. In some species, territory sizes in different habitats correlate with the densities of available food in these habitats (see Schoener, 1968b). Stenger (1958) has come close to a direct demonstration of this relationship by sampling insect densities in the leaf litter of different habitats of ovenbirds *(Seiurus aurocapillus)*. In red grouse *(Lagopus lagopus)*, differences in territory sizes among populations correlate with the nutrient content of growing heather, the principal food of the adult grouse (Miller, Jenkins, and Watson, 1966; Miller, Watson, and Jenkins, 1970; Moss, 1969). Year-to-year changes in territory densities of any one grouse population are also correlated with changes in heather quality but with a one-year lag in the response. Indirect evidence suggests that differences in territory size among populations of other species might also correlate with densities of available food. Moreover, individuals of some species, like the white wagtail *(Motacilla alba)* in winter, switch from a relatively unaggressive state to vigorous defense of small territories in the presence of concentrated food sources (Zahavi, 1971). In some nectar-feeding birds, aggressive interactions decrease at high food densities when food becomes superabundant (Gill and Wolf, 1975a; Carpenter and MacMillen, 1976b). However, food densities do not always regulate agonistic tendencies, since seasonal changes in territorial behavior in some bird populations are not synchronized with seasonal changes in food availability or dispersion (see Watson and Moss, 1970).

If individuals adjust their spacing to the available food, their tendencies to avoid, threaten, approach, and attack conspecifics at different locations or separations must change when food supplies change. These adjustments do not require direct responses to the ease or frequency of finding food or to the individual's hunger, but such responses would provide a mechanism for regulating spatial relationships in relation to food availability.

Experimental studies have explored the effects of acute food deprivation on the frequency of aggression between individuals in small groups. Such studies and anecdotal reports of field observations usually provide evidence that rates of aggression increase with hunger. However, according to more careful analyses of interactions in small flocks of finches and buntings, hunger increases the frequency of close approaches between individuals by reducing individuals' tendencies to avoid more dominant individuals, so that circumstances provoking threat and attack occur more frequently, yet the probability of attacks from a given separation remains unchanged (Marler, 1956b; Andrew, 1956). Rohles and Wilson (1974) have similarly shown that food deprivation increases the frequency of aggression among laboratory mice by increasing the frequency of close approach.

The effects of chronic hunger might differ from those of acute deprivation. Field studies of a North American bunting *(Junco hyemalis)* suggest that hunger, as a result of low temperatures during winter, reduces the frequency of aggression at localized food sources (Sabine, 1959; Pulliam, 1974). Pulliam's observations show that during colder weather, frequencies of threat and attack decrease for any separation of individuals. Sabine suggested that dominant individuals in these circumstances become habituated to the persistent, close approaches of subordinates. These field studies thus indicate that hunger reduces aggressive tendencies

PETER M. WASER
AND R. HAVEN
WILEY

for any specified separation of opponents, although temperature might directly affect activity. The changes in agonistic behavior of sunbirds and wagtails around concentrated food sources (see above) also suggest that in some circumstances a full stomach, rather than hunger, can encourage sedentariness and aggression.

AGONISTIC INTERACTIONS AND INDIVIDUAL DIFFERENCES IN TERRITORY SIZE. Within a population, individuals often differ in the sizes of their territories, and these differences are often thought to reflect individuals' differences in aggressiveness. Attempts to relate territory size to the resident's agonistic behavior, however, indicate that this relationship is complex.

Among red grouse in Scotland, territory size within one population correlated with an index of aggression based on both the frequency and the outcome of a resident's agonistic interactions (Watson and Miller, 1971). Although these authors inferred that greater aggression causes the larger territories, this causality is not certainly established. If larger territories had more frequent intruders, residents would engage in more frequent agonistic interactions. If intruders normally withdrew, holders of large territories would also have more frequent interactions in which the opponent withdrew. The greater index of aggression might thus result from, rather than cause, the larger territories. Since males implanted with testosterone enlarge their territories (Watson, 1970), a resident's aggressiveness clearly influences territory size, at least when neighbor's tendencies are not manipulated. In natural circumstances, territory size is likely to result from an interaction of the resident's and the neighbors' tendencies. Available evidence, however, does not establish the nature of this interaction. The finding that the sizes of territories in any one area and year correlate with the quality of food they contain (Lance, 1978b) suggests either that males adjust their aggressiveness in inverse relation to the quality of available food (Watson and Moss, 1972) or that competition for territories is greater in locations with better food. Variation in territory size from year to year also admits of alternate explanations. When breeding success is high, more young males subsequently establish territories, these territories are smaller, and aggression is lower than when breeding success is low (Watson and Miller, 1971). This situation could result from differences in the intrinsic aggressiveness of males reared in good and bad years (Watson and Moss, 1972) or from differences in the intensity of competition for territories in accordance with the numbers of young males reared. To establish the relative effects of residents' and neighbors' tendencies in the determination of territory sizes, it would help to study the responses of territorial males to standard stimuli.

To investigate the probability and intensity of attack or threat by an individual toward a standard opponent in a controlled location, Spurr (1974) presented realistic models to territorial Adélie penguins *(Pygoscelis adeliae)* in a dense nesting colony. Individuals with high rates of pecking tended to have more central locations in the colony and higher breeding success than did individuals with lower rates of pecking. The central location of the more aggressive individuals is probably only partly caused by their aggressiveness, as the older central individuals tend to return to the nesting area before the younger, peripheral penguins. Thus, younger individuals occupy larger territories in less desirable areas, and although they have lower aggressive tendencies in an experimental situation, they encounter more intruders and engage in more frequent agonistic encounters.

When neighboring territories differ in their attractiveness for residents, territory sizes are determined as much by neighbors' tendencies as by the residents'. On leks of sage grouse *(Centrocercus urophasianus),* where most copulations occur at the center of an aggregation of males' territories, a male spends most of its time on the side of its territory nearest this mating center. Among pairs of neighbors with territories along a radius from the center, the more central individual initiates most boundary interactions by dashing across his territory, from his preferred place closest to the center, to confront his neighbor encroaching centripetally. Consequently, residents initiate most of their encounters with more peripheral neighbors and parry the challenges received from their more central neighbors (Wiley, 1973). The central territories are smaller, presumably owing both to the greater preoccupation of the residents with females and the greater pressure of more peripheral neighbors toward the mating center. The behavioral regulation of an individual's isolation field in these sage grouse, as in red grouse and penguins, most likely depends on the external pressure from intruders as well as on the internal resistance from the resident.

Categories of Individuals That Engage in Spacing Behavior

Differentiation of the Sexes. In species as diverse as weasels (*Mustela* species) (Lockie, 1966), parrotfish *(Scarus croicensis)* (Buckman and Ogden, 1973), and dragonflies, *Odonata* (Campanella and Wolf, 1974), the sexes differ in their spacing behavior. In polygamous species of both birds and mammals, aggression between members of the limiting sex is reportedly infrequent. In many polygynous ungulates, females are gregarious while males tend to be solitary and mutually aggressive (Jarman, 1974; Geist and Walther, 1974). Among tenrecs, prosimians, and other "solitary" mammals, females' home ranges often overlap more than do males' (Charles-Dominique, 1974; Eisenberg, 1975, 1977). In most monkey species, males play the primary role in intergroup conflicts (Clutton-Brock and Harvey, 1976). When both sexes are involved in spacing interactions, aggression is generally intrasexual; in the red-winged blackbird, females have been reported to defend small territories among themselves within the larger territories of a male (Nero, 1956).

Among monogamous species, females vary from showing almost no participation in territorial defense to participating as extensively as males. In the American robin (*Turdus migratorius*), a monagamous species with extensive territories, quantitative information is available on agonistic behavior of both sexes (Young, 1951). The activity fields of neighboring pairs overlap extensively in this species, although the areas used most intensively by each pair (core areas) overlap much less. Both sexes are more likely to engage in intrasexual than intersexual interactions. Females have greater success in both intra- and intersexual interactions within their own core areas than outside them, but location seems not to influence the success of males.

TABLE II. SOME EXAMPLES OF SEXUAL ROLES IN TERRITORIAL DEFENSE AMONG
MONOGAMOUS PASSERINE BIRDS

A. Both Sexes Regularly Defend Territory against Intruders
   1. Species with sexually monomorphic plumage; territorial defense both intra- and intersexual
         Wheatear *Oenanthe oenanthe*
            (Conder, 1956)
         Wrentit *Chamaea fasciata*
            (Erickson, 1938)
         Black-capped chickadee *Parus atricapillus*
            (Stefanski, 1967)
         European robin *Erithacus rubecula*
            (Lack, 1943)
   2. Species with sexually dimorphic plumage; territorial defense intrasexual only
         American redstart *Setophaga ruticilla*
            (Ficken, 1962)
          Galapagos finches, Geospizinae[a]
            (Lack, 1954)
         Chaffinch *Fringilla coelebs*
            (Marler, 1956a)
         Snow bunting *Plectrophenax nivalis*
            (Tinbergen, 1939)
         American robin *Turdus migratorius*[b]
            (Young, 1951)
B. Male Only Defends Territory against Intruders; Territorial Defense Both Intra- and Intersexual
         House wren *Troglodytes aedon*
            (Kendeigh, 1941)
         Ovenbird *Seiurus auricapillus*
            (Stenger and Falls, 1959)
         Great tit *Parus major*
            (Hinde, 1952)
         Meadowlarks *Sturnella magna, S. neglecta*
            (Lanyon, 1957)
         Song sparrow *Melospiza melodia*[c]
            (Nice, 1943)

[a]Males defend territories against intruders of both sexes, females only against other females.
[b]Species with weakly developed dimorphism in plumage; territorial defense primarily but not exclusively intrasexual (see text).
[c]Defense primarily intrasexual.

    Though quantitative data for other avian species are lacking, the degree to which females regularly confront intruding individuals appears to correlate with sexual dimorphism (Table II). In monogamous dimorphic species, females are normally involved in territorial defense, but, as in American robins, they normally engage only other females. In some monogamous, monomorphic species, like the European robin *(Erithracus rubecula),* both sexes regularly defend the territory; in others, like the meadowlarks *(Sturnella* species), only males do so. In both cases, however, defense is inter- as well as intrasexual.

    Among mammals, spacing is commonly intrasexual, and male and female activity fields are often not congruent. In many carnivores, especially Felidae and Mustelidae, males have large, mutually exclusive ranges that overlap the smaller ranges of females (Lockie, 1966; Erlinge, 1968; Hornocker, 1969; Muckenhirn and Eisenberg, 1973; Kleiman and Eisenberg, 1973).

    Among dikdiks *(Madoqua kirki),* elephant shrews *(Elephantulus rufescens* and

Rhyncocyon chrysopygus), and red fox *(Vulpes vulpes)*, male and female home ranges become completely overlapping, so that mating occurs exclusively within pairs even though individuals are only occasionally associated spatially (Hendrichs and Hendrichs, 1971; Kleiman, 1977; Rathbun, in press). Among dikdiks, males defend largely exclusive territories against intruders of both sexes (Hendrichs and Hendrichs, 1971).

On the other hand, mammals with strong tendencies for long-term hetero-sexual associations combine monogamous bonds with sex-specific aggression. Among certain species of gibbon *(Hylobates)*, marmoset *(Callithrix)*, titi monkey *(Callicebus)*, and jackals *(Canis)*, members of a pair are nearly always found together, and aggression between pairs is primarily intrasexual (Chivers *et al.*, 1975; Epple, 1975; Kleiman, 1977; Moehlman, 1977; Robinson, in press; Tenaza, 1975)—a situation resembling that among monogamous, dimorphic birds.

Even among monogamous animals, mates' activity fields are not always congruent. In some species, mates never achieve a close match in the limits of their activity fields. Kendeigh (1941) reported that female house wrens *(Troglodytes aedon)* persistently venture beyond their mates' boundaries in spite of regular eviction by the neighboring males. In contrast, female tree sparrows have substantially smaller activity fields than males (Weeden, 1965).

Observers often note that females seem unaware of their mates' boundaries at first but that their activity fields eventually become more similar. Congruence between the activity fields of mates requires either (1) that one match its activity field to the other's by direct experience with its movements independent of agonistic interactions with neighbors or (2) that each develop corresponding relationships between its movements and agonistic interactions with neighbors. As reviewed previously, males sometimes modify their activity and aggression fields when their mates select nest sites near or beyond their previous territorial borders. These males appear to adjust their spacing behavior as a result of direct experience with their mate's movements. Agonistic interactions with neighbors, on the other hand, seem likely to influence the movements of females as well as males. Among some birds that are monomorphic in plumage, females maintain individual territories during the winter but join a male on his territory for breeding (Lack, 1943; Miller, 1931; Michener and Michener, 1935). During the process of pairing, when the female shifts her activity and aggression fields to coincide with those of her mate, both sexes defend the pair's territory against intruders. Similar trends have been found among monogamous mammals, for instance, gibbons (Tenaza, 1975) and some carnivores (Kleiman and Eisenberg, 1973). These considerations suggest that congruent activity fields of mates in monogamous species often require agonistic interactions of both males and females with neighbors, rather than adjustment of one member's activity field to the other's through direct experience with others' movements.

OTHER CATEGORIES OF OPPONENTS. An individual's agonistic behavior varies with attributes of an opponent other than its sex, particularly special behavior of the opponent and the opponent's familiarity. Field studies and some laboratory studies suggest that the probability or intensity of an individual's aggressive behavior often depends on the opponent's behavior. Early descriptions of territorial behavior in birds noted that intruding individuals often evoke the resident's aggression only after they sing (Tinbergen, 1939; Lack, 1943), and subsequent field studies have often reported similar observations. The European robin's red breast, the male chaffinch's orange underparts, and the orange opercular patch of of male cichlids *(Haplochromis burtoni)* increase the aggression evoked from other individuals (Lack, 1943; Marler, 1955b, 1956b; Heiligenberg, 1965; Leong, 1969). Among fish, coloration can change within seconds, so that a trespassing individual can adopt alternative color patterns quickly. In *Haplochromis,* a male that retains its nonterritorial coloration would escape much of a territorial resident's aggression even when detected. Among certain amphibians, birds, and mammals, specific behavior patterns of certain males allow them to coinhabit territorial males' activity fields. Cessation of calling and adoption of the "low" posture allows "satellite" male bullfrogs *(Rana catesbiana)* to remain within a few meters of calling males (Emlen, 1976). Ovenbirds tethered to the forest floor do not sing and are not attacked by the territory owner (Zach and Falls, in press). Tolerance by male white rhinos of other "nonterritorial" males is associated with their abandonment of spray-urination and dung-scattering behavior (Owen-Smith, 1975). Do transitory advertising displays, such as singing or scent marking, increase a resident's aggressive tendencies toward the signaler, or do they only increase the probability of detection?

Opponents' familiarity with each other usually decreases aggression. In studies of macaques, hens, rats, and mice, in which prior familiarity with an opponent reduced aggression, the establishment of familiarity included the establishment of a polarized, dominance–subordination relationship (e.g., Craig, Biswas, and Guhl, 1969; Southwick, Farooqui, Siddiqi, and Pal, 1974). During reunion after a period of separation, this relationship was evidently remembered and went unchallenged. In experiments with bobwhite quail *(Colinus virginianus)*, a reduction in aggression as a result of prior exposure to opponents did not even require that the initial exposure include physical contact (Garreffa, 1969). Relatively solitary species often fight bitterly without cessation when individuals are confined together (e.g., Lorenz, 1952). In natural circumstances, however, even solitary mammals become less aggressive toward each other with familiarity. Raccoons *(Procyon lotor)* and foxes *(Vulpes fulva)* engage in less aggression when conspecifics trapped at localities near each other are confined together than when conspecifics from more widely separated localities are paired (Barash, 1974).

Among territorial birds and fish, agonistic interactions between neighbors wane in frequency and intensity after territory establishment. Studies of convict cichlids *(Cichlasoma nigrofasciatum)* and three-spined sticklebacks *(Gasterosteus aculeatus)* have demonstrated the similarity between this phenomenon and other forms of habituation (Peeke, Herz, and Gallagher, 1971; van den Assem and van der Molen, 1969). Perhaps the most striking demonstrations of waning responses to neighbors have employed playbacks of advertising song to territorial passerines. Such experiments have shown that a wide variety of species respond much less reliably and intensely to playbacks of neighbors' songs than to strangers' songs. This difference apparently results in part from habituation of territorial residents' responses to advertising vocalizations heard regularly. Several studies have documented waning responses to repeated playbacks of advertising songs (Verner and

Milligan, 1971; Brooks and Falls, 1975); territorial male white-throated sparrows *(Zonotrichia albicollis)* respond more intensely to playbacks of neighbors' songs early in the season than later, while responses to playbacks of strangers' songs do not decrease (Brooks and Falls, 1975). On the other hand, a recent study of towhees *(Pipilo erythrophthalmus)* with abnormal songs demonstrated that neighbor–stranger discrimination can result from associative learning rather than habituation to familiar songs (Richards, in press).

Of special significance for the control of spacing are cases in which recognition of neighbors' vocalizations is specific to the usual direction from which the neighbor sings. This feature of neighbors' interactions has so far been demonstrated only for two species of passerines: white-throated sparrows, a species that establishes individual territories, and stripe-backed wrens *(Campylorhynchus nuchalis),* which maintain group territories and perform duets and choruses as advertising vocalizations (Falls and Brooks, 1975; Wiley and Wiley, 1977). At least in the latter species, residents do not attend to the differences between neighbors' vocalizations in the correct and the wrong places as promptly as they do to the differences between neighbors' and strangers' vocalizations. If neighbors rarely sang from outside their own territories, an ability to recognize neighbors out of place promptly would confer little selective advantage. Individual recognition of opponents and association of each with its usual locations are especially important when individuals' ranges overlap substantially.

Conclusion

Our review of the behavioral mechanisms of spacing began by emphasizing the importance of site-dependent agonistic behavior. Although changes in agonistic tendencies in accordance with the proximity of opponents influence the simultaneous locations of individuals, site-dependent agonistic behavior can more reliably generate evenly distributed activity fields. Yet, ethology so far has little clear evidence about the behavioral mechanisms that generate spatial variation in tendencies to approach, avoid, or attack opponents. A similar lack of precision or interest has also hampered our understanding of the behavioral mechanisms that produce individual and population differences in spacing behavior or the mechanisms that control spatial relationships of the sexes. The time seems ripe for a full integration of laboratory and field experimentation on aggression and spacing.

Communication of Advertisement or Threat

Analysis of spacing mechanisms is complicated by the existence of advertising behavior that influences the movements of a conspecific at locations or times removed from the performance of the behavior. Clearly, if an organism can elicit avoidance by its neighbors by means of a long-range or persistent signal rather than a physical contest, it stands to reduce both its risk of injury and its expenditure of energy by doing so. Because conspicuousness is an expected characteristic of such signals, it is not surprising that "distance-increasing" behaviors (Marler, 1968) have been widely described. They range from the urination of mice and the dung-piling of rhinoceroses to the bright colors of reef fish and the vocal choruses of bullfrogs, songbirds, and forest primates.

GENERAL CONSIDERATIONS

Spacing signals can modify the relationships between activity, aggression, and isolation fields in a number of ways. For instance, signals influence the distance and the locations at which neighbors detect each other and thus the degree to which they may penetrate each other's ranges without a face-to-face encounter. Perhaps even more important is the influence of signals on the means by which aggression fields regulate spatial relationships. Agonistic tendencies underlying overdispersed activity fields might emphasize either avoidance or aggression; overdispersion could result either from aggressive reactions to stealthy opponents or from avoidance of advertising signals. On the continuum between aggression and advertisment, on the one hand, and stealth and avoidance, on the other, species have struck different balances.

Environmental factors that alter neighbors' probabilities of detecting each other can have pronounced effects on their isolation fields. In laboratory situations, partial physical barriers within an enclosure sometimes allow two individuals to establish areas of dominance where only one becomes established in the absence of barriers (Sale, 1972; Jenni, 1972). Habitats with dense vegetation might have similar effects (Burger and Beer, 1975). By reducing movements, barriers might limit individuals' activity fields even in the absence of opponents and thus make it easier for a second individual to establish itself. In addition, the obstruction of communication by the barriers reduces the frequency of encounters across the barrier and consequently might permit the establishment of two individuals at closer spacing.

The costs as well as the efficacy of spacing signals vary between species. Perched hummingbirds *(Eulampis jugularis)* broadcast a continuous visual spacing signal at little caloric cost (Wolf and Hainsworth, 1971). When male black-and-white colobus bask in the sun in emergent trees, their conspicuous coat may even provide a net energy gain (Oates, 1976). Olfactory spacing signals used by mammals frequently involve the metabolic by-products sometimes produced by commensal bacteria (Gorman, Nedwell, and Smith, 1974). On the other hand, in singing katydids, metabolism can increase by an order of magnitude over resting rates (Stevens and Josephson, 1977). Even when the broadcasting of a spacing signal is energetically cheap, any conspicuous signal potentially carries an increased risk of predation. The magnitude of such risks remains to be investigated, but their presence suggests that the use of long-range signals should not be universal.

The possibility of substituting threats or long-distance signals for overt attacks also introduces two new behavioral alternatives not otherwise open to the contestants: bluffing, in essence suggesting a greater likelihood of detecting or evicting an intruder than actually exists; and calling bluffs, by ignoring spacing signals and attempting to avoid detection (Maynard Smith and Price, 1973; Parker, 1974; Maynard Smith and Parker, 1976). Consider a long-distance spacing call: it is advantageous for the sender to increase its range as long as this increases the area from which neighbors are excluded. But neighbors hearing the call can also use it to determine into which areas intrusion is unlikely to be detected, a possibility that increases with distance from the sender. How accurately, and over what distance, should an individual broadcast its location?

CHANNELS FOR SPACING SIGNALS

Presumed spacing signals have employed all sensory modalities, even electrical (Hopkins, 1974). For long-range transmission, the modalities of choice are usually auditory and olfactory: the former where separation of individuals in space at any one time is of primary importance; the latter especially for separation in time of activities at any one place. The channel of choice thus depends in part on the spatial and temporal distribution of the resources at issue and on their renewal rates.

The optimal modality for spacing communication also varies with the amount of interference in the available communication channels. Many forest primates, from lemurs to apes, possess long-range vocalizations with presumed spacing functions, whereas these have not been described in patas monkeys, baboons, geladas, or other primates of open country, where long-range visual communication is possible. The forest-living, nocturnal tree hyrax broadcasts its location several times nightly with deafening, long-distance screams, while the diurnal rock hyraxes have no comparable vocalizations. Reef fish in clear shallow water are brightly colored and possess conspicuous visual displays; fish in deeper or more turbid waters are more likely to be drab but acoustically or electrically conspicuous. Constraints placed by various environments on visual signals are at least qualitatively obvious to us; comparable acoustic and olfactory constraints are much less well known.

The size of the area within which exclusion of competitors is worthwhile could also influence the choice of a modality. Considering that smaller animals usually maintain smaller mean interindividual distances, one might expect a general trend toward visual signals in smaller animals, auditory or olfactory in larger ones. Exaggerated visual-spacing displays are most common in small, closely spaced diurnal animals such as lizards, coral reef fish, and intertidal crabs, while elaborate olfactory marks or acoustic signals characterize larger, mobile mammals and birds.

Finally, the modalities differ in the precision with which the sender can be located. Visual signals completely specify the current location of the signal source; acoustic and olfactory signals may not. When the interests of sender and receiver are opposed, as in the long-distance spacing call discussed above, this characteristic may also affect the sender's choice of modality.

The formulation of specific hypotheses concerning the expected modality of spacing signals is only beginning. One approach to the problem, the computer simulation of animal movements and interactions, has been initiated by Montgomery (1974). Taking distributions of rates of movement and rates of turn from radio-tracking data, Montgomery determined the potential frequencies of contact between individual foxes on the same home range that would result from a variety of hypothetical visual, auditory, and olfactory signals. Simulation models could readily be extended to investigate efficiencies of communication between individuals in adjacent ranges.

ADAPTATIONS OF SIGNAL STRUCTURE

The range of many acoustic spacing signals is impressively long: the drumming of ruffed grouse *(Bonasa umbellus)* (Archibald, 1974); the roar of lions *(Panthera leo)* (Schaller, 1972); and the loud calls of many forest primates (Altmann, 1967; Marler, 1968). Sound propagation in different vegetation types has been investigated with a view toward understanding the evolution of signal form (Chappuis, 1971; Morton, 1975; Marten, Quine, and Marler, 1977; Marten and Marler, 1977) for long-range communication. In both West African (Chappuis, 1971) and Central American (Morton, 1975) forests, there is at least a general tendency for the dominant frequencies of avian songs to match frequency bands with superior transmission characteristics and for tonal signals to replace the complex spectra or rapid frequency modulations characteristic of avian songs in open habitats.

The hypothesis that spacing calls are specialized for long-distance transmission has been directly investigated only for some forest primates. Audible range is influenced by source sound levels, background noise levels, rates of signal degradation, and the perceptual abilities of the receiver. Waser and Waser (1977) have investigated the first three parameters for primate species in a Ugandan rain forest. Relative to other calls in their vocal repertoires, the long-distance vocalizations of *Colobus guereza, Cercopithecus mitis, C. ascanius,* and *Cercocebus albigena* show significantly lower rates of attenuation when broadcast and rerecorded after passage through the forest canopy. Transmission experiments using pure tones suggest that the spectral distribution of energy in these calls is a primary factor responsible for their decreased attentuation rates; temporary transmission "windows" at intermediate frequencies (500–2000 Hz), as well as efficient transmission at low frequencies (125 Hz), were characteristic of the forest canopy. Long-distance calls were also found to have less variable attenuation rates than either nonspacing calls or pure tones. Evidently, aspects of signal structure other than modal frequency are of importance in their transmission. Sound propagation experiments carried out at different heights and times of day also indicated that calling from heights of 15–20 m (normal for a monkey) can more than double the audible range of the call over that at 1.5 m, and that primate species tend to concentrate their long-distance vocalizing either before dawn, when background noise was found to be lowest, or in early morning, when attenuation rates for those calls dropped by several db/100 m.

In contrast to their specialization of form and timing, the long-distance vocalizations of these primates were not characterized by unusually high sound levels at the source; frequently these did not exceed the levels of other calls in the repertoire. Moreover, sound levels of long-distance primate calls are equaled by those produced by much smaller animals, including cicadas and Orthoptera (Dumortier, 1963), frogs (Gerhardt, 1975), and birds (Morton, 1975). One possible explanation for this phenomenon lies in the physical nature of sound attenuation. Attenuation losses from spherical spreading of energy from a point source—losses that can generally be overcome only by an increase in source sound level—fall off logarithmically with distance, roughly 6 db for each doubling of distance from the source. On the other hand, losses from sound absorption—which can be reduced by modifying signal structure—are related to distance in an approximately linear fashion. As distance from the source increases, absorption accounts for an increasing proportion of the total attenuation.

Long-distance transmission of acoustic signals near the ground is affected by interference from sound reflected by the ground. This ground attenuation, confirmed repeatedly in transmission experiments with pure tones (Marten and Marler, 1977; Marten *et al.*, 1977; reviewed by Wiley and Richards, 1978), depends on the height of the source and the receiver in relation to the wavelength of the sound and on the acoustic impedance of the ground, which in turn varies with features of the soil and the ground vegetation. As the height of the transmission path above the ground increases, the wavelength for maximum ground attenuation also increases (see Wiley and Richards, 1978). For transmission within a few meters of the ground, a well-marked transmission "window" occurs for intermediate frequencies (1–3 kHz) (Morton, 1975; Marten and Marler, 1977; Marten *et al.*, 1977); lower frequencies are subject to greater attenuation from ground reflection, higher ones to greater attenuation from atmospheric absorption and scattering. In addition, reverberation in forests is minimal between 1 and 3 kHz (Richards and Wiley, in press). Most territorial birds in forests use this frequency band for their long-range acoustic signals (Morton, 1975; Richards and Wiley, in press).

Sound transmission in natural habitats has other properties, in addition to frequency-dependent attenuation, that affect the evolution of signal structure. Rapid variations in background noise, reverberation, and random fluctuations in amplitude from turbulence (Knudsen, 1946; Ingard, 1953; Wiener and Keast, 1959; Marten and Marler, 1977; Richards and Wiley, in press; Waser, personal observation) limit the use of intensity patterns and rapid, repetitive frequency patterns for long-range transmission of information (Wiley, 1976b; Wiley and Richards, 1978). Greater reverberation in forests, in comparison to open habitats, probably explains why many forest-dwelling birds avoid rapid repetitive frequency modulation in their advertising songs (Chappuis, 1971; Morton, 1975; Richards and Wiley, in press).

A vocalizer also faces different problems in communicating his direction and distance in different habitats. Mangabeys are able to localize single experimentally broadcast spacing calls with a median accuracy of 6° from a distance of several hundred meters (Waser, 1977b), despite the fact that many of the classical cues for direction (Konishi, 1973) are greatly degraded at that distance. High frequencies have been differentially attenuated, and scattering has blurred sharp onsets. Of course, these types of degradation also provide a listener with information on source distance (Griffin and Hopkins, 1974; Coleman, 1963; Wiley and Richards, 1978).

The constraints operating on spacing signals in other sensory modalities are

PETER M. WASER
AND R. HAVEN
WILEY

much less well understood. Background noise from distant lightning, as well as rapid signal attenuation, is a constraint on the electrical signals used by some tropical fish (Hopkins, 1974). Olfactory signals have two characteristics of obvious relevance to their use in spacing: fade-out time and active space. The flank marks of male golden hamsters *(Mesocricetus auratus)* elicited responses for 25–50 days after their deposition, the first measurement of fade-out time for presumptive olfactory spacing signals (Johnston and Lee, 1976). Fade out time and active space vary with rate or frequency of deposition, sensitivity of receptors, and rates of diffusion of the chemical signal (Bossert and Wilson, 1963; Wilson and Regnier, 1971). Rate of odorant release depends not only on such chemical properties of the signal as molecular weight and functional groups but also on environmental factors such as adsorptivity of substrate, ambient humidity, and local wind speed. The fade-out time of a nonpolar molecule can also depend on whether or not it is deposited in conjunction with a lipid (Regnier and Goodwin, 1977). The deposition of a fixed proportion of both polar and nonpolar molecules in a lipid (or any other combination of molecules with different diffusion rates) allows detection of the age of an olfactory mark.

Although adaptations for communication between individuals in the end determine the possibilities for spacing without close-range encounters, studies of the properties of signals that permit the transmission of information to long distances or over long time periods have just begun.

Evolution of Spacing Behavior

Regardless of the behavioral mechanisms of spacing, natural selection should adjust these mechanisms to maximize the propagation of individuals' genes. For over a quarter of a century after Howard's (1920) seminal treatment of territoriality, discussions of the evolution of spacing centered on the "functions" of territoriality: the importance of this behavior for securing a reserve of food, for isolation from interference in pair formation, and for protection from predators or epidemics (reviewed by Hinde, 1956). This discussion revolved in part around the distribution of various activities with respect to an individual's defended area. Few firm conclusions could be reached, in part because of the variety of relationships among feeding, pair formation, and territories in different species or even different populations of the same species. In retrospect, much of this literature suffers from the allied shortcomings of failing to analyze in detail the variable spatial relationships of individuals' activities and agonistic tendencies and seeking to explain the evolution of territoriality as a unitary phenomenon, rather than attempting to identify differences in selection pressures that might explain variations in activity, isolation, and aggression fields.

The appearance of Wynne-Edwards's book (1962) changed the emphasis in studies of territoriality. He contended that territorial behavior, and indeed many forms of social behavior, had the effect of limiting population densities and evolved because of the adaptedness of limitations on density that would prevent excessive exploitation of food resources. In contrast, Lack has long argued that territorial behavior does not limit population densities but only disperses individuals once settled (Lack and Lack, 1933; Lack, 1966) and that, in general, populations, whether territorial or not, are limited directly by the food available.

There are several differences between Lack's and Wynne-Edwards's positions. To begin with, they differ with regard to the behavioral mechanisms of territoriality. Two questions are pertinent here. First, to what extent do territorial individuals exclude newcomers? Second, do the behavioral mechanisms of territoriality permit adjustments to immediate or recent experience with the food supply? As has been discussed in the second section, the relationships of activity fields and agonistic behavior to isolation fields differ among species, so that neither Lack's nor Wynne-Edwards's view permits unqualified generalization.

Lack's and Wynne-Ewards's positions also differ on evolutionary questions: How important is competition between demes in the evolution of the larger population's gene pool? Can any selection regime favor the evolution of behavior that limits population density below maximum exploitation of resources? The first question has received thorough debate. The consensus agrees with Lack in minimizing the importance of interdemic selection (Williams, 1966, 1971; Maynard Smith, 1958; see Wilson, 1975, for a review of recent literature). The latter question hinges on the proper balance of short- and long-term advantages in the evolution of density-dependent reproduction. We are not aware of any formal treatment of this problem.

In retrospect, both Lack and Wynne-Edwards seem to have overlooked significant variations in spacing behavior among species and consequently proposed oversimplified explanations for the evolution of spacing mechanisms.

Costs and Benefits of Spacing

The evolutionary advantages of spacing behavior, most of them enumerated early in the study of territoriality, are probably never without qualifications. Both wide dispersion and aggregation confer conflicting advantages and disadvantages. Thus, predators are in some cases more reliably detected or repelled by groups of individuals, yet groups more often catch a predator's attention. Aggregation can have advantages for individuals in finding or capturing food (Krebs, this volume), yet aggregation increases the demands on locally available resources.

Spacing behavior, like most social interaction, takes time and energy and involves some risk of injury or exposure to predators. The advantages of the social relationship achieved by these interactions must thus compensate the participants for the costs of the interactions. Brown (1964) and Brown and Orians (1970) introduced such an economic analysis of the costs and benefits to individuals in terms of changes in their fitnesses, or the rates of propagation of their genes.

The evolution of territorial defense, as Brown indicated, requires that the individual obtain some benefit as a result of increased access to a limiting resource and that the costs of defense be less than the benefits. Because cost and benefit are decreases or increases in the fitnesses of genes associated with the expression of territorial defense, a resource is limiting if its availability influences an individual's survival or reproduction. Brown's formulation suggests particular questions about the evolution of spacing. What, for any given population of animals, are the limiting resources? And what, in general terms, are the attributes of a resource that make it defensible?

Because ephemeral aggregations of food are difficult to defend, many seabirds that feed on schools of fish and swallows that locate aggregations of flying insects nest in colonies and do not defend territories. Conversely, territorial defense occurs in many animals that feed on relatively evenly dispersed and temporally stable populations of prey, such as birds taking insects on foliage or monkeys feeding on leaves (see Crook, 1961; Eisenberg, Muckenhirn, and Rudran, 1972). Larger areas become more difficult to defend, and animals requiring them, like patas monkeys *(Erythrocebus patas)* in open savanna and nomadic ungulates, often lack elaborate spacing behavior (Hall, 1965; Jarman, 1974). Beyond these gross generalizations, the "defensibility" of resources is related to the availability, spatiotemporal dispersion, and turnover rates of resources in complex and as yet poorly understood ways. Schoener (1971) has developed a formal expression of the net benefit of territorial defense as a function of the area defended and the effectiveness of defense, but we still lack a model with sufficiently few and accessible parameters to allow reliable predictions for most species in the field.

Despite these difficulties, the territorial behavior of certain nectarivorous birds is predicted remarkably well by cost–benefit analyses (Wolf and Hainsworth, 1971; Gill and Wolf, 1975a,b; Carpenter and MacMillen, 1976a,b). For some hummingbirds, sunbirds, and depranid honeycreepers, one can measure the amount of food in a territory and its rate of production by determining the density of flowers, their nectar content, and their rates of nectar production. Individuals defend feeding territories when the metabolic costs of defense are compensated by a gain in nectar availability (Gill and Wolf, 1975b; Carpenter and MacMillen, 1976b). In particular, territoriality occurs neither when food densities are very low, so that the gain in available food (in calories) does not compensate the costs of defense (in calories), nor when food densities are very high, so that the presence of competitors has little effect on available food. In addition, increased numbers of competitors raise the costs of defense and can result in abandonment of territoriality (Stiles and Wolf, 1970). In species like nectarivores, for which food occurs in patches that vary markedly in richness across time and locations, individuals change from nonterritorial to territorial behavior in accordance with food availability in defended and undefended areas and the intensity of competition for rich sites.

An inherent difficulty with cost–benefit analyses is that the behavior of intruders, as well as residents, is likely to depend on the distribution and abundance of a limiting resource. Because properties of the resource that make it beneficial for a resident are likely to make it attractive for an intruder, the benefits and the costs of defense are likely to vary jointly with the characteristics of the resource. Moreover, because the behavior during encounters depends on both individuals' cost–benefit ratios, a general theory will need to consider the relative advantages of different agonistic tactics by both opponents. The key is probably in identifying those circumstances in which the benefits of a resource for a resident outweigh its attraction to intruders. Along these lines, in "Spacing in Relation to Resources" below, we consider conditions that make the benefits of a resource greater for a resident than for intruders.

Analysis of Contingencies in Social Interactions

An approach that explicitly analyzes agonistic behavior as an interaction, in which the effect of an individual's behavior is contingent on its opponent's behavior, employs game theory and the concept of an evolutionarily stable strategy (ESS) (Maynard Smith and Price, 1973). An ESS is one invulnerable to invasion by any mutant strategy; the expected benefit from a strategy when matched against itself must exceed the benefit when matched against any other strategy.

Particularly relevant to spacing behavior are contests with "uncorrelated asymmetry" (Maynard Smith and Parker, 1976; Maynard Smith, 1974b, 1976), in which the opponents differ in some way not associated with the "payoff" (the benefits that accrue to the winner of an interaction) or the "resource-holding potential" (an individual's inherent ability to win if it tries, as opposed to its strategy of how much and when to try). In particular, Maynard Smith analyzed a situation in which the asymmetry of opponents might involve ownership of a resource. In this situation, an ESS could result from conventional settlement of contests by escalating a contest ("hawk" strategy) when an owner and retreating immediately ("dove" strategy) when not, provided that all individuals are equally likely to play either role and provided that the escalating strategy is continued to a sufficient degree of risk (the expected gain in encounters between escalators must be negative). Thus, territorial defense by conventional behavior could evolve in spite of a lack of correlation between prior residence and either the benefits of ownership or inherent abilities to win encounters.

Advantages of prior ownership could also explain the evolution of conventional behavior in territorial interactions (Maynard Smith, 1976). Consequently, the occurrence of conventional interactions does not necessarily establish that they are "uncorrelated asymmetric" interactions. In fact, territorial and nonterritorial individuals in a population, or early and late arrivers, or residents in optimal and in suboptimal areas, often differ in age, so that one might expect correlations between prior residence and inherent abilities to win encounters. In stable populations of relatively long-lived animals, older individuals tend to invest more energy in reproduction than younger ones, and their additional experience might also favor them. Furthermore, residents might reap greater benefits from an area, at least for the immediate future, than newcomers, provided that an individual's experience in an area increases its benefit. The stipulation that individuals are equally likely to play either role in asymmetrical contests also seems unlikely to apply; age in particular often correlates with prior residence in territorial contests. In fact, the example cited by Maynard Smith and Parker (1976) to illustrate conventional behavior in territorial interactions, Krebs's (1971) study of great tits *(Parus major),* illustrates well the correlation of age with residence in an optimal, as opposed to a less advantageous, location. The failure of young birds in poorer habitats to challenge older birds in better habitats might well result from the correlations of this asymmetry.

Relationships between territorial neighbors might meet the requirements for an uncorrelated, asymmetrical contest better, although Maynard Smith and Parker (1976) dismiss the possibility. Here, individuals might take the roles of intruder and resident equally frequently, and this asymmetry might in fact lack association with payoffs or resource-holding potentials. Purely conventional behavior seems to be the rule in encounters between an intruding neighbor and a resident. At the boundary, or when a boundary has not yet been established by new neighbors, the contest is no longer asymmetrical, and in these circumstances, encounters between neighbors seem closer to Maynard Smith's "war of attrition."

Game theory is notably successful in predicting the global properties of animal conflicts and holds considerable promise for formulating more precise predictions about differences in spacing behavior between species and populations. It remains unclear, however, just what form of "game" animals are really playing in spacing interactions. Certainly, they are not playing repeatedly against the same opponent with the same payoffs and resource-holding potentials. Instead, they are playing a series of individuals with differing resource-holding potentials and differing payoffs, and even their own resource-holding potential varies with age or experience in past interactions.

Perhaps of special importance is the problem of treating games in which information is imperfect (Maynard Smith and Parker, 1976). Real animals almost never know their opponent's payoffs or resource-holding potentials precisely and have to estimate them from indirect information transmitted by the opponent. It seems likely that many spacing behaviors—and spacing signals, in particular—serve to obtain the information necessary to refine estimates of payoff and opponent's resource-holding potentials or to confound an opponent's attempt to do the same. Strategies for obtaining this information are surely an integral part of the "game." Intuitively, it seems clear that evolutionarily stable strategies depend on the accuracy of such estimates, yet only a beginning has been made on this difficult problem (Maynard Smith and Parker, 1976). What factors determine, in any real case, where the balance lies between bluffing and calling bluffs or between mutual avoidance and overt aggression? What factors determine the optimal area or effectiveness of defense? Game theory remains to be applied to these questions.

SPACING IN RELATION TO A RESOURCE: INDIVIDUALS WITH BASES OF OPERATION

In another approach to the evolution of spacing patterns, the spatial relationships optimal for resident individuals in a population at saturation density are derived from the spatial distribution of food in the environment. Two related calculations along these lines have shown that dispersed, stable resources, exploited by animals foraging radially from a base of operations, such as a nest or cache, favor dispersed ranges without overlap, rather than aggregations. Horn (1968) imagined an environment in which food occurred predictably in equal amounts at regular intervals. He could easily show that the distance a bird traveled to bring a given amount of food to its nest was less when individuals had ranges without overlap than when several individuals foraged from the same base. A similar demonstration by Smith (1968) showed that squirrels collecting seeds for caching at a central location traveled shorter distances if each occupied exclusive ranges than if two shared the same range. In essence, when individuals aggregate under these conditions, an individual must travel farther to collect the food to replace that already removed by others from locations close by.

The inverse theorem, however, seems not to follow, in spite of Horn's (1968) deductions. Clumped resources that vary in space and time are not necessarily more efficiently exploited by aggregated individuals foraging from a base than by dispersed ones, at least from the sole standpoint of the expected distance traveled per unit of resource. Horn's deductions for a habitat with a variable distribution of food pertain only to habitats with dimensions similar to the maximum ranges of foraging individuals. Horn imagined a habitat of 16 locations for food, at each of which enough food for 16 individuals appears with a probability of $1/16$ in each unit of time. In these circumstances, individuals travel the least distance per unit of food on the average if they all are based in the center of the habitat (Horn, 1968). A base near one edge requires that an individual spend some of its time foraging near the opposite edge; with a base near the center, an individual never has to travel that far for food. In essence, a resource with high spatiotemporal variation is not efficiently exploited from a base near one edge of a block of habitat.

Consider a similar habitat, in which enough food for 16 individuals appears at each location with a probability of $1/16$ per unit of time, but extending indefinitely, unlike Horn's example. When the dimensions of the habitat greatly exceed the foraging ranges (F) of individuals, all locations greater than a distance F from an edge have equal accessibility to the patches of food. In this case, widely overlapping but dispersed activity fields have the same efficiency as aggregations.

Brewer's blackbirds *(Euphagus cyanocephalus)* in central Washington nest beside lakes, around which they feed on concentrations of emerging odonates (Horn, 1968). The aggregation of their nests, insofar as access to food is the determining selection pressure, is as much a consequence of the large-scale restriction of a predictable food source to the shores of one moderate-sized lake as of the small-scale unpredictability in the location around the lake shore at which food accumulates on any one day. Aggregation, as Horn (1968) suggested, might also confer evolutionary advantages in protection from predators and in communication about the locations of patches of food.

These calculations suggest three principles about the dispersion of individuals in relation to the dispersion of a resource, when individuals forage from a base of operations and no selection pressures affect the dispersion of individuals other than the effort necessary to transport the resource to the base:

1. If the availability of the resource does not vary appreciably in space and time, evenly dispersed activity fields without overlap provide the most efficient spacing.

2. If the availability of the resource varies appreciably in space and time and if the habitat has dimensions approximating the foraging ranges of individuals, then

PETER M. WASER
AND R. HAVEN
WILEY

aggregated bases of operation near the center of the habitat provide the most efficient spacing.

3. If the availability of the resource varies as above and the habitat has dimensions greatly exceeding the foraging ranges of individuals, then *either* aggregated bases of operation *or* evenly dispersed but widely overlapping activity fields provide equally efficient spacing.

The distinction between the conditions for Principles 2 and 3, which hinges on the relationships between the dimensions of a patch of habitat and the foraging ranges of individuals, depends on the distribution of the shortest distance between sites at which the resource is simultaneously available. This distribution determines how large the diameter of an individual's activity field must be to encompass a productive site with a sufficiently high probability in any unit of time.

The distinction between stable and variable resources, which differentiates Principle 1 from the other two, hinges on the relationship between an individual's needs (N) in some appropriate time period (Δt) and both the amount of resource available at a particular site (R) and the variation in R from one interval Δt to the next. The central question is whether or not an individual, in an environment at saturation density, can get by on a fixed set of sites equal to its own share of the environment. If so, evenly dispersed bases are most efficient. An individual can manage in this way only if its own share of sites has a sufficiently high probability of having enough resource to meet its needs continually. For some simple conditions, the sufficiency of each individual's share of sites increases as the availability of the resource becomes more evenly distributed across sites and time periods (appendix).

This discussion is well illustrated in qualitative terms by a comparison of two species of birds that consume insects of the litter on forest floors: ovenbirds *(Seiurus aurocapillus)* (Stenger, 1958; Stenger and Falls, 1959; Zach and Falls, in press) and bicolored antbirds *(Gymnopithys bicolor)* (Willis, 1967). Ovenbirds, which remain primarily within their own territories, search for insects scattered in the forest litter. The food available (R) at any one site is certainly less than an individual's needs during a foraging bout, but at any one time, numerous locations within a territory have food. Sizes of territories vary from habitat to habitat in accordance with the abundance of insects in the litter.

Bicolored antbirds catch insects flushed from the litter by advancing columns of army ants in neotropical forests. Because they rely entirely on this food supply, their food is available only in small patches widely scattered in the forest in locations that are relatively unpredictable from week to week. At an army ant raid, though, there is enough food for many individuals $(R > N)$, and, in fact, several pairs of this species and individuals of many other species often gather. Pairs of bicolored antbirds occupy regularly spaced activity fields with extensive overlap. The dimensions of the habitat are clearly greater than the sufficient diameter of an activity field, so Principle 3 applies. Evidently, some other selection pressure, perhaps an advantage of dispersed, cryptic nests in avoiding predation, favors dispersed spacing rather than aggregations. Note that the demand for resources within relatively large areas is set by the distances between the centers of individuals' activity fields as well as by the degree of overlap (Willis, 1967).

In summary, an extensive habitat with unpredictable patches of food places no constraints on the dispersion of individuals' bases of operations: overdispersed and aggregated bases are equally efficient in minimizing travel time. Other factors affect the spacing of bases in such an environment. A habitat with sparse, evenly distributed food, on the other hand, specifically favors overdispersed bases of operation, because regular spacing minimizes travel time from the base to locations with food. For such populations to evolve aggregated bases, selection for aggregation for other reasons must more than compensate for the disadvantage of increased travel time.

SPACING IN RELATION TO RESOURCES: A GENERAL PERSPECTIVE

The preceding principles depend strongly on the assumption that each individual has a fixed base of operation from which it forages, such as a nest, a den, or a cache. These principles relate the optimal dispersion of individuals' bases of operation to the dispersion of a limiting resource. In this situation, animals adjust one constraint on their activity fields, the locations of their bases, to another constraint, the dispersion of a limiting resource. In fact, this situation is a special case of the problem of multiple constraints on individuals' spacing.

S. Altmann (1974) has analyzed multiple constraints on activity and isolation fields, including the effects of two or more limiting resources with different dispersions, such as sleeping sites, food, and water, in a comparison of baboons *(Papio)* in Amboseli and Nairobi National Parks, Kenya. He suggested, among other principles, that overlap of home ranges is determined by the spacing of those essential resources most restricted in their distribution. For instance, baboon troops overlap at large but scarce waterholes or sleeping groves. In Amboseli, where sleeping groves and water holes are less evenly distributed than at Nairobi, baboon troops occupy activity fields with more overlap than do troops in Nairobi. This principle, however, specifies only a *minimum* extent of home range overlap.

Consider what might influence the spacing of individuals in relation to a resource, without other constraints on movements. If regular dispersion is favored, what influences the degree of isolation within individuals' activity fields? In particular, what favors exclusive activity fields as opposed to overlapping ones?

Individuals with no other constraints on their movements would minimize their travel times if they could match their activity fields to the dispersion of food in their environment. When R (the amount of resource available at a site) is not much greater than N (an individual's needs), individuals should forage independently from one food item or patch to the next. However, when clumps of food contain amounts subtantially greater than N, individuals should aggregate; the number of individuals per clump of food should vary from population to population or from time to time with the expected amount of food per clump. Spider monkeys *(Ateles belzebuth)* show such adaptability in spacing (Klein and Klein, 1975).

Thus, when the availability of a limiting resource varies appreciably across locations and time, individuals should occupy widely overlapping activity fields. This prediction resembles Principle 3 above: either with or without bases of

PETER M. WASER
AND R. HAVEN
WILEY

operation, individuals exploiting a variable resource should occupy widely over-lapping activity fields (see also Waser, 1976, and appendix). The analog of Principle 1, when individuals lack bases of operation, is less clear.

What might favor exclusive activity fields for individuals foraging solitarily in an environment with an evenly dispersed, stable resource? Consider an animal that has traveled a certain distance in one direction and now faces a decision of whether to proceed or turn back. The optimal decision depends in part on what it "knows" about the current state of the area it just passed through in comparison to the area ahead. If it knows that the availability of the resource is low in the area behind, then proceeding would be preferable.

There are several ways that a foraging animal could know that the availability of a resource is low in an area just searched: the animal might already have removed most of the resource and know that renewal rates are low; it might have encountered little and know that rates of encounter are correlated at nearby locations or in successive time intervals at any one location; or it might know that the behavior of prey individuals changes to reduce their vunerability for a while after detecting a predator. Of course, these sorts of "knowledge" could result either from the animal's own experience or from inheritance of adapted behavioral tactics. The first and third of the preceding possibilities have been termed exploitation depression and behavioral depression of a resource as a consequence of an animal's foraging activities (Charnov, Orians, and Hyatt, 1976).

Any persistent depression or scarcity of the resource in the area immediately to the rear favors continuing forward. The animal's optimal procedure thus depends on whether some advantage of turning around can compensate. On the other hand, if the availability of food fluctuates rapidly at any one site or renews rapidly after exploitation, rates of encounter with food might have little serial correlation over relatively brief periods. In this case, moving ahead or to the rear could prove equally fruitful.

Consider first the case in which turning around has no sufficient advantage. If it is disadvantageous for an individual to backtrack, it will probably also prove disadvantageous for two individuals to search near each other. The optimal spacing would consist of widely overlapping activity fields, regular olfactory marking or acoustic advertisement while moving, and immediate avoidance of other individuals' paths or locations, behavior like that of cheetahs (see the second section). If the cumulative searching by all individuals at a locality were disproportionately low in relation to the availability of the resource there, it would prove advantageous for one or more individuals to shift their activity fields to include more time there. In such cases, regular dispersion of the widely overlapping activity fields would equalize the demands on resources at different sites over large areas.

In contrast, consider the consequences when turning back has advantages. Suppose, for instance, that an individual can find food more rapidly in familiar areas than in strange ones. Then knowledge of good places to find food farther to the rear could compensate for the disadvantages of backtracking through recently searched areas immediately to the rear. Furthermore, if familiarity with an area enhances ability to find food reliably, an individual might face the disadvantage of competing with a more efficient individual in the area ahead. So when familiarity with an area increases an individual's efficiency in exploiting the limiting resource there, an individual would do best to stick near familiar areas and avoid areas more familiar to another individual.

Few studies have explicitly investigated the effects of an animal's familiarity with an area on its ability to find food there, although such an effect is likely to influence foraging efficiencies for many species that search for cryptic or sparsely distributed food. "Search images" or spatial restrictions on searching (see Krebs, 1973, and this volume) would permit individuals to concentrate on the kinds of food or locations that maximize foraging success in local areas. Individuals familiar with an area could monitor small patches of renewing resources (Zach and Falls, 1976c). Individual differences in prey selection, as Southern (1954) reported for neighboring tawny owls *(Strix aluco)* in the same wood, suggest these consequences of familiarity with an area. One direct confirmation that familiarity increases foraging success in an area comes from a study of pinioned ovenbirds confined to fenced enclosures on the forest floor (Zach and Falls, 1976a,b). On introduction to an enclosure, individuals with earlier experience there returned immediately to the previous locations of patches of food.

When familiarity with an area increases foraging success, it would prove advantageous for neighboring individuals to establish clear boundaries and avoid each other's areas. Of course, these areas must reliably include enough of the limiting resource to sustain an individual or group of individuals (see appendix). Consequently, optimal spacing in this case would consist of activity fields with little overlap and isolation fields with pronounced convexity. The less the advantage of familiarity in exploiting the resource, the more often excursions across the boundary might occur, and avoidance would have less importance in the isolation of individuals from their neighbors.

Renewal rates of a limiting resource also influence the relative advantages of proceeding ahead or turning back. As noted above, the costs of backtracking are low when renewal rates are high. Consequently, a slight advantage of familiarity with an area would favor exclusive activity fields when renewal rates are high, while much greater advantages would be necessary when they are low.

These considerations lead to the major conclusion that a stable, evenly dispersed resource does not necessarily favor exclusive activity fields for animals without bases of operation. This conclusion stands in contrast to our earlier one for animals with bases. In the absence of bases of operation, exclusive activity fields evolve only when each individual realizes an advantage from confining itself to a set of sites equal to its share at saturation density. This stipulation normally requires an advantage to turning around while foraging. In a sense, a base of operations—a nest, den, or cache—creates the clearest sort of advantage for turning back. Our reasoning above suggests that any advantage of site attachment, such as an advantage of familiarity with an area in exploiting a limiting resource, could favor returning after an individual had proceeded some distance in one direction.

For animals whose spacing is constrained by a single limiting resource, the following two principles apply, in place of those stated above:

4. If the availability of the resource varies appreciably in space and time, then

widely overlapping activity fields provide the most efficient spacing; individuals or cohesive groups might aggregate temporarily, depending on the amount of resource in a particular clump.

5. If the availability of the resource does not vary appreciably in space and time, then *either* overlapping *or* exclusive activity fields provide the most efficient spacing, depending on whether or not a sufficient turning-around advantage exists; individuals or cohesive groups should forage solitarily.

This approach to understanding the evolution of spacing has focused on the relations of neighboring, resident individuals. Our reasoning has suggested that either overlap or exclusiveness of neighbors' activity fields could prove mutually advantageous for neighbors, depending on spatiotemporal variability in the resource and any turning-around advantage. The argument has proceeded in two steps. The first question is whether or not an individual, in a population at saturation density, can get by on its share of sites or area. If it can, a second question is whether or not there are reasons for an individual to confine itself to this minimal set of sites. These arguments suggest that established neighbors should engage only in ritualized encounters, with outcomes predictable in advance, either mutual avoidance or ritualized encounters at established boundaries. Once residents have occupied the environment at saturation density, strangers should evoke greater hostility than established neighbors, a phenomenon verified by field experiments (see the second section).

SPACING IN RELATION TO RESOURCES: EXAMPLES

The preceding conclusions apply well to the arboreal primates of the Kibale Forest in Uganda (Struhsaker, 1975, 1978; Struhsaker and Oates, 1975; Oates, 1976; Rudran, 1976; Waser, 1976), five species that differ widely in the characteristics of their movements, their group size, the overlap of activity fields, and intergroup encounters (Table III; Struhsaker, 1975).

Of these five species, the mangabey uses the most clearly patchy resource; it feeds primarily at fruiting fig trees *(Ficus)*, which at any one time are widely and irregularly scattered in the forest. Information on the density and fruiting of fig trees in the Kibale Forest suggests that the activity field of a mangabey group includes enough trees to ensure, with negligible risk, a continuous supply of food. As expected for a resource with high temporal and spatial variability (see appendix and Waser, 1976), activity fields that are large enough to ensure a continuous supply for one individual or a cohesive group will often include enough for others as well.

The two species of colobus in the same area contrast in their spacing (Struhsaker and Oates, 1975; Struhsaker, 1975). The red colobus *(Colobus badius)* takes a diet of growing leaves and shoots plus some fruit and flowers. These items tend to be available in abundance on a given tree or species of tree for a short period during the year, so that red colobus groups must exploit a variety of food sources. In addition, this species seems to prefer a varied diet even when one kind of food is locally abundant (Clutton-Brock, 1975). Although the temporal and spatial variation in the food sources of red colobus are not so clear as in the figs that mangabeys depend on, some of the important food trees are clumped within the habitat, and their phenologies suggest substantial temporal variation in availability (Struhsaker, 1975). Red colobus seem to provide a second example of a species with variable resources and widely overlapping activity fields. Moreover, to the extent that this species concentrates on short-lived resources with low renewal rates, there is little premium on turning back.

Black-and-white colobus, in contrast, consume a less diverse diet, mostly leaves of a few species of common trees, which are continuously available in relatively small areas throughout the year (Oates, 1976). In addition, they can subsist during lean periods primarily on mature leaves. Although neighboring groups have appreciable overlap in their activity fields, the overlap is much less than for red colobus or mangabeys. A group probably depletes the available food in one place only slightly before moving on, so there is probably little disadvantage to turning back. Consequently, for black-and-white colobus, only a slight turning-around advantage, perhaps from familiarity with the best shelter, paths, or food trees, would compensate for the slight disadvantage of crossing recently exploited areas.

The two species of *Cercopithecus* in the Kibale Forest have largely exclusive activity fields and include insects as an important component of their diets (Rudran, 1976; Struhsaker, 1975, 1978). Groups of blue monkeys *(C. mitis)* move more or less straight ahead during any one day, over a route that amounts to

TABLE III.   SUMMARY OF MOVEMENTS, SPACING, GROUP SIZE, AND INTERACTIONS BETWEEN GROUPS FOR FIVE ARBOREAL PRIMATES IN THE KIBALE FOREST, UGANDA[a]

Species	Usual group size	Approximate mean area of activity field (ha)	Extent of overlap by neighboring groups	Nature of encounters between groups
Gray-cheeked mangabey (*Cercocebus albigena*)	6–28[b]	400	Wide	Short-term avoidance independent of location
Red colobus (*Colobus badius*)	12–80[b]	35–50	Wide	Intergroup supplantations independent of location
Black-and-white colobus (*C. guereza*)	3–15	15	Intermediate	Long-range acoustic communication; infrequent short-range interaction
Blue monkey (*Cercopithecus mitis*)	10–28	100	Little	Long-range acoustic communication; infrequent short-range interaction
Red-tailed monkey (*C. ascanius*)	15–35	25	Very little	Regular short-range interactions

[a]After Struhsaker, 1975.
[b]Usually two or more adult males per group.

appreciably less than the diameter of a typical activity field. Red-tail monkeys (*C. ascanius*) move back and forth in any one day, over a route that is generally much longer than the diameter of a typical activity field. Both species take a highly diverse diet, but the inclusion of insects might mean that groups familiar with their foraging areas would have a distinct advantage. These two species thus exemplify the case of exclusive activity fields in association with evenly dispersed resources and an advantage of familiarity with foraging areas.

The diets and foraging techniques of blue and red-tailed monkeys suggest a plausible explanation for the differences in their daily movements. Blue monkeys take large, apparently sedentary insects from foliage without special movements, while red-tails take many smaller, active insects, which they often catch with a sudden grab. The lower abundance of large items suitable for blue monkeys and the lower renewal rates of these items could favor lower rates of return to particular areas within the monkeys' activity fields. For red-tails, the renewal of suitable items in accessible locations probably proceeds much more rapidly, so that more frequent returns to a particular area become possible.

The differences in daily movements of these two species might, in turn, explain the differences in the nature of agonistic interactions between neighboring groups. Blue monkeys only infrequently engage in short-range encounters with their neighbors, while red-tails regularly encounter their neighbors at short range (Rudran, 1976; Struhsaker and Leland, 1979). A species with short daily movements in relation to the diameter of its activity field would incur a substantial cost in traveling to and from boundaries especially to encounter neighbors at short range, a circumstance that might favor long-range acoustic interactions for maintaining exclusive activity fields. In addition, acoustic advertisement at long range for a restricted period each day can provide reliable information on the positions of groups with respect to their boundaries throughout the day. In contrast, when a group's movements take it near boundaries repeatedly during the day, short-range interactions with visual contact become necessary to define boundaries, yet they incur little extra cost in travel.

With the possible exception of red colobus, none of the primates of Kibale seems to exemplify the evolution of overlapping activity fields for a dispersed resource without a sufficient turning-around advantage. Possibly, long residence in an area normally results in sufficient advantages from familiarity with foraging sites, shelter, or routes of travel, so that exclusive activity fields would prove optimal for dispersed resources.

The situation might be different for transient individuals. The shorebirds studied by Goss-Custard (1970) in migration and winter exemplify widely overlapping movements in exploiting a dispersed resource, invertebrates of intertidal mudflats. This resource might also change in its microdistribution from one tide to the next, a circumstance that would further reduce the possibility of a bird's familiarizing itself with foraging areas. Although migrant sandpipers sometimes defend small areas or localized food sources (Hamilton, 1959), most species on migration or in winter, including those studied by Goss-Custard, do not. As Goss-Custard demonstrated, organisms living near the surface withdraw into the mud and become unavailable to surface-feeding sandpipers for a period of three to five minutes after a bird walks past. Goss-Custard did not determine the extent of this effect on either side of a walking sandpiper beyond a minimum distance of 4 cm. This temporary reduction in the availability of prey behind a foraging sandpiper favors dispersion of individuals, in order to minimize mutual interference, and also discourages turning around by a foraging individual. In fact, species that feed on organisms near the surface tend to scatter more widely while foraging. Those that probe deep into the mud standardly form tight flocks while foraging.

Species feeding on organisms near the surface do not consistently turn less frequently than those feeding on deeper organisms; however, the former species move much faster. Consequently, although Goss-Custard did not analyze his data in this way, species feeding on organisms near the surface apparently make fewer turns per meter as they forage.

Thus, wintering sandpipers that exploit a dispersed, gradually renewing resource avoid each other, seldom backtrack while foraging, and use widely overlapping areas. They exemplify overlapping activity fields for utilizing a dispersed resource in the absence of a sufficient turning-around advantage. Those sandpipers that exploit a less predictable resource avoid each other less and turn more per distance traveled.

OTHER INFLUENCES ON THE EVOLUTION OF SPACING BEHAVIOR

The spatial and temporal distribution of a limiting resource in an environment, as we have seen, determines the disadvantages of foraging near other individuals or in areas used by others. The possibilities of such interference, however, are not the only consideration in predicting the optimal spacing of individuals. In addition, opportunities for cooperation in obtaining food and avoiding predation might vary with individuals' spatial relationships. The optimal spacing for individuals in a particular population might thus require a compromise between possibilities for reducing interference and increasing cooperation among individuals.

If nearby individuals can cooperate in locating resources or capturing prey, aggregation rather than dispersion would have advantages (see Krebs, this volume). Aggregations also sometimes have advantages in detecting cryptic predators or surprise attacks and in reducing the risk of mortality once a predator is detected by means of coordinated activities of the group, such as mobbing the predator to repel it (Kruuk, 1964; Hamilton, 1971a; Vine, 1971; Pulliam, 1973; Siegfried and Underhill, 1975).

On the other hand, aggregations often attract a predator's attention more than solitary individuals and carry the risk of disproportionate loss when predators can easily attack several individuals at once or in close succession. Tinbergen and his collaborators (Patterson, 1965; Tinbergen, Impekoven, and Franck, 1964; Tinbergen, 1967) have clearly shown the counteracting effects of aggregation and dispersion of nests in reducing predation within colonies of birds.

Recent evidence suggests that kinship, a factor rarely considered in the control of spacing patterns, can affect spacing behavior in some striking ways. As would be expected from theoretical arguments (Hamilton, 1971b), sea anemones

PETER M. WASER
AND R. HAVEN
WILEY

display aggression between clones but not within them (Francis, 1973). At the opposite end of the phylogenetic array, among siamang *(Symphalangus syndactylus),* the territory of a male offspring is often carved out of the parents' range without obvious interference from them (Aldrich-Blake and Chivers, 1973). The inheritance of part of the natal home range by offspring has been suggested as a major evolutionary route to sociality (Brown, 1964; Eisenberg, 1977; Woolfenden and Fitzpatrick, 1978). The phenomenon is increasingly reported in organisms traditionally regarded as solitary, including white-crowned sparrows (Baker and Mewaldt, 1978), sloths (Montgomery, in press), bears (Herrero, 1978), and leopards (Bertram, 1974). The persistence of kin as neighbors in solitary species will require explicit consideration in future evolutionary discussions of spacing phenomena.

CONCLUSION

A general theory of adaptations in spacing behavior must predict not only the distribution of activity fields in space but also the optimal form of an individual's activity, aggression, and isolation fields. For some species or populations, one or a few ecological parameters accurately predict the optimal parameters of spacing behavior. For other species, the ecological parameters undoubtedly have complex correlations among themselves and interacting effects on spacing behavior. Adaptations in spacing behavior depend on at least the following ecological variables: the dispersion in space and time of one or more limiting resources; the effects of familiarity with an area on an individual's ability to exploit a limiting resource; the existence or not of a base of operations, such as a nest, a den, or a cache; the effects of proximity to other individuals on an individual's ability to exploit a limiting resource; and the effects of proximity to other individuals on the risks of predation.

APPENDIX

In considering the optimal spacing of animals, either with or without bases of operation, we encountered the question of whether or not an individual's share of sites at saturation density is enough to provide a reliable supply of a limited resource. If a set of locations equal to an individual's share at saturation density can provide, with a sufficiently high probability, the individual's needs in any one time period, then any form of site attachment, either a base of operation or some other sufficient turning-around advantage, would favor individuals that restricted their foraging to that minimal set of locations.

Our task, then, is to analyze the relationship between the temporal and spatial variability of a resource and the probability that an individual's share of sites will include enough resource in any one time period. First, following Horn (1968), choose a spacing of sites (or dimensions of quadrats) and duration of time intervals Δt, so that the availability of the resource varies independently across sites and time intervals. Then let D = the density of sites, $\overline{R}$ = the mean availability of the resource across sites at any one time and across time at any one site, and N = an individual's needs (in the same units as R) in one time period. Then, the saturation density of individuals will be $\overline{R}D/N$, and an individual's share of sites at saturation density will equal $N/\overline{R}$. Over the long term, regardless of whether resources are stable or variable, $N/\overline{R}$ sites will average an amount N of resource, enough for one individual in one time period.

The average availability of the resource is not our principle concern; instead, we want to know the probability that $N/\overline{R}$ sites will have enough resource for an individual *in any one time period*. Assume for simplicity, as Horn (1968) did, that each site has either an amount of resource R or nothing at any time period Δt. Then, each site has a probability of $\overline{R}/R$ that resource is available in any Δt. The probability that a set of $N/\overline{R}$ sites will include A sites with resources available in any Δt is specified by the binomial distribution for A successes in $N/\overline{R}$ trials when the probability of success per trial is $\overline{R}/R$.

The number of sites that will satisfy an individual's needs in any Δt depends on whether R is greater or less than N. When $R > N$, an individual needs to visit, in any Δt, only one site with the resource available. The question then is whether or not $N/\overline{R}$ sites, an individual's share at saturation density, will include *at least one* with the resource during any Δt. This probability, available from the cumulative binomial distribution, approaches 1.0 as $\overline{R}/R$ approaches 1.0. In contrast, when $\overline{R}/R$ is small, an individual's share of sites at saturation density would have a low probability of including enough resource during any one time period. Yet, if R is greater than N, when the resource is present at a site, there is more than enough for one individual. In addition, the probability that two or more sites will have the resource, among a set of $N/\overline{R}$ sites, would be appreciable. Under these conditions, overlapping ranges would prove most efficient, whether or not individuals had bases of operation.

When $R < N$, then no one site can provide enough resource for an individual in any Δt. Each individual needs to collect the resource at N/R sites in each Δt. For

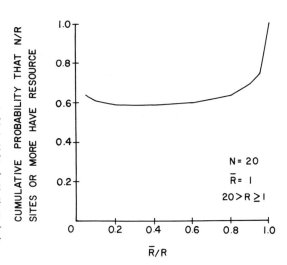

Fig. 6. Effects of spatiotemporal variation in the availability of a limiting resource on the probability that an individual's share of sites will include at least enough resource in a time period, Δt. N/R, an individual's share of sites at saturation density; $\overline{R}/R$, the probability that an amount R of resource is available at a site in Δt; N, an individual's needs in Δt; $R < N$. For this example, N is held constant, while R varies. See text for further explanation.

N = 20

$\overline{R}$ = 1

20 > R ≥ 1

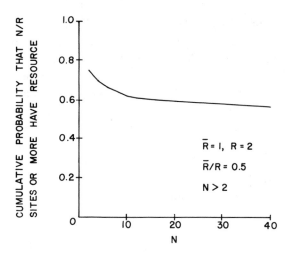

Fig. 7. Effects of N, an individual's or a cohesive group's needs in any time period, on the probability that the individual's or group's share of sites will include at least enough resource in a time period. N/R and $\overline{R}/R$, as in Figure 6; $R < N$. Here R is held constant, while N varies. See text for further explanation.

any given $\overline{R}$ and N, which specify an individual's share of sites $N/\overline{R}$, a decrease in R will increase both the probability of a resource at any one site, $\overline{R}/R$, and the number of sites with resource needed to support an individual in any Δt, N/R. These changes have counteracting effects on the cumulative probability of at least N/R successes in $N/\overline{R}$ trials when each trial has a probability of success $\overline{R}/R$. Examples taken from tables of the cumulative binomial distribution indicate that the probability of having enough resource within an individual's share of sites varies remarkably little over wide ranges of $\overline{R}/R$, for a given N and $\overline{R}$, or over wide variation in N, for a given $\overline{R}/R$. The probabilities vary between 0.5 and 0.75, until $\overline{R}/R$ approaches very close to 1.0 (Figures 6 and 7). Consequently, when an individual must collect the resource from a number of locations to fill its needs, wide variation in the predictability of resource at each site has little effect on the probability that an individual's share of sites will include enough in any one time period. Overlapping activity fields would prove necessary unless the presence of the resource were *highly* predictable.

References

Adams, L., and Davis, S. D. The internal anatomy of home range. *J. Mammal.,* 1967, *48,* 529–536.

Aldrich-Blake, F. P. G., and Chivers, D. J. On the genesis of a group of siamang. *Am. J. Physic. Anthropol.,* 1973, *38,* 631–636.

Altmann, J. Observational study of behavior: Sampling methods. *Behaviour,* 1974, *49,* 227–267.

Altmann, S. Field observations of a howling monkey society. *J. Mammal.,* 1959, *40,* 317–330.

Altmann, S. The structure of primate social communication. In S. Altmann (ed.), *Social Communication in Primates.* University of Chicago Press, Chicago, 1967, pp. 325–362.

Altmann, S. Baboons, time, space and energy. *Am. Zool.,* 1974, *14,* 221–248.

Altmann, S., and Altmann, J. *Baboon Ecology.* University of Chicago Press, Chicago, 1970.

Andrew, R. J. Influence of hunger on aggressive behaviour in certain buntings of the genus *Emberiza. Physiol. Zool.,* 1956, *30,* 177–185.

Archibald, H. L. Directional differences in the sound intensity of ruffed grouse drumming. *Auk,* 1974, *91,* 517–521.

Archibald, H. L. Temporal patterns of spring space use by ruffed grouse. *J. Wildl. Manage.* 1975, *39*, 472–481.

Assem, J. van den. Territory in the three-spined stickleback *Gasterostus aculeatus* L. *Behavior, Suppl.,* 1967, *16*, 1–164.

Assem, J. van den, and Molen, J. N. van der. Waning of the aggressive response in the three-spined stickleback upon constant exposure to a conspecific. I. A preliminary analysis of the phenomenon. *Behaviour,* 1969, *34*, 286–324.

Baerends, G. P., and Baerends-van Roon, J. M. An introduction to the study of the ethology of cichlid fishes. *Behaviour, Suppl.,* 1950, *1*, 1–243.

Bailey, T. N. Social organization in a bobcat population. *J. Wildl. Manage.,* 1974, *38*, 435–446.

Baker, M. C., and Baker, A. E. M. Niche relationships among six species of shorebirds on their wintering and breeding ranges. *Ecol. Monogr.,* 1973, *43*, 193–212.

Baker, M. C., and Mewaldt, L. R. The use of space by white-crowned sparrows. Juvenile and adult ranging patterns and home range vs. body size comparisons in an avian granivore community. *Evolution,* 1978, *38*, 712–722.

Banerjee, U. An inquiry into the genesis of aggression in mice induced by isolation. *Behaviour,* 1971, *40*, 86–99.

Barash, D. P. The social biology of the Olympic marmot. *Anim. Behav.* Monogr., 1973, *6*, 172–245.

Barash, D. P. Neighbor recognition in two "solitary" carnivores: The raccoon *(Procyon lotor)* and the red fox *(Vulpes fulva). Science,* 1974, *185*, 794–796.

Barnett, S. A. *The Rat.* Aldine, Chicago, 1963.

Bearder, S., and Randall, R. Comparative olfactory marking in the spotted hyaena and civets. *Carnivore,* 1978, *1*, 32–48.

Beeler, M. Paterson's worm. *M.I.T. Artificial Intelligence Memo,* 1973, 290.

Bennett-Clark, H. C. The mechanism and efficiency of sound production in mole-crickets. *J. Exp. Biol.,* 1970, *52*, 619–652.

Bertram, B. R. Radiotracking leopard in the Serengeti, *African Wildlife Leadership Foundation News,* 1974, *9*, 8–10.

Black, C. H., and Wiley, R. H. Spatial variation in behavior in relation to territoriality in dwarf cichlids *Apistogramma ramirezi. Z. Tierpsychol.,* 1977, *45*, 288–297.

Bossert, W. H., and Wilson, E. O. An analysis of olfactory communication among animals. *J. Theor. Biol.,* 1963, *5*, 443–469.

Braddock, J. C. The effect of prior residence upon dominance in the fish *Platypoecilus maculatus. Physiol. Zool.,* 1949, *22*, 161–169.

Bramley, P. S., and Neaves, W. B. The relationship between social status and reproductive activity in male impala *Aepyceros melampus. J. Reprod. Fert.,* 1972, *31*, 77–81.

Brian, M. V., Hibble, J., and Kelly, A. F. The dispersion of ant species in a southern English heath. *J. Anim. Ecol.,* 1966, *35*, 281–290.

Brooks, R. J., and Falls, J. B. Individual recognition by song in white-throated sparrows. I. Discrimination of songs of neighbors and strangers. *Can. J. Zool.,* 1975, *53*, 879–888.

Brown, J. L. Aggressiveness, dominance and social organization in the Steller jay. *Condor,* 1963, *65*, 460–484.

Brown, J. L. The evolution of diversity in avian territorial systems, *Wilson Bull.,* 1964, *6*, 160–169.

Brown, J. L., and Orians, G. H. Spacing patterns in mobile animals. *Ann. Rev. Ecol. System.,* 1970, *1*, 239–262.

Brown, L. E. Home range in small mammal communities. *Surv. Biol. Prog.,* 1962, *4*, 131–179.

Buchler, E. A chemiluminescent tag for tracking bats and other small nocturnal animals. *J. Mammal.,* 1976, *57*, 173–176.

Buckman, N. S., and Ogden, J. C. Territorial behavior of the striped parrotfish *Scarus croicensis* Bloch (Scaridae). *Ecology,* 1973, *54*, 1377–1382.

Burger, J., and Beer, C. G. Territoriality in the laughing gull *(L. atricilla). Behaviour,* 1975, *55*, 301–320.

Burt, W. H. Territoriality and home range concepts as applied to mammals. *J. Mammal.,* 1943, *24*, 346–352.

Calhoun, J. B. *The Ecology and Sociology of the Norway Rat.* U.S. Public Health Service, Washington, D.C., 1962 (Publication No. 1008).

Calhoun, J. B., and Casby, J. U. *Calculation of Home Range and Density of Small Mammals.* U.S. Public Health Service, Washington, D.C., 1958 (Monograph 55).

Campanella, P., and Wolf, L. L. Temporal leks as a mating system in a temperate zone dragonfly *(Odonata: Anisoptera)*. I. *Plathemis lydia* (Drury). *Behaviour*, 1974, *51*, 49–87.

Carpenter, F. L., and MacMillen, R. E. Energetic cost of feeding territories in an Hawaiian honeycreeper. *Oecologia*, 1976a, *26*, 213–233.

Carpenter, F. L., and MacMillen, R. E. Threshold model of feeding territoriality and test with a Hawaiian honeycreeper. *Science*, 1976b, 194, 639–641.

Caryl, P. G. Aggressive behaviour in the zebra finch *Taeniopygia guttata*. I. Fighting provoked by male and female social partners. *Behaviour*, 1975, *52*, 226–252.

Cashner, F. M. The ecology of *Cercocebus albigena* and *Cercocebus torquatus* in Rio Muni, Republic of Equatorial Guinea, West Africa. Ph.D. dissertation, Tulane University, 1972.

Chalmers, N. Group composition, ecology, and daily activities of free living mangabeys in Uganda. *Folia Primatol.*, 1968a, *8*, 247–262.

Chalmers, N. The social behavior of free-living mangabeys in Uganda. *Folia Primatol.*, 1968b, *8*, 263–281.

Chappuis, C. Un exemple de l'influence du milieu sur les émissions vocales des oiseaux: L'évolution des chants en forêt équatoriale. *Terre et Vie*, 1971, *25*, 183–202.

Charles-Dominique, P. Aggression and territoriality in nocturnal prosimians. In R. L. Holloway (ed.), *Primate Aggression, Territoriality, and Xenophobia*. Academic Press, New York, 1974, pp. 31–48.

Charnov, E. L., Orians, G. H., and Hyatt, K. Ecological implications of resource depression. *Am. Natur.*, 1976, *110*, 247–259.

Chivers, D. J. On the daily behaviour and spacing of howling monkey groups. *Folia Primatol.*, 1969, *10*, 48–102.

Chivers, D. J., Raemakers, J. I., and Aldrich-Blake, F. P. G. Long-term observations of siamang behaviour. *Folia Primatol.*, 1975, *23*, 1–49.

Clark, P. J., and Evans, F. C. Distance to nearest neighbor as a measure of spatial relationships in populations. *Ecology*, 1954, *35*, 445–453.

Clark, P. J., and Evans, F. C. On some aspects of spatial pattern in biological populations. *Science*, 1955, *121*, 397–398.

Clutton-Brock, T. H. Ranging behaviour of red colobus *(Colobus badius tephrosceles)* in the Gombe National Park. *Anim. Behav.*, 1975, *23*, 706–722.

Clutton-Brock, T. H., and Harvey, P. H. Evolutionary rules and primate societies. In P. P. G. Bateson and R. A. Hinde (eds.), *Growing Points in Ethology*. Cambridge University Press, Cambridge, 1976, pp. 195–238.

Cody, M. L. Finch flocks in the Mojave Desert. *Theor. Pop. Biol.*, 1971, *2*, 142–158.

Cody, M. L. Optimization in ecology. *Science*, 1974, *183*, 1156–1164.

Coleman, P. D. An analysis of cues to auditory depth perception in free space. *Psychol. Bull.*, 1963, *60*, 302–315.

Collias, N. E. Statistical analysis of factors which make for success in initial encounters between hens. *Am. Natur.*, 1943, *77*, 519–538.

Colwell, R. K., and Futuyma, D. J. On the measurement of niche breadth and overlap. *Ecology*, 1971, *52*, 567–576.

Conder, P. J. Individual distance. *Ibis*, 1949, *91*, 649–655.

Conder, P. J. The territory of the wheatear *Oenanthe oenanthe*. *Ibis*, 1956, *98*, 453–459.

Courchesne, E., and Barlow, G. W. Effect of isolation on components of aggressive and other behavior in the hermit crab, *Pagurus samuelis*. *Z. Vgl. Physiol.*, 1971, *75*, 32–48.

Craig, J. V., Biswas, D. K., and Guhl, A. M. Agonistic behavior influenced by strangeness, crowding and heredity in female domestic fowl *(Gallus gallus)*. *Anim. Behav.*, 1969, *17*, 498–506.

Crook, J. H. The basis of flock organisation in birds. In W. H. Thorpe, and O. L. Zangwill (eds.), *Current Problems in Animal Behaviour*. Cambridge University Press, Cambridge, 1961, pp. 125–149.

DeVore, I., and Hall, K. R. L. Baboon ecology. In I. DeVore (ed.), *Primate Behavior*. Holt, Rhinehart, and Winston, New York, 1965, pp. 20–52.

Dhondt, A. A. A method to establish boundaries of birds' territories. *Giervalk*, 1966, *56*, 404–408.

Dice, L. R., and Clark, P. J. The statistical concept of home range as applied to the recapture of the deermouse *(Peromyscus)*. *Contributions of the University of Michigan Laboratory of Vertebrate Biology*, Contribution 62, 1953.

Diebschlag, E. Psychologische Beobachtungen über die Rangordnung bei der Haustaube. *Z. Tierpsychol.*, 1941, *4*, 173–187.

Dixon, K. L. Some aspects of social organization in the Carolina chickadee. *Proc. XIII Ornithol. Cong.,* 1963, 240–258.

Dixon, K. L. Dominance–subordination relationships in mountain chickadees. *Condor,* 1965, *67*, 291–299.

Dumortier, B. The physical characteristics of sound emission in Arthropoda. In R. G. Busnel (ed.), *Acoustic Behavior of Animals.* Elsevier, Amsterdam, 1963.

Dunford, C. Behavioral aspects of spatial organization in the chipmunk, *Tamias striatus. Behaviour,* 1970, *36*, 215–231.

Dunn, J. E., and Gipson, P. S. Analysis of radiotelemetry data in studies of home range. *Biometrics,* 1977, *33*, 85–101.

Eaton, R. L. Group interactions, spacing and territoriality in cheetahs. *Z. Tierpsychol.,* 1970, *27*, 481–491.

Eisenberg, J. F. Phylogeny, behavior, and ecology in the Mammalia. In P. Luckett, and F. Szaley (eds.), *Phylogeny of the Primates.* Plenum Press, New York, 1975, pp. 47–68.

Eisenberg, J. F. The evolution of the reproductive unit in the class Mammalia. In J. S. Rosenblatt and B. R. Komisaruk (eds.), Reproductive Behavior and Evolution. Plenum Press, New York, 1977, pp. 39–71.

Eisenberg, J. F., Muckenhirn, N. A., and Rudran, R. The relation between ecology and social structure in primates. *Science,* 1972, *176*, 863–874.

Ellefson, J. O. Territorial behavior in the common white-handed gibbon, *Hylobates lar* Linn. In P. Jay (ed.), *Primates: Studies in Adaptation and Variability.* Holt, Rinehart and Winston, New York, 1968, pp. 180–199.

Emlen, J. T., Jr. Flocking behavior in birds. *Auk,* 1952, *69*, 160–170.

Emlen, J. T., Jr. Defended area? A critique of the territory concept and of conventional thinking. *Ibis,* 1957, *99*, 352.

Emlen, J. T., Jr., and Lorenz, F. W. Pairing responses of free-living valley quail to sex-hormone pellet implants. *Auk,* 1942, *59*, 369–378.

Emlen, S. T. Lek organization and mating strategies in the bullfrog. *Behav. Ecol. Sociobiol.,* 1976, *1*, 283–313.

Epple, G. The behavior of marmoset monkeys. In L. A. Rosenblum (ed.), *Primate Behavior,* Vol. 4. Academic Press, New York, 1975, pp. 195–239.

Erickson, M. M. Territory, annual cycle, and numbers in a population of wren-tits *(Chamaea fasciata). Univ. Calif. Publ. Zool.,* 1938, *42*, 247–321.

Erlinge, S. Territoriality of the otter *Lutra lutra* L. *Oikos,* 1968, *19*, 81–98.

Estes, R. D. Territorial behavior of the wildebeest *(Connochaetus taurinus,* Burchell, 1823). *Z. Tierpsychol.,* 1969, *26*, 284–370.

Evans, J., and Griffith, R. E. A fluorescent tracer and marker for animal studies. *J. Wildl. Manage.,* 1973, *37*, 73–81.

Evans, L. T. A study of a social hierarchy in the lizard *Anolis carolinensis. J. Gen. Psychol.,* 1936, *48*, 88–111.

Ewer, R. F. *Ethology of Mammals.* Logos, London, 1968.

Fagen, R. M., and Goldman, R. N. Behavioral catalog analysis methods. *Anim. Behav.,* 1977, *25*, 261–274.

Falls, J. B., and Brooks, R. J. Individual recognition by song in white-throated sparrows. II. Effects of location. *Can. J. Zool.,* 1975, *53*, 1412–1420.

Feynman, R. P., Leighton, R. B., and Sands, M. *The Feynman Lectures on Physics.* Addison-Wesley, Reading, Mass., 1964.

Ficken, M. S. Agonistic behavior and territory in the American redstart. *Auk,* 1962, *79*, 607–632.

Fitch, H. S. A field study of the growth and behavior of the fence lizard. *Univ. Calif. Publ. Zool.,* 1940, *44*, 151–172.

Francis, L. Intraspecific aggression and its effect on the distribution of *Anthopleura elegantissima* and some related sea anemones. *Biol. Bull.,* 1973, *144*, 73–92.

Frantz, S. C. Fluorescent pigments for studying movements and home ranges of small mammals. *J. Mammal.,* 1972, *53*, 218–223.

Fredericson, E., Story, A. W., Gurney, N. L., and Butterworth, K. The relationships between heredity, sex, and aggression in two inbred mouse strains. *J. Gen. Psychol.,* 1955, *87*, 121–130.

Frey, D. F., and Miller, R. J. The establishment of dominance relationships in the blue gourami, *Trichogaster trichopterus* (Pallas). *Behaviour,* 1972, *42*, 8–62.

Garreffa, L. F. Aggression reduced by prior experience in bobwhite quail *(Colinus virginianus). Commun. Behav. Biol.,* 1969, *4*, 251–254.

Gautier-Hion, A. L'écologie du talapoin du Gabon. *Terre et Vie,* 1971, *25*, 427–490.

Geist, V., and Walther, F. (eds.). *The Behavior of Ungulates and Its Relation to Management.* I.U.C.N., Morges, Switzerland, 1974, (Publication No. 24).

Gerhardt, C. Sound pressure levels and radiation patterns of the vocalizations of some North American frogs and toads. *J. Comp. Physiol.,* 1975, *102*, 1–12.

Gill, F. B., and Wolf, L. R. Economics of feeding territoriality in the golden-winged sunbird. *Ecology,* 1975a, *56*, 333–345.

Gill, F. B., and Wolf, L. R. Foraging strategies and energetics of East African sunbirds at mistletoe flowers. *Am. Natur.,* 1975b, *109*, 491–510.

Glase, J. C. Ecology of social organization in the black-capped chickadee. *Living Bird,* 1973, *12*, 235–268.

Goodall, D. W. Statistical plant ecology. *Ann. Rev. Ecol. System.,* 1970, *1*, 99–123.

Gorman, M. L. A mechanism for individual recognition by odour in *Hespestes auropunctatus* (Carnivora: Viverridae). *Anim. Behav.,* 1976, *24*, 141–145.

Gorman, M. L., Nedwell, D. B., and Smith, R. M. An analysis of the contents of anal scent pockets of *Hespestes auropunctatus* (Carnivora: Viverridae). *J. Zool. Lond.,* 1974, *172*, 24, 141–145.

Goss-Custard, J. D. Feeding dispersion in some overwintering wading birds. In J. H. Crook (ed.), *Social Behaviour in Birds and Mammals.* Academic Press, London, 1970, pp. 3–35.

Gottfried, B. M., and Franks, E. C. Habitat use and flock activity of dark-eyed juncos in winter. *Wilson Bull.,* 1975, *87*, 374–383.

Griffin, D. R., and Hopkins, C. D. Sounds audible to migrating birds. *Anim. Behav.,* 1974, *22*, 672–678.

Guhl, A. M., and W. C. Allee. Some measureable effects of social organization in flocks of hens. *Physiol. Zool.,* 1944, *17*, 320–347.

Hall, C. S., and Klein, L. L. Individual differences in aggressiveness in rats. *J. Comp. Psychol.,* 1942, *33*, 371–383.

Hall, K. R. L. Behavior and ecology of the wild patas monkey. *Erythrocebus patas,* Uganda. *J. Zool. Lond.,* 1965, *148*, 15–87.

Hamilton, W. D. Geometry for the selfish herd. *J. Theor. Biol.,* 1971a, *31*, 295–311.

Hamilton, W. D. Selection of selfish and altruistic behavior in some extreme models. In J. F. Eisenberg and W. S. Dillon (eds.), *Man and Beast: Comparative Social Behavior.* Smithsonian, Washington, D.C., 1971b, pp. 57–91.

Hamilton, W. J. Aggressive behavior in migrant pectoral sandpipers. *Condor,* 1959, *61*, 161–179.

Harding, R. S. O. Ranging patterns of a troop of baboons *(Papio anubis)* in Kenya. *Folia Primatol.,* 1976, *25*, 143–185.

Harris, V. A. *The Life of the Rainbow Lizard.* Hutchinson, London, 1964, p. 174.

Harrison, J. L. Range of movement of some Malayan rats. *J. Mammal.,* 1958, *39*, 190–206.

Hartzler, J. E. Winter dominance relationships in black-capped chickadees. *Wilson Bull.,* 1970, *82*, 427–434.

Hayne, D. W. Calculation of size of home range. *J. Mammal.,* 1949, *30*, 1–18.

Hazlett, B. A. Individual distance in the hermit crabs *Clibanarius tricolor* and *Clibanarius antillensis. Behaviour,* 1974, *52*, 253–265.

Hediger, H. *Wild Animals in Captivity.* Butterworth, London, 1950.

Heiligenberg, W. The effect of external stimuli on the attack readiness of a cichlid fish. *Z. Vgl. Physiol.,* 1965, *49*, 459–464.

Heiligenberg, W., and Kramer, U. Aggressiveness as a function of external stimulation. *J. Comp. Physiol.,* 1972, *77*, 332–340.

Hel, G. S. The ecological context of aggression in the coconut crab, *Birgus latro* (L.) *Abs. Anim. Behav. Soc. Meeting,* May 1975.

Hendrichs, H., and Hendrichs, U. *Dikdik und Elephanten.* Piper, München, 1971.

Herrero, S. A comparison of some features of the evolution, ecology, and behavior of black and grizzly bears. *Carnivore,* 1978, *1*, 7–16.

Heuts, B. A., and Boer, J. N. de. Territory choice guided by familiar object cues from earlier territories in the jewel fish *Hemichromis bimaculatus* Gill 1862 (Pisces, Cichlidae). *Behaviour,* 1973, *45*, 67–82.

Hinde, R. A. The behavior of the great tit *(Parus major)* and some other related species. *Behav. Suppl.,* 1952, *2*, 1–201.

Hinde, R. A. The biological significance of the territories of birds. *Ibis,* 1956, *98*, 340–369.

Holgate, P. Random walk models for animal behavior. *Int. Symp. Statist. Ecol.,* 1969, *2*, 1–12.

Holmes, R. T., and Pitelka, F. A. Food overlap among coexisting sandpipers on northern Alaskan tundra. *System. Zool.*, 1968, *17*, 305–318.

Hopkins, C. D. Electric communication in fish. *Am. Sci.*, 1974, *62*, 426–437.

Horn, H. S. Measurement of "overlap" in comparative ecological studies. *Am. Natur.*, 1966, *100*, 419–424.

Horn, H. S. The adaptive significance of colonial nesting in the Brewer's blackbird *(Euphagus cyanocephalus)*. *Ecology*, 1968, *49*, 682–694.

Hornocker, M. G. Winter territoriality in mountain lions. *J. Wildl. Manage.*, 1969, *33*, 457–464.

Howard, E. *Territory in Bird Life*. Collins, London, 1920.

Hutchinson, G. E. The concept of pattern in ecology. *Proc. Nat. Acad. Sci.*, 1953, *105*, 1–12.

Huxley, J. S. A natural experiment on the territorial instinct. *Br. Birds*, 1934, *27*, 270–277.

Ickes, R. A., and Ficken, M. S. An investigation of territorial behavior in the American redstart utilizing recorded songs. *Wilson Bull.*, 1970, *82*, 167–176.

Iersel, J. J. A. van. Some aspects of territorial behaviour of the male three-spined stickleback. *Arch. Néer. Zool. 13, Suppl*, 1958, *1*, 384–400.

Ingard, U. A review of the influence of meteorological conditions on sound propagation. *J. Acoust. Soc. Am.*, 1953, *25*, 405–411.

Janzen, D. H. Euglossine bees as long-distance pollinators of tropical plants. *Science*, 1971, *171*, 203–205.

Jarman, P. J. The social organisation of antelope in relation to their ecology. *Behaviour*, 1974, *48*, 215–267.

Jenni, D. A. Effects of conspecifics and vegetation on nest site selection in *Gasterosteus aculeatus* L. *Behaviour*, 1972, *42*, 97–118.

Jennrich, R. I., and Turner, F. B. Measurement of non-circular home range. *J. Theor. Biol.*, 1969, *22*, 227–237.

Jewell, P. A. The concept of home range in mammals. In P. A. Jewell and C. Loizos (eds.), *Play, Exploration, and Territory in Mammals. Symp. Zool. Soc. Lond.*, 1966, *18*, 85–109.

Johnston, R. E., and Lee, N. A. Persistence of the odor deposited by two functionally distinct scent marking behaviors of golden hamsters. *Behav. Biol.*, 1976, *16*, 199–210.

Jorgensen, C. D. Home range as a measure of probable interaction among populations of small mammals. *J. Mammal.*, 1968a, *49*, 104–112.

Jorgensen, C. D. Spatial relationships of *Perognathus longimembris* (Coues) in southern Nevada. *Proc. Utah Acad. Sci. Arts, Lett.*, 1968b, *45*, 118–125.

Justice, K. E. A new method for measuring home ranges of small mammals. *J. Mammal.*, 1961, *42*, 462–470.

Kendeigh, S. C. Territorial and mating behavior of the house wren. *Ill. Biol. Monogr.*, 1941, *18*, 1–120.

Kleiman, D. G. Monogamy in mammals. *Q. Rev. Biol.*, 1977, *52*, 39–69.

Kleiman, D. G., and Eisenberg, J. F. Comparisons of canid and felid social systems from an evolutionary perspective. *Anim. Behav.*, 1973, *21*, 637–659.

Klein, L. L., and Klein, D. J. Social and ecological contrasts between four taxa of neotropical primates *(Ateles belzebuth, Alouatta seniculus, Saimiri sciurensis, Cebus apella)*. In. R. Tuttle (ed.), *Socioecology and Psychology of Primates*. Mouton, The Hague, 1975.

Klopfer, P. H., and Jolly, A. The stability of territorial boundaries in a lemur troop. *Folia Primatol.*, 1970, *12*, 199–208.

Knapton, R. W., and Krebs, J. R. Settlement patterns, territory size, and breeding density in the song sparrow *(Melospiza melodia)*. *Can. J. Zool.*, 1974, *52*, 1413–1420.

Knudsen, V. The propagation of sound in the atmosphere—Attenuation and fluctuations. *J. Acoust. Soc. Am.*, 1946, *18*, 90–96.

Konishi, M. Locatable and nonlocatable acoustic signals for barn owls. *Am. Natur.*, 1973, *107*, 775–785.

Krebs, J. R. Territory and breeding density in the great tit, *Parus major* L. *Ecology*, 1971, *52*, 1–22.

Krebs, J. R. Behavioral aspects of predation. In P. P. G. Bateson and P. H. Klopfer (eds.), *Perspectives in Ethology*. Plenum, New York, 1973, pp. 73–111.

Kruuk, H. Predators and anti-predator behaviour of the black-headed gull *(Larus ridibundus* L.). *Behav., Suppl.*, 1964, *11*, 1–130.

Kummer, H., Götz, W., and Angst, W. Triadic differentiation: An inhibitory process protecting pair bonds in baboons. *Behaviour*, 1974, *49*, 62–87.

Lack, D. *The Life of the Robin*. Witherby, London, 1943.

Lack, D. The Galapagos finches (*Geospizinae*): A study in variation. *Occasional Papers of the California Academy of Sciences*, 1945, *21*, 1–159.

Lack, D. *Population Studies of Birds*. Clarendon, Oxford, 1966.

Lack, D., and Lack, L. Territory reviewed. *Br. Birds*, 1933, *27* 179–199.

Lagerspetz, K. M. J. Genetic and social causes of aggressive behavior in mice. *Scand. J. Psychol.*, 1961, *2*, 167–173.

Lagerspetz, K. M. J., and Hautojarvi, S. The effect of prior aggressive or sexual arousal on subsequent aggressive or sexual reactions in male mice. *Scand. J. Psychol.*, 1967, *8*, 1–6.

Lance, A. N. Survival and recruitment success of individual young cock red grouse *Lagopus l. scoticus* tracked by radio-telemetry. *Ibis*, 1978a, *120*, 369–378.

Lance, A. N. Territories and the food plant of individual red grouse. II. Territory size compared with an index of nutrient supply in heather. *J. Anim. Ecol.*, 1978b, *47*, 307–313.

Lanyon, W. E. The comparative biology of the meadowlarks (Sturnella) in Wisconsin. *Publications of the Nuttall Ornithological Club*, 1957, *1*, 1–67.

Leong, C. Y. The quantitative effect of releasers on the attack readiness of the fish *Haplochromis burtoni* (Cichlidae, Pisces). *Z. Vgl. Physiol.*, 1969, *65*, 29–50.

Leyhausen, P. The communal organization of solitary mammals. *Symp. Zool. Soc. Lond.*, 1965, *14*, 249–263.

Leyhausen, P., and Wolff, R. Das Revier einer Hauskatze. *Z. Tierpsychol.*, 1959, *16*, 666–670.

Lighter, F. J. The social use of space in the Hawaiian ghost crab *Ocypode ceratophthalmus* and *O. laevis. Abstr., Anim. Behav. Soc. Meeting*, May 1975.

Lockie, J. D. Territory in small carnivores. *Symp. Zool. Soc. Lond.*, 1966, *18*, 143–165.

Lorenz, K. *King Solomon's Ring*. Crowell, New York, 1952.

Marler, P. Studies of fighting in chaffinches. I. Behaviour in relation to the social hierarchy. *Br. J. Anim. Behav.*, 1955a, *3*, 111–117.

Marler, P. Studies of fighting in chaffinches. II. The effect on dominance relations of disguising females as males. *Br. J. Anim. Behav.*, 1955b, *3*, 137–147.

Marler, P. Behaviour of the chaffinch *Fringilla coelebs. Behaviour, Suppl.*, 1956a, *5*, 1–184.

Marler, P. Studies of fighting in chaffinches. III. Proximity as a cause of aggression. *Br. J. Anim. Behav.*, 1956b, *4*, 23–30.

Marler, P. Territory and individual distance in the chaffinch *Fringilla coelebs. Ibis*, 1956c, *98*, 496–501.

Marler, P. Studies of fighting in chaffinches. IV. Appetitive and consummatory behaviour. *Br. J. Anim. Behav.*, 1957, *5*, 29–37.

Marler, P. Aggregation and dispersal: Two functions in primate communication. In P. C. Jay (ed.), *Primates: Studies in Adaptation and Variability*. Holt, Rhinehart, and Winston, New York, 1968, pp. 240–438.

Marler, P. Vocalizations of East African monkeys. II. Black and white colobus. *Behaviour*, 1972, *42*, 175–196.

Marler, P. On animal aggression: The roles of strangeness and familiarity. *Am. Psychol.*, 1976, *31*, 239–246.

Marten, K., and Marler, P. Sound transmission and its significance for animal vocalization. I. Temperate habitats. *Behav. Ecol. Sociobiol.*, 1977, *2*, 271–290.

Marten, K., Quine, D., and Marler, P. Sound transmission and its significance for animal vocalization. II. Tropical forest habitats. *Behav. Ecol. Sociobiol.*, 1977, *2*, 291–302.

Mason, W. A. Use of space by Callicebus groups. In P. Jay (ed.), *Primates: Studies in Adaptation and Variability*. Holt, Rinehart, and Winston, New York, 1968, pp. 200–216.

May, R. M. Some notes on estimating the competition matrix α. *Ecology*, 1975, *56*, 737–741.

Maynard Smith, J. *The Theory of Evolution*. Penguin, Baltimore, 1958.

Maynard Smith, J. *Models in Ecology*. Cambridge University Press, New York, 1974a.

Maynard Smith, J. The theory of games and the evolution of animal conflicts. *J. Theor. Biol.*, 1974b, *47*, 209–221.

Maynard Smith, J. Evolution and the theory of games. *Am. Sci.*, 1976, *64*, 4145.

Maynard Smith, J., and Parker, G. A. The logic of asymmetric contests. *Anim. Behav.*, 1976, *24*, 159–175.

Maynard Smith, J., and Price, G. R. The logic of animal conflicts. *Nature*, 1973, *246*, 15–18.

Mazurkiewicz, M. Size, shape, and distribution of home ranges of *Clethrionomys glareolus. Acta Theriol.*, 1971, *16*, 23–60.

McNab, B. Bioenergetics and determination of home range size. *Am. Natur.*, 1963, *97*, 133–140.

Metzgar, L. H. The measurement of home range shape. *J. Wildl. Manage.*, 1972, *36*, 643–645.

Metzgar, L. H. A comparison of trap- and track-revealed home ranges in *Peromyscus*. *J. Mammal.*, 1973a, *54*, 513–515.

Metzgar, L. H. Home range shape and activity in *Peromyscus leucopus*. *J. Mammal.*, 1973b, *54*, 383–390.

Metzgar, L. H., and Hill, R. The measurement of dispersion in small mammal populations. *J. Mammal.*, 1971, *52*, 12–20.

Michener, H., and Michener, J. R. Mockingbirds, their territories and individualities. *Condor*, 1935, *37*, 97–140.

Miller, A. H. Systematic revision and natural history of the American shrikes (*Lanius*). *Univ. Calif. Publ. Zool.*, 1931, *38*, 11–242.

Miller, G. R., Jenkins, D., and Watson, A. Heather performance and red grouse populations. I. Visual estimates of heather performance. *J. Appl. Ecol.*, 1966, *3*, 313–326.

Miller, G. R., Watson, A., and Jenkins, D. Responses of red grouse populations to experimental improvement of their food. In A. Watson (ed.), *Animal Populations in Relation to Their Food Resources*. Blackwell, Oxford, England, 1970, pp. 323–335.

Miller, R. S., and Stephen, W. J. D. Spatial relationships in flocks of sandhill cranes (*Grus canadensis*). *Ecology*, 1966, *47*, 323–327.

Moehlman, P. D. Jackal social organization and ecology. *Ann. Rep. Serengeti Res. Inst.*, 1977, 112–117.

Montgomery, G. G. Communication in red fox dyads: A computer simulation study. *Smithson. Contrib. Zool.*, 1974, *187*, 1–30.

Montgomery, G. G. (ed.). *Arboreal Folivores*. Smithsonian Institution Press, Washington, D.C., in press.

Montgomery, G. G., Cochran, W. W., and Sunquist, M. E. Radiotracking arboreal vertebrates in tropical forest. *J. Wildl. Manage.*, 1973, *37*, 426–428.

Morse, D. H. Ecological aspects of some mixed species foraging flocks of birds. *Ecol. Monogr.*, 1970, *40*, 119–168.

Morse, D. H. Variables affecting the density and territory size of breeding spruce-woods warblers. *Ecology*, 1976, *57*, 290–301.

Morton, E. S. Ecological sources of selection on avian sounds. *Am. Natur.*, 1975, *109*, 17–34.

Moss, R. A comparison of red grouse (*Lagopus l. scoticus*) stocks with the production and nutritive value of heather (*Calluna vulgaris*). *J. Anim. Ecol.*, 1969, *38*, 103–112.

Muckenhirn, N. A., and Eisenberg, J. F. Spacing and predation by the Ceylon leopard. In R. Eaton (ed.), *The World's Cats*. Unimark, Seattle, 1973.

Mugford, R. A. Inter-male fighting affected by the home cage odors of male and female mice. *J. Comp. Physiol. Psychol.*, 1973, *84*, 289–295.

Nero, R. W. A behavior study of the red-winged blackbird. II. Territoriality. *Wilson Bull.*, 1956, *68*, 129–150.

Nero, R. W., and Emlen, J. T., Jr. An experimental study of territorial behavior in breeding red-winged blackbirds. *Condor*, 1951, *53*, 105–116.

Neville, M. K. The population structure of red howler monkeys (*Alouatta seniculus*) in Trinidad and Venezuela. *Folia Primatol.*, 1972, *17*, 56–86.

Nice, M. M. The role of territory in bird life. *Am. Midl. Natur.*, 1941, *26*, 441–487.

Nice, M. M. Studies in the life history of the song sparrow. *Trans. Linn. Soc. N.Y.*, Vol. 2, 1943, *6*, 1–328.

Nicholls, T. H., and Warner, D. W. Barred owl habitat use as determined by radiotelemetry. *J. Wildl. Manage.*, 1972, *36*, 213–224.

Oates, J. F. The guereza and its food. In T. Clutton-Brock (ed.), *Primate Ecology*. Academic Press, London, 1976, pp. 276–371.

Odum, E. P. Winter homing behavior of the chickadee. *Bird-Banding*, 1941, *12*, 113–119.

Odum, E. P., and Kuenzler, E. J. Measurement of territory and home range size in birds. *Auk*, 1955, *72*, 128–137.

Owen-Smith, R. N. Territoriality: The example of the white rhinoceros. *Zool. Afr.*, 1972, *7*, 273–280.

Owen-Smith, R. N. The social ethology of the white rhinoceros *Ceratotherium simum* (Burchell 1817). *Z. Tierpsychol.*, 1975, *38*, 337–384.

Parker, G. A. Assessment strategy and the evolution of fighting behaviour. *J. Theor. Biol.*, 1974, *47*, 223–243.

Patterson, I. J. Timing and spacing of broods in the black-headed gull, *Larus ridibundus*. *Ibis*, 1965, *107*, 433–460.

Peeke, H. V. S., Herz, M. J., and Gallagher, J. E. Changes in aggressive interaction in adjacently territorial convict cichlids (*Cichlasoma nigrofasciatum*): A study of habituation. *Behaviour*, 1971, *40*, 43–54.

Peters, R. P., and Mech, L. D. Scentmarking in wolves. *Am. Sci.,* 1976, *63*, 628–637.

Pianka, E. R. Niche relations of desert lizards. In M. L. Cody and J. M. Diamond, (eds.), *Ecology and Evolution of Communities.* Belknap Press, Cambridge, Mass., 1975, pp. 292–314.

Pielou, E. C. *An Introduction to Mathematical Ecology.* Wiley, New York, 1969.

Pitelka, F. A. Numbers, breeding schedule, and territoriality in pectoral sandpipers in northern Alaska. *Condor,* 1959, *61*, 233–264.

Post, W. Functional analysis of space-related behavior in the seaside sparrow. *Ecology,* 1974, *55*, 564–575.

Preston, F. W. The canonical distribution of commonness and rarity. *Ecology,* 1962, *29*, 254–283.

Pulliam, H. R. On the advantages of flocking. *J. Theor. Biol.* 1973, *38*, 419–422.

Pulliam, H. R., Anderson, K. A., Misztal, A., and Moore, N. Temperature-dependent social behaviour in juncos. *Ibis,* 1974, *116*, 360–364.

Rasa, O. A. E. Appetence for aggression in juvenile damsel fish. *Z. Tierpsychol.,* 1971, *Beiheft 7*, 1–20.

Rathbun, G. The social behavior and ecology of elephant shrews. *Z. Tierpsychol.,* in press.

Regnier, F. E., and Goodwin, M. On the chemical and environmental modulation of pheromone release from vertebrate scent marks. In D. Muller-Schwarze (ed.), *Chemical Signals in Vertebrates.* Plenum Press, New York, 1977.

Richards, D. G. Recognition of neighbors by associative learning: An experiment with interspecific imitation in rufous-sided towhees. *Auk,* in press.

Richards, D. G., and Wiley, R. H. Reverberations and amplitude fluctuations in the propagation of sound in a forest: Implications for animal communication. *Am. Natur.,* in press.

Ritchey, F. Dominance–subordination and territorial relationships in the common pigeon. *Physiol. Zool.,* 1951, *24*, 167–176.

Robinson, J. G. Vocal regulation of use of space by groups of titi monkeys *Callicebus moloch. Behav. Ecol. Sociobiol.,* in press.

Robinson, W. L., and Falls, J. B. A study of homing in meadow mice. *Am. Midl. Natur.,* 1965, *73*, 188–224.

Rohles, F. H., Jr., and Wilson, L. M. Hunger as a catalyst in aggression. *Behaviour,* 1974, *48*, 123–130.

Rohlf, F. J., and Davenport, D. Simulation of simple models of animal behavior with a digital computer. *J. Theor. Biol.,* 1969, *23*, 400–424.

Rudran, R. Socioecology of the blue monkey *(Cercopithecus mitis stuhlmanni)* in the Kibale forest, Uganda. Ph.D. dissertation, University of Maryland, 1976.

Sabine, W. S. The winter society of the Oregon junco: Intolerance, dominance, and the pecking order. *Condor,* 1959, *61*, 110–135.

Sale, P. F. Effect of cover on agonistic behavior of a reef fish: A possible spacing mechanism. *Ecology,* 1972, *53*, 753–758.

Sanderson, G. C. The study of mammal movements: A review. *J. Wildl. Manage.,* 1966, *30*, 215–235.

Schaller, G. *The Mountain Gorilla.* University of Chicago Press, Chicago, 1963.

Schaller, G. *The Seregenti Lion.* University of Chicago Press, Chicago, 1972.

Schleidt, W. M. Localization of sound-producing animals by means of arrival-time differences of their signals at an array of microphones. *Experientia,* in press.

Schoener, T. W. The Anolis lizards of Bimini: Resource partitioning in a complex fauna. *Ecology,* 1968a, *49*, 704–726.

Schoener, T. W. Sizes of feeding territories among birds. *Ecology,* 1968b, *49*, 123–142.

Schoener, T. W. Nonsynchronous spatial overlap of lizards in patchy habitats. *Ecology,* 1970, *51*, 408–418.

Schoener, T. W. Theory of feeding strategies. *Ann. Rev. Ecol. System.,* 1971, *2*, 369–404.

Scott, J. P., and Fredericson, E. The causes of fighting in mice and rats. *Physiol. Zool.,* 1951, *24*, 273–309.

Siegfried, W. R., and Underhill, L. G. Flocking as anti-predator strategy in doves. *Anim. Behav.,* 1975, *23*, 504–508.

Siniff, D. B., and Jessen, C. R. A simulation model of animal movement patterns. *Adv. Ecol. Res.,* 1969, *6*, 185–219.

Smith, C. C. The adaptive nature of social organization in the genus of tree squirrels *Tamiasciurus. Ecol. Monogr.,* 1968, *38*, 31–63.

Smith, J. N. M. The food searching behaviour of two European thrushes. II. The adaptiveness of the search patterns. *Behaviour,* 1974, *49*, 1–61.

Southern, H. N. Tawny owls and their prey. *Ibis,* 1954, *96*, 384–410.

Southwick, C. H., Farooqui, M. Y., Siddiqi, M. F., and Pal, B. C. Xenophobia among free-ranging Rhesus groups in India. In R. L. Holloway (ed.), *Primate Aggression, Territoriality, and Xenophobia.* Academic Press, New York, 1974, pp. 185–209.

Spencer, J., Gray, J., and Dalhouse, A. Social isolation in the gerbil: Its effect on exploratory or agonistic behavior and adrenocortical activity. *Physiol. Behav.,* 1973, *10*, 231–237.

Spurr, E. B. Individual differences in aggressiveness of Adelie penquins. *Anim. Behav.,* 1974, *22*, 611–616.

Stefanski, R. A. Utilization of the breeding territory in the black-capped chickadee. *Condor,* 1967, *69*, 259–267.

Stenger, J. Food habits and available food of ovenbirds in relation to territory size. *Auk,* 1958, *75*, 335–346.

Stenger, J., and Falls, J. B. The utilized territory of the ovenbird. *Wilson Bull.,* 1959, *71*, 125–140.

Stevens, E. D., and Josephson, R. K. Metabolic rate and body temperature in singing katydids. *Physiol. Zool.,* 1977, *50*, 31–42.

Stickel, L. F. Populations and home range relationships of the box turtle *Terrapene c. carolina. Ecol. Monogr.,* 1950, *20*, 353–378.

Stiles, F. G., and Wolf, L. L. Hummingbird territoriality at a tropical flowering tree. *Auk,* 1970, *87*, 467–491.

Struhsaker, T. T. Social structure among vervet monkeys *(Cercopithecus aethiops). Behaviour,* 1967, *29*, 83–121.

Struhsaker, T. T. *The Red Colobus Monkey.* University of Chicago Press, Chicago, 1975.

Struhsaker, T. T. Food habits of five monkey species in the Kibale Forest, Uganda. In D. J. Chivers (ed.), *Recent Advances in Primatology.* Academic Press, New York, 1978, pp. 225–248.

Struhsaker, T. T., and Leland, L. Socioecology of five sympatric monkey species in the Kibale Forest, Uganda. In press.

Struhsaker, T. T., and Leland, L. Socioecology of five sympatric monkey species in the Kibale Forest, Uganda. In J. S. Rosenblatt, R. A. Hinde, E. Shaw, and C. Beer (eds.), *Advances in the Study of Behavior* (Vol. 9). Academic Press, New York, 1979.

Struhsaker, T. T., and Oates, J. F. A comparison of the behaviour and ecology of red colobus and black-and-white colobus monkeys in Uganda: A summary. In R. H. Tuttle (ed.), *Socioecology and Psychology of Primates.* Mouton, The Hague, 1975, pp. 103–124.

Taber, R. D., and Cowan, I. McT. Trapping and marking wild animals. In R. H. Giles (ed.), *Wildlife Management Techniques.* The Wildlife Society, Washington, D.C., 1971, pp. 277–318.

Tenaza, R. R. Territory and monogamy among Kloss' gibbons *(Hylobates klossii)* in Siberut Island, Indonesia. *Folia Primatol.,* 1975, *24*, 60–80.

Tinbergen, N. The behavior of the snow bunting in spring. *Trans. Linn. Soc. N.Y.,* 1939, *51*, 1–94.

Tinbergen, N. *The Herring Gull's World,* rev. ed. Basic Books, New York, 1960.

Tinbergen, N. Adaptive features in the black-headed gull. *Proc. XIV Inter. Ornithol. Cong.,* 1967, 43–60.

Tinbergen, N., Impekoven, M., and Franck, D. An experiment on spacing-out as a defense against predation. *Behaviour,* 1964, *28*, 307–321.

Tinkle, D. W. Home range, density, dynamics, and structure of a Texas population of the lizard *Uta stansburiana.* In W. W. Milstead (ed.), *Lizard Ecology.* University of Missouri Press, Kansas City, 1965.

Turner, F. B., Jennrich, R. I., and Weintraub, J. D. Home ranges and body size of lizards. *Ecology,* 1969, *50*, 1076–1081.

Ulrich, J. The social hierarchy in albino mice. *J. Comp. Physiol. Psychol.,* 1938, *25*, 373–413.

Valzelli, L. Aggressive behaviors induced by isolation. In S. Garattini and E. B. Sigg (eds.), *Aggressive Behaviour.* Excerpta Medica, Amsterdam, 1969, pp. 70–76.

Verner, J., and Milligan, M. M. Responses of male white-crowned sparrows to playback of recorded songs. *Condor,* 1971, *73*, 56–64.

Vine, I. Risk of visual detection and pursuit by a predator and the selective advantage of flocking behavior. *J. Theor. Biol.,* 1971, *30*, 405–422.

Waser, P. M. Experimental playbacks show vocal mediation of intergroup avoidance in a forest monkey. *Nature,* 1975a, *255*, 56–58.

Waser, P. M. Spatial associations and social interactions in a "solitary" ungulate: The bushbuck *Tragelaphus scriptus* (Pallas). *Z. Tierpsychol.,* 1975b, *37*, 24–36.

Waser, P. M. *Cercocebus albigena:* Site attachment, avoidance, and intergroup spacing. *Am. Natur.,* 1976, *110*, 911–935.

Waser, P. M. Individual recognition, intragroup cohesion, and intergroup spacing: Evidence from sound playback to forest monkeys. *Behaviour,* 1977a, *60,* 28–74.

Waser, P. M. Sound localization by monkeys: A field experiment. *Behav. Ecol. Sociobiol.,* 1977b, *2,* 427–431.

Waser, P. M., and Floody, O. Ranging patterns of the mangabey *Cercocebus albigena* in the Kibale forest, Uganda. *Z. Tierpsychol.,* 1974, *35,* 85–101.

Waser, P. M., and Waser, M. S. Experimental studies of primate vocalization: Specializations for long-distance propagation. *Z. Tierpsychol.,* 1977, *43,* 239–263.

Watkins, W. A. Biological sound-source locations by computer analysis of underwater array data. *Deep-Sea Res.,* 1976, *23,* 175–180.

Watson, A. Territorial and reproductive behaviour of red grouse. *J. Reprod. Fertil.,* 1970, *Suppl. 11,* 3–14.

Watson, A., and Miller, G. R. Territory size and aggression in a fluctuating red grouse population. *J. Anim. Ecol.,* 1971, *40,* 367–383.

Watson, A., and Moss, R. Dominance, spacing behaviour and aggression in relation to population limitation in vertebrates. In A. Watson (ed.), *Animal Populations in Relation to Their Food Resources.* Blackwell, Oxford, 1970, pp. 167–218.

Watson, A., and Moss, R. A current model of population dynamics in red grouse. *Proc. XV Internat. Ornithol. Cong.,* 1972, 134–149.

Weeden, J. S. Territorial behavior of the tree sparrow. *Condor,* 1965, *67,* 193–209.

White, J. E. An index of range activity. *Am. Midl. Natur.,* 1964, *71,* 369–373.

Wiener, F. M., and Keast, D. N. Experimental study of propagation of sound over ground. *J. Acoust. Soc. Am.,* 1959, *31,* 724–733.

Wiley, R. H. Territoriality and non-random mating in sage grouse *Centrocercus urophasianus. Anim. Behav. Monogr.,* 1973, *6*(2), 85–169.

Wiley, R. H. Affiliation between the sexes in common grackles. I. Specificity and seasonal progression. *Z. Tierpsychol.,* 1976a, *40,* 59–79.

Wiley, R. H. Communication and spatial relationships in a colony of common grackles. *Anim. Behav.,* 1976b, *24,* 570–584.

Wiley, R. H., and Richards, D. G. Physical constraints on acoustic communication in the atmosphere: Implications for the evolution of animal vocalizations. *Behav. Ecol. Sociobiol..* 1978, *3,* 69–94.

Wiley, R. H., and Wiley, M. S. Recognition of neighbors' duets by stripe-backed wrens *Campylorhynchus nuchalis. Behaviour,* 1977, *62,* 10–34.

Williams, G. C. *Adaptation and Natural Selection.* Princeton University Press, Princeton, N.J., 1966.

Williams, G. C. (ed.). *Group Selection.* Aldine-Atherton, Chicago, 1971.

Willis, E. O. The behavior of bicolored antbirds. *Univ. Calif. Publ. Zool.,* 1967, *79,* 1–132.

Willis, E. O, The behavior of spotted antbirds. *Am. Ornithol. Un.,* 1972, Ornithological Monograph *10.*

Wilson, E. O. *Sociobiology: The New Synthesis.* Harvard University Press, Cambridge, Mass., 1975.

Wilson, E. O., and Regnier, F. E., Jr. The evolution of the alarm-defense system in the formicine ants. *Am. Natur.,* 1971, *105,* 279–289.

Winkle, W. van. Comparison of several probabilistic home-range models. *J. Wildl. Manage.,* 1975, *39,* 118–123.

Wolf, L. L., and Hainsworth, F. R. Time and energy budgets of territorial hummingbirds. *Ecology,* 1971, *52,* 980–988.

Woolfenden, G. E., and Fitzpatrick, J. W. The inheritance of territory in group-living birds. *Bioscience,* 1978, *28,* 104–108.

Wrangham, R. W. Artificial feeding of chimpanzees and baboons in their natural habitat. *Anim. Behav.,* 1974, *22,* 83–93.

Wynne-Edwards, V. C. *Animal Dispersion in Relation to Social Behaviour.* Oliver and Boyd, Edinburgh, 1962.

Young, H. Territorial behavior in the eastern robin. *Proc. Linn. Soc. N.Y.,* 1951, *58–62,* 1–37.

Zach, R., and Falls, J. B. Foraging behavior, learning, and exploration by captive ovenbirds (Aves: Parulidae). *Can. J. Zool.,* 1976a, *54,* 1880–1893.

Zach, R., and Falls, J. B. Influence of capturing a prey on subsequent search in the ovenbird (Aves: Parulidae). *Can. J. Zool.,* 1976b, *55,* 1958–1969.

Zach, R., and Falls, J. B. Ovenbird (Aves: Parulidae) hunting behavior in a patchy environment: an experimental study. *Can. J. Zool.,* 1976c, *54,* 1863–1879.

Zach, R., and Falls, J. B. Foraging and territoriality of male ovenbirds (Aves: Parulidae) in a heterogeneous habitat, in press.

Zahavi, A. The social behaviour of the white wagtail *Motacilla alba alba* wintering in Israel. *Ibis,* 1971, *113*, 203–211.

Zayan, R. C. Défense du territoire et reconnaissance individuelle chez *Xiphophorus* (Pisces, Poeciliidae). *Behaviour,* 1975, *52*, 266–312.

Zayan, R. C. Modification des effets liés à la priorité de résidence chez *Xiphophorus* (Pisces, Poeciliidae): Le rôle de l'isolement et des différences de taille. *Z. Tierpsychol.,* 1976, *41*, 142–190.

Zucker, N. Shelter building as a means of reducing territory size in the fiddler crab *Uca terpsichores* (Crustacea: Ocypodidae). *Am. Midl. Natur.,* 1974, *91*, 224–235.

5

Foraging Strategies and Their Social Significance[1]

John R. Krebs

Introduction

My aim in this paper is to discuss foraging behavior from a functional point of view. I will review the attempts to construct general rules about the design of predator behavior based on the theory of natural selection. The general approach in this type of work is to work out in theory how an ideal predator ought to behave and to test these rules against observations or experiments. Since natural selection is an optimizing process, it should be possible to formulate the rules for the decisions of an ideal predator based on the principle of optimization. A completely independent argument for using optimality models is that many aspects of decision making (in both nonbiological and biological contexts) can be understood by assuming that there is a maximizing principle and that the decision maker trades off the benefit of alternative courses of action. One point that follows from this argument is that using optimality theory to study decisions does not necessarily assume in a Panglossian way that animals are perfectly adapted to their environment (Krebs, Houston, and Charnov, 1979). Optimality models form the basis of a considerable body of literature on foraging, and a similar approach has been used in some discussions of group size and territorial defense.

The first step in developing a theory of optimal foraging-decision rules is to choose a goal for the optimal predator. This is essentially a problem of translating the ultimate currency of natural selection, changes in gene frequency measured as

[1]This article was written in December 1976 and was updated in February 1979.

JOHN R. KREBS   Edward Grey Institute of Field Ornithology, Zoology Department, Oxford University, Oxford. The work was supported by the Science Research Council.

inclusive fitness, into a shorter-term, measurable objective that can then be subjected to a cost–benefit analysis. In the literature on optimal foraging, the usual solution has been to consider only costs and benefits directly associated with harvesting food and to assume that the predator, regardless of its species-characteristic specialization for food gathering, should aim to maximize its net rate of food intake during the period in which it is foraging. This approach ignores the question of how the predator allocates its time between foraging and other activities, and it also does not take into account the possibility that during a foraging bout, a predator might aim to achieve an alternative goal, such as minimizing the risk of predator attack or minimizing the variance in rate of food intake (Thompson, Vertinsky, and Krebs, 1974). The arguments in favor of choosing maximal net rate of food intake as the short-term index of maximal fitness are twofold. On the one hand, many predators are probably limited in their ability to survive by the availability of food: a graphic example is Gibb's (1960) observation that a coal tit *(Parus ater)* in winter has to capture an insect about once every two seconds just in order to stay alive. This is strong support for the choice of maximum intake as the goal of an optimal predator. In contrast, some predators do not spend a large proportion of their time hunting and do not appear to be directly food-limited. Here, the argument for maximizing net rate of food intake is that feeding always competes for time with other, incompatible, activities, such as avoiding enemies, defending a territory, and so on. For example, woodpigeons *(Columba palumbus)* feeding on brassicae in winter spend a considerable time resting, because they are limited in their rate of assimilation of food by a digestive bottleneck (Kenward and Sibly, 1977). Nevertheless, the pigeons do not reduce their rate of pecking while actually feeding on brassicae; they feed quickly on the ground and then retreat to the safety of trees in order to digest their food. Whether predators that are not limited by their rate of food intake still follow the design rules based on maximizing rate has to be determined empirically, but at least, one can put forward an intuitive argument as to why they should.

An alternative method of translating the long-term goal of maximizing fitness into a short-term goal is taken by Sibly and McFarland (1976) (see also McFarland, 1976, 1977, 1978). They define the fitness over a short time period as the integral over that period of birthrate minus death rate, and then, they define the *cost* of any particular behavior per unit time period in similar terms: the death rate minus the birthrate. The cost depends on the internal state of the animal (e.g., the risk of a particular level of hunger) and the effectiveness of a behavior in changing the internal state (which in the case of hunger might include the influence of food availability) and the cost of the behavior itself (e.g., the risk of attack from a predator while feeding). The optimal choice of which behavior to do next is that which minimizes the cost over the next time period. Sibly and McFarland suggested that in general, costs increase as power functions of both the physiological needs of an animal and the rate of performing a particular activity, and they described a method for calculating which choice of behavior minimizes the cost function. There are several advantages to this method of tackling the optimization problem: the model provides a method of combining on a common scale different types of cost, for example, the physiological cost of dehydration and the risk of predator attacks, but the model requires a detailed knowledge of both the physiological state of the animal and the cost function, although a knowledge of the decision rules could be substituted for one of these in estimating the optimal choice of behavior. While Sibly and McFarland (1976) provided a convincing example of the application of their model in the laboratory, it remains to be seen whether the same approach can be used in more elaborate environments. In the subsequent discussion, I will sidestep the issue of how an animal decides whether or not to forage (which could in theory be predicted from the Sibly and McFarland model) and assume, as have other authors on optimal foraging, that the decision to forage has already been taken.

If we accept, for the moment, that the goal of the optimal predator is to maximize its net rate of intake while foraging, the next step in formulating the theory is to extract the bare essentials of foraging behavior that might be common to a variety of predators. Any predator (using the term in a broad sense) can be viewed as making a series of decisions when it is foraging: it chooses where to forage within its home range or activity space, which type of prey to capture once encountered, and what sort of movement path to follow within and between areas (Figure 1). Each of these decisions may in turn be influenced by, or influence, whether the predator forages solitarily or in a group. An example of the influence of a group on the choice made by individuals comes from the work of Murton (1971), who found that the choice of seeds by individual woodpigeons was influenced by the preference of other members of the same flock.

In addition to the choice of a goal, any cost–benefit analysis has to identify the constraints. I am referring here to historical constraints rather than to the immediate physical constraints, such as the maximum rate at which a bird can peck. Historical constraints may be short-term: Heinrich (1976) showed that bumblebees unused to foraging on monkshood flowers are inefficient at nectar extraction, but that efficiency goes up rapidly with experience; or they may be long-term: learning abilities that might enhance foraging efficiency are obviously to a great extent determined by phylogenetic heritage. There is no hard-and-fast rule for deciding on the historical constraints limiting the performance of a particular species; it is more a matter of intuition.

I have now discussed a possible basis on which to formulate design rules for an optimal predator, and I have briefly indicated that these rules might be applied

CHOICE OF PREY ITEMS

SEARCH STRATEGY

GROUP SIZE

ALLOCATION OF TIME BETWEEN AREAS

Fig. 1. A summary of the foraging decisions facing a typical predator. From Krebs and Cowie, 1976, based on Charnov, 1973.

in the context of predator decisions about allocation of foraging time between area, choice of prey, choice of search path, and group size. In the following sections, I will examine each of these decisions in more detail, concentrating on attempts to test theoretical ideas with some rigor. Much of the work on optimal foraging has been concerned with weak evidence: the prediction that an optimal predator should become more selective in its choice of diet in richer habitats (MacArthur, 1972) is neither surprising nor unique to an optimal foraging model. On the other hand, the prediction that a predator should completely ignore certain prey, regardless of their availability, under certain quantitatively specified conditions (Krebs, Erichsen, Webber, and Charnov, 1977) is powerful because in making it, the model sticks its neck out.

ALLOCATION OF FORAGING TIME BETWEEN AREAS

SIMPLE RULES OF ALLOCATION

Food is rarely distributed in a completely uniform fashion throughout a mobile predator's home area, and frequently, it is likely to be clumped or patchy in distribution. These patches may be associated with broad-scale heterogeneities in the physical environment, or at the other extreme, they may reflect microhabitat preferences or social groupings of the prey. Regardless of their cause, if the heterogeneities in distribution are sufficiently small in relation to the predator's foraging range, an individual needs to have rules for allocating its time between areas. The optimal rules for this situation have been discussed by many authors, for example, MacArthur and Pianka (1966), Royama (1971), Tullock (1971), Charnov (1973, 1976b), Cook and Hubbard (1977), and Hubbard and Cook (1978).

In qualitative terms, an optimal predator should allocate most of its time to the more profitable areas. In fact, in the extremely simple case in which the food resource is never depleted and the environment is in equilibrium (the relative quality of different areas is constant), the predator should simply choose the most productive patch and spend all its time foraging there. This situation is well known in the psychological literature on probability learning, in which a pigeon or other test animal is offered a simultaneous choice of two keys with different reward rates. The rewards are on a variable-ratio schedule, which means that a certain proportion of pecks are rewarded, rather than a certain proportion of time. The optimal choice is clearly to learn which key gives the higher reward rate and then to respond exclusively to this key. Results show that rats and pigeons (but perhaps not cold-blooded vertebrates) behave in this manner (which is termed *maximizing*) (Shimp, 1969; Herrnstein and Loveland, 1975; Mackintosh, 1974). Figure 2 shows two examples in which even a fairly small deviation from equal reward rates on the two keys leads to a strong preference for the majority key. Even when an animal is maximizing, it occasionally pecks at the alternative key. The mechanism postulated to account for this is that the animal sometimes attends to an irrelevant cue, such as position of the key, instead of reward rate. A functional explanation of the behavior could be that the animal always invests a small amount of effort in sampling alternative patches (see also below, under "Sampling"): although the experiments refer only to equilibrium conditions, the pigeon or rat may be designed to cope with changing environments in which there is a payoff for sampling.

The real world is rarely in such a stable equilibrium. Changes in the relative profitability of patches are likely to face the predator. They may result either from the predator's own activity (depletion) or from seasonal, diurnal, and other factors

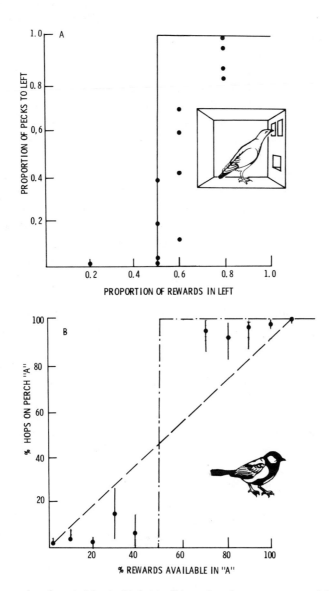

Fig. 2. Two examples of maximizing by birds in a Skinner box, in a concurrent variable-ratio experiment. The birds tend to direct all their foraging effort to the key offering the higher reward rate. This is the optimal strategy in an equilibrium environment. From Krebs, 1978b; Herrnstein and Loveland, 1975.

external to the predator. Optimal foraging models designed to deal with the situation in which a predator gradually depletes the patch in which it is foraging involve both an analog of memory and flexibility on the part of the predator, since it has to behave as if it can compare its immediate success with its expected success in other patches (Charnov, 1973, 1976b). However, before going on to discuss these models, I will mention two simpler mechanisms requiring no flexibility in the predator's behavior, which will enable the animal to concentrate its foraging effort in more profitable patches and perhaps approximate an optimal pattern of time allocation.

Hassell and May (1974) discussed these two ideas. They gave several examples of how predators ranging from insects to birds distribute their searching effort, measured as the proportion of total hunting time, according to prey density when offered a simultaneous choice of patches. They concluded that there is usually a sigmoid "aggregative response." Predators tend to spend little time in areas of low prey density and do not discriminate strongly between such areas; they discriminate very strongly at intermediate prey densities, and rather little again at very high prey density. This is roughly what one would expect according to an optimal time-allocation model (Royama, 1970). Hassell and May suggested that the sigmoid response could come about by two mechanisms: area-restricted searching and a fixed giving-up time. Area-restricted search means that the predator adjusts its search path immediately after a capture, so as to concentrate its search effort near the last prey. For example, Murdie and Hassell (1973) showed that houseflies *(Musca domestica)* increase their rate of turning after encountering a sugar droplet, an effect that decays after a few seconds. Area-restricted searching is probably widespread in invertebrate and vertebrate predators (Krebs, 1973a), and it has been most thoroughly studied by Smith (1974a,b) in birds and by Thomas (1974) in fish. The latter author also found that sticklebacks tend to move away from areas in which they have just had an unsuccessful encounter with a prey (so-called area-avoided search). Smith (1974b) found that blackbirds *(Turdus merula)* modify their search path after a find by making several successive turns in the same direction, rather than by increasing the rate of turning or the size of individual turns.

The second hypothesis discussed by Hassell and May, and also independently by Murdoch and Oaten (1975), is based on the idea that after a find, a predator searches in the immediate vicinity for a fixed time and leaves if it does not have another success. If it does find another prey, it simply "resets its clock" and searches again until the waiting time has elapsed with no capture. Although this "fixed giving-up time" rule enables the predator to concentrate its effort in more profitable patches, as Charnov (1976b) showed, an optimal predator would have a variable giving-up time rule. For a short-lived predator such as an insect, a fixed rule may be sufficient, as seasonal changes in the environment may not occur within the lifetime of an individual.

An example of the way in which simple short-term changes in behavior of the type I have discussed so far may influence the allocation of time between patches of different profitability is Harwood's (1974) study of grazing in blue geese *(Anser caerulescens)*. Harwood observed blue geese foraging in large enclosures that contained a checkerboard arrangement of fertilized and unfertilized squares, the former having more grass and a higher nitrogen content per unit weight. The birds concentrated their effort in the fertilized squares, which were quantitatively and qualitatively more profitable, and the allocation of searching effort was achieved through three short-term responses by the geese: they walked more slowly, pecked faster, and pecked for longer bouts in the fertilized squares. It is possible that in addition, the geese showed some longer-term modification of their search behavior in relation to the overall quality of the habitat, since the birds in a good-quality environment seemed to be more selective than those in a poorer area.

OPTIMAL TIME ALLOCATION: THEORY

I have already indicated that in deciding how to allocate its time between depleting patches, an optimal predator has to adjust its rules according to the overall quality of habitat. Although this does not imply any particular *type* of memory mechanism, it does imply flexibility on the part of the predator. (It is worth emphasizing that optimal foraging models in general do not imply any particular behavioral mechanisms [Cowie and Krebs, 1979]). A graphical model of optimal time allocation is shown in Figure 3 (from Charnov, 1973, 1976b). The model assumes that the predator does not know the quality of a patch before

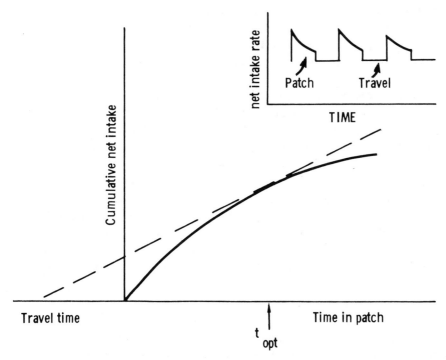

Fig. 3. A graphical representation of the model of optimal time allocation of Charnov (1976b). The predator gradually depletes each patch, so that the capture rate gradually declines with time in a patch (hence, the curve of cumulative intake decelerates). The inset shows how the bird might estimate its average intake over a series of patches.

arriving, so the decision of how to allocate time between patches is one of choosing a criterion for leaving each patch.

When the predator first arrives in a patch, its rate of food intake is likely to be quite high, but as the patch is gradually depleted, the rate of intake falls, and eventually the net rate may even become negative. Figure 3 shows the *cumulative* net intake as a function of time, the rate being given by the slope of the graph. The predator has to choose a point on this curve of diminishing returns at which to give up and move to another patch. The optimal rule is to give up when the expected net rate of food intake would be higher as a result of moving than it is in the present patch. This expected rate of intake could be estimated by the bird from its recent experience (inset in Figure 3): the last few patches visited would give an estimate of both the travel costs and the average quality of a patch.

In Figure 3, the travel time between patches is plotted on the abscissa to the left of the ordinate. By drawing the tangent from the point on the x-axis representing the travel time, which just intersects the curve of cumulative net intake, one can obtain a triangle that represents the overall net gain per unit time from an average patch, the gain being the vertical and the time the base of the triangle. Since the optimal giving-up rule is to leave a patch when the rate of intake within a patch is such that the overall average rate of gain for the environment is maximized, the giving-up threshold is given by the maximum slope attainable of the broken line in Figure 3. This maximum slope is, of course, constrained by travel time and the cumulative gain curve. Its point of intersection with the gain curve is the optimal time spent in a patch. The same optimal giving-up threshold should apply to all patches in a particular environment, no matter what the starting density of prey in the patch. In other words, the predator should reduce all patches to the *same marginal value* (Charnov, 1976b), this value being equal to the predator's expected average rate of intake from the whole environment (I will return later to discuss what I mean by the "environment").

Obviously, patches in which the initial density of prey is so low that they are below the giving-up threshold for that environment should not be visited at all, although the predator may have to sample them if there is no advance indication of patch quality, so that the model predicts that predators should become more selective in their choice of patches as the overall quality of the environment increases (MacArthur and Pianka, 1966). Although the model does not make any specific assumption about the shape of the curve depicted in Figure 3, it does assume that the predator's foraging time is spent either traveling between patches or foraging within them. While this division might be clear-cut in some cases—for example, the one for which the model was originally developed (titmice foraging for insect larvae hidden in groups of pine cones)—in other instances, the recognition of patches by an observer may not be straightforward. One possible approach may be to use the technique described by Cody (1974a). He plotted on a cumulative graph, for a variety of different species of birds, distance traveled while foraging as a function of time. Most of the species he studied tended to move in "steps," with pauses between. It is possible that the pause lengths and step lengths are an indication of the time spent within and traveling between patches, respectively. In order to test this behavioral method of defining patch size, it would be necessary to sample the food supply and test for heterogeneities in its distribution.

The giving-up threshold rule, which has been developed independently in the context of male mating strategies in dungflies by Parker and Stuart (1976), is very robust. Although I have only discussed a deterministic model, similar conclusions emerge from a stochastic version (Charnov, 1973; A. Barber, personal communication; but see Oaten, 1977, for a critique).

One of the implications of the model is that the predator should behave as if it compared two rates: the rate of intake within a patch and the rate for the whole environment. It is possible that a predator could approximate this result without any comparison of rates (see below), but at least the bird predators that have been studied experimentally do seem to assess the average capture rate in an environment (Krebs, Ryan, and Charnov, 1974; Cowie, 1977). In an experimental setup, the "environment" is usually defined in terms of a particular experimental treatment, in which the overall availability of prey is fixed at a chosen level (Krebs *et al.*, 1974), but in the real world, the "environment" for which the predator takes an average might reflect some time period preceding the current patch, which constitutes the predator's effective memory ("memory window"—Cowie, 1977). There may in fact be an optimal length of memory. Increasing the number of patches over which the average is estimated increases the accuracy of the estimate, but this increase follows a curve of diminishing returns (Figure 4A). There is also

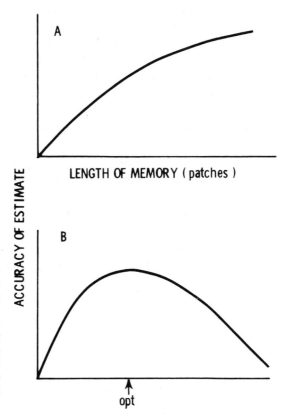

Fig. 4. The problem of an optimal memory length for averaging rate of intake in an environment. (A) With increasing memory length, the accuracy of any estimate of average quality of the environment increases at an ever-decreasing rate. (B) By assuming a penalty for averaging over too long a threshold period (the predator fails to adjust its giving-up threshold), an optimal memory span can be found.

likely to be a penalty for averaging over too long a time period, because by so doing, the predator tends to "smooth out" potentially important fluctuations in habitat quality. At the upper extreme, if the predator averaged over its whole lifetime, it would in effect operate according to a "fixed giving-up time" rule of the type described by Hassell and May (1974). The conclusion is that there must be an intermediate optimal memory span, but it is not possible to find an explicit solution to this optimum without making some highly specific and therefore probably unrealistic assumptions about the penalty for averaging over too long a time period. In Figure 4B, I have drawn a curve for one instance in which I have calculated an optimal solution: I assumed that the average quality of the habitat fluctuates up and down in a sinusoidal fashion, and that superimposed upon this long-term fluctuation there are local fluctuations in the quality of individual patches. The optimal memory span is one in which the predator achieves the best trade-off in assessing the average quality of the habitat at any one instant in time. The specific solution is of little importance, but the general point is that there might be an optimum length of memory for a predator to assess the average quality of the environment.

OPTIMAL TIME ALLOCATION: EVIDENCE

There are two types of evidence in the literature for optimal time allocation. One comes from observing the density of prey in patches before and after predation, and the other comes from direct measurements of time allocation or giving up thresholds of individual predators, usually in the laboratory.

Some of the most striking field evidence comes from the work of Gibb (1958), reanalyzed by Tullock (1971), Solomon *et al.,* 1976, and Heinrich (1976), all of whom measured the initial and final density of prey in individual patches or groups of patches but did not record the giving-up thresholds of predators directly. Gibb studied the predation by titmice on the larvae of a eucosmid moth that lives inside pine cones. He divided his study area, an extensive pine planta-tion, into 16-ha plots and estimated the initial density in each plot before the winter predation, as well as the final density of larvae in the spring. Although the initial density of larvae (measured as larvae per cone) varied considerably between areas, the final density at the end of the winter was similar in all plots (Tullock, 1971). This finding is in agreement with the optimal time allocation model, since it implies that all patches were reduced to the same marginal value, but the pattern of predation may well have reflected the fact that more birds searched in the better-quality plots, rather than optimal foraging by each individual. (Note that Gibb's conclusion about the pattern of predation on a finer scale—that the birds were exploiting individual groups of cones by searching for a fixed number of larvae—is quite different from the optimal time allocation rule. However, the evidence for this idea of "hunting by expectation" was not very clear cut [see Krebs, 1973a]).

Heinrich (1976) measured the nectar content of flowers of a variety of species both before and after exploitation by bumblebees. As Figure 5 shows, he found that the different species (which can be considered analogs of different-quality patches) started off with widely varying nectar levels, but they were all reduced to the same final level. In Heinrich's study, the optimal pattern of exploitation seemed to be a result of the population of bees distributing their foraging effort among the flower species according to their initial nectar content, while each individual bee concentrated on only one or two species of flower. In another study of nectivorous predators, Wolf, Hainsworth, and Stiles (1972) noted in passing that individuals of three species of hummingbird reduced the nectar volume of *Heliconia* flowers to the same final nectar volume in spite of initially different levels.

The first direct experimental test of the giving-up threshold model was the study of Krebs *et al.* (1974), who investigated the behavior of black-capped chickadees *(Parus atricapillus)* hunting for mealworm pieces hidden in artificial pine cones (blocks of wood) hanging on "trees" in a large aviary. This experimental arrangement was based on Gibb's observations, which I discussed above. Individual birds were allowed to search (by hanging on the cones and peeling off small round paper stickers covering holes in which mealworms could be hidden) for several short test periods in the aviary, and estimates of the giving-up threshold were made by measuring the time interval between the last find in a patch (a group of four pine cones) and the moment of departure, the "giving-up time." As predicted by the model, when three different patch types, with different initial prey densities, were offered during the same test, the giving-up time was similar in

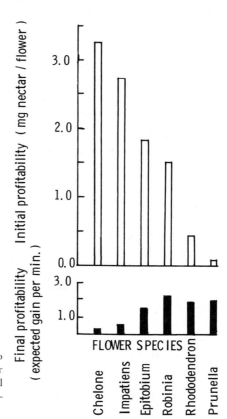

Fig. 5. Bumblebees exploit different flower species so as to leave a similar amount of nectar in each type after exploitation (Heinrich, 1976). Upper graph: initial nectar volume. Lower graph: final profitability—expected reward rate in grams of sugar/min.

all three types. Also in agreement with the model was the finding that the giving-up threshold, estimated by the reciprocal of the giving-up time, was directly proportional to the average capture rate experienced by the birds in an experimental treatment. In four different treatments, the average capture rate was manipulated by changing the number of prey per patch, and the giving-up time changed as predicted by the model. In fact, there is no reason to expect the relationship between giving-up time and the average capture rate to be as close as found, since the giving-up time is only an estimate of the giving-up threshold, based on the fact that all the prey were small and had negligible handling times. One might expect that a measure such as the average of the giving-up time and the previous intercatch interval to provide a better estimate of the giving-up threshold, but Krebs *et al.* (1974) did not discuss this possibility.

As Cowie and Krebs (1979) pointed out, there is a problem with giving-up times; if the predator leaves patches at random, it has shorter giving-up times when the capture rate is high. They suggested that a better way to test the model is to measure the gain curve and the travel time and to use these to predict the optimal time in a patch. This has been done by Cowie (1977). He worked with great tits *(Parus major)* hunting in a large aviary for small pieces of mealworm hidden in small plastic cups filled with sawdust and fixed on the branches of artificial trees similar to those used by Krebs *et al.* (1974). The experiment involved manipulating travel time and predicting how time spent in a patch should change. Travel time was manipulated as follows. In one treatment, the birds had to remove a loose fitting cardboard lid from each patch before searching in the sawdust, and in the other, they had to prize off a tight-fitting lid. In the former situation, the time spent after leaving one patch before starting to forage in the next one was about 5 seconds, while in the latter experiment, it was about 15 seconds. By measuring the curve of cumulative food intake within a patch and the travel time, it was possible to construct the graph drawn in Figure 6. As shown, the observed relationship between travel time and time in patch was close to that predicted. Similar results have also been obtained by Cook and Cockrell (1978), who worked with *Notonecta glauca* feeding on the larvae of *Culex.* They treated the individual prey as patches and were able to calculate the extraction rate by the *Notonecta* as a function of time spent feeding on a patch by interrupting feeding bouts after varying lengths of time. Using five different prey densities (producing five different "travel times"), they were able to show that the observed and predicted giving-up thresholds on a larva were correlated.

The most detailed field test of the marginal value model is the work of Parker (1978) on dungflies *(Scatophaga stercoraria).* He applied the model to males searching for females, which is exactly analogous to foraging, except that the fitness consequences are directly observable. Parker showed that both the time spent in copulation by a male with a single female and the time spent by males hunting for females on a particular dungpat could be accurately predicted by the marginal value model. The predictions of stay times on dungpats were particularly interesting because there is no single optimal solution. Females arrive continuously, but in decreasing numbers with time, after a dungpat has been laid. The males very soon assemble at fresh pats, and within a pat, there is competition between males to mate with newly arriving females and for takeovers *in copula.* The gain rate (eggs fertilized per minute) for any one male thus depends on the number of other males on the pat and the arrival rate of new females. Parker showed that under these conditions, there is no single optimal emigration threshold: as soon as one male leaves, the rest expect to do slightly better. The result is that there should be a phased emigration. The males should leave one after the other, each expecting the same fitness gain (a mixed evolutionary stable strategy), because the intensity of competition declines in parallel with the declining input of new females. This is exactly what happened. Parker's work is a brilliant example of how the principles of optimal foraging theory can be tested in the field.

There are numerous other studies in which giving-up thresholds have been measured (e.g., Ware, 1971; Krebs, 1974; Croze, 1970), but without any attempt to relate giving-up thresholds to the average rate of intake from the environment, so one cannot use these data to test the optimal foraging model. Zach and Falls (1976a) attempted to test the giving-up time model in a laboratory experiment in which ovenbirds *(Seiurus aurocapillus)* foraged for small pieces of mealworm hid-

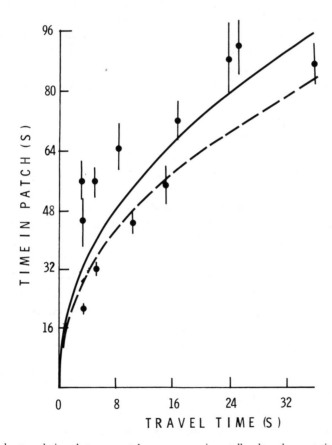

Fig. 6. When the travel time between patches was experimentally altered, great tits adjusted the average time per patch approximately as predicted by the model. The predictions were obtained from an exponential fit to the depletion curve within a patch. The dotted line is the prediction when the energy cost of traveling between patches is taken into account (using standard metabolic-rate equations). This gives a better fit than the uncorrected curve (solid line).

den in holes drilled in large boards (patches). They failed to find any supporting evidence for the optimal foraging model, but their data show that the capture rate within a patch (one of the boards) did not decrease as a function of time spent searching in the patch. This means that the giving-up threshold model is not applicable to their data.

The experiments discussed so far have involved predators encountering a series of patches, the quality of which could not be predicted by the predator in advance. Differences in quality between areas in the field may, however, persist over a relatively long time period as a result of renewal of the food supply, so that a predator can gradually accumulate experience and allocate its foraging time according to the experience gained in an initial sampling period (Royama, 1970). In an aviary study designed to investigate this possibility, Smith and Sweatman (1974) showed how individual great tits gradually learned during a series of tests to concentrate their searching effort in the most profitable of six possible foraging patches. A patch consisted of 256 plastic cups covered by small lids and glued onto a large board. The birds removed the lids when searching for prey hidden inside the cups. A very similar experiment, yielding similar results, has been carried out by Zach and Falls (1976b,c) working with ovenbirds hunting for mealworms in leaf litter on the floor of a large enclosure (see also Simons and Alcock, 1971). Alcock (1973) also found that captive redwinged blackbirds (*Agelaius phoenicus*) can learn to search for food in a particular place where they have previously been successful. Several field studies have also shown that predators allocate their time to different areas according to the prey availability (e.g., Goss-Custard, 1970a; Hartwick, 1976), one of the most detailed being the work of Tinbergen (1976) on starlings (*Sturnus vulgaris*) foraging for tipulid larvae in a pasture. Tinbergen sampled the availability of tipulids in the soil and found that the starlings made longer and more frequent visits to areas of high prey density. These results, in agreement with the laboratory studies discussed above, show that predators can learn the difference between areas of different profitability and allocate their time mainly to areas of high prey density, but does this mean that the predators are allocating their time in the optimal manner?

A version of the optimal time allocation model that is suitable for analyzing the experimental results of Smith and Sweatman (1974) and Zach and Falls (1976b) has been described by Cook and Hubbard (1977). Their model is based on the assumption that within a patch, the relationship between the number of prey eaten, or the number of hosts parasitized in the case of an insect parasite, and the initial density is described by the random predator or random parasite models of Rogers (1972).

Cook and Hubbard used this equation to calculate the number of hosts parasitized per patch in relation to host density in the patch and the number of searching parasitoids. They found the optimal time allocation pattern by summing the equation over all patches and solving to maximize the hosts parasitized over a fixed time. This is essentially a "group optimization" rather than an "individual optimization" result when more than one parasite is searching. The results are similar if solved for individual optima (Comins and Hassell, in press).

Cook and Hubbard used the model to analyze the data of Hassell (1971) describing the parasitism of *Ephestia cantella* by *Nemeritis*. In these experiments, the parasites were confronted with a choice of 15 patches of six types, containing between 4 and 128 hosts concealed in plastic dishes and covered with sawdust. Hassell found that the *Nemeritis* spent more time in patches with high host density, producing the aggregative response discussed earlier. Figure 7A shows that the predicted time allocation is close to the observed. Cook and Hubbard's model uses the marginal value conclusion that the *Nemeritis* should leave a patch when the current gain drops below a critical level that is the same for all patches. Figure 7B shows that the terminal encounter rates in all patches in an experiment (Hubbard and Cook, 1978) were in fact very similar in spite of initial big differences.

Although these results suggest that *Nemeritis* is capable of approximating the optimal solution, Waage (1977) has suggested that the underlying mechanism is very simple. He showed in an elegant series of experiments that the decision made by an individual to leave a patch of hosts depends on a mechanism involving habituation to host scent. Waage (1977) went on to show that the habituation

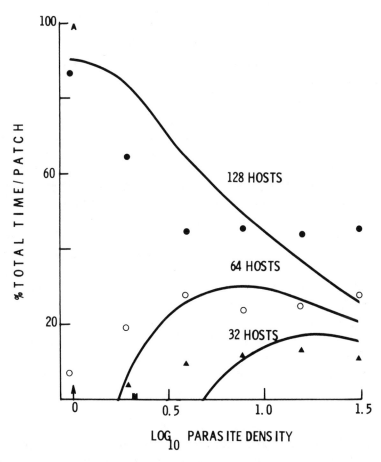

Fig. 7. (A) Observed (symbols) and predicted (lines) time budgets for *Nemeritis* hunting for patches of different host density and at different parasite densities. From Cook and Hubbard, 1977.

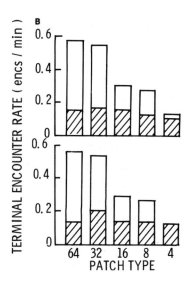

Fig. 7. (B) Terminal encounter rates in five different patches (solid bars) compared with initial rates (open bars). The upper graph refers to experiments with one searching parasite and the lower graph to experiments with two parasites. From Hubbard and Cook 1978.

mechanism in any one patch is relatively little influenced by experience in previous patches. The implication is that *Nemeritis* are less flexible in their foraging than birds, and that they cannot adjust their giving-up threshold in relation to overall environmental quality. This implication has not yet been critically tested.

Cook and Hubbard's model can be modified to predict the optimal time allocation for predators by using the "random predator" equation of Rogers (1972) (see Krebs and Cowie, 1976). Figure 8 shows the predicted and observed results for the studies of great tits and ovenbirds. In both cases, but especially in the great tit, there is an appreciable deviation from the predicted result. The birds spent more time in low-density areas than expected from the model, and Smith and Sweatman, in discussing this point, followed Royama in suggesting that the birds may sacrifice short-term efficiency for a longer-term payoff from time spent in sampling alternative food sources. An additional factor in both the great tit and the ovenbird experiments may have been the proximity of the different patches. Since the patches were close together, it is possible that the birds did not clearly recognize the boundaries between areas of different prey density.

Smith and Sweatman (1974) were able to show that the birds had in fact accumulated knowledge through sampling. After a sequence of about 30 trials lasting five minutes each, in which the relative qualities of the patches had been maintained at a constant level by replenishing the mealworms, the positions of the best and worst areas were reversed. The tits immediately concentrated their search effort in the second-best area, showing that the birds had stored up information about the relative quality of the different patches and that they used the information when the environment changed. The birds managed to maintain a more-or-less constant rate of intake during the switch period, which suggests that the profitability of a patch is, as Royama (1971) suggested and as implied by the model of Cooke and Hubbard (1977), a negatively accelerating function of prey density.

Murdoch, Avery, and Smyth (1975) also studied the ability of a predator, the guppy *Lebistes reticulata,* to switch from one area to another when the relative profitabilities changed. They offered the guppies a choice of foraging at the top of a tank for *Drosophila* larvae or near the bottom for *Tubifex* worms. The two prey types were offered in different proportions on different trials, and some individuals switched their foraging effort when the relative profitabilities changed, while others did not. The nonswitchers, which did not take advantage of changes in profitability, had a lower rate of capture than the switchers, and it seemed that the main contributing factor to this difference was that the latter group spent less time in transit between the two areas.

GROUP FORAGING AND TIME ALLOCATION

Several authors have emphasized the role of group foraging in the exploitation of patchily distributed food (Ward and Zahavi, 1973; Krebs, 1974; Horn, 1968). The most widely discussed idea is that social feeding is a mechanism by which individuals increase their foraging success by learning from others the location or nature of good feeding places. This type of copying is known to take place on a fine scale—for example, within one tree—in single- and mixed-species flocks of titmice (*Parus* spp.) (Krebs, MacRoberts, and Cullen, 1972; Krebs, 1973b). These studies showed that if one member of a group finds a piece of food, nearby individuals in the flock quickly change their searching behavior so as to concentrate near the site of the find or in the same type of place. Krebs *et al.* (1972) also showed that as a consequence of this copying, each individual in a flock

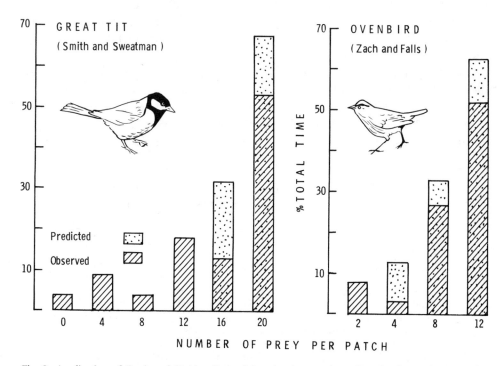

Fig. 8. Application of Cook and Hubbard's model to the data on time allocation by captive great tits and ovenbirds. From Krebs and Cowie, 1976.

of four birds had a higher probability of finding and eating food, during a short experiment, than when foraging alone or in a pair. This experiment was done with a highly clumped and abundant (within the clump) source of food. Intuitively, one would predict that any advantage of being in a flock that results from copying would vary according to the dispersion of the food. This idea was subsequently tested in a laboratory experiment with black-capped chickadees by Krebs (unpublished). In this experiment, eight birds were allowed to search, in flocks of four and in pairs, for food that was either clumped (one patch containing 30 mealworms) or dispersed (five patches, each containing six mealworms). The worms were hidden in plastic cups fixed onto the branches of trees in the manner described by Krebs (1973b). The results are summarized in Table I, which shows the median latency to find food for an individual in a flock of four and in a pair, when hunting for clumped or dispersed food. As predicted, the flock birds are at an advantage when searching for clumped food, but not when the food is dispersed.

Social learning of feeding places on a much larger scale is also well known at a descriptive level (e.g., Ward and Zahavi, 1973), but there is relatively little quantitative evidence to show that predators may learn from one another about large patches of food and enjoy an increase in foraging success as a consequence. Krebs (1974) studied the foraging success of great blue herons (*Ardea herodias*) in flocks of different sizes and found that foraging success, measured either as gross intake per minute or as intake per unit effort, increased with group size up to a flock of about 20 and then declined again. It appeared that the flock birds did better mainly because flocks occur only in good feeding places or, in other words, because birds locate good feeding sites by copying other individuals (see also Murton, 1965). There was no further positive enhancement of feeding success as a result of intraflock interactions within the feeding area.

Other studies in which foraging success as a function of group size has been measured include those of Smith (1977) on great-tailed grackles (*Cassidix mexicanus*); Smith and Evans (1973) on bar-tailed godwits (*Limosa lapponica*); Goss-Custard (1976) on redshank; Barnard (1978) on house sparrows; and the work of Kruuk (1972) and Schaller (1972) on hyenas and lions, respectively.

TABLE I. THE FORAGING SUCCESS OF BLACK-CAPPED CHICKADEES HUNTING FOR CLUMPED OR DISPERSED FOOD IN GROUPS OF TWO OR FOUR BIRDS[a]

	Flock of four		Pair
Dispersed food	51.5		46.5
Clumped food	150.5	[b]	304.5

[a]From Krebs, unpublished data. The figures are median times in seconds between the start of a trial and the first successful find by an individual. Six birds were used in the experiments, each bird being tested in both treatments (a total of 8 trials for the group of four and 16 trials with pairs). The "clumped" food source was one patch of 30 mealworms; the "dispersed" was five patches, each containing 6 worms.

[b]$p < 0.05$ (median test).

In the mammal studies, it is clear that hunting success increases with group size as a result of cooperative maneuvers by the predators in capturing large prey. In terms of the payoff for individuals, Caraco and Wolf (1975) pointed out that the optimal group size (defined by prey weight per lion times percentage of success) for a lion hunting for both Thomson's gazelle and large prey such as wildebeest or zebra is two individuals. Lions do in fact hunt gazelles in groups of two, but they hunt wildebeest in groups of up to seven, which is a larger number than the optimum, perhaps because there is some other advantage of being in large groups that outweighs the cost in terms of hunting (Bertram, 1975).

Goss-Custard (1976) showed a negative influence of flock density (he did not report on flock size as such) on foraging success, measured as prey captured per unit time in redshank hunting by sight, and he showed no correlation between flock density and feeding rate for birds feeding at night. The redshank feeding by day use visual cues to locate prey and apparently interfere with one another by causing their prey *(Corophium)* to retreat beneath the mud surface. At night, the birds hunt by touch, probing into the mud, so that this sort of interference is less important.

Smith and Evans (1973) showed that bar-tailed godwits feeding in flocks had a higher peck rate and percentage of success than solitary individuals in the same area, although they did not discuss any possible mechanism underlying this difference. Smith (1977) was unable to show any consistent correlation between flock density (an index of flock size) and peck rate in grackles. In a detailed study of sparrow *(Passer domesticus)* flocks, Barnard (1978) showed that birds peck faster when in larger groups. In one area with low predation rates and highly clumped food, this behavior could be attributed to birds' copying each other to find the best food clumps. In another area with less clumped food but high predation risk, the effect of flock size on peck rate seemed to be mediated through a decrease in time spent scanning for predators (see also Powell, 1974).

Many flock-feeding birds also roost or nest in groups, and Ward and Zahavi (1973), among others, have suggested that this is an extension of the role of flocking as a feeding adaptation. They hypothesized that unsuccessful foragers may find food by following successful individuals from the roost or nesting colony to good feeding areas, and that in species in which the food is patchy and unpredictable, the net benefit to each individual from this form of reciprocal copying may be large. The evidence for this hypothesis, together with a discussion of some of its ramifications, may be found in Krebs (1978b).

Cody has proposed a totally different role for bird flocks in exploiting patchily distributed food. He suggested that the effect of flocking is to increase the patchiness of food, because when a flock moves through an area it depletes the food supply more thoroughly than would a single individual and hence makes it easier for birds to recognize, and avoid revisiting, depleted areas. One problem with the idea seems to be that in depleting the food to a lower level, the birds in a flock must suffer to some extent from increased competition in comparison with solitary individuals.

So far, my discussion of foraging groups has concentrated on single-species aggregations, and one point to be considered is whether or not the same arguments about location of good feeding places can apply to mixed groups. Some authors have argued that the species in mixed groups often eat rather similar types of food, or at least food types that occur in the same places (e.g., Kushlan, 1976), so that interspecific social learning of feeding sites may be important in enhancing foraging success (Krebs, 1973b, 1978b). Krebs (1973b) showed experimentally that in mixed-species groups of chickadees (*P. atricapillus* and *P. rufescens*), the two species converge in their foraging stations as a result of social learning, and that this can enhance the learning of novel feeding sites. Rubinstein, Barnett, Ridgeley, and Klopfer (1977) supported this conclusion with field data on mixed-species flocks of seed eaters (*Tiaris olivacea* and the two species of *Sporophila*). They showed that all three species increase their feeding rate in the presence of heterospecifics (by having longer feeding bouts). They concluded that this advantage comes about through social learning of good feeding sites. On the other hand, Morse (1970) suggested that the various species in mixed insectivorous flocks of temperate zones actually increase their niche separation when in mixed groups, indicating that there may be competition in these flocks. Although it has been argued that avoidance of competition is a function of mixed flocks, it is not easy to see why competition should lead to flocking, and it is probably better to view competition as a cost of flocking to be offset against some other, perhaps antipredator, advantage, as demonstrated by Powell (1974) and Siegfried and Underhill (1975). In tropical mixed flocks, there seems to be a totally different food-related advantage, resulting from the flushing of insects (Swynnerton, 1915), but this is not likely to be of much importance in winter flocks of temperate zones that fed on nonmoving prey.

The question of the optimal size of foraging groups has not been the subject of much study, at either the empirical or the theoretical level (Schoener, 1971). As I mentioned above, in a study of flock feeding in great blue herons, I found that foraging success was highest in groups close to but below the observed maximum size, which might indicate an optimum group size, with competition perhaps setting the upper limit. Similarly, Caraco and Wolf (1975) showed that an intermediate group size is optimal for foraging in lions. Thompson *et al.* (1974) analyzed optimal foraging group size in a simulation model, in which they allowed predators to search for food in a large grid, the movements of each individual being determined by complex rules involving an individual's own search strategy, modified to some extent by interbird attraction and repulsion. All three components of movement could be influenced by immediately preceding foraging success, individuals tending to stay in areas where they were successful (area-restricted search) and approaching other individuals that had just found a food item (copying). The results of the simulation showed that for a wide variety of prey distributions, and especially those that were judged to approximate natural distributions. the optimal group size for maximizing an individual's rate of food intake was about 4 individuals. In contrast, the optimal group size in terms of an alternative measure of foraging success was about 12–16 individuals. This second measure of success was the probability of an individual's not finding a food item during a certain time period of the simulation, the optimum group size being the one producing the lowest value of "risk." The model was largely designed around data on the searching pattern of tit flocks, which commonly occur in sizes closer to the second optimum than to the first. This pattern at least suggests that tits may be minimizing risk as well as maximizing rate (of food intake) in their flocking strategies.

Finally, as Krebs and Barnard (in press) have pointed out, if flocking has costs (e.g., interference) as well as benefits (e.g., increased predator awareness), it might be expected that birds would distribute themselves in flocks of different sizes so that net benefit is equalized over all flocks (an "ideal free distribution"). If this happens, it may not be possible to observe a relationship between flock size and benefit.

Time Allocation without Prey Depletion

Predators must often reduce the availability of prey in a small area as a result of their own foraging activities, by exploiting the readily available prey first, by straightforward depletion of the prey stock, or by frightening mobile prey and thus making them less accessible (see earlier discussion of redshank feeding on *Corophium*). Sometimes, however, changes in the quality of a patch may result from changes independent of the predator's own activity. In a field study of spotted flycatchers *(Muscicapa striata)*, Davies (1977a) has investigated one such situation. The flycatcher has to make the choice of whether or not to return to the same perch (analog of a patch) after each foraging sally. Figure 9 shows that successive intercatch intervals from a perch are roughly constant, indicating that there is no gradual depletion of prey. The major factor determining the profitability of a particular perch is whether or not there happens to be a swarm of flies within striking distance, since capture success declines rapidly with length of sally made by the bird. Davies found that a flycatcher changes to another perch if it waits for longer than about 1.5 times the average intercatch interval. The optimal choice of this giving-up time involves a trade-off between the disadvantage of

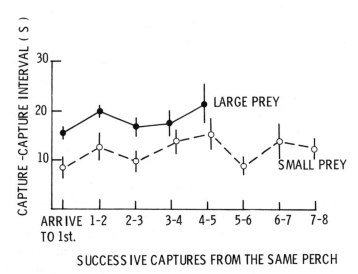

Fig. 9. Successive intercatch intervals from the same perch by spotted flycatchers. From Davies, 1977a.

leaving while the current swarm is still within striking distance and the cost of waiting for a long time for a next swarm to arrive if the current one has moved away. Although Davies did not measure the arrival rate of swarms and was thus not able to quantify the second cost directly, he was able to show in a simulation model that the observed giving-up time was close to the minimum possible for achieving maximum capture rate within a swarm. Thus, the flycatchers appear to be making an optimal trade-off between captures within a swarm and waiting between swarms.

SEARCH PATHS

OPTIMAL SEARCH PATHS

Many ecological models of parasite and predator searching behavior assume random encounters between predator and prey, or parasite and hosts, within a patch, and models based on this assumption give a good fit to experimental results (Rogers, 1972). However, the assumption of random encounters does not necessarily imply random search, since if the prey are distributed at random within a patch, random encounters could result from nonrandom search. Random search is in fact highly inefficient, at least when the prey do not renew themselves extremely rapidly, so it seems rather unlikely that any predators or parasites do search in a truly random fashion.

There have been a number of investigations of searching efficiency using simulation models (Cody, 1971; Pyke, 1978; Cullen, cited in Smith, 1974b; Gilbert, Guitterez, Frazer, and Jones, 1976). In Pyke's simulation, the predator could move from one point to any of the four neighbouring positions on a lattice grid, the total area of the grid (number of points) being varied from one simulation to another. The probabilities of moving in the four possible directions—forward, backward, left, and right (Pf, Pb, Pl, and Pr)—were varied in order to find the movement rules for the optimal search path. The optimal path is one in which the maximum number of grid points (which are, in effect, prey items) are visited during a set number of moves or, in other words, the path that minimizes revisiting depleted places if there is no replacement of prey. An important variable in the simulation was the rule for changing behavior at the boundary of the grid, and Pyke considered two possibilities; a reflecting boundary, in which the rule is simply to reverse direction at the boundary ($Pb = 1$), and a partially reflecting boundary, in which the predator moves with approximately equal probability to the left, to the right, and backward when at the boundary. Pyke considered the most realistic boundary conditions either an effectively infinite grid (for example, a bumblebee foraging in a large meadow) or a grid with a partially reflecting boundary (the pattern of behavior shown by hummingbirds hunting on an artificial grid). If the searching path is symmetrical ($Pl = Pr$), then the path can be characterized by one measure ($Pf - Pb$), which Pyke calls "directionality." On an infinite grid, the optimal directionality is obviously 1, and the results of Pyke's simulation model showed that with a partially reflecting boundary, the optimal directionality was somewhere between 0.8 and 1.0, depending on the size of the grid. Pyke computed the directionality for a number of real search paths (e.g., Sinniff and Jessen, 1969; Kleerekoper, Timms, Westlake, Davy, Malar, and Anderson, 1970; Smith, 1974a) and found that the observed directionalities lay between 0.1 and 0.8. Although it is not clear that all of the examples analyzed by Pyke were in fact search paths as opposed to other types of movement, the conclusion is clear: Pyke's simulation does not adequately account for observed search patterns, unless, of course, the real search paths are all well away from the optimum. Pyke suggested two reasons for the discrepancy between his results and the real world, the most important being that as his simulated predators did not have any sense organs, they did not detect a prey until hitting it by landing on a grid point. A second factor influencing real search paths is that predators often, as I have discussed earlier, modify their search path after a capture by decreasing the directionality.

The simulation model cited in Smith (1974b) is somewhat more realistic than Pyke's in that it includes both sensory abilities of the predator, represented as a "domain of danger" around each prey, and a greater flexibility in the choice of directions open to the predator for each move. The model is less realistic in other respects: it assumes a very restricted prey universe and has no prey depletion, or rule for staying within the boundary of the prey universe. In the model, the predator starts at a central point surrounded by a ring of prey, and the optimal search path is one that maximizes the "hit rate" of prey by the predator. The optimal path was, as in Pyke's simulation, far from random, but it had a directionality somewhat lower than the 0.8 of Pyke's model.

Many of the real search plans that were analyzed by Pyke have a slight asymmetry; that is, the mean direction deviates significantly from zero (counting left turns as positive and right turns as negative), and Cody (1971), in a simulation model similar to that of Pyke's, concluded that a slight asymmetry increases search efficiency. Cody also concluded that his observed directionality of 0.64 for finch flocks was optimal, but as Pyke showed, it is optimal only under the particular grid and boundary conditions chosen by Cody for his simulation.

In summary, there are no quantitative conclusions that can be drawn from these simulation studies, but they all reach the qualitative conclusion that directional search paths are more efficient than random ones and that to specify an optimum more precisely one needs to know about the predator's sensory abilities, the effective grid size, the boundary rules, and the prey distribution.

Pyke (1974) also discussed an analytical model of optimal search paths for bumblebees gathering nectar in a large meadow. The model assumes that food is distributed at discrete points and is nonrenewable and that the bee uses memory only in recording its arrival direction at a flower and the amount of nectar extracted from a particular plant. The hypothesis is that a bee chooses its departure direction from a point by "aiming" in a particular direction and then scanning for flowers within a given "scanning sector" distributed about this aiming direction (Figure 10). The model is designed to investigate the optimal choice of aiming direction and the optimal width of the scanning sector. Pyke used the results of his simulation model to make the assumption that the optimal aim on an effectively infinite grid should be straight ahead (continuing the direction of arrival), and

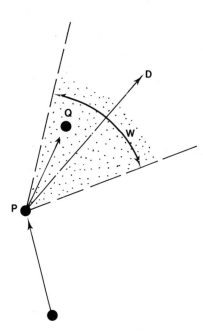

Fig. 10. Pyke's model of the optimal search path in bumblebees. The bee leaves a resource point, P, and "aims" in a direction, D, with scanning sector, W. It then heads for the nearest resource point within W (Q). From Pyke, 1974.

then he went on to show that if the optimal aim involves a turn angle of zero, the observed distribution of turn angles, which are not in themselves a measure of the aimed direction, would have a mean of zero. This assumption is in agreement with the data he collected on bumblebees. The optimal scanning angle depends on the quantity of nectar extracted from the current resource point: the poorer the quality of the current plant, the smaller the scanning angle should be. This idea is somewhat similar to that of area-restricted search, since a smaller scanning angle results in a narrower distribution of turn angle about the mean of zero. If the predator has just exploited a poor-quality resource point, it should move out of the areas as fast as possible (area-avoided search), since it might be crossing the path of a previous forager. Pyke estimated the width of scanning angle by angular deviation of the observed angles of turn between successive flowers, and he showed that the angular deviation increases asymptotically as a function of the amount of nectar extracted from the current plant, the latter being estimated by the time spent on the flowers. This result is in good qualitative agreement with the model, although it was not possible to make a more quantitative test.

Modification of Search Path through Experience

In the models I have discussed above, the predators were capable of rather simple modifications of their search path, such as area-restricted searching, but many predators probably use longer-term memory in modifying their search paths. For example, both Smith (1974b) and Pyke (1974) found that blackbirds and bumblebees, respectively, tend to alternate left and right turns in their search paths.

Beukema (1968) investigated the ability of sticklebacks (*Gasterosteus aculeatus*) to improve their search efficiency by learning to exploit a particular distribution of prey in an artificial environment consisting of a large tank divided into 18 small hexagonal cells. The fish could travel between cells through gates, and once within a cell, they could detect any prey immediately, so that the optimal search path involved visiting as few cells as possible per prey encountered. In an experiment, Beukema placed a single prey item in one of the 12 outer cells of his tank, so that a fish, starting from a randomly chosen point in the outer ring, could in theory encounter the prey after visiting an average of 6 cells. This path would result from a strategy of swimming directly around the outer ring of cells. Beukema calculated the encounter efficiency (number of prey encountered per cell visited) of a variety of search strategies, varying from random to the optimal. The sticklebacks performed well above random, mainly because they tended to search in a directional manner, and they also gradually improved their performance over a series of trials (Table II) but did not reach anything like the optimal value of 0.17. This result shows that sticklebacks are capable of adaptively modifying their search path in response to a particular distribution of prey, and the fact that they did not reach the optimum path may be a reflection of the rather artificial task with which they were faced.

A second example of a long-term modification of search paths in response to experience of a particular prey distribution was reported by Smith (1974b) and Zach and Falls (1977). They showed that the overall tortuosity of search paths increases in areas of high prey density. Zach and Falls, following Williamson and Gray (1975), described the tortuosity of search paths by the "meander ratio," which is defined as the actual distance traveled between two points divided by the beeline distance. An increase in the meander ratio, together with an increase in the number of visits, accounts for the fact that the ovenbirds tested by Zach and Falls allocated most of their foraging time to more profitable patches (see above, Figure 8). Zach and Falls (1977) showed that the overall change in search path is not merely a consequence of changes in tortuosity after a find. Since the predator is likely to make more captures in a high-density area, it would be expected to show more area-restricted searching, which could involve turning through bigger angles, making successive turns in the same direction, or decreasing move lengths

TABLE II. THE EFFICIENCY (PREY ENCOUNTERED PER CELL VISITED) OF DIFFERENT HYPOTHETICAL SEARCH PATHS IN AN 18-CELL MAZE[a]

Type of search path	Encounter efficiency (e)
1. Random	0.04
2. Random, but outer cells only	0.02
3. Ongoing (no reverse moves)	0.13
4. Outer cells only and ongoing	0.17
5. Actual fish: naive	0.07
6. Actual fish: experienced	0.10

[a]From Beukema, 1968. The predators (sticklebacks) were searching for a single prey item in one of the 12 outer cells of the maze: they were more efficient than if searching at random, but less than optimal.

between turns (Smith, 1974b), all of which would produce an increase in tortuosity.

Zach and Falls showed that after an ovenbird had become accustomed to searching in a large arena for a single patch of prey, it would continue to show an increase in tortuosity of its search path when entering the patch even when tested with no prey present; probably at least part of the effect was due to partially reflecting boundary behavior. Although Zach and Falls referred to this response of increased meander ratio in areas of high prey density as "area-restricted search," it falls outside the more usual definition of this phenomenon. The important point is that the birds showed a long-term change in search behavior in response to heterogeneities in the distribution of prey.

Smith (1974b) also found that his predators had more tortuous search paths in areas of high prey density. He showed that this pattern results partly from boundary behavior (the birds tended to turn back at the edge of the area) and partly from the fact that the birds made bigger turns between successive steps in high-density areas. In contrast, area-restricted search after a find, which results at least in blackbirds from the tendency to make several successive turns in the same direction, was if anything less marked in the high-density area than in an area of low prey density. Area-restricted search was quantified by a decrease in the beeline distance between the bird and the point of capture in pairwise comparisons of various numbers of moves before and after the catch (Figure 11), and as Smith pointed out, the fact that search paths were more convoluted before a capture in the high-density area makes it more difficult to show a decrease in beeline distance after a find.

Smith investigated the ability of blackbirds to increase or decrease the amount of area-restricted searching in response to changes in the dispersion of artificial prey consisting of pastry caterpillars. At low overall prey densities (0.064 prey/m²), the birds showed no area restriction when hunting for regularly distributed prey, but they did when hunting for random or clumped prey. At high prey density (0.3 prey/m²), the birds showed no restricted search with random and regular distributions and only a slight tendency with clumped prey. As I discussed above, the fact that the search paths in the high-density areas were highly convoluted before a capture makes it difficult to positively show area restriction. Further, at high prey density, search efficiency is not so likely to limit the rate of food intake, so that one might expect the birds to be more finely tuned to making adaptive changes in search paths at low prey densities (Smith, 1974b; Krebs, 1973a).

OPTIMAL RETURN TIMES

In the discussion of search paths, I have been assuming that prey are essentially nonrenewing, but if one assumes not only that a predator might deplete food stocks during its foraging but also that the food replenishes itself rapidly, one can consider how rapidly a predator ought to return to a particular place for forage (Cody, 1971; Charnov, Orians, and Hyatt, 1976). In theory, one could imagine that a predator is selected to travel around its foraging area in a pattern that maximizes the harvest from a particular patch on each visit. As Charnov *et al.*

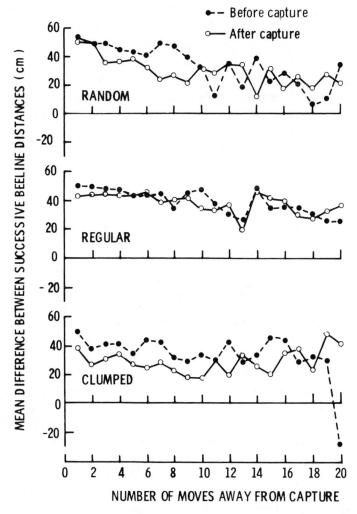

Fig. 11. Area-restricted search in European thrushes (*Turdus* spp.) (Smith, 1974b). The graphs show changes in the beeline distance betwen the bird and the capture point for various numbers of moves before and after the capture. When prey are clumped in distribution, the changes in beeline distance are consistently smaller after than before capture for about the first 10 moves (bottom graph). This pattern indicates that the birds are searching near the capture point. With regular prey distributions (middle graph), there is no such effect, and with randomly distributed prey, the results are intermediate (top graph).

(1976) discussed, an "optimal return time" in searching strategy requires that the predator have exclusive use of an area, since otherwise, there may be interference with the recovery of prey after depletion. This reduction of interference could be achieved by territorial exclusion (Charnov *et al.,* 1976) or by group foraging: if all the predators in an area forage in one group, there will be no interference between individuals in return time harvesting (Cody, 1971). In his discussion of mixed flocks of finches, Cody (1971, 1974b) regarded one of the major benefits of flocking as its enabling the birds to optimize their return times, although he did not actually show that the flocks he studied had exclusive ranges, an essential prerequisite for the hypothesis. Cody studied flock movements in two areas, one close to a mountain range and one further away toward a desert. The former, wetter, area had a more abundant but less rapidly renewing food supply (ripening seeds), while the dry desert had sparse but rapidly renewing supplies of seed. Cody's data suggest that flocks in the desert area moved faster and took bigger turns than the birds close to the mountains. These two factors together would decrease the return time in response to the sparser but more rapidly renewing food. It is unfortunate that in Cody's study, two variables—food density and renewal rate—were confounded, so that one cannot tell which factor influenced the birds' movement pattern. It would be interesting to find out how the flocks behave when both food density and renewal rate are low. The same problem arises in the study of Bernstein (1975) on foraging columns of ants. Seed-harvesting ants of the genera *Veromessor* and *Pogonomyrmex* can forage either individually or in columns radiating out of the nest, and they tend to do the latter when food is scarce, as Bernstein showed by food addition experiments. The foraging column gradually rotates like a spoke of a wheel around the central colony, and the speed of rotation varies according to food availability and renewal rate, being faster when the food is scarce and quickly renewing. Bernstein suggested that the column foraging method enables the ants to avoid searching the same area twice within a short time, to choose the best rotation speed (return time), and to find food at a greater distance from the colony. It would be interesting to separate out the influence of renewal rate and food density on the behavior of a foraging column. Drent and van Eerden (in press) have recently obtained convincing evidence that goose flocks act as return time maximizers. They showed that barnacle geese (*Branta leucopsis* and *B. bernicla*) moved around an area of salt marsh cropping the vegetation at regular intervals. The cropping interval was shown to be near the optimum for stimulating plant growth and maximizing yield to the geese.

Although there is little direct evidence on the role of exclusive territories as return time optimizers, Kamil (1978) has shown that territorial amakihis (*Loxops vireus*) avoid revisiting recently exploited flowers. He also showed that intruders do not avoid exploited flowers and therefore do less well than residents when foraging in the same general area. Clutton-Brock (1975), in his study of a Troop of red colobus (*Colobus badius*), which contained about 80 individuals and occupied a range of about 114 ha, noted that the group patrolled around the home range in a rather systematic fashion, so that it avoided revisiting the same area more rapidly than the limit imposed by the size of the range. Since the red colobus feeds to a large extent on shoots, fruit and flowers, it is quite likely that the monkeys are maximizing their return time so as to allow recovery of their food. Another anecdotal observation of a territorial species avoiding recently exploited patches is in Wolf, Hainsworth, and Gill's (1975) report of territorial sunbirds. The limpet *Lottia gigantea* is also a likely candidate for return time optimizing. As Stimson (1970) showed, *Lottia* grazes on algal film, defends a territory, and adjusts its territory size according to the thickness of the algal film. The growth rate of *Lottia* is well correlated with the depth of algae in its territory, and by maintaining an exclusive territory against members of its own and other, smaller, species, it prevents the film from being cropped close enough to depress the its own growth.

Thus, territoriality in *Lottia* enables the limpet to "farm" the algae film and maintain it at the maximal depth. Part of the strategy of farming might well include avoidance of recently grazed areas.

The most detailed investigations of the ability of predators to optimize return times have been those involving a choice between two concurrent variable-interval schedules (Shimp, 1969; Herrnstein, 1970; Mackintosh, 1974). In these experiments, the animal was offered a choice of two keys or levers that yielded rewards at different rates per unit time (*not* per unit effort, as in the variable ratio schedules discussed earlier). The interreward intervals were distributed with either a pseudorandom or a peaked-probability distribution about a mean, which differed for the two keys. The animal could not increase the reward rate per unit time by responding faster to a key, but if it failed to respond for too long, it might miss an opportunity when the reward system was briefly enabled. This means that the animal faced a trade-off problem closely analogous to that of optimal return times: responding too soon after the last reward resulted in wasted effort, but waiting too long resulted in lost opportunities.

In a natural setting, predators may often decrease the availability of food in a very short-term manner. For example, Davies (1977a) has described how yellow wagtails (*Motacilla flava*) feeding on dungflies (*Scatophaga*) scare the flies off a dungpat and snatch them as they land on the surrounding grass and before they disperse. The flies eventually reassemble at a dungpat, but before they do so, the wagtail cannot forage successfully in the area. Similarly, Goss-Custard (1976) reported that the amphipod *Corophium* retreats into the mud when a redshank walks over it and becomes less easily available to the bird until it moves back up to the surface.

To return to variable-interval schedules, one can see intuitively, in contrast to the variable-ratio schedule discussed earlier, that the optimal strategy is no longer to respond exclusively to the key with the higher reward rate, even if the difference between the two is large. If it has just obtained a reward, the animal should switch to the other key for a short time interval, the length depending on the exact variable interval schedule. The results of studies of concurrent variable-interval schedule show that animals such as rats and pigeons tend to match. That is, they distribute their responses in proportion to the availability of rewards: if the left key offers twice the reward rate of the right key, it receives twice the number of responses (Herrnstein, 1970; see also Herrnstein and Loveland, 1975, for a discussion of matching in relation to maximizing—they argue that the two are not fundamentally different).

Shimp (1969) has argued that matching is an optimal strategy by which animals maximize reward rate. He showed this by simulating a variety of alternative possible rules for the allocation of responses. The optimization theory would also explain why animals march according to "prey size" (length of access to food) when offered two variable-interval schedules that are otherwise identical (Catania, 1963). Although most of the work on matching has involved only two concurrent schedules, Miller and Loveland (1974) have reported matching in a situation where a pigeon is confronted with a choice of five keys, although it is not clear if Shimp's optimization result holds for this more complex environment.

Zach and Falls (1976a) studied revisiting of patches (blocks of wood drilled with holes) by ovenbirds in an aviary experiment. In this experiment, patches were clearly distinct, and the birds tended to avoid revisiting, but in another experiment (Zach and Falls, 1976b), where the patches were not so distinct, the sequence of visits to four patches did not deviate from random.

THE CHOICE OF PREY TYPES

OPTIMAL CHOICE: THEORY

Each prey type (species, or size class within a species) that a predator encounters has a potential reward (in terms of the net food intake) and a cost (the handling time). By measuring the gain as net food (e.g., calories or weight) intake, one can take into account factors such as digestibility and the energy cost of subduing the prey. The handling time is considered to be a cost, because it reduces the time available for searching for alternative prey. A number of authors have derived models to show how an optimal predator, aiming to maximize its net rate of intake while foraging, should select prey (Schoener, 1971; Emlen, 1966; Charnov, 1976a). Although the models differ in detail, they all reach essentially the same conclusions. Clearly, an optimal predator should be able to recognize prey types of different profitability (net yield per unit handling time) and should choose prey of high profitability in preference to others. Further, an ideal predator should rank different prey types according to their profitabilities and should prefer them according to their rank order. The more interesting predictions of optimal diet models are concerned with the consequences of changes in the availability of different prey types. When all types are scarce, the searching time is high, so that a predator can less easily afford to be selective, since selective hunting for profitable prey increases the search time even further. However, when profitable prey are common, search time contributes less to the total, so that a predator will increase its net rate of intake by feeding only on the more profitable prey. Thus, the models predict that predators should be more selective when food availability (more precisely, availability of high-quality prey) is high than when food is scarce. Rather more surprising is the prediction that whether or not low-ranking prey should be included in the diet depends only on the availability of high-ranking types, and not on the encounter rate with the low-ranking prey themselves. In other words, if good-quality prey are common enough, the predator should never "take time out" to eat unprofitable prey, even if they are very abundant. This prediction is perhaps the most interesting, since it is hard to imagine the same prediction arising from other models. In order to make these predictions quantitative (i.e., to specify the exact points at which the predator should switch from including to excluding a particular type of prey), it is necessary to know not only the profitability of each prey but also the predator's encounter rate with each type. Encounter rate is not the same as abundance; it includes the effect of such things as crypsis of prey, search images, and so on. The necessity of measuring these components of the model makes it difficult to test the model directly and quantitatively (Krebs et al., 1977). If one interprets the model in a quantitative way, a further prediction can be made, namely, that the inclusion or exclusion of a particular prey type from the diet should be a step function; that is, the predator should switch from no selection to selection in an all-or-nothing manner. This is true because a prey type must either decrease or increase the predator's net rate of intake by its inclusion in the diet. If it would decrease intake, it should be totally ignored; if it would increase intake, it should always be eaten.

As pointed out by Charnov (1973), Elner and Hughes (1978), and Hughes (in press), if prey cannot be recognized instantaneously, the optimal diet model makes different predictions. Most important, if there is a time cost associated with rejecting unprofitable prey, such prey may be included in the optimal set when they are common. This is true simply because the rejection cost has to be paid each time an unprofitable item is encountered, and a large number of rejection times might lower the selective predator's intake rate sufficiently to bring less profitable prey into the optimal set. Tests of this version of the model have been done by Elner and Hughes (1978), Houston, Krebs, and Erichsen, (in press), and Erichsen, Krebs, and Houston (in press). They confirm that when there is a time cost of rejection, the inclusion of less profitable prey in the diet is no longer independent on the encounter rate with them.

OPTIMAL DIETS: EVIDENCE

The basic assumption of optimal diet models—that predators prefer prey of high profitability—has been verified in many different studies. Gill and Wolf (1975b) found that the sunbird (*Nectarinia kilimensis*) prefers closed mistletoe flowers (ones in which the corolla tube has not been split open by a bird during a previous visit), and that these flowers yield 2.6 times more nectar per unit handling time than the open flowers. (However, in a more recent laboratory study, Hainsworth and Wolf [1976], investigating the choice by hummingbirds of different nectar concentrations with various handling times, found that the birds preferred high concentrations [high-quality prey] even when the energy yield per unit handling time was higher from low nectar concentrations. It is likely that for a hummingbird, the energy cost of carrying around a large bulk of fluid in the stomach is so high that low-concentration nectar is virtually never a profitable food). Davies (1977a) offered a choice of different-sized flies to a captive yellow wagtail and found that the bird preferred the most profitable prey (Figure 12), and a similar result was obtained by Kear (1962), who offered captive chaffinches (*Fringilla coelebs*) a choice of seed types. The rank order of preference for six types correlated almost perfectly with the rank of profitability. Other studies showing a preference for more profitable prey include those of Menge (1972) on starfish and Smith (1970) on *Tamiasciurus* squirrels.

There are also a number of studies in which it has been found that the degree of selectivity of a predator increases when overall food availability is high. These results may come from comparing populations living in productive and unproductive environments. For example, Herrera (1975), comparing the width of diet of barn owls in northern and southern Europe, showed that in the latter, more productive environment, the owls were more selective. In a comparison between

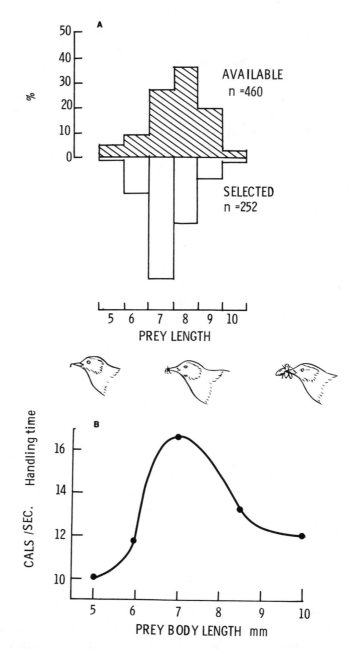

Fig. 12. A demonstration that yellow wagtails prefer flies of a size that yield the highest return per unit handling time. (A) shows the percentage of frequency distributions of available and consumed dung-flies of different size. (B) shows the profitability of various size classes, measured as gross calories per unit handling time. From Davies, 1977a.

seasons, Menge (1972) found that the starfish *Leptasterias* was less selective in winter than in summer, when food was abundant. Charnov (1976a) reanalyzed the data of Holling (1966) on the response of preying mantids to prey of different profitability, and he showed that mantids become less selective when they are hungrier, hunger being a proximate indication to the mantid of overall prey availability. The different prey types were houseflies presented at different distances, the distant ones being less profitable. Holling's data reveal that the mantids responded to increasing hunger, as measured by how much food was left in the gut, by attacking flies at successively greater distances. This pattern is analogous to a predator's adding prey to its diet in rank order of profitability. Davidson (1978) showed experimentally that harvester ants of the genus *Pogonomyrmex* rank barley seed particles on the basis of size (caloric content) and that the preference for profitable size becomes most marked as total prey availability increases.

While these observations lend qualitative support to the optimal diet model, they are not strong evidence because they are open to alternative interpretation. Predators may become less selective at low food abundances because they are more willing to expose themselves to predators (Charnov, 1976b).

Experiments aimed at testing the predictions of optimal diet models more precisely have been carried out by Werner and Hall (1974), Goss-Custard (1977a), and Krebs *et al.* (1977) (see also Elner and Hughes, 1978; Houston *et al.*, in press; Erichsen *et al.*, in press). All these studies have involved predators choosing between size classes of the same prey species, and in all cases, there was a correlation between size and profitability, so that in effect, the tests were of size selection by the predator. Further, in these experiments, profitability was assumed to be equal to gross intake per unit handling time, thus ignoring differences between prey types in digestibility or energy cost of capture.

Werner and Hall (1974) studied the choice by bluegill sunfish *(Lepomis macrochirus)* of different size classes of *Daphnia magna.* Their experiments consisted of putting mixtures of different proportions of four size classes of *Daphnia* in a tank and allowing the fish to forage for a short time. In order to overcome the problem of assessing the encounter rates of the predator with the different-sized classes of prey, Werner and Hall measured the "reaction distance" of the fish to each size class, and they used these data to correct for differences in visibility. By making a few assumptions about the shape of the fish's visual field, they could estimate encounter rates. In three experimental treatments, Werner and Hall exposed fish to three levels of encounter rate with the largest, most profitable, size class of prey, and from measurements of handling times and weights of each size class, they could predict which prey the fish should choose. The predictions were that the fish should not select at all in the "low-density" experiment, should select the two largest size classes in the next treatment, and should select only the largest prey in the "high-density" treatment. The results conformed quite well to this pattern, although Werner and Hall did not find out exactly how closely the model could predict switch points from no selection to selection.

Although Werner and Hall's results appear to provide strong support for the optimal diet model, they might be open to an alternative interpretation. If the fish obeyed a rule that simply said, "After a capture, chase the next prey entering the visual field," then selectivity for the large (most conspicuous) prey would increase as the encounter rate with these prey increased, although the quantitative pattern of selection might not be as predicted by the optimal foraging model (O'Brien, Slade, and Vinyard, 1976). This hypothesis is, of course, a proximate explanation, while the optimal diet model is an ultimate explanation of prey choice, so the two are not really alternatives. However, the optimal diet predicts that once it is above the "selection threshold," the predator should continue to ignore small prey, regardless of the encounter rate with them. This outcome would not be predicted by the proximate hypothesis I have just described, but Werner and Hall did not test this prediction of the model.

Krebs *et al.* (1977) also tested the optimal diet model in short-term laboratory experiments, using great tits as predators, and they specifically set out to test the prediction that the encounter rate with unprofitable prey has no effect on selectivity. They used only two prey types, large and small pieces of mealworm. These differed in profitability by approximately twofold, but the exact value varied from one bird to another (five birds were tested). The problem of measuring encounter rates was surmounted by presenting the prey at intervals on a moving belt to a waiting predator. In this way, the bird was confronted with a sequential choice of prey at differing encounter rates in different experimental treatments.

When the two prey types were presented at low encounter rates, the birds were nonselective, but when the encounter rate with large prey was high, most individuals were selective, and they maintained their preference for large prey in the face of a sixfold change in the encounter rate with small prey. Furthermore, one of the five birds failed to show any selection, and the relative profitabilities of the two prey types for this individual were such that the model predicted no selection. These results provide strong support for the optimal diet model, although the experimental design had a drawback: the prey were not presented in a random sequence (for logistic reasons), which means that the model had to be modified, since the usual model assumes random encounters. One way in which the results of Krebs *et al.* (1977), as well as the results of other studies, do not support the optimal diet model is that the change from no selection to selection of more profitable prey is not, as predicted, an all-or-nothing switch but a gradual change. Although Pulliam (1975) has produced a model with nutrient constraints predicting a gradual change in selection, this model is not likely to be relevant to the selection of profitable size classes within a species. More probable is that the predator invests a certain amount of time in sampling alternative prey. Krebs *et al.* (1977) discussed this point and described how they estimated the slope of the transition from no selection to selection.

The best published attempt to test the optimal diet models in detail in the field is the work of Goss-Custard (1977a) on the selection of different-sized classes of polychaete worms *(Nereis, Nephthys)* by redshank. Goss-Custard's data consisted of detailed information on the prey chosen by individual redshank and on the density of different-sized worms in the mud. Although he did not directly measure the availability of the worms to the redshank—and hence, the encounter rate—Goss-Custard examined the relationship between the feeding rate of the redshank on a particular size class and its density in the mud. In order to eliminate the complication of the bird's pausing to handle one prey and interrupting its search for the next prey, Goss-Custard expressed both feeding rates and prey densities as prey per linear meter searched. He found that the largest prey-size classes, with the highest profitability, were taken in direct proportion to their own density, but that the smallest, least-profitable size class of worms were taken not in relation to their own density but at a rate inversely proportional to the density of large prey in the mud. Hence, when the birds were feeding at a high rate on profitable prey, they ignored small prey regardless of the latter's density. Goss-Custard discounted the possibility that this pattern could be due to small prey's being less available (e.g., deeper in the mud) where large prey are common, on the grounds that a similar pattern of predation was shown by captive redshank in controlled laboratory conditions. Associated with the tendency to select only large prey where these are common, the redshank walk faster but have a lower percentage of success and a longer peck time when feeding on large prey. In fact, Goss-Custard suggested that the proximate mechanism by which redshank achieve the change in their selection behavior is the alteration of their walking speed. In order to test for optimal prey selection, Goss-Custard incorporated his empirically determined relationships between prey density, prey choice, and search behavior into a simulation model. By varying the pattern of selection in the model, he showed that the choice made by the redshank maximized gross returns per unit time (or per meter searched).

Discussion

The three studies I have discussed that were designed specifically to test the optimal diet model have been remarkably consistent in showing the predictions to be reasonably good. However, none of these studies specifically examined the energetic costs of handling and digesting different prey types, nor did they look at selection between prey species. In fact, Goss-Custard (1977b) found that red-shank, while they select the optimal diet within one prey type—namely, worms—prefer a suboptimal prey species, *Corophium,* which has a smaller gross energy return for unit effort than *Nereis.* Goss-Custard suggested that this preference may reflect some crucial difference between the two prey types in nutrient value. Whatever the reason, the moral seems to be that optimal diet models will have to become more sophisticated to deal with complex choice situations (Krebs, 1978b; Pulliam, 1975). One laboratory that failed to support the optimal diet model is that of Emlen and Emlen (1975). They studied selection of seeds by laboratory mice supplied with *ad lib* alternative food, which does not seem to be a situation in which the predators would be pressured enough to forage very efficiently.

Sampling and Optimal Foraging

I have referred several times to the fact that one weakness of simple optimal foraging models is that they do not include any provision for sampling. The predator is considered omniscient, choosing patches, prey, or search paths without any trial and error. In fact, one might expect sampling to be important both in the initial period in which a predator becomes familiar with an environment and at later stages as a hedge against changes in the environment. As I discussed earlier, in at least one study, a payoff for sampling was demonstrated directly (Smith and Sweatman, 1974).

Oster and Heinrich (1976) presented a theoretical discussion of sampling by a foraging animal. Heinrich (1976) had observed that different individual bumble-bees specialize in harvesting nectar from different species of flowers. Bees are most efficient at foraging on their specialist flower (see below), but each individual bee consistently visits a few flowers of an alternative species (which Heinrich calls its "minor"). If a bee could predict reliably which flower species would be the most profitable for it, the optimum strategy would be to choose the most profitable plant and forage only on that species. However, Oster and Heinrich (1976) showed that if nature is unpredictable, a pure strategy of foraging only in the most profitable flowers is no longer optimal. In the most extreme case, with two alternative flower species, in which nature obeys Murphy's law and whatever the bee thinks is best immediately becomes the worst, a "mixed strategy" is best because it insures against a sudden change. If we assume that nature is perverse, but not too perverse, then the best strategy is somewhere between the mixed and pure alternatives.

This model shows qualitatively why pure specialization on the best prey or patches may not be the best foraging rule in the longer run, and it fits well with the data on bees. The bees could be induced to switch their specialization by supplementing the nectar supply with sugar droplets in one of the "minor" flower types, which seems to indicate that sampling knowledge is used. However, the model does not produce an easily testable quantitative prediction of how much time a predator should allocate to sampling—in other words, how much sampling the predator should do before it decided on which is the most profitable foraging patch or prey type. This problem has been tackled in a preliminary way by Krebs, Kacelnik, and Taylor (1978). They studied the sampling strategy of great tits faced with a choice of two patches of unknown quality. The patches were operant devices that offered rewards on a variable-ratio schedule, and the schedule differed for the two patches by different amounts in different experimental treatments. The tits started by sampling the two patches approximately equally but later switched to almost exclusive foraging in the more profitable place. Krebs *et al.* (1978) calculated the optimal trade-off between exploration and exploitation, using a Bayesian model based on classical "two-armed bandit" theory. The birds' behavior was remarkably close to that predicted by the model.

The Cost of Alternative Foraging Activities

Although in the optimal foraging models so far discussed the payoffs have been measured in net rate of food intake, which implies that the energy costs of foraging are known, most experimental studies of optimal foraging have measured gross intake. Evans (1976) and Norberg (1977) have analyzed the problem of how a predator should choose between alternative foraging methods that have different gross returns per unit time and different energy costs. Consider two alternative foraging methods, one a "high-return, high-cost" tactic and the other a "low-return" tactic with a low energy cost per unit searching time. At high prey densities, the search time is very small, so that the foraging method that yields a large gain per capture but has a high searching cost is more advantageous in terms of net gain than the cheaper method, which has a low return per capture. When prey density is low, and search time increases correspondingly, the high search costs of the former method outweigh its benefit, and the net intake drops below that achieved by the cheaper method. The conclusion is that predators should use high-return, high-cost methods of foraging when prey are abundant and low-cost methods with lower gross returns when prey are scarce. For example, insectivorous birds such as titmice often take prey by hovering (a high search cost method) or by gleaning branches (low cost), and given that hovering yields more energy per capture, one might expect birds to switch from hovering to gleaning as prey density drops. Neither Evans, who developed the argument graphically, nor Norberg, who presented an algebraic model, had any direct evidence for the hypothesis, but Evans mentioned that bar-tailed godwits search progressively smaller areas of mudflat and become less selective in their food intake as the temperature falls and the cost of walking increases. Under some adverse weather conditions, when the energy cost of foraging would be extremely high and prey availability low, the godwits stop foraging altogether.

MacArthur and Pianka (1966) developed an analogous line of reasoning, when they suggested that in general, animals with high searching costs should be less selective in their choice of diet at a given level of prey abundance than sit-and-wait predators, which spend little time in searching. By decreasing selectivity of prey or patches, the searching predator decreases the average interprey search time and thus decreases the costs of foraging.

Specialists and Generalists

One of the classical hypotheses in ecological theories of resource partitioning is that specialists, species that concentrate on exploiting a narrow range of resources, are more efficient than generalists in exploiting the same type of resource (e.g., Cody, 1974a; Levins, 1968; Pianka, 1976). One of the results is that specialists may replace generalists through competition. On islands, where competition may be reduced because fewer species arrive, specialists tend to increase their niche width (competitive release), and sometimes one intermediate jack-of-all-trades may replace two specialists (e.g., Schoener, 1974). However, although the observations of increased niche width on islands are compatible with the idea that specialists can outcompete generalists, there is rather little direct evidence for this assumption.

Clearly, morphological adaptations to deal with particular prey lead to an increase in foraging efficiency on that type of food, so that species differing in the morphology of their feeding apparatus differ in the type of prey that they exploit most efficiently. For example, Kear (1962) showed that finches with larger bills are more efficient at dehusking large seeds (efficiency was measured as food intake per unit handling time), and in general, she found a correlation between the preference of a species and the type of seed on which it could feed most efficiently. Partridge (1976b) studied the ability of blue tits and coal tits to exploit different types of foraging stations. She showed that blue tits are more efficient at hacking and pulling movements as well as in exploiting food that requires greater agility, and that coal tits are better at probing and extracting food from small crevices. These differences between the two species are correlated with differences in their preferences for different feeding stations in the wild.

These sorts of differences between species have almost certainly evolved over a long time period, and therefore they do not reveal much about the immediate role of competition between specialists and generalists in the evolution of niche width. Comparisons between individuals within a species, to test whether specialists on a particular part of a resource spectrum are more efficient than generalists, or to test whether specialists on different food types are efficient in their preferred type, would be a more directly relevant observation.

Two studies in which the efficiency of individual specialists has been measured are those of Partridge (1976b) on great tits and Heinrich (1976) on bumblebees. Heinrich compared the efficiency of individual bumblebees that had specialized in extracting nectar from *Aconitum* with a control group that had not experienced this flower, the *Aconitum* flowers in the foraging range of the latter group having been covered with an exclosure up to the time of the experiment. *Aconitum* is unusual in having its nectar hidden in two modified petals. The experienced specialist bees were highly efficient in extracting nectar, while the naive "generalist" bees were often unsuccessful in extracting any nectar at all. Partridge (1976a) studied the efficiency with which eight individual captive great tits extracted food from four different types of feeding place. She found that different individuals differed in the efficiency with which they exploited the different plates (the places involved tasks such as peeling bark off a tree, probing for food in sawdust, and so on) and furthermore, that the birds specialized in the foraging niche where they as individuals had the highest efficiency, some being specialist probers, others hackers, and so on. In contrast to the bees studied by Heinrich, the tits did not specialize first and increase their efficiency as a consequence, nor did they increase their specialization through experience of their efficiency in exploiting the four types of place. Instead, the tits seemed to have acquired during their development (or from their genes) a match between profitability and preference.

In these studies, no measurements were made of the influence of specialization on competitive ability, but in both cases, it follows from the results that a specialist would be more efficient than a nonspecialist in exploitation competition for its own preferred resource type.

FEEDING DISPERSION: COST–BENEFIT ANALYSES

I have already discussed how group foraging might increase the efficiency with which individuals allocate their time to different patches. The same sort of argument—that groups make more accurate choices than solitary individuals—could in theory be equally well applied to choice of prey types and sampling strategies, although to my knowledge this application has not yet been made (with the possible exception of Murton's [1971] work on prey selection in pigeon flocks).

If group foraging is on the whole advantageous, because it enables individuals to make more accurate foraging decisions, why is solitary foraging so common? The factors favoring group or solitary living are numerous (Waser and Wiley; this volume), and I will mention only briefly some examples of cost–benefit analyses applied to foraging groups or territoriality.

Horn (1968) and Smith (1968) have both produced cost–benefit models of feeding dispersion based on the travel costs of bringing food to a central place. Horn considered whether solitary or colonial nesting would be more economical for predators exploiting an unpredictable food supply. He showed by simple geometry that in order to minimize the average travel distance from all the possible food sites to the nest, assuming that during the whole nesting period food will at one time or another occur at all the designated sites in an area with roughly equal frequency, the predators should nest in the geometric center of the feeding sites. If all pairs attempted to do this, the result would be a nesting aggregation. In order to test Horn's idea, it would be necessary to show: (1) that nesting colonies occur roughly in the center of all the feeding sites (with appropriate weighting for differential use of feeding sites) and (2) that colonies have exclusive feeding ranges. This second point is significant since the implication of Horn's model in its simplest version is that there is little interference between colonies. Horn also showed that if food occurs predictably at each feeding site, nesting pairs can minimize travel distance by nesting solitarily and excluding others from their feeding areas.

Smith's (1968) model is designed to show why *Tamiasciurus* squirrels hold separate, rather than pair feeding territories in the winter. The squirrels harvest pine cones from within their territory and store them in a central cache, and territorial defense in this species seems to be of survival value in excluding competitors from the food supply both before and after harvesting. Smith showed in a model that if food is initially uniformly dispersed over the territory, the distance traveled to harvest cones and store them in a cache is smaller for a single territory-holder than for a pair on a territory of twice the area. Smith also found that the average territory size in more productive areas (hemlock) is smaller than that in less productive lodgepole pine forests, so that the squirrels compensate for an increase in food density by decreasing the distance over which they travel, supporting Smith's argument that travel distance is important. This may have been a *direct* response to the food supply or an *indirect* consequence of greater pressure on territories in good habitats (Krebs, 1971). The fact that *within* one habitat, territory size was not related to food density suggests the latter. Although a relationship between food density and territory size (Slaney and Northcote, 1974; Simon, 1975; Stenger, 1958) does not necessarily show that territorial behavior is primarily concerned with defense of food, it lends support to Smith's argument that territory size is influenced by a cost–benefit balance in which the benefits are related to food (Figure 13).

One of the first attempts to discuss the economics of territory defense was that of Brown (1964), who introduced the idea of the "defendability" of a resource, referring to the fact that the costs of territorial defense and advertisement must be more than offset by the gain in resources for territoriality to be economically

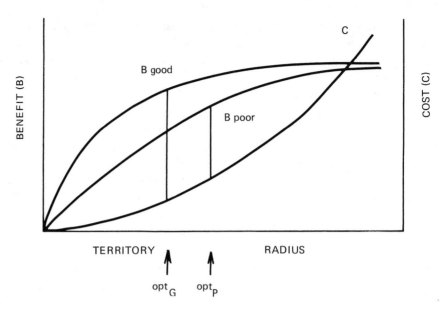

Fig. 13. A graphical cost–benefit model suggesting that territory size might decrease when food density is high. The costs of territory defense are shown as an accelerating function of territory radius (assuming costs are proportional to area of territory; if they are proportional to perimeter the function would be linear). Benefits (in terms of food) rise more sharply in a good habitat than in a poor one. The benefit curve flattens off when the territory contains a surfeit of food. The optimal territory size (maximizing B–C) is smaller in the good-quality habitat.

advantageous. Two studies in which this intuitively obvious notion has been examined in a quantitative manner both involve nectivorous birds (Gill and Wolf, 1975a; Carpenter and MacMillen, 1976).

Gill and Wolf (1975a) studied the defense of *Leonotis* flowers by the golden-winged sunbird *(Nectarinia reichenowi)*. Their main conclusions were that the efficiency (net gain per unit time) of the birds in extracting nectar is a function of nectar volume in the flowers, and that by defending flowers against nectar thieves, a bird can maintain the nectar level in flowers within its territory at a higher level than in undefended flowers. Gill and Wolf were able to show that the benefit in terms of time saved by having a higher nectar level in the territory more than compensated for the time involved in territory defense. The Hawaiian honey-creeper *(Vestiaria coccinea)* studied by Carpenter and MacMillen (1976) occasion-ally, but not often, defends a feeding territory centered on the flowers of *Metrosi-deros* trees. Using the same argument as Brown (1964), Carpenter and MacMillen developed a simple model predicting that territorial defense of flowers should occur only at a specifiable intermediate range of nectar production. At very high rates of nectar production, the extra gain in nectar volume by excluding compet-itors would be negligible, since there is more than enough nectar to go round. At very low levels of nectar production, no amount of exclusion of rivals could produce an increase in nectar levels sufficient to pay for the cost of territorial defense. By measuring or estimating the nectar production, energy costs of main-tenance and territorial defense, and the efficiency of exclusion of intruders, Car-penter and MacMillen were able to predict whether or not particular individuals should be territorial. Ten birds were studied, six territorial and four nonterritorial, and nine of these supported the prediction. Although the Carpenter and MacMillen model contains some surprising simplifications (for example, defense costs are assumed to be independent of invader pressure), it does seem to be successful in its predictions, and it represents a good example of how a cost–benefit analysis can be done.

CONCLUSIONS

Are predators designed to make foraging decisions that maximize their net rate of food intake? This survey of the literature suggests that they are, at least under laboratory and some simple field conditions. The question of whether other goals, such as optimizing whole sequences of behavior (Sibly and McFarland, 1976) or optimization of foraging behavior with the goal of minimizing the variance in the rate of food intake (Thompson *et al.*, 1974), are more important in many complex natural situations has not been answered. However, even if other factors often override or modify the goal of optimal foraging, we can still conclude that this goal must be important at least some of the time, since predators have been designed by natural selection to be capable of following the appropriate rules.

Arguments based on the theory of natural selection tend to be tautologous (Popper, 1976), and it may appear that the optimization approach falls into this trap: after making the assumption that evolution is an optimizing process, it attempts to show that predators are indeed optimal. The argument is, however, not a tautology because the cost function or the goal of the optimization process is chosen out of a number of alternative hypotheses, and any one cost function could be rejected on experimental or observational grounds. There is, however, a technical difficulty in rejecting a particular hypothesis, namely, that if an animal is observed failing to optimize according to a particular goal, we can only conclude either that the hypothesis about the goal was wrong or that the animal was in an inappropriate environment. To give an example, when Nelson (1964) apparently showed that Lack's hypothesis of the optimal clutch size in nidicolous birds was wrong with reference to the gannet *(Sula bassana)*, a species that can successfully rear more than its normal brood, Lack (1966) concluded that the environment and not the hypothesis was wrong. This conclusion, which might have seemed like an *ad hoc* escape clause, was later vindicated by the work of Jarvis (1974), showing that the gannet *(Sula capensis)* in an environment relatively undisturbed by man is not capable of rearing to full weight more than their normal brood.

Even though natural selection inevitably pushes toward optimal solutions, it can be argued that true optima, even optimal compromises, are rarely achieved. For example, if selection is frequency-dependent, at any instant in time the majority of the population will not have the optimal genotype. Further, even when selection is directional, so that one could view the adaptive landscape as having one peak higher than all others, we do not know how easily selection will succeed in pushing animals from suboptimal adaptive peaks (local optima) to the global optimum.

Acknowledgments

I thank the following for very kindly showing me unpublished manuscripts and for allowing me to quote from their work: Ric Charnov, Barbara Cockrell, Robin Cooke, Richard Cowie, John Harwood, Steve Hubbard, Graham Pyke, Jamie Smith, Jeff Waage, and Reto Zach.

References

Alcock, J. Cues used in searching for food by redwinged blackbirds *Agelaius phoenicus. Behaviour,* 1973, *46*, 174–188.

Barnard, C. J. Aspects of winter flocking and food fighting in the house sparrow. D.Phil. thesis, 1978, Oxford.

Bernstein, R. A. Foraging strategies of ants in response to variable food density. *Ecology,* 1975, *56*, 213–219.

Bertram, B. C. R. Social factors influencing reproduction in wild lions. *J. Zool. Lond.,* 1975, *177*, 463–482.

Beukema, J. J. Predation by the three-spined stickleback (*Gasterosteus aculeatus* L.): The influence of hunger and experience. *Behaviour,* 1968, *31*, 1–126.

Brown, J. L. The evolution of diversity in avian territorial systems. *Wilson Bull.,* 1964, *6*, 160–169.

Caraco, T., and Wolf, L. L. Ecological determinants of group sizes in foraging lions. *Am. Natur.,* 1975, *109*, 343–352.

Carpenter, F. L., and MacMillen, R. E. Threshold model of feeding territoriality and test with a Hawaiian Honeycreeper. *Science,* 1976, *194*, 639–641.

Catania, A. C. Concurrent performances: A baseline for the study of reinforcement magnitude. *J. Exp. Anal. Behav.,* 1963, *6*, 299–300.

Charnov, E. L. Optimal foraging: Some theoretical explorations. Ph.D. thesis, 1973, University of Washington, Seattle.

Charnov, E. L. Optimal foraging: Attack strategy of a mantid. *Am. Natur.,* 1976a, *110*, 141–151.

Charnov, E. L. Optimal foraging: The marginal value theorem. *Theor. Popul. Biol.,* 1976b, *9*, 129–136.

Charnov, E. L., Orians, G. H., and Hyatt, K. The ecological implications of resource depression. *Am. Natur.,* 1976, *110*, 247–259.

Clutton-Brock, T. H. Ranging behaviour of red colobus (*Colobus badius tephrosceles*) in the Gombe National Park. *Anim. Behav.,* 1975, *23*, 706–722.

Cody, M. L. Finch flocks in the Mohave desert. *Theor. Pop. Biol.,* 1971, *2*, 142–148.

Cody, M. L. Competition and the structure of bird communities. *Princeton Monographs in Population Biology,* 1974a, *7*, 318 pp.

Cody, M. L. Optimisation in ecology. *Science,* 1974b, *183*, 1156–1164.

Comins, H. N., and Hassell, M. P. The dynamics of optimally foraging predators and parasitoids. *J. Anim. Ecol.,* in press.

Cook, R. M., and Cockrell, B. J. Predator ingestion rate and its bearing on feeding time and the theory of optimal diets. *J. Anim. Ecol.,* 1978, *47*, 529–548.

Cook, R. M., and Hubbard, S. F. Adaptive searching strategies in insect parasites. *J. Anim. Ecol.,* 1977, *46*, 115–125.

Cowie, R. J. Optimal foraging in great tits (*Parus major*). *Nature,* 1977, *268*, 137–139.

Cowie, R. J., and Krebs, J. R. Optimal foraging in patchy environments. In R. M. Anderson, B. D. Turner, and L. R. Taylor (eds), *Population Dynamics*. Blackwell Scientific Publications, Oxford, 1979.

Croze, H. J. Searching image in carrion crows. *Z. Tierpsychol. Beiheft.,* 1970, *5*, 1–85.

Davidson, D. W. Experimental tests of optimal diet in the social insects. *Behav. Ecol. Sociobiol.,* 1978, *4*, 35–41.

Davies, N. B. Food, flocking and territorial behaviour of the pied wagtail (*Motacilla alba yarrellii* Gould) in winter. *J. Anim. Ecol.,* 1976, *45*, 235–253.

Davies, N. B. Prey selection and social behaviour in wagtails (Aves: Motacillidae). *J. Anim. Ecol.,* 1977a, *46*, 37–57.

Davies, N. B. Prey selection and the search strategy of the spotted flycatcher (*Muscicapa striata*): A field study in optimal foraging. *Anim. Behav.*, 1977b, *25*, 1016–1033.

Drent, R., and van Eerden, M. Goose flocks and food exploitation: How to have your cake and eat it. *Proc. XVII Int. Orn. Cong.*, in press.

Elner, R. W., and Hughes, R. N. Energy maximisation in the diet of the shore crab *Carcinus maenas* (L). *J. Anim. Ecol.*, 1978, *47*, 103–116.

Emlen, J. M. The role of time and energy in food preference. *Am. Natur.*, 1966, *100*, 611–617.

Emlen, J. M., and Emlen, M. G. R. Optimal choice in diet: Test of a hypothesis. *Am. Natur.*, 1975, *109*, 427–435.

Erichsen, J. T., Krebs, J. R., and Houston, I. A. Optimal foraging and cryptic prey. *J. Anim. Ecol.*, in press.

Evans, P. R. Energy balance and optimal foraging strategies in shorebirds: Some implications for their distributions and movements in the non-breeding season. *Ardea*, 1976, *64*, 117–139.

Gibb, J. A. Predation by tits and squirrels on the eucosmid *Ernarmonia conicolana* (Heyl.). *J. Anim. Ecol.*, 1958, *27*, 375–396.

Gibb, J. A. Population of tits and goldcrests and their food supply in pine plantations. *J. Anim. Ecol.*, 1960, *35*, 43–53.

Gilbert, N., Guitterez, A. P., Frazer, B. D., and Jones, R. E. *Ecological Relationships*. Freeman, San Francisco, 1976.

Gill, F. B., and Wolf, L. L. Economics of territoriality in the golden-winged sunbird. *Ecology*, 1975a, *56*, 333–345.

Gill, F. B., and Wolf, L. L. Foraging strategies and energetics of East African sunbirds at mistletoe flowers. *Am. Natur.*, 1975b, *109*, 491–510.

Goss-Gustard, J. D. Factors affecting the diet and feeding rates of the redshank (*Tringa totanus*). *Symp. Br. Ecol. Soc.*, 1970a, *10*, 101–110.

Goss-Custard, J. D. The responses of redshank (*Tringa totanus* (L.)) to spatial variations in their prey density. *J. Anim. Ecol.*, 1970b, *39*, 91–113.

Goss-Custard, J. D. Variation in the dispersion of redshank *Tringa totanus* on their winter feeding grounds. *Ibis*, 1976, *118*, 257–263.

Goss-Custard, J. D. Optimal foraging and the size selection of worms by redshank *Tringa totanus*. *Anim. Behav.*, 1977a, *25*, 10–29.

Goss-Custard, J. D. Predator responses and prey mortality in the redshank *Tringa totanus* (L.) and a preferred prey *Corophium volutator* (Pallas). *J. Anim. Ecol.*, 1977b, *46*, 21–36.

Hainsworth, F. R., and Wolf, L. L. Nectar characteristics and food selection by hummingbirds. *Oecologia*, 1976, *25*, 101–113.

Hartwick, E. B. Foraging strategy of the black oystercatcher (*Haemotopus bachmanni* Audubon). *Can. J. Zool.*, 1976, *54*, 142–155.

Harwood, J. Grazing strategies of blue geese *Anser caerulescens*. Ph.D. thesis, 1974, University of Western Ontario, London, Ontario.

Hassell, M. P. Mutual interference between searching parasites. *J. Anim. Ecol.*, 1971, *40*, 473–486.

Hassell, M. P., and May, R. M. Aggregation of predators and insect parasites and its effect on stability. *J. Anim. Ecol.*, 1974, *43*, 567–594.

Heinrich, B. Foraging strategies of individual bumblebees. *Ecol. Monogr.*, 1976, *46*, 105–128.

Herrera, C. M. Trophic diversity of the barn owl *Tyto alba* in continental western Europe. *Ornis. Scand.*, 1975, *5*, 181–191.

Herrnstein, R. J. On the law of effect. *J. Exp. Anal. Behav.*, 1970, *13*, 243–266.

Herrnstein, R. J., and Loveland, D. H. Maximising and matching on concurrent ratio schedules. *J. Exp. Anal. Behav.*, 1975, *24*, 107–116.

Holling, C. S. The functional response of invertebrate predators to prey density. *Mem. Entomol. Soc. Can.*, 1966, *48*, 1–86.

Horn, H. S. The adaptive significance of colonial nesting in the Brewer's blackbird (*Euphagus cyanocephalus*). *Ecology*, 1968, *49*, 682–694.

Houston, I. A., Krebs, J. R., and Erichsen, J. T. Optimal choice and discrimination time in the great tit. *Behav. Ecol. Sociobiol.*, in press.

Hubbard, S. F., and Cook, R. M. Optimal foraging by parasitoid wasps. *J. Anim. Ecol.*, 1978, *47*, 593–604.

Hughes, R. N. Optimal diets under the energy maximisation premise: The effect of recognition time and learning. *Amer. Natur.* (in press).

Jarvis, M. J. F. The ecological significance of clutch size in the South African gannet (*Sula capensis* (Lichtenstein)). *J. Anim. Ecol.*, 1974, *43*, 1–17.

Kamil, A. C. Systematic foraging by a nectar feeding bird, the amakihi *(Loxops virens)*. *J. Comp. Physiol. Psychol.*, 1978, *92*, 388–396.

Kear, J. Food selection in finches with special reference to interspecific differences. *Proc. Zool. Soc. Lond.*, 1962, *138*, 163–204.

Kenward, R. E., and Sibly, R. M. A woodpigeon *Columba palumbus* (L.) feeding preference explained by a digestive bottleneck. *J. Appl. Ecol.*, 1977, *14*, 815–826.

Kleerekoper, H., Timms, A. M., Westlake, G. F., Davy, F. B., Malar, T., and Anderson, V. M. An analysis of locomotor behaviour of the Goldfish *(Carasius auratus)*. *Anim. Behav.*, 1970, *18*, 317–330.

Krebs, J. R. Territory and breeding density in the great tit *Parus major* (L.). *Ecology*, 1971, *52*, 2–22.

Krebs, J. R. Behavioural aspects of predation. In P. P. G. Bateson and P. H. Klopfer (eds.), *Perspectives in Ethology*, Vol. 1. Plenum Press, New York, 1973a.

Krebs, J. R. Social learning and the significance of mixed-species flocks of chickadees *(Parus spp.)*. *Can. J. Zool.*, 1973b, *51*, 1275–1288.

Krebs, J. R. Colonial nesting and social feeding as strategies for exploiting food resources in the Great Blue Heron *(Ardea herodias)*. *Behaviour*, 1974, *50*, 99–134.

Krebs, J. R. Colonial nesting in birds, with special reference to the Circoniiformes. *Wading Birds* (Research Report No. 7) National Audubon Society, New York, 1978a, pp. 299–314.

Krebs, J. R. Optimal foraging: decision rules for predators In J. R. Krebs and N. B. Davies (eds), *Behavioural Ecology: An Evolutionary Approach*, Chapter 2. Blackwell Scientific Publications, Oxford, 1978b.

Krebs, J. R., and Barnard, C. J. Comments on the function of flocking in birds. *Proc. XVII Int. Orn. Cong.*, in press.

Krebs, J. R., and Cowie, R. J. Bird foraging strategies. *Ardea*, 1976, *64*, 98–116.

Krebs, J. R., Erichsen, J. T., Webber, M. I., and Charnov, E. L. Optimal prey selection in the great tit *(Parus major)*. *Anim. Behav.*, 1977, *25*, 30–38.

Krebs, J. R., Houston, I., and Charnov, E. L. Some recent developments in optimal foraging. In A. C. Kamil and T. D. Sargent (eds), *Foraging Behaviour*. Garland Press, New York, 1979.

Krebs, J. R., Kacelnik, A., and Taylor, P. J. Test of optimal sampling by foraging great tits. *Nature*, 1978, *275*, 27–31.

Krebs, J. R., MacRoberts, M. H., and Cullen, J. M. Flocking and feeding in the great tit: An experimental study. *Ibis*, 1972, *114*, 507–530.

Krebs, J. R., Ryan, J. C., and Charnov, E. L. Hunting by expectation or optimal foraging? A study of patch use by chickadees. *Anim. Behav.*, 1974, *22*, 953–964.

Kruuk, H. *The Spotted Hyena: A Study in Predation and Social Behavior.* University of Chicago Press, Chicago, 1972.

Kushlan, J. Wading bird predation in a seasonally fluctuating pond. *Auk*, 1976, *93*, 464–476.

Lack, D. *Population Studies of Birds.* Oxford University Press, Oxford, 1966.

Levins, R. Evolution in changing environments. *Princeton Monographs in Population Biology* 2. Princeton University Press, Princeton, N.J., 1968.

MacArthur, R. H. *Geographical Ecology.* Harper & Row, New York, 1972.

MacArthur, R. H., and Pianka, E. R. On the optimal use of a patchy environment. *Am. Natur.*, 1966, *100*, 603–609.

Mackintosh, N. J. *The Psychology of Animal Learning.* Academic Press, New York, 1974.

McFarland, D. J. Form and function in the temporal organisation of behaviour In P. P. G. Bateson and R. A. Hinde (eds.), *Growing Points in Ethology.* Cambridge University Press, Cambridge, England, 1976.

McFarland, D. J. Decision making in animals. *Nature*, 1977, *269*, 15–21.

McFarland, D. J. Optimality considerations in animal behaviour. In N. G. Blurton-Jones (ed.), *Human Behaviour and Adaptation.* Academic Press, New York, 1978, pp. 53–76.

Menge, B. A. Foraging strategy of a starfish in relation to actual prey availability and environmental predictability. *Ecol. Monogr.*, 1972, *42*, 25–50.

Miller, H. L., Jr., and Loveland, D. H. Matching when the number of response alternatives is large. *Anim. Learning Behav.*, 1974, *2*, 106–110.

Morse, D. H. Ecological aspects of some mixed-species foraging flocks of birds. *Ecol. Monogr.*, 1970, *40*, 119–168.

Murdie, G., and Hassell, M. P. Food distribution, searching success and predator prey models. In M. S. Bartlett and R. W. Hiorns (eds.), *The Mathematical Theory of the Dynamics of Biological Populations.* Academic Press, New York, 1973.

Murdoch, W. W., Avery, S., and Smyth, M. E. B. Switching in predatory fish. *Ecology,* 1975, *56*, 1054–1105.

Murdoch, W. W., and Oaten, A. Predation and population stability. *Adv. Ecol. Res.,* 1975, *9*, 1–131.

Murton, R. K. *The Woodpigeon.* Collins, New York, 1965.

Murton, R. K. The significance of a specific search image in the feeding behaviour of the woodpigeon. *Behaviour,* 1971, *40*, 10–42.

Nelson, J. B. Factors influencing clutch size and chick growth in the North Atlantic gannet *(Sula bassana). Ibis,* 1964, *106*, 63–77.

Norberg, R. A. An ecological theory on foraging time and energetics and choice of optimal food-searching method. *J. Anim. Ecol.,* 1977, *46*, 511–530.

Oaten, A. Optimal foraging in patches: A case for stochasticity. *Theor. Pop. Biol.,* 1977, *12*, 263–285.

O'Brien, W. J., Slade, N. A., and Vinyard, S. L. Apparent size as a determinant of prey selection by Bluegill sunfish *(Lepomis macrochirus). Ecology,* 1976, *57*, 1304–1311.

Oster, G., and Heinrich, B. Why do bumblebees major? A mathematical model. *Ecol. Monogr.,* 1976, *46*, 129–133.

Parker, G. A., and Stuart, R. A. Animal behaviour as a strategy optimiser: Evolution of resource assessment strategies and optimal emigration thresholds. *Am. Natur.,* 1976, *110*, 1055–1076.

Parker, G. A. Searching for mates. In J. R. Krebs and N. B. Davies (eds.), *Behavioural Ecology: An Evolutionary Approach.* Blackwell Scientific Publications, Oxford, 1978.

Partridge, L. Field and laboratory observations on the foraging and feeding techniques of blue tits *(Parus caeruleus)* and coal tits *(Parus ater)* in relation to their habitats. *Anim. Behav.,* 1976a, *24*, 534–544.

Partridge, L. Individual differences in feeding efficiencies and feeding preferences of captive great tits. *Anim. Behav.,* 1976b, *24*, 230–240.

Pianka, E. R. Competition and niche theory. In R. M. May (ed.), *Theoretical Ecology.* Blackwell, Oxford, 1976.

Popper, K. *The Unended Quest.* Fontana, London, 1976.

Powell, G. Experimental analysis of the social value of flocking by starlings *(Sturnus vulgaris)* in relation to predation and foraging. *Anim. Behav.,* 1974, *22*, 501–505.

Pulliam, H. R. Diet optimisation with nutrient constraints. *Am. Natur.,* 1975, *109*, 765–768.

Pyke, G. H. Studies in the foraging efficiency of animals. Ph.D. thesis, 1974. University of Chicago.

Pyke, G. H. Are animals efficient harvesters? *Anim. Behav.,* 1978, *26*, 241–250.

Pyke, G., Pulliam, H. R., and Charnov, E. L. Optimal foraging: A selective review of theory and test. *Q. Rev. Biol.,* 1977, *52*, 137–154.

Rogers, D. Random search and insect population models. *J. Anim. Ecol.,* 1972, *41*, 369–383.

Royama, T. Factors governing the hunting behaviour and selection of food by the Great Tit *(Parus major* L.). *J. Anim. Ecol.,* 1970, *39*, 619–668.

Royama, T. A comparative study of models of predation and parasitism. *Res. Popul. Ecol. Kyoto, Suppl.,* 1971, *1*, 1–91.

Rubinstein, D. I., Barnett, R. J., Ridgeley, R. S., and Klopfer, P. H. Advantages of mixed-species feeding flocks among seed-eating finches in Costa Rica. *Ibis,* 1977, *119*, 10–21.

Schaller, G. *The Serengeti Lion.* University of Chicago Press, Chicago, 1972.

Schoener, T. W. Theory of feeding strategies. *Ann. Rev. Ecol. Syst.,* 1971, *2*, 369–404.

Schoener, T. W. Resource partitioning in ecological communities. *Science,* 1974, *185*, 27–39.

Shimp, C. Optimal behaviour in free-operant experiments. *Psychol. Rev.,* 1969, *76*, 97–112.

Sibly, R. M., and McFarland, D. J. On the fitness of behaviour sequences. *Am. Natur.,* 1976, *110*, 601–617.

Siegfried, W. R., and Underhill, L. G. Flocking as an antipredator strategy in doves. *Anim. Behav.,* 1975, *23*, 504–508.

Simon, C. A. The influence of food abundance on territory size in the iguanid lizard *Scleropus jarrovi. Ecology,* 1975, *56*, 993–998.

Simons, S., and Alcock, J. Learning and the foraging persistence of white-crowned sparrows *Zonotrichia leucophrys. Ibis,* 1971, *113*, 477–482.

Sinniff, D. B., and Jessen, C. R. A simulation model of animal movement patterns. *Adv. Ecol. Res.,* 1969, *6*, 185–219.

Slaney, P., and Northcote, T. G. The effects of prey abundance on density and territorial behaviour of young rainbow trout *Salmo gairdneri* in laboratory stream channels. *J. Fish. Res. Bd. Can.,* 1974, *31*, 1201–1209.

Smith, C. C. The adaptive nature of social organisation in the genus of tree squirrels *Tamiasciurus. Ecol. Monogr.,* 1968, *38*, 31–63.

Smith, C. C. The coevolution of pine squirrels *(Tamiasciurus)* and conifers. *Ecol. Monogr.,* 1970, *40*, 349–371.

Smith, J. N. M. The food searching behaviour of two European thrushes. I. Description and analysis of search paths. *Behaviour,* 1974a, *48*, 276–302.

Smith, J. N. M. The food searching behaviour of two European thrushes. II. The adaptiveness of the search patterns. *Behaviour,* 1974b, *49*, 1–61.

Smith, J. N. M. Feeding rates, search paths and surveillance for predators in great-tailed grackle flocks. *Can. J. Zool.,* 1977, *55*, 891–898.

Smith, J. N. M., and Sweatman, H. P. A. Food searching behaviour of titmice in patchy environments. *Ecology,* 1974, *55*, 1216–1232.

Smith, P. C., and Evans, P. R. Studies of shorebirds at Lindisfarne, Northumberland. I. Feeding ecology and behaviour of the bar-tailed godwit. *Wildfowl,* 1973, *24*, 135–139.

Solomon, M. E., Glen, D. M., Kendall, D. A., and Milsom, N. F. Predation of overwintering larvae of codling moth *(Cydia pomonella* (L.) by birds. *J. Appl. Ecol.* 1976, *13*, 341–352.

Stenger, J. Food habits and available food of ovenbirds in relation to territory size. *Auk,* 1958, *75*, 335–346.

Stimson, J. Territorial behaviour of the owl limpet *Lottia gigantea. Ecology,* 1970, *51*, 113–118.

Swynnerton, C. F. M. Mixed bird parties. *Ibis,* 1915, *3*, 346–354.

Thomas, G. The influences of encountering a food object on subsequent searching behaviour in *Gasterosteus aculeatus* (L.). *Anim. Behav.,* 1974, *22*, 941–952.

Thompson, W. A., Vertinsky, I., and Krebs, J. R. The survival value of flocking in birds: a simulation model. *J. Anim. Ecol.,* 1974, *43*, 785–820.

Tinbergen, J. M. How starlings *(Sturnus vulgaris)* apportion their foraging time in a virtual single-prey situation on a meadow. *Ardea,* 1976, *64*, 155–170.

Tullock, G. The coal tit as a careful shopper. *Am. Natur.,* 1971, *105*, 77–79.

Ward, P., and Zahavi, A. The importance of certain assemblages of birds as "information centres" for food finding. *Ibis,* 1973, *115*, 517–534.

Waage, J. K. Behavioural aspects of foraging in the parasitoid *Nemeritis canescens* (Grav.). Unpublished Ph.D. thesis, London University, 1977.

Ware, D. The predatory behaviour of rainbow trout. Ph.D. thesis, 1971, University of British Columbia.

Werner, E. E., and Hall, D. J. Optimal foraging and the size selection of prey by the bluegill sunfish *(Lepomis macrochirus). Ecology,* 1974, *55*, 1216–1232.

Williamson, P., and Gray, L. Foraging behaviour of the starling *(Sturnus vulgaris)* in Maryland. *Condor,* 1975, *77*, 84–89.

Wolf, L. L. Energy intake and expenditure in a nectar-feeding sunbird. *Ecology,* 1975, *56*, 92–104.

Wolf, L. L., Hainsworth, F. R., and Gill, F. B. Foraging efficiencies and time budgets in nectar-feeding birds. *Ecology,* 1975, *56*, 117–128.

Wolf, L. L., Hainsworth, F. R., and Stiles, F. G. Energetics of foraging: Rate and efficiency of nectar extraction by hummingbirds. *Science,* 1972, *176*, 1351–1352.

Zach, R., and Falls, J. B. Do ovenbirds (Aves: Parulidae) hunt by expectation? *Can. J. Zool.,* 1976a, *54*, 1894–1903.

Zach, R., and Falls, J. B. Foraging behaviour, learning and exploration by captive ovenbirds (Aves: Parulidae). *Can. J. Zool.,* 1976b, *54*, 1880–1893.

Zach, R., and Falls, J. B. Ovenbird (Aves: Parulidae) hunting behaviour in a patchy environment. *Can. J. Zool.,* 1976c, *54*, 1863–1879.

Zach, R., and Falls, J. B. Influence of capturing a prey on subsequent search in the ovenbird *(Aves: Parulidae). Can. J. Zool.,* 1977, *55*, 1958–1969.

Zach, R., and Falls, J. B. Area restricted searching in ovenbirds (Aves: Parulidae). *Can. J. Zool.,* in press.

The Evolution of Mating Systems in Birds and Mammals

JAMES F. WITTENBERGER

INTRODUCTION

The evolution of sex created a fundamental problem for nearly all plants and animals; namely, the need to fertilize eggs. Numerous types of mating systems have evolved as solutions to this problem, each molded by particular environmental circumstances and particular species attributes. Various hypotheses have been advanced to explain each type of mating system, but an integrated theory is only now beginning to emerge. Since mating behavior is affected by nearly all other aspects of an organism's behavioral adjustments to its environment, such a theory must fit within a composite view of animal social behavior and hence must include explicit points of contact with related bodies of theory. In particular, mating system theory must mesh with theoretical advances concerning the evolution of territoriality, parental behavior, and animal sociality. By including the appropriate theoretical work from these other areas, an integrated theory of vertebrate mating systems can be developed.

Understanding the evolution of mating systems requires a type of thinking that is not widely familiar. An analogy with human economic decision-making is illustrative. Economic decisions are made with the aim of maximizing monetary profits. Evolutionary decisions are made to maximize lifetime production of mature offspring. Both kinds of decisions depend on three key variables: the costs entailed by each available option, the benefits expected from adopting each option, and the element of uncertainty. Imperfect knowledge and the passage of time introduce the risk of incurring unexpected losses or failing to realize

JAMES F. WITTENBERGER   Department of Zoology, University of Washington, Seattle, Washington 98195.

expected benefits. One available option in every decision-making process is therefore to acquire more information before deciding between options. Since taking this course always entails costs of its own, reducing uncertainty is not always the best tactic. Thus, one can imagine animals making decisions between alternative behavioral options on the basis of costs, benefits, and uncertainties. These decisions may or may not be based on conscious and rational thought, as they often are in humans, but they can be examined as if they were. It is often easier to formulate theory in terms of decision-making processes rather than in terms of genetic processes, and the conclusions reached at the behavioral level are generally the same. Thinking in economic terms, with lifetime reproductive output as the common currency, is a useful conceptual tool for comprehending the often complex behavioral strategies involved in animal mating systems.

Focusing on the options available to each individual within a social system is imperative in studies of animal social behavior. Animal behavior has evolved to maximize the inclusive fitness of individuals (as defined by Hamilton, 1964), not the average fitness of groups. A social system therefore cannot be understood until the costs, benefits, and uncertainties faced by each individual member are identified and evaluated. However much we as humans value altruistic acts, the behavior of animals is for the most part selfish (Wilson, 1975; Dawkins, 1976; Barash, 1977). The rare instances of altruism in animals are really just alternative ways of propagating genes when opportunities for producing direct progeny are limited. Altruism in animals, as far as is now known, involves close relatives who share a substantial fraction of genes with the altruist, and helping a relative is simply an alternative way of propagating one's own genes.

The more common situation is for individuals to share overlapping but conflicting reproductive interests. Overlapping interests may promote the evolution of cooperation, but the remaining element of conflict introduces some degree of competition into every social interaction.

An important component of behavioral competition entails actions that affect the decision-making processes of others, either by constraining their future options or by increasing their costs of continued competition (e.g., see Popp and DeVore, 1979). Much of mating behavior involves these tactics, and they are best understood in terms of the partially conflicting interests of males and females. The conflict of interests between males and females is fundamental and arises directly from the differentiation and specialization of organisms into two sexes. The origin of this conflict and its evolutionary consequences are the central topics of this chapter.

Any discussion of a topic as broad as vertebrate mating systems must necessarily be selective. I have chosen to emphasize research on avian mating systems, where much of the theory has originated, and mammalian mating systems, where attempts at applying the theory have been most controversial. The mating systems of other vertebrates are equally fascinating, but I will not consider them here. I am less familiar with these groups, and much of the research concerning them has focused on spacing behavior, parental care patterns, egg cannibalism, and other topics rather than mating relationships *per se*. For further information on the lower vertebrates, the reader is referred to Duellman (1966, 1967), Barlow (1974),

Brattstrom (1974), Myrberg and Thresher (1974), Reese (1975), Wilson (1975), Stamps (1977), Wells (1977), Rohwer (1978), and Perrone and Zaret (1979). I have also excluded from discussion the evolution of cooperative and communal breeding systems in birds for lack of space. The interested reader is referred to Brown (1974), Brown and Balda (1977), Fry (1977), Vehrencamp (1977), Emlen (1978), and Rowley (1978).

Male Competition and Female Choice

The conflicting interests of males and females are made evident by the differing roles taken by each sex in reproductive behavior. As a general rule, males compete among themselves for mating opportunities and make little attempt to discriminate between appropriate and inappropriate mating partners, while females take little part in competing for mates and instead are often highly selective in choosing mates (Darwin, 1871; Williams, 1966, 1975; Trivers, 1972). This difference results from the differing parental investments contributed by each sex, where *parental investment* refers to any immediate investment in offspring that diminishes immediate or future investments in other offspring (Trivers, 1972).

Female gametes have evolved large size to improve their probability of survival (Parker, Baker, and Smith, 1972), but their larger size increases the initial investment of energy and nutrients required to produce each one. Fertilization often obligates females to provide additional parental investment as well, especially in mammals, which are committed to prolonged periods of gestation and lactation. Since obligatory parental investments are high for females, the lifetime reproductive output of females is limited by the amount of time and energy they can devote to offspring production and not by the number of mates they can acquire (Bateman, 1948). Females therefore gain little by copulating with more than one male during each reproductive effort. In addition, females face considerable risk each time they reproduce. Both males and females suffer reduced fitness whenever they waste parental investments, but the risk of wastage is much higher for females because of their higher parental commitments. Copulation itself entails a risk, since the male may father inviable or competitively inferior offspring. To minimize this risk, females are selective when choosing mates and base their choices on male attributes that are indicative of low-risk matings (reviewed by Trivers, 1972).

The reproductive strategy of males has evolved to exploit the relatively large parental investment of females (Parker *et al.*, 1972). Male gametes are small, energetically cheap, and specialized for seeking out eggs. The lifetime reproductive output of males depends on the number of eggs they can fertilize and not on the number of sperm they can produce (Bateman, 1948; Trivers, 1972). Even though numerous sperm are invested with each copulation, males risk little when they copulate with a female because wasted gametes are easily replaced. Taking the time to be selective of mates usually gains them little, and it reduces the time available for seeking additional mates or conducting other activities. Thus, males generally compete for mating opportunities without being selective of mates. Only under unusual circumstances should males be selective of mates. These will be discussed in the next section.

Mate selection is only part of the larger problem facing females at the onset of a breeding season. The quality of a prospective mate is just one of several factors contributing to a female's risk of failure. Females should take into account all factors affecting their success, including habitat quality and the number of other males and females associated with a breeding situation, before making a choice (Orians, 1969; Wittenberger, 1976a, in press, a). They should choose to breed where their *expectations* of success are highest. This may not be where their *actual* success is highest because females face many uncertainties at the time they make their choices. In choosing among potential breeding situations, females are faced with a difficult sampling problem. They must depend on an array of predictive cues, each with differing reliability, and the use of one set of cues may often preclude the use of another. The actual criteria used by females to make their choices depends on how reliable potential cues are as predictors of success and on how costly they are to assess. Females may opt for breeding within social groups or in particular habitats or with particular males. Each choice limits the options remaining available to other females and males in a social system, and the consequences of these choices determine the makeup of the mating system.

FEMALE COMPETITION AND MALE CHOICE

In a very small number of vertebrates, females take the aggressive role in competing for mates while males take the passive role of selecting mates. Sexual dimorphism is often associated with this role reversal, and when it is, the female is larger and more brightly colored than the male. The roles of the sexes in caring for offspring is also reversed, with males assuming most or all parental responsibilities normally performed by females.

The evolution of sex role reversal is a major unsolved problem. It has occurred in seahorses and pipefish (Syngnathidae), cassowaries *(Casuarius casuarius)*, jacanas (Jacanidae), phalaropes (Phalaropidae), button quails (Turnicidae), the plains wanderer (Pedionomidae), the variegated tinamou *(Crypturellus variegatus)*, painted snipes (Rostratulidae), and Bensch's rail *(Monias benschi)* (Lack, 1968; Jenni, 1974; Williams, 1975; Crome, 1976). Sex role reversal should evolve only when male reproductive output is limited by time or energy constraints and female output is limited by mate availability (Trivers, 1972). The problem is to identify the conditions that cause this to occur.

Female seahorses and pipefish deposit their eggs in specialized brood pouches of the male (Fiedler, 1955; Takai and Mizokami, 1959). In at least pygmy seahorses *(Hippocampus zosterae),* males can brood the eggs from only one female at a time, and it takes them about two weeks to rear each brood (Strawn, 1958). Thus, male reproductive success is limited by the time available for rearing broods, and any time wasted because of low viability or genetic inferiority of eggs reduces their fitness. Females commit more energy and nutrients to gamete production than males, but their fecundity is limited by the availability of males with empty brood pouches and not by their ability to produce eggs. The major unanswered question for these species is how obligatory male brood care evolved in the first place.

Sex role reversal in birds is closely related to female desertion of clutches immediately after laying (Jenni, 1974; Graul, Derrickson, and Mock, 1977). Trivers (1972) originally maintained that whichever sex contributed the largest prior parental investment should be most likely to desert, but in fact, desertion should evolve when the benefits gained by deserting exceed the costs, regardless of prior investments (Dawkins and Carlisle, 1976; Boucher, 1977; Maynard Smith, 1977). Trivers (1976) concurred with this modification of his theory. As Maynard Smith put it, desertion decisions should be prospective rather than retrospective.

In birds, female desertion is possible only if conditions predispose deserted males to remain behind and rear the female's offspring unaided (Graul *et al.*, 1977). Of course, males must also be capable of rearing offspring successfully without female assistance. Any environmental conditions or population attributes that severely limit mating opportunities for deserted males will predispose males to rear deserted clutches and hence will facilitate female desertion. Most of the data on this point stem from studies of polyandrous birds and will be discussed in the section pertaining to polyandry. The important point here is that female desertion of clutches and male care of offspring create a situation that can favor sex role reversal.

Female desertion does not always lead to sex role reversal. For example, it occurs in the absence of sex role reversal in rheas and in various arctic shorebirds (Bruning, 1974; Pitelka, Holmes, and MacLean, 1974). The reason is that the reproductive success of males in these species is still limited by their ability to obtain mates, while the reproductive success of females is still limited by the rate they can produce eggs. In rheas, male success depends to a large extent on how early the male can acquire a harem of females, and in Arctic shorebirds, males delay incubation to continue competing for females until the short mating season ends.

Sex role reversal has evolved whenever the reproductive output of females is limited by their ability to obtain mates. This fact has been documented to date only in spotted sandpipers and American jacanas (*Jacana spinosa*) (Hays, 1972; Jenni and Collier, 1972; Oring and Knudsen, 1972), but most of the remaining species exhibiting sex role reversal have not been adequately studied. In phalaropes, this relationship does not seem to hold because most species are monogamous (see Jenni, 1974). Female phalaropes do not defend territories, and why the sex roles are reversed is still unknown (Höhn, 1967; Johns, 1969; Howe, 1975a, b; Kistchinski, 1975). Desertion by female phalaropes has probably evolved to recoup the energetic losses entailed by egg production, thereby enhancing female survival prospects (Graul *et al.*, 1977). Female phalaropes may therefore gain important energetic advantages by finding mates as early as possible.

Theoretically, female competition and male choice can evolve even in the absence of sex role reversal. Superior males in a population are likely to attract many females and thus have the option of choosing among potential mates. Males should usually not exercise this option because they can increase their reproductive success by mating with as many females as possible, but if males are limited in the number of mates they can accept, they may benefit from being selective. Male choice would be most likely to evolve in monogamous species, although even then the advantages of early breeding may be more important than the advantages of selectively choosing mates. Several conditions must hold before female competition for superior males and mate selection by these males can evolve. First, females must be able to identify which males are superior. Second, the number of mates a male can accept must be less than the number of females competing to mate with him. Finally, the benefits for males that can be gained by being selective must exceed the costs of being selective. When these conditions hold, female competition for superior males and mate choice by those males may occur simultaneously with male competition and female choice. It is perfectly plausible for males to compete in demonstrating their superiority (i.e., increasing their attractiveness to females) and then, having competed successfully, to choose the best female(s) from among those attracted.

Proving the existence of female competition and male choice in animals lacking sex role reversal is difficult. Female competition for mates frequently does not entail overt aggression and may primarily involve gaining prior access to the best males. Male choice of mates is equally difficult to detect because female mate selection is occurring simultaneously in the same population. Males of monogamous birds often court several females in succession before acquiring a mate, but it is usually difficult to prove which sex terminated an aborted courtship sequence. For these reasons, careful behavioral studies will be needed before the existence of female competition and male choice is unequivocally demonstrated in species lacking sex role reversal.

Terminology

The terminology adopted here follows that of Lack (1968) and Selander (1972), with several modifications (Table I). For present purposes, each type of mating system is most usefully subdivided according to its spatial characteristics. Monogamous mating systems are here divided into those associated with defense of resources, those based on male sequestering of females, and those based on female dominance within social groups. Polygynous mating systems are divided into those based on male territoriality and those based on male defense of female social groups. Promiscuous mating systems are divided into those involving the release of gametes into the surrounding environmental medium, those resulting from overlapping home ranges, those based on male territoriality, and those based on male dominance hierarchies. A temporal classification based on the timing of pair formation and the duration of pair bonds is also presented because it is useful for some purposes, but this classification will not be used extensively here. The term *polygamy* is used by most authors to include polygyny and polyandry only, but its usage is extended here to include promiscuity as well because an all-inclusive term for nonmonogamous mating systems has greater utility than an inclusive term for those nonmonogamous mating systems that are based on prolonged pair-bonding.

A second way of classifying mating systems is used by some authors (e.g., Wiley, 1974; Payne and Payne, 1977; Ralls, 1977). In this schema, polygyny occurs when more females than males contribute gametes to zygotes in a population; polyandry occurs when more males than females contribute gametes to zygotes; and monogamy occurs when equal numbers of males and females contribute gametes to zygotes. Usage of the same terminology for these population attributes could lead to confusion, but no alternative terms have been suggested. Hence, the classification system adopted should always be explicitly stated. Since this second classification system is most appropriate for analyzing the population genetics of mating systems, it will not be used in the ensuing discussion.

TABLE I.   A CLASSIFICATION OF MATING SYSTEMS

General classification	Spatial classification	Temporal classification
I. *Monogamy:* Prolonged association and essentially exclusive mating relationship between one male and one female at a time.	A. *Territorial Monogamy:* The monogamous pair shares a common territory. B. *Female-Defense Monogamy:* Each male defends access to a female instead of defending a territory. C. *Dominance-Based Monogamy:* Females maintain monogamous pair bonds within social groups by dominating more subordinate females.	A. *Serial Monogamy:* Individuals of both sexes usually pair with a new mate each year or in each breeding cycle. B. *Permanent Monogamy:* Mated pairs usually remain together for life, though sometimes they change mates after failed breeding attempts.
II. *Polygyny:* Prolonged association and essentially exclusive mating relationship between one male and two or more females at a time.	A. *Territorial Polygyny:* Several females are paired with at least some territorial males. B. *Harem Polygyny:* A single male defends access to each social group of females.	A. *Successive Polygyny:* Polygynous males acquire each of their mates in temporal succession. B. *Simultaneous Polygyny:* Polygynous males acquire all their mates at the same time.
III. *Polyandry:* Prolonged association and essentially exclusive mating relationship between one female and two or more males at a time.	A. *Territorial Polyandry:* Several males are paired with at least some territorial females. B *Nonterritorial Polyandry:* Females desert their first males and pair with new males elsewhere.	A. *Successive Polyandry:* Polyandrous females acquire each of their mates in temporal succession. B. *Simultaneous Polyandry:* Polyandrous females acquire all their mates at the same time.
IV. *Promiscuity:* No prolonged association between the sexes and multiple matings by members of at least one sex.	A. *Broadcast Promiscuity:* Gametes are shed into the surrounding environmental medium so that sperm competition is prevalent. B. *Overlap Promiscuity:* Promiscuous matings occur between solitary individuals with overlapping home ranges or during brief visits by one sex to the home range or territory of the other. C. *Arena Promiscuity:* Males defend a display area or territory that is used exclusively or predominantly for attracting mates. D. *Hierarchical Promiscuity:* Males establish dominance hierarchies that affect their ability to inseminate females.	

JAMES F.
WITTENBERGER

THEORY

Most early ornithologists attributed polygyny in territorial birds to unbalanced sex ratios, but more recent evidence fails to support this interpretation. Many species are polygynous despite 50/50 adult sex ratios, and in some species, territorial males regularly obtain multiple mates while neighboring males remain unmated (Verner, 1964; Wittenberger, 1976a). In these species, a shortage of males cannot explain why some females pair with already mated males.

The importance of resource availability in favoring polygyny was first recognized by Armstrong (1955) and Crook (1964, 1965), who argued that superabundant food resources would emancipate males from parental duties and allow them to seek additional mates. Male emancipation is only a partial explanation, however, because it fails to account for female decisions in selecting breeding situations. Territorial polygyny cannot evolve unless males can attract more than one female to their territories, a capability that is possible only when some females benefit by pairing with already mated males.

Several costs potentially accrue to females who select already mated males as their mates, including the loss or reduction of male parental assistance, increased competition for food resources with other females on the territory, and increased attractiveness of the territory to predators. An unmated female should therefore pair with an already mated male only if she receives benefits that outweigh these costs. One possible benefit is the opportunity to breed on a higher-quality territory (Verner, 1964). A second-mated female could reproduce more successfully on a high-quality territory despite the costs of polygyny if the quality of all remaining territories held by unmated males is low enough. The difference between the high- and low-quality territories needed for a female to reproduce more successfully as a second mate has been termed the *polygyny threshold* (Verner and Willson, 1966).

A graphic model illustrates the polygyny-threshold concept (Figure 1) (Orians, 1969). The upper curve in the model represents the fitness a monogamous female can expect by breeding on each territory within a habitat continuum. The lower curve represents the fitness an unmated female can expect should she choose to breed as a second mate on each territory along the same continuum. The habitat continuum along the abscissa need not correspond to any recognizable environmental gradient. It simply represents a rank ordering of territories according to their quality, with quality measured in terms of female fitness. At the polygyny threshold, an unmated female is most fit by becoming a second mate on a high-quality territory instead of a monogamous mate on a marginal territory.

Each component of the model requires some elaboration. Labeling the abscissa "environmental quality" oversimplifies the general model. Unmated females should base their decisions on the overall quality of each potential breeding situation and not solely on environmental quality (Emlen, 1957; Orians, 1969; Wittenberger, 1976a; Weatherhead and Robertson, 1977). One important component of the quality gradient may be male quality. If male quality is strongly correlated with territory quality, it should cause a quantitative change in the polygyny threshold but not a relative change in the rank ordering of territories along the abscissa. If it is weakly correlated with territory quality and females respond to male quality more than to territory quality, male quality would change the rank ordering of territories along the abscissa.

The actual effect of male quality on the polygyny threshold is uncertain. It may be particularly important in fish, where male size often affects the quality of male parental care (Perrone, 1975; Downhower, 1977). Male quality may be less important in birds, but evidence is still lacking for most species. Weatherhead and Robertson (1977) argued that male quality is important in red-winged blackbirds (*Agelaius phoeniceus*) because they found no correlation between harem size and an index of territory quality, but their index was based entirely on nest site attributes and may not have been a good measure of overall territory quality. Other studies have shown correlations between territory quality and harem size in redwings (Holm, 1973; Lenington, 1977; Monahan, 1977), and attempts to demonstrate correlations between male attributes and harem size have been unsuccessful (Searcy, 1977). Yasukawa (1977) has shown that male age and male reproductive success in previous years correlates with the number of females attracted to territories, but the males in his study exhibited high site fidelity, so it is not possible to separate the effects of male attributes from territory attributes. Vasectomy experiments and direct observations have demonstrated that female redwings and female yellow-headed blackbirds (*Xanthocephalus xanthocephalus*) regularly copulate with territorial males other than their mates (Bray, Kennelly, and Guarino, 1975;

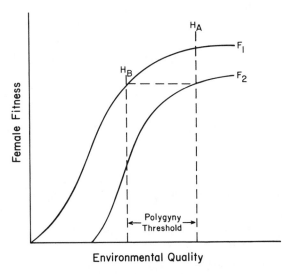

Fig. 1. The polygyny-threshold model (modified from Orians, 1969). Polygyny should occur when unmated females must choose between mated territorial males in H_A and unmated territorial males to the left of H_B. F_1 = fitness of monogamous females; F_2 = fitness of second-mated females; H_A = the best available habitat; H_B = marginal habitats located at the polygyny threshold; and the polygyny threshold = the difference in quality between H_A and H_B just sufficient to make polygyny advantageous for unmated females.

Emily Davies, unpublished data). This behavior is difficult to explain if female choices of breeding situations are based primarily on male attributes.

Labeling the ordinate "female fitness" is somewhat misleading because it ignores the temporal component of breeding situations. Females should base their decisions on the fitness that they can expect to attain, given the information available to them at the time they make their choice. They certainly cannot base their decisions on realized fitness (i.e., the success attained at the end of breeding). Opportunities for predicting realized fitness vary between environments and between various factors affecting it, and this variation should affect the criteria used by females in making their choices. Some components of female success (e.g., food availability versus predation pressure) may be more predictable than others and hence play a greater role in female decision-making. To ignore the model's temporal component is to ignore several of its more interesting theoretical attributes. These attributes are explored further in a later section.

Also important is the meaning of "female fitness." The polygyny-threshold model has usually been interpreted in terms of annual reproductive success, but female fitness is actually related to lifetime reproductive success. A more general form of the model is based on lifetime reproductive output and raises the possibility of polygyny evolving to increase female longevity at the expense of immediate reproductive success (Altmann, Wagner, and Lenington, 1977; Wittenberger, in press, a; see also Elliott, 1975).

Orians (1969) inadvertently introduced one ambiguity into the model by labeling the lower curve in Figure 1 as the average fitness of both females mated to a bigamous male (see Altmann *et al.*, 1977). This definition of the lower curve implies that polygyny evolves to maximize the fitness of a group of females rather than that of individual females, thus implicating group selection. The hypothesis proposed by Verner (1964) and extended by Orians (1969) is based on individual selection and depends only on the interests of individual unmated females. Hence, Orians's original labeling does not correctly depict Verner's hypothesis. Orians (personal communication) agrees that the lower curve should refer solely to the fitness of secondary (i.e., second-mated) females and not to the average fitness of both (or all) females on a territory. The distinction is crucial in conceptualizing the model and has an important effect on data analysis whenever a female's success is affected by her rank (i.e., order of mating).

The upper curve of the model represents the fitness of monogamous females, not primary (i.e., first-mated) females. The fitness of a primary female who is mated to a polygynous male may be a poor estimate of the fitness expected on the same territory by a monogamously mated female. The presence of additional females on a territory may depress the fitness of the primary female because second and subsequent mates can usurp resources, divert male parental allocations, and attract predators. The response of primary females to these deleterious effects may increase the costs of polygyny for other females electing to settle on the territory and hence lower the curve for secondary females.

Primary females should try to exclude unmated females from the territory whenever the net benefits of trying and sometimes succeeding exceed the costs incurred by not trying. In most polygynous birds, primary females are not aggressive, possibly because aggression reduces the energy available for egg production and the time available for incubation (Orians, 1979), but in a few species, they are. For example, female red-winged blackbirds partition male territories in Wisconsin and exclude other females from their holdings (Nero and Emlen, 1951; Nero, 1956). This behavior is most prevalent early in the nesting season and subsides as the season progresses. Female aggressiveness may alleviate competition for food on the territory, but the extent to which females obtain food on their territories was not studied. Orians (1979) reported that female redwings do not partition male territories in the potholes of eastern Washington, but his observations were largely begun well after breeding commenced. More recent observations in the same area indicate that females are aggressive toward intruding females early in the season, with the result that each male initially attracts only one female to his territory (Orians and Wittenberger, personal observation). During the next few weeks, females partition male territories and actively defend them from intruding females (Emily Davies and Carla D'Antonio, unpublished data). Only later do these partitions dissolve. The extent that females forage on male territories early in the season has not been investigated in the potholes either. Female aggression also leads to partitioning of male territories in the long-billed marsh wren *(Telmatodytes palustris)* (Welter, 1935). Since female marsh wrens forage almost entirely on their territories, this aggression may serve to reduce competition for food. It is probably also critical in preventing other females on the territory from entering a female's nest and puncturing her eggs (Picman, 1977b). Female yellow-headed blackbirds are aggressive in the immediate vicinity of their nests. Nevertheless, they often nest within a few meters of each other, and their aggression does not delay nesting by subsequent mates on a territory (Fautin, 1940; Willson, 1966; Orians, 1979). Female yellowheads sometimes also chase off encroaching females from neighboring territories during the nestling period, but this behavior occurs only sporadically (Wittenberger, personal observation). Finally, severe fighting has been described between resident females and newly arriving females in several species where polygyny is rare (Haartman, 1969). In some cases, these fights prevent polygynous matings, but in others, they do not. The absence of female aggression in other polygynous birds does not imply an absence of deleterious effects on primary females. Attempts to exclude unmated females may simply cost more than they are worth. In mammals, female aggression conflicts less with other reproductive activities and hence is more prevalent. Its effects will be discussed in a later section.

The fitness curve for monogamous females need not lie below the curve for secondary females. A model based on female cooperation rather than competition is fully compatible with the polygyny-threshold model and should be considered as one of its possible formulations (Altmann *et al.*, 1977). Placing the curve for secondary females below that of monogamous females is appropriate when females on each territory compete for resources, but placing it above the curve for monogamous females is more appropriate when females breed in groups on a territory to obtain cooperative benefits. Because the advantages of cooperation can be counteracted by increased competition, the curve for secondary females may lie above that of monogamous females on high-quality territories and below that of monogamous females on low-quality territories (Figure 2). The intersection point would occur where the advantages of cooperation equal the costs of competition.

The shape of the fitness curves is also important for another reason. If the fitness curves are continuous, polygyny results when habitat heterogeneity and population size are large enough to exceed the polygyny threshold (Figure 1). If the fitness curves are discontinuous or drop sharply at the edge of discrete habitat patches (Figure 3), polygyny results when a fraction of the total male population can exclude the remaining males from all suitable habitat patches.

EFFECTS OF POLYGYNY ON MALE PARENTAL BEHAVIOR

The prospect of attracting a second mate has an important effect on male behavior, which in turn changes the positions of the female fitness curves in the model. Since males can generally expect higher reproductive success if they attract additional mates, they should allocate more effort to mate attraction and less to parental care when the prospects for polygyny increase. Males of many monogamous passerine birds, for example, continue singing after they become mated, possibly on the chance that they may acquire second mates (McLaren, 1972). Advertising for females requires time and energy that could be allocated to other activities such as parental care, so opportunities for obtaining additional mates should affect how males allocate their reproductive efforts. When females select mates only during a short mating period, males gain little from continued efforts to attract females and should be more prone to care for offspring instead (Willson, 1966; Emlen and Oring, 1977). When mating periods are longer, males should continue advertising for females at the cost of expending less parental care on their early nests.

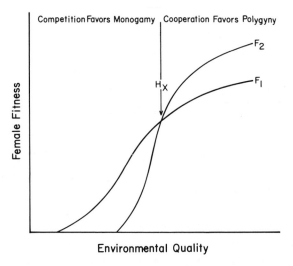

Fig. 2. A cooperative version of the polygyny-threshold model. In environments higher in quality than H_X, the benefits of cooperation exceed the costs of competition and polygyny should occur. In environments lower in quality than H_X, the costs of competition exceed the benefits of cooperation and monogamy should occur. F_1 and F_2 are defined as in Figure 1.

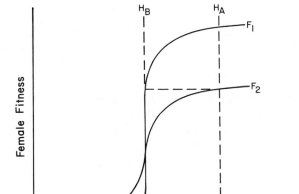

Fig. 3. The polygyny-threshold model for species with clumped nesting distributions that breed in discrete habitat patches. Symbols are defined as in Figure 1.

Male parental care is prevalent in all polygynous birds studied to date that have relatively short mating seasons, including pied flycatchers *(Ficedula hypoleuca)* (Haartman, 1951b; Lack, 1966), bobolinks *(Dolichonyx oryzivorus)* (Martin, 1971, 1974), tricolored blackbirds *(Agelaius tricolor)* (Lack and Emlen, 1939; Orians, 1961), Brewer's blackbirds *(Euphagus cyanocephalus)* (Williams, 1952), and lark buntings *(Calamospiza melanocorys)* (Pleszczynska, 1978). All these species rear a single brood each year, and there is little or no overlap between mating and nestling periods. In yellow-headed blackbirds, the mating season is more prolonged and overlaps the nestling period of early mates considerably (Willson, 1966). In this species, males do not begin feeding nestlings until they are 5–7 days old, and they deliver less food relative to that delivered by females than in the other species.

The long mating seasons associated with double-broodedness or frequent remating by females following nest failure favor continued efforts by males to attract mates and hence reduced male parental care. This occurs in Australian bell-magpies *(Gymnorhina)* (Wilson, 1946; Robinson, 1956), great-tailed grackles *(Quiscalus mexicanus)* (McIlhenney, 1937), oropendolas and caciques (Icteridae) (Chapman, 1928; Skutch, 1954; Tashian, 1957; Drury, 1962), red-winged blackbirds (Orians, 1961), polygynous weaver finches (Ploceinae) (Crook, 1964), dickcissels *(Spiza americana)* (Zimmerman, 1966), corn buntings *(Emberiza calandra)* (Ryves and Ryves, 1934), and indigo buntings *(Passerina cyanea)* (Carey and Nolan, 1975; Carey, 1977). The result is a lowering of the fitness curves for all females and a narrowing of the difference in success between monogamous and low-ranking females on any given territory.

In a few double-brooded species, including house wrens *(Troglodytes aedon)* (Kendeigh, 1941), European wrens *(T. troglodytes)* (Armstrong, 1955; Armstrong and Whitehouse, 1977), prairie warblers *(Dendroica discolor)* (Nolan, 1963, 1978), "Ipswich" sparrows *(Passerculus sandwichensis princeps)* (Stobo and McLaren, 1975), savanna sparrows *(Passerculus sandwichensis)* (Welsh, 1975), and probably meadow-larks *(Sturnella)* (Lanyon, 1957), the nesting cycles of successive mates overlap less, and males make some parental contributions to each brood. In European wrens, males provide more parental assistance on barren islands where polygyny is absent than in forests where it is prevalent (Armstrong, 1955), and in long-billed marsh wrens, they provide more parental care in marshes where polygyny is rare than in marshes where it is common (Kale, 1965; Verner, 1965).

Opportunities for polygynous matings also intensify intermale competition for the best territories or breeding sites, which in turn often generates pronounced sexual dimorphism and delayed plumage maturation. These effects are well known and will not be elaborated upon here (see Selander, 1965, 1972; Orians, 1969; Crook, 1972; Trivers, 1972; Alexander, Hoogland, and Sherman, 1978).

Evidence for the Polygyny-Threshold Model

The approach most commonly taken in attempts to test the polygyny-threshold model has been to document the predicted relationship between polygyny and territory quality. Two types of studies have demonstrated correlations between the incidence of polygyny in birds and vegetation structure, food availability, or both. Some studies show that polygynous species occupy habitats with different structural attributes or exploit food resources with different spatial or temporal distributions than closely related monogamous species (e.g., Crook, 1964, 1965; Pitelka *et al.*, 1974), while others show that polygynous males hold territories with different attributes than monogamous males or polygynous males with fewer females within the same population (e.g., Verner, 1964; Willson, 1966; Zimmerman, 1966, 1971; Martin, 1971; Holm, 1973; Harmeson, 1974; Stobo and McLaren, 1975; Wittenberger, 1976b; Armstrong and Whitehouse, 1977; Carey, 1977; Lenington, 1977; Monahan, 1977; Nolan, 1978; Orians, 1979). These studies clearly document the relationship between habitat quality and polygyny, but they provide little real support for the concept of a polygyny threshold. The crucial and as yet poorly tested point of the model is that polygyny represents the optimal choice for unmated females that pair with already mated males. None of the above studies provide evidence on this question.

To test the polygyny-threshold model adequately, the expected fitness of second-mated females in optimal habitat must be compared to that of monogamous females in marginal habitat. Using actual reproductive success to estimate the polygyny threshold is often not sufficient, especially when predictability of realized success is low at the time females choose their mates. Female choices must be based on expected success, not on realized success, and hence the polygyny threshold must stem from variations in expected success between territories. The importance of this distinction can be made clear with a hypothetical example. Suppose that a major factor contributing to nest failure is predation but that females cannot predict with any degree of reliability how vulnerable their nests will be to predation in any particular habitat. Females consequently base their choices on food availability, even though starvation is a much less important cause of nestling mortality. Haphazard predation patterns could then mask female choices based on food availability if predation losses are included in the data analysis. This is especially true when predation is nonrandomly distributed because of the spatial distribution of predators. Most studies do not cover large enough areas or last long enough to obtain unbiased estimates of predation effects as a function of vegetation structure, and the results of data analysis can then easily reflect predator hunting patterns rather than female habitat choices. The appropriate comparison in this example would be nestling starvation rates on various territories and not overall reproductive success. Studies of habitat variables must therefore take into account the extent to which the effects of these variables on female success are predictable at the time females make their choices.

A second problem in testing the model is to identify the most marginal habitats, especially when monogamous matings occur over a broad range of habitats. The most promising approach is to estimate expected reproductive success on each territory with multiple regression techniques (see Lenington, 1977) and then use these estimates to rank-order territories with respect to habitat quality. The realized success achieved by secondary females can then be compared to that achieved by monogamous females on the poorest territories. Only those components of realized female success that are predictable at the time females select habitats should be used for making this comparison. The first study to provide evidence on this question is that of Pleszczynska (1978), who found that secondary female lark buntings have nesting success equal to that of monogamous females breeding in marginal habitats.

A second approach has been to test various predictions drawn from the model. Orians (1969) predicted that polygyny should be less prevalent in altricial birds than in either precocial birds or mammals because females of altricial birds suffer higher costs by forgoing male parental assistance. Polygamy is somewhat more prevalent in precocial birds than in altricial birds (Lack, 1968), but many of the precocial species are promiscuous rather than polygynous. Since the relevance of the polygyny-threshold model and even the importance of female choice are questionable for promiscuous birds (see below), the greater incidence of polygamy in precocial species does not provide convincing support for the prediction. Similarly, polygamy is much more prevalent in mammals than in altricial birds (Eisenberg, 1966; Wilson, 1975), but many polygamous mammals are again promiscuous rather than polygynous. Any broad comparisons between birds and mammals are further confounded by the greater prevalence of social grouping behavior in mammals, which generates very different selective pressures than those expected in territorial systems.

The prediction that increased heterogeneity in habitat quality should lead to an increased incidence of polygyny is supported by better evidence. Habitat heterogeneity appears especially high and niche widths appear especially broad in two-dimensional habitats, and polygyny is most common among birds inhabiting grasslands and marshes (Verner and Willson, 1966). The correlation is clear for North American and African species but is less evident for the most conspicuously polygynous European species (Haartman, 1969). Two of these species are hole-nesting flycatchers of forested areas, but neither species is encompassed by the polygyny-threshold model because the males are polyterritorial (see below). Of the remaining European species, all inhabit cultivated lands, open brush, or marshes except the European wren, which breeds in a wide range of habitats, from dense forests to open moors and even reed beds (see Armstrong, 1955). Thus, the general correlation does seem to hold in Europe as well as elsewhere. The weak point of this evidence is that the higher habitat heterogeneity assumed to exist in two-dimensional habitats has not been adequately documented.

Orians (1972) argued that habitat heterogeneity for red-winged blackbirds is higher in the western United States than in the East because aridity in the West greatly reduces the quality of uplands relative to marshes. He then showed that territorial male redwings average more mates in the West than in the East, presumably because the low quality of arid uplands causes a greater proportion of females to pack into western marshes. Similarly, Wittenberger (1978a) found a lower incidence of polygyny among bobolinks in Oregon than Martin (1971) found in Wisconsin and attributed the difference to greater physiognomic hetero-geneity on Martin's study area. Finally, Carey and Nolan (1975) predicted and verified the occurrence of polygyny in indigo buntings from observations that this species utilizes an unusually broad range of nesting habitats that are likely to vary considerably in quality. However, since their prediction was also based on the existence of strong sexual dimorphism and the lack of male participation in feeding nestlings, it does not provide strong evidence for the relationship between habitat heterogeneity and polygyny.

Orians's (1969, 1972) prediction that harem size should not be negatively correlated with female reproductive success is contradicted by some evidence. Downhower and Armitage (1971) found that the average reproductive success of female yellow-bellied marmots *(Marmota flaviventris)* decreases as harem size increases, and consequently they rejected the polygyny-threshold model for mar-

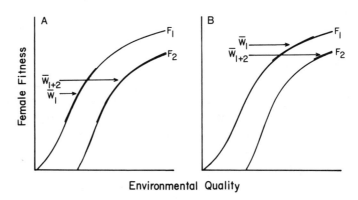

Fig. 4. Relationship between female fitness and mean harem size (after S. Lenington, personal communication). Heavy lines indicate range of habitats occupied by harems of one and two females, respectively. $\overline{W}_1$ = mean fitness of monogamous females; $\overline{W}_{1+2}$ = mean fitness of females in harems of two females (fitness of primary female is assumed here to be depressed by presence of the secondary female, so that fitnesses of both females are equal). Other symbols are defined as in Figure 1. A: A positive correlation is predicted between mean female fitness and harem size. B: A negative correlation is predicted between mean female fitness and harem size.

mots. This oft-cited study has been accepted by many subsequent authors as strong evidence against the model.

Before accepting this conclusion, the validity of Orians's prediction should be examined. Compare, for example, two hypothetical populations with identical fitness functions (Figure 4). In the first population (Figure 4A), males attract two mates in a broad range of superior habitats, and the average success of polygynous females exceeds that of monogamous females, just as Orians predicted. But in the second population (Figure 4B), males attract two mates in only a narrow range of superior habitats, and the relationship is reversed. This example was based on the assumption that female rank does not influence reproductive success. When female rank is important, as in species where males help feed primary nestlings but not secondary nestlings, a negative correlation between harem size and mean female reproductive success is highly likely because all monogamous females receive male help, while only half of all bigamous females receive male help. This effect explains why the mean reproductive success of monogamous females averages higher than that for polygynous females in bobolinks (see Martin, 1971, 1974; Wittenberger, 1978a). Finally, changing the shape of the fitness functions can also yield a negative correlation between harem size and mean female success. When habitat quality drops sharply outside suitable habitat patches, as is likely in species that breed in discrete habitats such as marshes or isolated trees, a negative correlation is easy to predict (Figure 5). This effect can readily explain the results obtained by Downhower and Armitage (1971), as will be shown in the next section. Clearly, any relationship can obtain when all data for a population are pooled. A consistently nonnegative correlation can be expected only when the average success of secondary females is compared to that of monogamous females who breed in the most marginal habitats occupied by the population and provided that habitat quality follows a continuous distribution, as depicted in Figure 4.

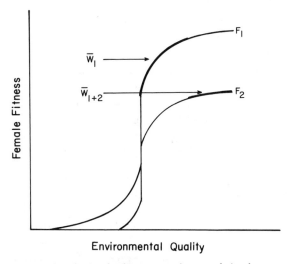

Fig. 5. Discontinuous habitat distribution leads to a negative correlation between mean female fitness and harem size. Heavy lines indicate range of habitats occupied by harems of one and two females, respectively. All symbols are defined as in Figure 4.

The above arguments are easily extended to cases where males attract more than two mates. The lower curve may then represent second and subsequent mates combined if they all have similar fitnesses, or additional curves may be added for tertiary, quaternary, etc., mates if they do not (see Altmann *et al.,* 1977).

The most compelling reason to date for accepting the polygyny-threshold model is the general validity of its two essential assumptions. The model follows directly from the assumptions that polygyny evolves through individual selection and results from female choice of optimal breeding situations. Individual selection is generally accepted as the best explanation for virtually all aspects of animal social behavior (Williams, 1966; Brown, 1969, 1975; Alexander, 1974; Wilson, 1975; Dawkins, 1976; Barash, 1977), and few authors question its applicability to polygynous mating systems (see Orians, 1969, for further discussion). The validity of the female choice assumption has been disputed by Downhower and Armitage (1971), but their argument was based on the erroneous prediction discussed above. Darwin's (1871) concept of females' choosing mates on the basis of an aesthetic sense akin to human beauty has been rightly criticized (Huxley, 1938), but the modern concept of females' choosing superior mates or breeding contexts to enhance their fitness is widely accepted (e.g., Fisher, 1958; Maynard Smith, 1958; Goss-Custard, Dunbar, and Aldrich-Blake, 1972; Selander, 1972; Trivers, 1972; Emlen and Oring, 1977). In territorial systems, polygyny can evolve only when already mated males attract additional females to their territories, so its evolution is clearly dependent on the choices made by unmated females. Nevertheless, validating these assumptions is not proof of the model. Such a proof must be based on tests of the polygyny-threshold concept itself, and as pointed out above, data supporting this concept are still inadequate.

COLONIAL RODENTS

The work by Downhower and Armitage (1971) on yellow-bellied marmots has made colonial rodents something of a test case for the polygyny-threshold model. It is therefore appropriate to consider in detail the various hypotheses advanced to explain polygyny in these species. Before discussing these hypotheses, a word on terminology is necessary. Other species of marmots are often referred to as *colonial* because several individuals breed together in a group, but they are not colonial in the sense used here. *Coloniality* refers here to the clumping of several breeding units (i.e., harems or extended-family groups) or territories into confined areas or discrete habitat patches and not to single, dispersed breeding units.

Setting group selection models aside, two different hypotheses have been proposed to explain polygyny in yellow-bellied marmots. Both assume that each unmated female maximizes her fitness, given the options left open to her, and hence, both fit the polygyny-threshold model. One hypothesis conforms to the cooperative version of the model, while the other conforms to the competitive version.

In the cooperative version, individual females sacrifice some of their immediate reproductive output to enhance survival and hence increase opportunities for future reproduction (Elliott, 1975). Females accomplish this by accepting the competitive costs of polygyny in return for the vigilance provided by other females on the territory. For a population with zero intrinsic rate of increase, polygyny should be advantageous when the percentage increase in a female's annual survival rate exceeds the percentage decrease in her annual reproductive rate (Wittenberger, in press, a). Optimal harem size is determined by the point where these percentages are equal, and females should try to become members of harems with that size. Since competition may vary between territories, optimal harem size may differ for each territory in a colony.

Several lines of evidence suggest that colonial rodents depend on cooperation to lessen their vulnerability to predation. In most species, females warn others by adopting conspicuous alert postures and giving specialized alarm calls (King, 1955; Armitage, 1962; Eisenberg, 1966; Waring, 1970; Carl, 1971; Smith, Smith, Oppenheimer, de Villa, and Ulmer, 1973; Nel, 1975; Owings and Ross, 1978). Their alarm calls evolved in at least some species by kin selection (Dunford, 1977; Sherman, 1977), and they act as a cooperative warning network. Carl (1971), for example, found that he could approach solitary Arctic ground squirrels (*Spermophilus undulatus*) more closely than he could approach colony members because the alarm was sounded earlier when he approached a colony. Cooperation also enables individuals to construct more elaborate burrow systems than would otherwise be possible, thus increasing the number of escape routes available for foraging females on each territory (King, 1955). Since coloniality has evolved only in diurnal rodents that inhabit open environments, cooperation in defending against predators seems to be an important advantage of living in groups (Eisenberg, 1966; see also Hoogland, 1977).

Cooperation may provide another survival advantage in addition to better protection from predators. In yellow-bellied marmots (and other colonial rodents), territory occupants usually hibernate together (Andersen, Armitage, and Hoffman, 1976). Hibernating in groups would reduce heat loss and may possibly increase both juvenile and adult survival. It may also be important in conserving female fat reserves for use the next spring. Overwintering survival of juveniles is not correlated with harem size in yellow-bellied marmots (Downhower and Armitage, 1971), but the effects of increased harem size on adult female survival have not been evaluated.

The advantages derived from cooperation could favor colonial breeding without favoring polygyny itself because females could theoretically rely on the vigilance of individuals from neighboring territories for protection. When the density of rodents in colonies is high enough for females to hear or see warnings given from neighboring territories, sharing a male's territory with other females may provide little additional benefit. The fact that female yellow-bellied marmots are highly aggressive and try to exclude unmated females from their home ranges (Armitage, 1965; Svendsen, 1974) indicates competition between resident females on each male territory. Female aggression might seem incompatible with the hypothesis that females form harems to enhance their survival prospects, but it would not contradict the hypothesis if it is most prevalent on poor territories where low habitat quality reduces optimal harem size to one female. The cooperative version of the model therefore predicts that polygyny should occur on high-quality territories in the colony but not on low-quality territories. Without data on the survival advantages gained by females as a result of joining harems, acceptance or rejection of the cooperation hypothesis would be premature.

The competitive version of the polygyny-threshold model explains the polygynous behavior of colonial rodents in a different way. The hypothesis is best viewed in terms of the options available to each unmated female (Figure 6). In yellow-bellied marmots and perhaps also in other colonial rodents, a female can reproduce most successfully by becoming the sole mate of a colony male (Downhower and Armitage, 1971; see also King, 1955). Once all males in a colony have a mate, the best choice remaining for an unmated female is to pair with an already mated male in the colony rather than breeding in isolation outside the colony (Downhower and Armitage, 1971). In yellow-bellied marmots, polygynous matings reduce the success of resident females, so resident females should try to prevent unmated females from entering their home ranges. Some resident females succeed and retain their monogamous status. Others fail and are joined by a second female to form a "harem." Once opportunities for mating with males having only one mate are exhausted, unmated females must choose between a bigamous colony male and breeding in isolation. Their best choice is to pair with a bigamous male. At some point, the combined aggressiveness of all resident females on each territory prevents further entry into the colony, and any remaining unmated females are forced into isolated areas. Thus, polygyny could result because relatively few males can exclude all other males from each colony site and many females must accept polygynous status to breed within a colony. In effect, males can defend larger territories in the colony than females.

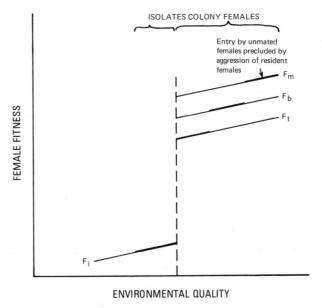

Fig. 6. A competitive version of the polygyny-threshold model for explaining polygyny in yellow-bellied marmots (modified from Wittenberger, 1979a). Heavy lines indicate territories containing harems of each size. F_m = fitness of monogamously mated females; F_b = fitness of bigamously mated females; F_t = fitness of trigamously mated females; F_i = fitness of females breeding alone in isolated areas. See text for further explanation.

All the evidence for yellow-bellied marmots fits the competitive model. The reproductive success of females breeding in isolation is substantially lower than that of any colony females, including those in the largest harems (Downhower and Armitage, 1971; Armitage and Downhower, 1974). Hence, females entering colonies as second or third mates are making a better choice than if they had chosen to breed in isolation. Since polygynous matings reduce the success of females already in the colony, resident females should be and are aggressive toward unmated females trying to enter their territories. The most aggressive females remain monogamously paired, while less aggressive females become members of harems (Svendsen, 1974). The reasons that some females are more aggressive than others have not been investigated, but they may be related to differing physical conditions of females in early spring or to variations in food availability, lengths of tenure, or prior experiences. Each female can allocate only so much time and effort to aggressive behavior before it detracts from her reproductive success, and females presumably differ in the amount of effort they can expend. The costs of female aggression should be lowest on territories with abundant food resources because energetic expenditures are more easily replenished, so females should be most aggressive on high-quality territories. This prediction is just the opposite of the one derived from the cooperative model earlier. Finally, females on each territory localize their movements to subsections of each male's territory and defend only that area (Armitage, 1965). Since each female defends less space as harem size increases, the combined efforts of several females can effectively limit harem size without entailing any cooperation.

The reason that increased harem size reduces female reproductive success in yellow-bellied marmots has recently been clarified. Litter sizes and birth dates are influenced by the female's fat reserves and the amount of food available to her in early spring (Andersen *et al.*, 1976). Fat reserves depend on how much time is available for foraging the preceding summer and on winter weather conditions (Armitage and Downhower, 1974). Competition for food does not seem important in mid or late summer (Kilgore and Armitage, 1978), and larger harem sizes may even conserve fat reserves during winter because all territory occupants huddle together while hibernating. On the other hand, food is scarce in spring, and the increased competition caused by larger harem sizes results in smaller litter sizes and delayed births (Andersen *et al.*, 1976). Delays in giving birth are especially detrimental to female success because the overwintering survival of juveniles depends on how much time they have available for growing before winter. Juveniles born late in the season are invariably small and consequently survive less well through their first winter. Thus, polygyny seems deleterious to resident females largely in early spring, and that is when resident females are most aggressive (Armitage, 1965).

The relevance of the competitive model to other colonial rodents is less clear. Female Richardson's ground squirrels *(Spermophilus richardsonii)* defend individual territories in each colony, with males defending territories that encompass the burrow systems of several females (Yeaton, 1972). Female territoriality is associated with defense of lush vegetation that is found in depressed areas and is used for food. Habitats do not appear limited, but the clumping of female territories enables males to defend more than one at a time. Quite probably, clumping of female territories has evolved as a defense against predation. Female aggressiveness within harems (i.e., coteries) of prairie dogs *(Cynomys)* is largely absent (King, 1955), but this absence is associated with high genetic relatedness among females on each territory. Females are aggressive toward individuals from neighboring territories. Competition for food within colonies is well documented for prairie dogs, and present evidence suggests that suitable breeding sites are in short supply (King, 1955; Koford, 1958). Prairie dogs live in early successional stages of prairies, which they maintain by their foraging activities. Because unoccupied areas are generally in a later successional stage, they are not easily invaded. Newly mature males therefore have difficulty establishing territories, and colony expansion usually results from the gradual extension of peripheral territories into unoccupied areas.

OTHER MAMMALS

The competitive version of the polygyny-threshold model can adequately explain the extreme polygyny of colonial pinnipeds. Breeding populations of pinnipeds concentrate into relatively few areas for a combination of reasons. Breeding is restricted to relatively flat coastal areas because marine adaptations preclude efficient locomotion on land (Bartholomew, 1970). Colonial species usually breed on rocky coastlines or sandy beaches, while many noncolonial species breed on ice floes. Suitable coastlines are limited in availability relative to population size because very large populations can be supported by the abundant food resources present in vast areas of open ocean and extensive continental shelf areas. This limitation is accentuated by the necessity to breed on islands where pups are not threatened by terrestrial predators (Orr, 1965; Peterson, 1968; Bartholomew, 1970). Gray seals *(Halichoerus grypus)* are further restricted to sites where protected channels and inland pools provide places to wallow (Coulson and Hickling, 1964). Most species can breed only where fish and other prey are abundant, and this factor alone may be a major reason why suitable sites are limited.

Once females breed in dense colonies, they represent a defensible "resource" for males. In fur seals *(Callorhinus, Arctocephalus)* and sea lions *(Eumetopias, Zalophus, Otaria, Neophoca)*, males defend territories adjacent to water, where females are especially prone to congregate (Bartholomew and Hoel, 1953; Orr, 1965, 1967; Orr and Poulter, 1967; Peterson and Bartholomew, 1967; Peterson, 1968; Stirling, 1971, 1972). Females prefer breeding near water because they periodically return to the ocean to forage while nursing, and they can minimize harassment from other males by not breeding further ashore. In elephant seals *(Mirounga)*, females often congregate away from shorelines, and males control access to female pods through dominance status rather than territoriality (Bartholomew, 1952; Carrick, Csordas, Ingham, and Keith, 1962; Le Boeuf, 1972, 1974; Le Boeuf, Whiting, and Gantt, 1972). Males defend dominance status along extensive stretches of beach instead of establishing fixed territories because females congregate in unpredictable locations on the beach. Females show no preference for shorelines because they do not leave to forage while nursing.

Scarcity of suitable habitat is only partially responsible for making female elephant seal pods defensible. Females form compact pods instead of dispersing randomly over the rookery because males are prone to crush or injure both females and pups during fights (Le Boeuf, 1972; Le Boeuf *et al.*, 1972; Le Boeuf and Briggs, 1977). Central females in a pod are also more likely to be inseminated by a dominant male, thus increasing the genetic quality of their male offspring (McLaren, 1967), and females even incite fights that break up copulation attempts by subordinate males in order to gain this advantage (Cox and Le Boeuf, 1977). Both factors have a strong centripetal effect that favors female clumping and enables a few dominant males to control access to large numbers of females.

Various mammals are polygynous because males defend the individual home ranges of several females at a time. In the white-lined bat *(Saccopteryx bilineata)*, males from each roosting colony defend individual territories that encompass the foraging "beats" of several females (Bradbury and Emmons, 1974; Bradbury and Vehrencamp, 1976, 1977). The association between a male and his harem of females is relatively long-lasting and is maintained even within the day roosts, although females sometimes move their foraging beats to another male's territory. Food resources (aerial insects) are spatially clumped and reliably available on a seasonal basis, allowing relatively few males to control the best sites within the area exploited by each roosting colony. In some prosimians, females defend individual territories, with each male defending a larger territory that overlaps those of several females (Charles-Dominique, 1972, 1974; see also Charles-Dominique and Martin, 1972; Martin, 1972). A similar pattern also occurs in the northern reedbuck *(Redunca redunca)* (Hendrichs, 1975b), in lyrebirds *(Menura novaehollandiae)* (Kenyon, 1972), and in the brown lizard *(Anolis segreyi)* of the Bahama Islands (T. W. Schoener, personal communication).

Territorial polygyny in most other mammals seems to fit the cooperative version of the model. In lions *(Panthera leo)*, single males or coalitions of several males patrol and actively exclude other males from the home ranges of female prides (Schaller, 1972; Rudnai, 1973; Bertram, 1975). Males are able to defend female groups because females depend on cooperation for capturing prey and rearing cubs (see Schaller, 1972; Caraco and Wolf, 1975). Defending the pride home range instead of the pride itself appears advantageous because prides are incohesive and normally fragment into subgroups for prolonged periods of time. Males can defend pride home ranges only when females are sedentary. In areas of seasonal food scarcity, females are nomadic, and then males only consort temporarily with receptive females (Schaller, 1972; Eloff, 1973).

Olympic marmots *(Marmota olympus)*, hoary marmots *(M. caligata)*, and alpine marmots *(M. marmota)* all breed as single-family groups on widely separated home ranges or territories (Barash, 1973, 1974b, 1976). These groups usually consist of one adult male, two related adult females, and their immature offspring. Polygyny is apparently one part of a behavioral syndrome associated with short growing seasons (Barash, 1974a). Because these marmots breed at high elevations or high latitudes, growing seasons are short and offspring require two years to mature. Females breed once every two years, with the two females associated with each male giving birth in alternate years. Only one female is therefore lactating each spring, which may reduce competition for food during the critical early spring months and thereby facilitate the evolution of cooperative behavior as a defense against predation. A second factor that may be important in favoring polygyny is the relatedness of females in harems. Harems are formed by the replacement of dead adult females with juveniles raised in the harem, so females in each harem are always related. Since dispersal is likely to result in high juvenile mortality (e.g., see Downhower and Armitage, 1971), each resident female may have higher inclusive fitness by tolerating a low level of competition with a relative rather than forcing her to disperse. The combination of breeding in alternate years and relatedness between harem females probably promotes sociability between females, and the resulting female groups are defensible by single males. Why these species have not formed colonies of several breeding units as in yellow-bellied marmots has not been explained, but the distribution of their breeding habitats is probably the most important factor.

Territorial polygyny has evolved in a few ungulates and primates because males control resources vital to female groups or because males defend the home ranges of female groups. Females form social groups to gain better protection from predators (Alexander, 1974; Altmann, 1974; Estes, 1974; Geist, 1974; Leuthold, 1977; Wittenberger, in press, a) and remain on male territories to exploit the resources available there. For example, on the high Andean plateaus of Peru, male vicuñas defend unusually favorable grazing areas where cohesive groups of females forage (Koford, 1957). Females remain on a single male territory and exclude strange females from their group, possibly to maintain an optimal balance between the cooperative advantages and the competitive disadvantages of sociality (see Wittenberger, in press, a). Groups consisting of a single male and several females also defend territories in several primates (Crook, 1972; Jolly, 1972). The environmental factors favoring this type of social organization in primates are still unclear. Crook (1972) argued that the spatial distribution and seasonal variability of food resources should be important factors. In black-and-white colobus monkeys *(Colobus guereza)* and gray langurs *(Presbytis senex)*, territoriality is associated with a diet consisting largely of mature leaves (Clutton-Brock, 1974, 1975; Hladik, 1975; Struhsaker and Oates, 1975; Oates, 1977). Mature leaves are readily available throughout the year, so individuals can confine their activities to a smaller area than in species dependent on spatiotemporally variable food sources such as fruiting trees. The related red colobus monkey *(C. badius)* and Hanuman langur *(P. entellus)* range over larger areas to find fruit and other nutritive plant parts, and these species form larger social groups which occupy large overlapping home ranges (Clutton-Brock, 1974, 1975; Hladik, 1975; Struhsaker, 1974, 1975; Struhsaker and Oates, 1975).

In several ungulates, males defend resources required by females but are able to retain only temporary control over female groups (Leuthold, 1977). Since individual females or female groups often move from one territory to another, mating relationships are promiscuous rather than polygynous. Nevertheless, males still gain control of females by defending territories in particularly favorable habitats. The nature of the defended resources varies among species. Male pronghorn antelopes *(Antilocapra americana)* defend areas containing waterholes and high-quality grazing sites (Kitchen, 1974). Male impala *(Aepyceros melampus)* defend territories in deciduous woodlands and savanna, where loosely integrated female groups forage (Leuthold, 1970; Jarman and Jarman, 1974). Male Grant's gazelles *(Gazella granti)* defend hilltops in open savanna, where females prefer to graze (Walther, 1965; Estes, 1967). By occupying hilltops they may control the best vantage points for spotting predators and perhaps also the best grazing areas [Grant's gazelles graze mainly on forbs, which become overgrown with tall grasses in wetter swales (Gwynne and Bell, 1968; Bell, 1971)]. Male defassa waterbucks *(Kobus defassa)* and Coke's hartebeests *(Alcelaphus buselaphus)* defend riverine thickets or scrub edges that provide dense cover near good foraging areas (Kiley-Worthington, 1965; Spinage, 1969; Gosling, 1974). In each case, relatively few males can control a disproportionate share of mating opportunities by excluding other males from the limited number of high-quality habitats sought by females.

To summarize, territorial polygyny evolves in colonial mammals when relatively few males can exclude all remaining males from colony sites and in noncolonial mammals when territorial males can defend the home ranges of several individual females or those of female groups from other males. Female spacing patterns therefore govern to a large extent the reproductive tactics adopted by males, and female spacing is in turn dependent on the utility of cooperative defenses against predation and on the distribution of resources in space and time.

Passerine Birds

Territorial polygyny in passerine birds has evidently evolved in two ways. Among species with a clumped nesting distribution, polygyny occurs when a fraction of the male population can exclude the remaining males from all suitable nesting sites. Among species with a dispersed nesting distribution, it occurs when habitat differences cause some territorial males to attract several females while others remain unmated. Support for this conclusion comes from a comparison of population attributes in species exhibiting these dispersion patterns (Wittenberger, 1976a). In the ensuing discussion of this evidence, the term *colonial* is used to refer to clumped nesting distributions, and the term *noncolonial* is used to refer to nonclumped or widely spaced nesting distributions. The essential distinction emphasized here is based on how suitable nesting habitats are distributed in space and not on semantic issues concerning definitions of coloniality. Because many authors prefer using criteria other than habitat distribution to define coloniality, I will qualify my usage with quotation marks.

In "colonial" passerines, territorial males rarely or never fail to attract at least one mate (Table II; Wittenberger 1976a). Yearling males (and even some adult males) do not establish territories, and as a result, males generally do not attain adult plumage in their first year. The only exceptions are certain tropical oropendolas and caciques that also lack sexual dichromatism. "Colonial" species usually exhibit a high degree of polygyny, meaning that most territorial males are polygynous and many attract four or even more females. Exceptions are tricolored blackbirds, in which the mating period in each colony is very short (Lack and Emlen, 1939; Orians, 1961; Payne, 1969), and Australian bell-magpies, in which groups of several males and their mates defend joint territories against intruders of both sexes (Wilson, 1946; Robinson, 1956; Carrick, 1963). The degree of polygyny is intermediate in yellow-headed blackbirds, as harem sizes often exceed four females in some areas or years but are generally smaller in other areas or years (Willson, 1966; Orians, 1979; Monnett and Wittenberger, unpublished data).

In "noncolonial" species, territorial males regularly fail to attract any mates. Since most males, including yearlings, establish territories, males generally attain full adult plumage in their first year. A partial exception is the indigo bunting, in which yearling males occasionally have a mottled appearance (Carey and Nolan, 1975; Rohwer, Fretwell, and Niles, in press). "Noncolonial" species exhibit a low degree of polygyny, meaning that many males obtain only one mate and few obtain more than three. The most important difference between "noncolonial" and "colonial" species is that many territorial males of the former species fail to attract mates to their territories.

No male should establish a territory where it has little prospect of attracting a mate, unless he can thereby improve his chances of acquiring a nearby suitable territory should it become vacant. Territorial defense is costly and must be accompanied by attendant benefits before it can evolve (Brown, 1964, 1975). Males should generally not establish territories in unsuitable habitats unless they cannot predict accurately where females will later settle. When territorial males in marginal habitats regularly remain unmated, their mating prospects should be relatively unpredictable at the time they establish their territories.

In the ensuing discussion, the term *predictability* refers to the extent to which males can reliably assess which habitats will or will not attract females at some future date in a breeding season. With respect to females, it refers to the extent to which females can reliably assess their prospects for successful reproduction in particular habitats. More precisely, *predictability* refers here to the probability that the rank ordering of habitats in terms of their quality will remain the same within any specified time interval during the breeding season.

TABLE II.   CORRELATES OF POLYGYNY IN "COLONIAL" AND "NONCOLONIAL" PASSERINES [a]

Nesting dispersion	Number of genera	Territorial males often remain unmated	Male age dimorphism	High degree of polygyny
"Noncolonial" (dispersed)	13	92–100% [c]	0%	0%
"Colonial" (clumped)	12 [b]	0%	82% [d]	73% [e]

[a]Data based on Wittenberger, 1976a; *Menura novaehollandiae* was deleted because matings are apparently promiscuous instead of polygynous (Lill, personal communication); *Passerina cyanea* and *Cistothorus platensis* were added on the basis of Carey and Nolan (1975), Carey (1977), and Crawford (1977) and *Calamospiza melanocorys* was added on the basis of Pleszczynska (1978).

[b]*Agelaius phoeniceus* has a clumped nesting distribution in marshes and a dispersed nesting distribution in uplands, but its preferred habitat is marshes so it is included in this category.

[c]The possible exception is *Emberiza calandra*.

[d]Exceptions are *Zarhynchus wagleri* and *Psarocolius montezuma*, both of which also lack sexual dichromatism.

[e]Exceptions are *Agelaius tricolor* and *Gymnorhina*. *Xanthocephalus* is intermediate but was treated as an exception.

Two factors probably contribute to the unpredictability of male mating prospects in marginal habitats. One of these is uncertainty in predicting where the end point of the polygyny threshold (H_B of Figure 1) will occur (Wittenberger, 1976a). Birds select habitats according to environmental parameters (proximate cues) that predict habitat conditions (ultimate factors) later influencing their reproductive success (Svärdson, 1949; Hildèn, 1965a). Since proximate cues are not perfectly predictive, the ultimate quality of the best habitats (H_A) must be uncertain to some extent (ΔH_A) at the time males select them (Figure 7). That is, the quality of H_A may fall anywhere within the range ΔH_A by the time females select mates. The expected fitness of secondary females in optimal habitat is therefore indeterminate by an amount Δw at the time males select habitats, and the result is uncertainty in locating the end point of the polygyny threshold H_B. If territory quality in optimal habitat turns out to be high, most males in the range of marginal habitats indicated by ΔH_B will remain unmated. If territory quality in optimal habitat turns out to be low, most males in ΔH_B will attract a mate. Since males do not know in advance which will occur, they should occupy territories within nearly the full range of habitats encompassed by ΔH_B.

The second source of uncertainty comes from the problems of predicting in advance which habitats will fall into ΔH_B. Males should accept almost any habitat that has some chance of falling into the range of ΔH_B later in the season. Adding a third dimension to the polygyny-threshold model illustrates the point (Figure 8). The quality of each habitat open to a male at time T_1 (when males select habitats)

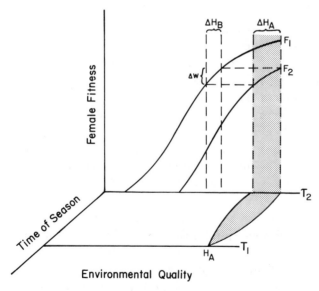

Fig. 7. Low predictability of habitat quality in the best areas creates a range of marginal habitats where territorial males have some probability of attracting mates but often remain unmated (modified from Wittenberger, 1976a). F_1 and F_2 are defined as in Figure 1. T_1 = time when males establish territories; T_2 = time when females select mates; H_A = best available habitat at time T_1. The conic projection on the horizontal plain delineates the amount of change in habitat quality that H_A can undergo by time T_2. The quality of a territory in H_A can fall unpredictably anywhere in the range ΔH_A (shaded area) by time T_2. Δw = unpredictability of the fitness of second-mated females caused by ΔH_A. ΔH_B = the resulting degree of uncertainty in predicting which marginal habitats are likely to attract females.

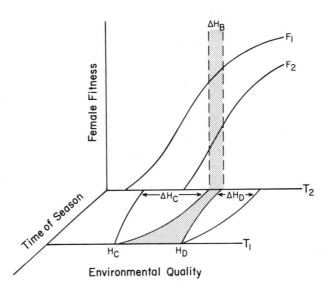

Fig. 8. High unpredictability of habitat quality causes some males to establish territories where they may later fail to attract mates. Symbols are defined as in Figure 7. H_C = the lowest-quality habitat that has some chance at time T_1 of attracting a female later in the season. H_D = the highest quality territory at time T_1 that has some chance of not attracting any females later in the season. ΔH_C and ΔH_D are defined similarly to ΔH_A of Figure 7. Shaded area is the range of habitats at any given time of season within which territorial males have uncertain prospects of attracting mates.

can be projected onto the axis at time T_2 (when females select mates). The width of each conic projection (e.g., ΔH_C, ΔH_D) indicates the degree of uncertainty involved in predicting the quality of a particular habitat. For instance, the quality of habitat H_C at time T_1 may change to any quality lying within the interval ΔH_C by time T_2, while the quality of habitat H_D at time T_1 may change to any quality lying within the interval ΔH_D by time T_2. The degree of uncertainty and hence the width of the projection may vary among habitats along the quality gradient. Any habitat between H_C and H_D has some chance of attracting a female and some chance of not attracting a female. Habitats near H_D in quality are almost certain to fall to the right of ΔH_B and hence are nearly certain to attract at least one female. Habitats near H_C have little chance of falling within ΔH_B and hence are not likely to attract any females. Males should accept most habitats between H_C and $H_{D,}$ although some habitats at the lower end of the quality gradient should not be accepted. The cutoff point should occur where the probability of attracting a mate is too low to offset the costs of maintaining the territory and advertising for females. The main point of the model is to show that uncertainties in predicting future habitat quality considerably expand the range of habitats in which males have some chance of remaining unmated.

Before leaving Figure 8, some additional complexities of the habitat selection problem merit attention. Males may select habitats at any time before or after T_1. For each point in time, one can visualize a set of conic projections corresponding to habitat unpredictability. Since the quality of each territory along the habitat continuum may change in a different direction as the season progresses, the rank order of habitats along the quality gradient may change through time. The probability that the rank order will change should decrease as the season advances because more information about habitat quality becomes available. Males are therefore continually faced with the trade-off between gaining more information about the ultimate rank order of habitats and losing the opportunity of selecting the habitats chosen earlier by competing males. Females face a similar problem, since the ultimate quality of habitats as it affects female fitness is determined at some future time, T_3, which is again related to the rank order of habitats present at time T_2 by a set of conic projections. Females can either delay their choice of habitats to gain more information or take advantage of whatever benefits accrue from earlier breeding.

The above argument depends on the assumption that habitat quality follows a continuous distribution. "Noncolonial" species breed in a broad range of environments, where a continuous model seems appropriate. Females depend on nest concealment or pendant nests for protection from predators, and a broad range of habitats can satisfy these requirements. Variations in the suitability of nesting substrate for concealing or suspending nests should be reasonably predictable for males, as they generally depend on differences in vegetation that are evident when territories are established. Hence, uncertainties in predicting habitat quality should arise largely because the future availability of food resources has relatively low predictability. Males generally select habitats according to physiognomic correlates of habitat quality (Lack, 1933, 1944; Miller, 1942; Svärdson, 1949; Hildèn, 1965a; Klopfer, 1969). If female habitat choices are more closely attuned to food availability, males would find it difficult to predict where females will settle. This uncertainty should result in many territorial males' remaining unmated. Since territorial males of "noncolonial" species often do remain unmated, food availability on territories should be important for these species in determining habitat quality. Polygyny should therefore evolve when differences in food availability, in conjunction with differences in other components of habitat quality, are large enough between territories to exceed the polygyny threshold. Only a low degree of polygyny is likely because a broad spectrum of habitats is suitable for breeding. In this situation, a relatively smaller proportion of territories is likely to fall above the polygyny threshold. Yearling males attain adult plumage and establish territories because relatively low habitat predictability allows them to defend potentially suitable breeding habitats.

For "colonial" species, a continuous distribution of habitats along the quality axis does not seem appropriate. Females depend to a considerable extent on the protection afforded by nesting in relatively inaccessible sites (Lack, 1968). Suitable sites are discrete habitat patches, such as marshes or isolated trees. Nesting success inside suitable patches should be markedly higher than in surrounding areas. The quality of potential nesting habitats for "colonial" species should therefore approximate a discontinuous distribution.

The discontinuous model predicts that males should have little difficulty in predicting where females will settle (Figure 9). All habitats to the right of H_B in the model attract at least one female, while none of the habitats to the left of H_B attract any females. Uncertainties in the quality of optimal habitat (ΔH_A) have little effect

JAMES F.
WITTENBERGER

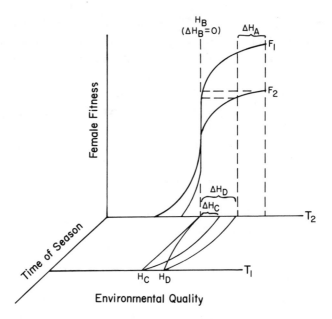

Fig. 9. In discontinuous habitats, male uncertainties in predicting habitat quality may affect harem size but not chances of attracting at least one mate. Symbols are defined as in Figure 7 and 8. All habitats to the right of H_B attract at least one female, and these habitats are distinguishable from habitats to the left of H_B throughout the breeding season (i.e., $\Delta H_B = 0$). All habitats between H_C and H_D at time T_1 will fall to the right of H_B at time T_2, and hence all will attract at least one female.

on where females in lower-quality areas will settle (i.e., $\Delta H_B = 0$) because virtually all areas within suitable patches lie above the polygyny threshold. In addition, the boundary between suitable and unsuitable habitats is readily identifiable throughout the breeding season because it is based on structural discontinuities in the environment or sometimes on the location of traditional colony sites. As a result, males rarely establish territories outside suitable habitat patches, and territorial males rarely remain unmated. Polygyny evolves when a fraction of the male population can control all suitable breeding sites, and this occurs when suitable habitat patches are scarce relative to population size. Since yearling males are the first to be excluded, age dimorphism in male plumage is a secondary result.

The fitness curves drawn for continuous and discontinuous habitat distributions represent the extremes of a single family of curves with varying steepnesses. Fitness curves with intermediate steepness are certainly possible, and these may lead to intermediate population attributes where males regularly but infrequently establish territories where they cannot attract females. However, present evidence is amenable only to comparisons between continuous and discontinuous distributions. More careful quantification of the regularity with which territorial males remain unmated and the steepness of habitat quality gradients will be needed before intermediate situations can be analyzed.

Perhaps the strongest support for the above theory comes from the correlations given in Table II. The relation between bachelor male territoriality and nesting dispersion was discovered as a result of the theory, and it provided general support from an unexpected quarter. The remaining evidence has been thoroughly discussed elsewhere (Wittenberger, 1976a) and will only be summarized here.

Most polygynous weaver finches are colonial and nest in isolated trees on open savanna (Crook, 1964). Many isolated trees are unoccupied, but at least some of these are probably too far from adequate seed resources. Nest sites appear limited because each colony has a finite size and new colonies are difficult to establish. Females can apparently nest more successfully in a large colony than in a small one, so newly established colonies attract few females (Collias and Collias, 1969). Both Orians (1961, 1969) and Lack (1968) attributed polygyny in weaver finches to the ability of relatively few males to control all nesting sites within each colony. Polygyny (or more accurately, promiscuity) has probably evolved for the same reason in *Quiscalus* grackles, oropendolas, and caciques (Selander, 1972; Wittenberger, 1976a).

Polygyny in marsh-breeding blackbirds was originally attributed to heterogeneity in food abundance (Willson and Orians, 1963; Verner and Willson, 1966; Willson, 1966; Orians, 1969), but subsequent evidence indicates that shortages of nesting substrate are more important. Several factors contribute to a shortage of suitable marsh nesting sites. Blackbirds have generalized winter diets that enable them to attain very high population densities relative to the number of available marshes (Orians, 1961). This imbalance has been greatly accentuated by large-scale grain production and extensive draining of marshes during the past century, but it was probably important even before these agricultural perturbations occurred. Marshes vary greatly in suitability because they differ in primary productivity and hence abundance of emergent insects (Orians, 1979). They also vary in suitability because different kinds of emergent vegetation provide differing degrees of protection against predation and adverse weather conditions (Fautin, 1940; Holm, 1973). Yellow-headed blackbirds are further restricted to the outer edges of reed beds in the more productive marshes (Willson, 1966; Orians, 1979), and red-winged blackbirds are excluded from some marshes by the interspecific territoriality of other blackbirds (Orians, 1961; Orians and Collier, 1963; Orians and Willson, 1964). Long-billed marsh wrens puncture blackbird eggs and kill nestlings, so the suitability of a marsh may be reduced if it contains marsh wrens (Picman, 1977a). Orians and Willson (1964), for example, noted that redwing nests invariably fail when built within marsh wren territories. For these reasons, many males are unable to establish territories in suitable marshes (see Orians, 1961; Peek, 1971; Holm 1973), and polygyny results because females can succeed better as second mates in marshes than as monogamous mates in surrounding uplands (see Robertson, 1972).

Females can breed more successfully in marshes than in uplands for at least two reasons. Marshes with high nutrient levels in the water produce much more abundant food resources for feeding nestlings than do surrounding uplands (Verner and Willson, 1966; Robertson, 1972; Orians, 1979), and females can make best use of these resources by nesting near them (see Orians and Pearson, 1978). Nevertheless, nesting in marshes is not a necessary prerequisite for exploiting emergent insects, because much of the emergence occurs along shorelines that lack reed beds. Brewer's blackbirds, for example, exploit these resources extensively even though they nest in sagebrush (Horn, 1968). Female redwings and yellowheads could conceivably nest in grass, sagebrush, or other types of vegetation near open shorelines, but they rarely do. In fact, they sometimes nest in low-productivity marshes and travel long distances to find food instead of nesting in uplands near their foraging areas (Holm, 1973). Female blackbirds evidently prefer nesting in marshes because they gain greater protection from predators. Robertson (1972) found that starvation rates of nestling redwings was similar in marshes and uplands but that predation rates averaged 60% lower in the marshes. Local site characteristics related to food availability and vulnerability of nests to predation, adverse weather, or destruction by marsh wrens may make some territories in marshes better than others, thus leading to variations in the number of females selecting each territory, but the fundamental reason for polygyny seems related to the advantage of nesting in marshes as a defense against predation and the ability of some males to exclude the remaining males from suitable marshes.

The theory is less well substantiated for "noncolonial" birds. Food availability on territories is apparently a major determinant of territory quality in bobolinks (Wittenberger, 1976b). The order in which females select territories and the number attracted to each are both correlated with food abundance. Males select habitats on the basis of physiognomic factors before most nestling food resources emerge, and they cannot distinguish areas of high food productivity from those of lower productivity within physiognomically similar habitats. Females forage outside male territories as well as on them while feeding nestlings, but food abundance on or near territories probably has an important effect on nesting success. Secondary females have lower success than primary females largely because more of their nestlings starve (Martin, 1971, 1974; Wittenberger, 1976b, 1978b), and they often depend on food resources near their nests to compensate for the loss of male parental assistance (Martin, 1974).

Martin (1971) attributed polygyny in bobolinks to variations in nesting cover between territories, but he did not measure food availability and his remaining evidence is not conclusive. Male pairing success was correlated with vegetation cover and density, but vegetation parameters may simply be secondary correlates of food productivity rather than direct determinants of nesting success. Evidence concerning the effects of vegetation structure on nesting success is needed for grassland birds before the role of this factor can be evaluated. The only relevant study is based on meadowlarks, which build domed nests, and in that study, Roseberry and Klimstra (1970) found no correlation between overhead cover and vulnerability of nests to predation. Gottfried and Thompson (1978) obtained a similar result for elevated nests placed in shrubbery within old fields, but their results cannot be generalized to ground-nesting species.

Nesting failure in dickcissels, another grassland species, results most often from predation or cowbird *(Molothrus ater)* brood parasitism (Zimmerman, 1966, 1971). Male pairing success is correlated with vegetation structure, and Zimmerman attributed polygyny in dickcissels to variations in nesting cover between male territories. The effects of vegetation cover on nest vulnerability are again unknown, and several inconsistencies in Zimmerman's data implicate the role of additional factors (Wittenberger, 1976a). Harmeson (1974) found a correlation between male pairing success and arthropod densities present on territories in June, so food availability may be an important component of territory quality. Female dickcissels regularly forage beyond territory boundaries, but the importance of food availability on their territories has never been assessed.

Polygyny is apparently associated with food availability in three species of polygynous wrens. In European wrens, polygyny is prevalent in productive forests but is absent on barren islands where food is scarce (Armstrong, 1955; Armstrong and Whitehouse, 1977). In house wrens, polygyny is infrequent and arises when males can devote time to seeking mates while feeding the nestlings of their first brood (Kendeigh, 1941). Since males should be better able to reduce their parental efforts and seek additional mates when food is more abundant on their territories, food availability seems implicated. In long-billed marsh wrens, male pairing success is correlated with the edge length of emergent vegetation on their territories, which in turn is correlated with the abundance of emergent insects (Verner, 1964).

EXCEPTIONS TO THE POLYGYNY-THRESHOLD MODEL

A few birds are polygynous because females cannot readily assess the true mated status of prospective mates (Lack, 1968; Haartman, 1969; Wittenberger, 1976a). In collared flycatchers (*Ficedula albicollis*), in pied flycatchers, and infrequently in several other European birds, males regularly establish two or three spatially separate territories, each of which may attract a female (Löhrl, 1949, 1959; Haartman, 1951a, 1956, 1969). Polyterritoriality is associated with hole nesting and not defense of food resources. The reason that some males are able to establish several territories is unclear, but it presumably relates to their physical condition and foraging efficiency. Since males help feed the offspring of only their first mates, females attracted to their second or third territories are at a disadvantage. Unmated territorial males are available at the time polygynous matings occur, but females have no easy way of distinguishing between unmated and mated males.

In California, late-pairing females have a similar problem within breeding colonies of Brewer's blackbirds (Williams, 1952). Males initially pair with females while still in winter flocks, and mated pairs establish a nest site in the colony tree together. Males defend females rather than territories, and they associate continuously with their first mates until incubation begins. Then, males temporarily leave their first mates and seek unmated females elsewhere in the colony. When a male finds an unaccompanied female who has chosen a nest site and has begun nest construction, he begins to accompany her and keep other males away. The female has little opportunity to distinguish between unmated and already mated males, so she accepts whichever male defends access to her. Since polygynous males divide their parental efforts about equally between their mates, each mate receives only half as much help as a monogamously mated female. Polygynous status therefore places females at a disadvantage, but they can do little to prevent it other than nesting away from the colony.

HAREM POLYGYNY

Male defense of female groups or harem polygyny becomes possible when females can survive and reproduce most successfully within social groups. Harem polygyny has evolved in a wide diversity of animals, including red jungle fowl *(Gallus gallus)* (Delacour, 1951), peafowl *(Pavo cristatus)* (Delacour, 1951; Sharma, 1969, 1970, 1972), coatimundis *(Nasua narica)* (Kaufmann, 1962), peccaries and some swine (Suidae) (Frädrich, 1965, 1974; Eisenberg and Lockhart, 1972; Sowls, 1974), red deer *(Cervus elephas)* and wapiti *(C. canadensis)* (Darling, 1937; Altmann, 1956; Franklin, Mossman, and Doe, 1975), horses and most zebras (Equidae) (Joubert, 1972; Tyler, 1972; Klingel, 1974a; Feist and McCullough, 1975), some bats (Bradbury, 1977a; Bradbury and Vehrencamp, 1977), patas monkeys *(Erythrocebus patas)* (Hall, 1968), and hamadryas baboons *(Papio hamadryas)* (Kummer, 1968, 1971). In each case, female groups are cohesive and relatively small, presumably because single males can defend only groups that have these attributes. Perhaps, the most interesting questions pertain to the determinants of group size and cohesiveness, but these are beyond the scope of the present discussion. The most important factors in that regard are probably predation pressure, intensity of competition for resources, proclivities for parasite or disease transmission, resource distribution, and in social carnivores, prey type and size (see Crook, 1970, 1972; Denham, 1971; Kruuk, 1972; Schaller, 1972; Kleiman and Eisenberg, 1973; Alexander, 1974; Altmann, 1974; Estes, 1974; Geist, 1974; Wilson, 1975; Eaton, 1976a; Wittenberger, in press, a).

When female groups are not cohesive, males cannot defend exclusive mating opportunities with group members. Males may attempt to keep females together by herding them, but they rarely succeed when females persistently try to leave (e.g., Buechner and Schloeth, 1963; Estes, 1967; Jarman and Jarman, 1974; Kitchen, 1974; Leuthold, 1977). Since defending groups is ineffective, males adopt a different tactic. In lions, female prides fragment into small subgroups that share a common home range, and males defend the pride range against other males (Schaller, 1972; Rudnai, 1973; Bertram, 1975). In several antelopes discussed earlier, females frequently move from one group to another, and males defend favorable habitats where females are prone to congregate (Leuthold, 1977). Thus, these mating patterns are intermediate between territorial polygyny and harem polygyny.

When females form large social groups, competition between males is too intense for single males to control access to entire groups. The usual result is multimale groups or mixed-sexual herds (e.g., Crook, 1970; Geist, 1971; Kelsall, 1968; Eisenberg, Muckenhirn, and Rudran, 1972; Jolly, 1972; Leuthold, 1977). In lions, males form coalitions to defend female prides if prides are large, but not if prides are small (Schaller, 1972; Rudnai, 1973). Males do not compete for females within coalitions, possibly because a large number of copulations are required to achieve fertilization (Bertram, 1975, Eaton, 1976b). In ungulates and primates, males organize into dominance hierarchies, within which dominant males consort temporarily with receptive females or defend territories associated with female groups. The factors determining which alternative evolves are unclear and will be discussed in a later section.

POLYANDRY

Polyandry is so unusual that virtually any mating system where a female pairs with more than one male during a single breeding season has been termed *polyandrous,* regardless of whether males also pair with more than one female. Both males and females form multiple pair bonds of relatively short duration in most polyandrous systems, and such systems are more accurately referred to as *polygyny–polyandry* (Jenni, 1974) or *serial polygamy* (Pitelka *et al.,* 1974). True polyandry, in which one female is the exclusive mate of several males, is exceedingly rare and has been documented in the wild only for spotted sandpipers *(Actitis macularis)*, Tasmanian native hens *(Tribonyx mortierii)*, and jacanas (Jacanidae) (Jenni, 1974).

POLYGYNOUS–POLYANDROUS SYSTEMS

One type of polygynous–polyandrous system is best illustrated by the greater rhea *(Rhea americana)* (Bruning, 1973, 1974). Female rheas form loose flocks during the nonbreeding season, perhaps to facilitate foraging by stirring up insects (cf. Rand, 1954), and hence represent a defensible "resource" for males. Shortly before breeding commences, males contest for dominance status. The large nonbreeding flocks of females split into smaller flocks of 2–15 females, and each flock is defended by a dominant male. Within a few days after copulations begin, the male constructs a nest near which all females of the group will lay. Nests containing early eggs are often abandoned, until finally all females are ready to lay synchronously. Once every 2 days for 7–10 days, each female deposits an egg near the nest, with the male then rolling the egg into his nest. Males remain on the nest almost continuously once laying begins, except for midday feeding trips of 10–60 minutes, but they do not start incubating until about the 3rd day. Males become increasingly aggressive toward laying females, culminating in termination of laying by the 10th day. About that time, the females attract the notice of another male and leave to repeat the cycle with him. Each group of females mates with 10–12 males in succession, with each male assuming all parental duties at his nest.

The rhea mating system is best examined by considering the individual interests of males and females separately. Since female groups are a defensible "resource," males can increase their success by defending access to them as in harem polygynous systems. Once females begin laying, males have two options. They can allow each female to lay in its own nest and let her assume parental duties, or they can take over parental duties themselves. The former pattern occurs, for example, in red jungle fowl and peafowl (Delacour, 1951; Sharma,

1969, 1970, 1972). The problem is to explain why male rheas chase away the females and undertake parental care without female assistance. By not taking over incubation duties, a male could remain with his original harem to fertilize replacement clutches, or he could abandon his harem to seek additional mates elsewhere. Opportunities for finding new mates seem high because many nests fail. Moreover, males accept a greater risk of failure, it seems, by incubating all the eggs in a single nest. Nests are often abandoned if even one egg rots and explodes (Bruning, 1973, 1974), so a male might achieve higher success by not putting all his eggs in one nest.

An important factor is the very low success rate for late clutches. Few late nests are successful because high daytime temperatures overheat eggs and cause nest abandonment (Bruning, 1973, 1974). Males deserting to find new mates therefore have little chance to augment their success. But why males should encourage laying in a single nest is less clear. One possibility is that females would not be able to attend their own nests adequately by themselves because of the energetic drain of egg production. Lower attendance by each female at her nest may lead to a higher rate of egg failure due to overheating than occurs when the male performs all incubation duties in a common nest. Since female energetics during laying has not been studied, this hypothesis remains to be tested.

Females clearly benefit by abandoning their first clutch. At best a female can lay only five or six hatchable eggs in a single nest (Bruning, 1973, 1974). With males assuming incubation duties, females can lay many more eggs than would otherwise be possible. Nevertheless, female desertion is evidently a response to male aggressiveness and not the cause underlying male assumption of parental duties. Desertion would obviously not be advantageous to females were it not for the propensity of males to provide the necessary parental care once they leave. The central and as yet unanswered question is therefore why males should chase off females and perform all parental duties by themselves. Perhaps a comparative study of rheas and ostriches (*Struthio camelus*) would be instructive, as the dominant female in each harem of ostriches remains and helps the male care for the eggs laid by the entire harem in a shared nest (Sauer and Sauer, 1966).

The polygynous–polyandrous systems of tinamous are less well studied, but they follow a similar pattern. In the brushland tinamou *(Nothoprocta cinerascens)* and Boucard's tinamou *(Crypturellus boucardi)*, territorial males attract a group of two to four females to their territories, and each female lays one egg in a common nest (Lancaster, 1964a,b). The female group then moves on to another male territory while the male incubates the eggs. In the variegated tinamou, a single female lays one egg for each territorial male before moving on to the next male, so the element of polygyny is absent (Beebe, 1925). In the highland tinamou *(Nothocercus bonapartei)*, each territorial male attracts a harem of two or three. Each female lays one egg in a common nest, which the male tends alone, but the females remain with the male to lay replacement clutches, so the element of polyandry is absent (Schäfer, 1954).

The tinamou pattern differs from that of rheas in at least three important respects. Male tinamous are territorial and advertise for females instead of defending female groups; the period of successful breeding is prolonged instead of relatively brief; and males do not aggressively chase females away from their nests. The costs and benefits associated with desertion may be very different for tinamous. Females gain substantial benefits by deserting *if* deserted males will incubate their eggs, because deserting minimizes the exposure of each egg to predation (since incubation begins immediately) and it may allow females to lay more eggs each season than would otherwise be possible. Deserted males can either advertise for a new female(s) or incubate the clutch left behind by the deserting female (or perhaps both). The reason that males choose the latter option is uncertain, but it is presumably related to a low probability of attracting new mates (note that in ancestral populations where female desertion is rare, new mates probably would not be deserters). Beebe (1925) found an 80/20 sex ratio among 40 specimens of variegated tinamous that he collected. If his sample is representative, males would indeed have difficulty finding new mates. The origin of such an imbalance in the sex ratio, if it exists, is unknown. Tinamous are exceedingly difficult birds to study in the wild because of their secretive habits, and as a result, very few data are currently available for testing hypotheses related to their mating systems.

   The other type of polygynous–polyandrous system appears quite different from the above. In several shorebird species, females lay a complete clutch for one male and then desert to produce a second and sometimes additional clutches with other males (Jenni, 1974). In sanderlings *(Calidris alba)*, Temminck's stints *(C. temminckii)*, mountain plovers *(Eupoda montana)*, northern phalaropes *(Lobipes lobatus)*, and rarely dotterels *(Eudromias morinellus)*, males incubate deserted clutches, though only after they spend several days seeking new mates, while females incubate their last clutches (Hildèn, 1965b; Parmelee, 1970; Hildèn and Vuolanto, 1972; Raner, 1972; Graul, 1973; Nethersole-Thompson, 1973; Parmelee and Payne, 1973). In spotted sandpipers, sex ratios are skewed toward excess males, and a polyandrous female's first mate incubates her first clutch alone, while her last mate helps her incubate her final clutch (Hays, 1972; Oring and Knudson, 1972; Oring and Maxson, 1978). Double-clutching with one sex caring for each nest also occurs in red-legged partridge *(Alectoris rufa)*, scaled quail *(Callipepla squamata)*, and California quail *(Lophortyx californicus)* (Goodwin, 1953; Jenkins, 1957; Schemnitz, 1961; McMillan, 1964; Francis, 1965; Anthony, 1970). Females of these species usually do not change mates between clutches, but Jenkins (1957) provided some evidence that one female red-legged partridge did change mates between successive clutches.

   The polygynous–polyandrous system of shorebirds evidently results from females' deserting their first clutches to lay a second one with a new mate. Two questions are of paramount interest. Under what environmental conditions should females desert, and why should deserted males assume parental responsibilities? The two questions are interrelated because the costs incurred by deserting females are always prohibitive unless deserted males are prone to rear abandoned clutches. The conditions favoring male assumption of parental duties will therefore be examined first.

   Graul *et al.* (1977) argued that males should be more likely to rear a deserted clutch if they have a low probability of attracting additional mates and a high

confidence of paternity, if females make a large initial investment in eggs, and if males have a high probability of raising the brood without assistance. However, confidence of paternity and the size of female investments are not crucial. If confidence of paternity is low, the benefits of remaining with a brood are less, but they could still exceed the benefits gained by leaving. In polyandrous American jacanas, for example, females copulate with several males on a single day, so confidence of paternity must be low (Jenni and Collier, 1972). The same argument applies to the size of a female's investment in eggs. Even if a male's chances of rearing a brood are reduced when a female lays small eggs, his best option may still be to remain and attempt to raise a deserted clutch. In most multiple-clutching shorebirds, females lay smaller clutches than strictly monogamous species, and yet deserted males remain with the first clutch (Hildèn, 1965b; Graul, 1973; Parmelee and Payne, 1973; Jenni, 1974).

Probably a critical factor for shorebirds is the limited opportunity for males to attract new mates (Parmelee and Payne, 1973). Mating seasons generally last only a couple of weeks in the Arctic, so males can delay incubation of the first clutch until most mating opportunities disappear. The polygynous–polyandrous system of Temminck's stints and sanderlings fits this pattern (Hildèn, 1965b; Parmelee, 1970; Parmelee and Payne, 1973). In mountain plovers, males also take advantage of additional mating opportunities by delaying incubation for several days (Graul, 1973), but the breeding season lasts longer for mountain plovers than it does for Arctic sandpipers (see Bailey and Niedrach, 1965). A potentially important factor in mountain plovers, as well as in quail and partridges, may be the propensity for females to remain with their original mates to lay their second clutches (Emlen and Oring, 1977). A female may be more prone to stay if the male has begun incubating her first clutch. Breeding seasons are even more prolonged in the spotted sandpiper. Polyandry in this species occurs in conjunction with female-biased sex ratios, and both the number of polyandrous females and the number of successive mates obtained by particular females are correlated with the degree of imbalance in the sex ratio (Hays, 1972; Oring and Knudson, 1972). A skewed sex ratio would limit mating opportunities for males, but the origin of this skew has not yet been determined.

Given a male propensity to rear deserted clutches, females should be most likely to desert when they can quickly recoup their energetic losses and garner energy for a second clutch or when they can add substantially to their survival prospects. In addition, female desertion should be likely only if single parents have a high probability of raising clutches unaided. Arctic shorebirds must attend eggs for most of the day to prevent chilling, especially during adverse weather (Norton, 1972), so adults must be able to find enough food for themselves in short foraging bouts if they are to succeed as single parents. Both preconditions suggest that female desertion and double-clutching should be associated with unusually abundant food resources. Indirect evidence indicates that polygynous–polyandrous systems based on double-clutching are usually associated with spatially clumped and locally abundant food resources in shorebirds, but direct measures of food availability are lacking (Graul, 1973, 1976; Pitelka *et al.*, 1974). Studies of food availability and the time–energy budgets of incubating adults are still needed to elucidate this problem.

Simultaneous Polyandry

309

EVOLUTION OF
MATING SYSTEMS IN
BIRDS AND
MAMMALS

The polyandrous mating system of Tasmanian native hens, a relative of rails and gallinules, is apparently unique among birds (Ridpath, 1972). One or two males (and sometimes even three or four males) defend a jointly held territory within the breeding marsh and pair with a single female. The males on each territory are usually siblings, although sometimes they are unrelated. Males remain with their parents for a year and then try to take over a neighboring territory as a group. Successful sibling groups usually pair with a young female that was raised on their newly acquired territory. Every male copulates with the female, and all participate in incubation and care of the chicks. Paternity is not spread equally, however, as one male usually dominates the other(s) and obtains a disproportionate share of the copulations. Since sex ratios are skewed toward excess males, several males can potentially associate with each female without leaving any females unmated.

The problem is to explain why the dominant male of each sibling group does not exclude the other(s). Males gain some benefit from the help of a second male, since trios rear more young than pairs (Ridpath, 1972), but they also suffer increased sperm competition. Maynard Smith and Ridpath (1972) calculated the threshold conditions that would favor toleration of related and unrelated subordinate males on the territory and concluded that the threshold is exceeded only when the males are related. The calculated threshold for related males is given by $n_2 > 1\frac{1}{3}n_1 + \frac{2}{3}n_3$, where n_2 = lifetime reproductive output of trios, n_1 = lifetime reproductive output of pairs, and n_3 = lifetime reproductive output of excluded males. The calculated threshold for unrelated males is given by $n_2 > 2n_1$. Annual reproductive rates for yearlings and adults are given in Table III. The replacement rate of territory occupants indicates that territory residency averages one to four years, so the ratio n_2/n_1 = 1.26 to 1.45. Since excluded males have little opportunity to breed elsewhere, n_3 is approximately zero. Thus, n_2/n_1 exceeds the calculated threshold for related males but not for unrelated males. These data therefore seem to support the conclusion that a dominant male tolerates another male on the territory only because the two males are related. However, the situation is probably not this simple.

Based on the data in Table III, the optimal male strategy should be to tolerate a brother for one year and then eject him from the territory. The ratio n_2/n_1 = 1.18 for adults, which no longer exceeds the calculated threshold for either related or unrelated males. Thus, an important factor has apparently been overlooked.

TABLE III. REPRODUCTIVE SUCCESS OF TASMANIAN NATIVE HENS IN RELATION TO MALE AGE WITHIN SIBLING GROUPS[a]

Number of adults	Mature groups		First-year groups	
	N	Surviving young	N	Surviving young
Pair	22	5.5 ± 0.63	15	1.1 ± 0.32
Trio	24	6.5 ± 0.72	7	3.1 ± 0.64

[a]Data are from Maynard Smith and Ridpath (1972).

In a system where habitats are in short supply and many males cannot breed, a coalition of two or more males has a better chance of obtaining and retaining a territory than a single male. The scarcity of breeding habitats available to Tasmanian native hens gives male coalitions a competitive advantage, and the prolonged association of male siblings on natal territories facilitates their formation. The situation is analogous to that of lions, except in native hens, increased competition between males is caused by habitat scarcity instead of increased size of female groups.

Selection for male coalitions may even explain why the sex ratio is skewed. Producing more sons increases the chances that at least two or three will survive to maturity, while producing fewer daughters has relatively little adverse effect on fitness because only one daughter can inherit the parental territory anyway and other daughters have little chance of breeding elsewhere. Since the sex ratio is skewed among juveniles as well as adults, the excess of males cannot be explained by differential mortality among breeding adults.

Polyandry in the American jacana has apparently evolved in a fashion comparable to territorial polygyny. Jacanas, or "lily trotters," are pond-dwelling "shorebirds" that glean insects by walking on top of floating vegetation in ponds and by searching in the grass of nearby lawns (Jenni and Collier, 1972). Breeding occurs only on territories around pond margins. Each male defends its own territory against other males and, with less success, against intruding females, while each female defends a larger territory that encompasses the territories of several males. The typical roles of the sexes are reversed, with females larger and more aggressive than males. Females lay a clutch for each male and replace clutches that are lost. Males incubate eggs and care for chicks with little or no aid from the female (Jenni and Betts, 1978). Breeding occurs all year at Turrialba, Costa Rica, where Jenni and Collier worked, but it is highly seasonal in most areas (Orians, personal communication). Suitable breeding habitat appears limited, as a sizable proportion of both the male and the female population is nonterritorial and hence not breeding at any given time. Polyandry in the Turrialba population seems to result because relatively few females can defend all suitable breeding habitats, a situation parallel to territorial polygyny in birds and mammals that breed in discrete habitat patches or colonies. Jenni and Collier (1972) conducted their study in a landscaped area, but Jenni and Betts (1978) have also observed polyandry in less disturbed areas.

The mating system of pheasant-tailed jacanas (*Hydrophasianus chirurgas*) may resemble that of American jacanas, but it is less well studied. Female pheasant-tailed jacanas lay clutches for several males in succession and replace lost clutches of previous mates (Hoffman, 1949, 1950), but details of spacing behavior and mating relationships are not yet known. Cursory observations of groups consisting of one female and two males suggest that polyandry also occurs in bronze-winged jacanas (*Metopidius indicus*) and the greater African jacana (*Actophilornis africana*), but copulations between the female and both males of each group have not been documented (Mathew, 1964; Vernon, 1973).

Since desertion enables female jacanas to lay more eggs, it could be advantageous if females can eliminate other mating opportunities open to males. Deserted male jacanas would have little chance of establishing new territories elsewhere because breeding sites are scarce, but they could theoretically attempt to attract a new mate to their territories. Advertising for a new mate instead of incubating a deserted clutch might be advantageous unless the deserting female can prevent her prior mates from obtaining other females. A female could do this by defending a large territory that encompasses the territories of all her mates. Defending a large territory and still laying successive clutches is energetically costly and would be prohibitive unless food is unusually abundant. Jacanas breed in ponds, where insect abundance is likely to be high, but the abundance of their food resources has not been measured. One might predict that jacanas are restricted to highly productive ponds or are monogamous in less productive ones. The latter possibility seems most likely since the wattled jacana (*Jacana jacana*) is monogamous in some areas and polyandrous in others (Osborne and Bourne, 1977).

In the population studied by Jenni and Collier (1972), females do limit male mating opportunities by defending larger territories than males, but this capability is based on the larger size and the more aggressive disposition of females. It is difficult to see how females could defend larger territories than males before sex role reversal evolved. Since breeding appears highly seasonal in most areas (Orians, personal communication), female desertion and sex role reversal may have originated because male mating opportunities were limited by short mating periods. Additional research in undisturbed environments will be needed before this possibility can be evaluated further.

PROMISCUITY

THEORY

The evolution of promiscuity *per se* has evoked little interest except for birds, because promiscuity in one form or another was the primordial mode of sexual reproduction. When neither sex contributes parental care following fertilization, prolonged pair bonding usually has little intrinsic value for either sex. Prolonged association of the sexes can evolve in the absence of parental care if the two sexes share a common territory, as occurs in some species of coral reef fish that broadcast their spawn into the pelagic zone (Federn, 1968; Low, 1971; Barlow, 1974; Reese, 1975), but the mating system apparently remains promiscuous when this occurs. The most interesting questions arise when parental contributions from at least one sex are obligatory for offspring survival. With the advent of obligatory parental care, females gain the potential for acquiring protection or direct energetic contributions from the male. Since female fecundity is generally limited by energetic constraints, females should take advantage of every opportunity to exploit male assistance. The problem in mammals and birds, which have obligatory parental care, is to identify the conditions that allow females to take advantage of male assistance. Promiscuity should evolve only when opportunities for gaining male assistance are absent or when the costs of taking advantage of them are too high. Such opportunities are generally lacking in amphibians and reptiles, with a few notable exceptions (e.g., Oliver, 1956; Lutz, 1960; Wells, 1977), and as a result these species are nearly all promiscuous.

From a female's point of view, the distinction between shareable and non-shareable parental assistance is vital. Shareable parental care can be distributed among several sets of offspring without detracting from the quality or quantity of care received by each set, while nonshareable parental care cannot (Figure 10). Male guarding of egg masses in fish appears to be a shareable form of parental care, while guarding of fry is not (Perrone, 1975). When males only guard eggs, fish are generally promiscuous, but when males also help guard fry, they are monogamous (Perrone and Zaret, in press). A female has little to gain by remaining with a male if only eggs are guarded, and by deserting the male, she can garner energy for laying another clutch. Male help in guarding fry, and hence monogamy, is associated with short breeding seasons, which preclude opportunities for breeding again elsewhere for both sexes.

A similar argument can be made for many mammals and precocial birds. When males contribute little more than vigilance for predators, a shareable type of parental care, females lose little by sharing a male with other females. When males make major contributions of nonshareable parental care, as in some carnivores, monogamy is more likely to prevail. Since in most mammals, the potential for nonshareable male parental contributions is less than in birds, the prevalence of promiscuity in mammals is not surprising. The most interesting problem in mammals concerns how the various kinds of promiscuity have evolved.

MAMMALS

Overlap promiscuity (see Table I) is a direct consequence of solitary habits and at least temporarily overlapping male and female home ranges. In rodents, insectivores, and various other mammals, solitary habits are associated with nocturnal activity patterns and densely vegetated habitats (Eisenberg, 1966). Females of these species depend on secretive behavior and concealment for protection, and

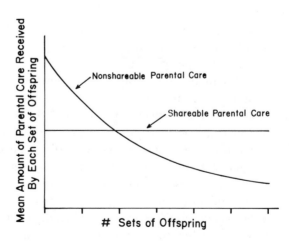

Fig. 10. The difference between shareable and nonshareable parental care. If parental care is shareable, the presence of additional sets of offspring does not reduce the amount of care received by the other sets of offspring.

the best way to maximize concealment is to remain solitary. Promiscuity appears advantageous because males can contribute little parental care or vigilance and their presence renders concealment tactics less effective.

Solitary habits and promiscuity have evolved in most cats for a similar reason (Kleiman and Eisenberg, 1973; Eaton, 1976a). The principal difference is that cats are ambush predators and depend on stealth for capturing prey rather than concealment for avoiding predators. In cheetahs *(Acinonyx jubatus)*, females remain solitary even though males are often social (Eaton, 1974, 1976a). Since male groups are more efficient at capturing prey, other factors must make solitary hunting advantageous for females. Cheetahs cannot prevent hyenas *(Crocuta crocuta)* from stealing kills, but they may reduce their chances of attracting hyenas by hunting alone. Competition for food at kills may also favor solitary hunting, especially when females are accompanied by cubs. Males apparently remain in (sibling) groups to enhance mating success, as males in groups enjoy higher success than single males. Female cats might potentially benefit from males' helping to feed cubs, but they have little opportunity for acquiring help. A female would have no way to prevent a male from deserting her except by accompanying him everywhere he goes, and this would reduce her hunting efficiency and interfere with caring for young cubs.

Overlap promiscuity may also arise in territorial species if energetic constraints make individual territories more advantageous than jointly held ones. Promiscuity is especially likely to evolve when males cannot contribute nonshareable forms of parental care. In tree squirrels *(Tamiasciurus)*, male and female territories are nonoverlapping for energetic reasons related to food-storing behavior, and males visit females only briefly to mate (Smith, 1968).

Arena promiscuity and hierarchical promiscuity are common mating systems in social mammals, but the conditions favoring one type over the other are poorly understood. Arena promiscuity is especially prevalent in African antelopes (Leuthold, 1977; Owen-Smith, 1977). Males of the most gregarious species commonly defend territories that serve only to attract mates. Their territories are not centered in habitats preferred by females, and males generally lose weight while defending them. The reasons that males defend territories instead of entering female groups are obscure. Owen-Smith (1977) suggested that territoriality might be a better strategy than establishing dominance hierarchies when large predators abound because males may be less susceptible to injury in territorial disputes. This argument is less than compelling. There is no evidence that territory defense is less injury-prone than status defense, and one might even expect males to survive better by remaining within the protective confines of a social group when predation pressure is high. Geist (1974) suggested that territory defense can evolve only when female groups have low mobility, but his evidence comes from species in which males defend favorable habitats where females forage. Males should have difficulty attracting nomadic females to static locations, but male wildebeest *(Connochaetes taurinus)* defend temporary territories while following nomadic female herds (Estes, 1969). Other factors must be involved in any case, since males of the sedentary Cape buffalo *(Syncerus caffer)* establish dominance hierarchies (Sinclair, 1974, 1977).

One factor may be the stability of group membership. Large ungulate herds tend to be incohesive, and stable male dominance hierarchies may be ineffectual in controlling access to receptive females when group composition is continually changing. When herd membership is transitory, females can identify a superior male more easily by selecting a territorial male than by selecting an unfamiliar male with uncertain status within the herd. A strong propensity for females to select territorial males would favor arena promiscuity even when territorial males survive less well than males remaining inside herds. The fact that Cape buffalo are unusual among African ungulates in forming both stable herds and male dominance hierarchies favors this hypothesis. The importance of group stability is also indicated by a comparison of equid mating systems. Feral horses and most zebras are harem polygynous, with females forming closed social groups that are defended by a dominant stallion (Joubert, 1972; Tyler, 1972; Klingel, 1974a; Feist and McCullough, 1975). However, in African and Asiatic wild asses *(Equus africanus* and *E. hemionus)*, females do not form stable social groups, and males defend territories instead of females (Klingel, 1977). This is also true of Grevy's zebra *(E. grevyi)* and feral donkeys (Klingel, 1974b; Moehlman, 1974). Mountain sheep *(Ovis canadensis)*, American bison *(Bison bison)*, and caribou *(Rangifer arcticus)* are exceptional, in that group membership is unstable and males defend receptive females within the herd one at a time instead of defending territories (McHugh, 1958; Lent, 1965; Kelsall, 1968; Geist, 1971). In at least mountain sheep, horn size acts as a highly visible signal of dominance rank that overcomes problems associated with unfamiliarity between group members. Territory defense may be prohibitively costly in mountain sheep because they depend on proximity to rock escarpments and early warning to escape wolves.

Hierarchical promiscuity has evolved in cohesive female groups that are too large for single males to defend (see earlier discussion). It is most prevalent in social primates (Crook, 1970; Jolly, 1972; Eisenberg *et al.,* 1972). Male reproductive strategies within social groups appear complicated. For example, in savanna baboons *(Papio cynocephalus)*, dominant males consort with females during periods of peak receptivity, while subordinate males consort with females in early and late stages of estrus (Hausfater, 1975). Infanticide is employed by males who have recently taken control of female groups in several species of primates and in lions (Blaffer Hrdy, 1974, 1977; Bertram, 1975; Angst and Thommen, 1977). Numerous studies show that male dominance status is correlated with copulatory success (e.g., DeVore, 1965, 1971; Geist, 1971; Hausfater, 1975; Bernstein, 1976), but recent evidence suggests that females exercise some choice in selecting mates within multimale primate troops (Dixson, Everitt, Herbert, Rugman, and Scruton, 1973; Eaton, 1973; Hausfater, 1975; Lindburg, 1975; Seyfarth, 1978).

PRECOCIAL BIRDS

The young of many precocial birds become capable of foraging for themselves soon after hatching, so males have less potential for contributing nonshareable parental investment than males of altricial birds. Nevertheless, males can assist in incubation and guarding of chicks. At least two general hypotheses for explaining why females accept the cost of losing male parental care are possible. They will be examined here with respect to grouse, the best studied of all promiscuous birds.

Wiley (1974) suggested that grouse are promiscuous when males and females have differing optimal life-history schedules. If delayed breeding is more advantageous for males than for females, a female-biased breeding sex ratio would develop, and females would have to mate promiscuously or not at all. Delayed breeding is most likely to evolve in long-lived species because high longevity provides more opportunities for future reproduction (Pianka, 1970; Stearns, 1976; Wittenberger, in press, b). Using a parallel argument, Wiley (1974) proposed that males of promiscuous grouse delay breeding longer than females, a condition he termed "sexual bimaturism," because males have higher expected longevity than females. He attributed the higher longevity of males to their larger body size. Large size could reduce male vulnerability to predation, since fewer predators are capable of capturing larger prey sizes, and it could create a better energy balance by reducing winter heat loss and lowering basal metabolic rates. Large size would not benefit females to the same extent because it would conflict energetically with egg production. The problems with Wiley's sexual bimaturism hypothesis are reviewed elsewhere (Wittenberger, 1978a) and will be summarized here.

The sexual bimaturism hypothesis reverses the usually accepted causal relationship between promiscuity and sexual size dimorphism. According to sexual selection theory, the larger size of males evolves as a response to the intensified competition for mates experienced by males of promiscuous and polygynous species and is deleterious to male survival (Amadon, 1959; Selander, 1965, 1972; Orians, 1969). The evidence for grouse conforms to the sexual selection theory and conflicts with Wiley's hypothesis. Several species of promiscuous grouse are no more dimorphic in size than monogamous grouse (data in Johnsgaard, 1973; Wiley, 1974), showing that sexual size dimorphism is not a necessary prerequisite for promiscuity to evolve. More importantly, males do not survive better than females in dimorphic species. Deviations from a 50/50 sex ratio are thought to reflect differential mortality rates between the sexes (Trivers, 1972), and nonjuvenile sex ratios in grouse are negatively correlated with the degree of sexual size dimorphism (Wittenberger, 1978a). This finding implies that increased male size is detrimental to male survival. Sex ratio data for grouse may be biased by hunter selectivity, but most of the data used for the analysis were not based on hunter kills.

Wiley's (1974) hypothesis also reverses the usually accepted causal relationship between promiscuity and sexual bimaturism. It implies that young male grouse defer breeding because the predation risks and energetic costs entailed in immediate breeding are too high and not because they cannot compete with older males for mates. If this interpretation is correct, removal of adult males should not induce young males to breed. Removal experiments have been performed on blue grouse *(Dendragapus obscurus)* (Bendell and Elliott, 1966, 1967; Bendell, King, and Mossop, 1972; Zwickel, 1972), ruffed grouse *(Bonasa umbellus)* (Boag and Sumanik, 1969; Rusch and Keith, 1971; Fischer and Keith, 1974), and sharp-tailed grouse *(Pedioecetes phasianellus)* (Rippin and Boag, 1974), and in every study, yearling males entered the removal area, established territories, and began advertising for mates. Even in the absence of experimental removals, yearling males have been reported breeding in ruffed grouse, sharp-tailed grouse, and greater prairie chickens *(Tympanuchus cupido)* (Marshall, 1965; Hjorth, 1970; Hamerstrom, 1972). The best interpretation of these data is that young males generally defer breeding because they cannot compete with older males and not because earlier breeding detracts from their survival prospects.

As an alternative hypothesis, Wittenberger (1978a) proposed that female grouse derive a net benefit from promiscuity. Males of monogamous grouse make two contributions to female success: they defend territories where females forage, and they provide continual vigilance while females forage. Females of monogamous species gain these benefits primarily during the early spring laying period, as males of most monogamous grouse are prone to desert during the incubation period. Males of monogamous grouse provide vigilance for incubating females in several populations, but they never incubate eggs and they help guard chicks in only a few populations.

Promiscuity might therefore evolve when the benefits gained by females from male defense of resources and male vigilance for predators are less than the costs of associating continuously with a male. Remaining with a male is likely to make a female more conspicuous to predators, especially during male disputes over females, so prolonged pair bonding could be deleterious to female survival (Braestrup, 1963; Crook, 1964). Male defense of food resources and male vigilance should allow females to garner energy for making eggs at a faster rate. Females should therefore benefit most from pair bonding when food resources are scarce during laying. Thus, monogamy might be expected when food resources are scarce during spring, especially in relatively open environments where concealment is a poor defense against predators, while promiscuity might be expected when food resources are more abundant and when cover is more available for foraging females.

Evidence on food availability is for the most part lacking, but the available evidence is consistent with this hypothesis. In the monogamous red grouse *(Lagopus l. lagopus),* both the quantity and the nutritive quality of heather food resources are limited for laying females, and both affect female reproductive success (Moss, 1969; Watson and Moss, 1972; Moss, Watson, and Parr, 1975). In comparison, all grouse that exploit conifer needles, an apparently superabundant food resource, are promiscuous. Several studies suggest that food availability for these species is not limited by the nutritive quality of conifer needles (Zwickel and Bendell, 1967, 1972; Ellison, 1976). Standard laboratory analyses for proteins, carbohydrates, fats, and numerous trace minerals revealed no differences between needles taken from preferred foraging sites and those taken from other parts of the same tree. Food intake rates may be limited by the rate at which conifer needles can be digested or by the accumulation of secondary plant toxins from the needles (cf. Rhoades and Cates, 1976). In either event, females would not be able to increase their food intake by associating with a male and relying on his vigilance. At present, the evidence is only suggestive. More data are needed concerning female energetics and food availability for both monogamous and promiscuous grouse, particularly those with more diversified diets.

Promiscuity has been reported in only a few other precocial birds. It occurs in the great snipe *(Gallinago media)* (Swanberg, 1965; Ferdinand, 1966), the American woodcock *(Philohela minor)* (Pitelka, 1943; Sheldon, 1967), the ruff *(Philoma-*

chus pugnax) (Hogan-Warburg, 1966), the pectoral sandpiper *(Calidris melanotos)* (Pitelka, 1959; Pitelka *et al.,* 1974), and the buff-breasted sandpiper *(Tryngites subruficollis)* (Pitelka *et al.,* 1974) among shorebirds, in Argus pheasants *(Rheinartia* and *Argusianus)* (Beebe, 1926; Delacour, 1951) among gallinaceous birds, in some populations of the great bustard *(Otis tarda)* (Gewalt, 1959; Lukschanderl, 1971) and little bustard *(O. tetrax)* (Dement'ev and Gladkov, 1967), and in Muscovy ducks *(Gairina moschata)* and musk ducks *(Biziura lobata)* among waterfowl (Delacour, 1954–1964; Johnsgaard, 1965; Lack, 1968). Pitelka *et al.* (1974) associated promiscuity in shorebirds with spatiotemporally variable food resources and an opportunistic breeding strategy. If food resources are indefensible, females would not be in a position to prevent males from deserting no matter how beneficial prolonged pair bonding might be. This argument will be developed more fully in the next section.

ALTRICIAL BIRDS

Aside from brood parasites, most promiscuous altricial birds are frugivorous, although one species eats seeds and another eats insects (Van Someren, 1945; Lack, 1968; Murray, 1969). Nearly three-fourths of all frugivorous species are monogamous (Lack, 1968), but many of these live in temperate environments. Fruiting seasons are generally more synchronous in temperate latitudes because of the greater seasonality of climate. In addition, the peak fruiting season generally occurs after most frugivorous birds are finished with nesting, so temperate frugivores usually feed insects to their nestlings (Morton, 1973). Tropical forests have more prolonged fruiting seasons, and the seasons for different trees are often staggered to alleviate competition for seed dispersers (Smythe, 1970; D. W. Snow, 1971a). As a result, tropical frugivores generally feed fruit as well as insects to their nestlings. This difference in nestling diet is crucial in explaining why promiscuity is prevalent only in tropical frugivores.

The problem in explaining promiscuity in altricial birds is that females seem to suffer a high cost from lost male parental assistance without gaining any apparent benefits in return. Some authors have therefore argued that the cost to females is actually minimal in frugivorous species. They argue that clutch sizes are limited by the low protein content of fruit rather than by the ability of the parents to feed nestlings and that the abundance of fruit enables females to feed nestlings adequately without male assistance (D. W. Snow, 1962a; Orians, 1969; B. K. Snow, 1970; see also Willis, Wechsler, and Oniki, 1978). Since males would gain little by helping females, they would be "emancipated" from parental responsibilities and free to seek additional mates. Females would also gain from promiscuity because they would then be able to mate with higher-quality males.

The male-emancipation hypothesis implies that clutch sizes are limited by the ability of parents to feed nestlings in monogamous species but not in promiscuous species. Otherwise, males should also be emancipated from parental duties in the monogamous species. The hypothesis therefore hinges on the factors limiting clutch sizes in tropical birds.

Clutch sizes are consistently lower in tropical birds than in related high-latitude species (Cody, 1966; Klomp, 1970). The underlying reasons for this trend are controversial. Skutch (1949) attributed the lower clutch size of tropical species to higher predation rates on nests. He argued that larger clutch sizes would necessitate more parental visits to the nest and hence make the nest more conspicuous to predators. However, the percentage of manakin nests lost to predators is the same during incubation and nestling periods despite a fourfold increase in parental visitation rates, suggesting that most predators find nests by searching in likely locations rather than by watching parent birds (D. W. Snow, 1962a; Lack, 1966). Similarly, Ricklefs (1969) found that predation rates averaged 1.2% lower per day during the nestling period than during the incubation period for the species studied by Skutch. This reduction during the nestling period undoubtedly resulted from the early destruction of the most easily found nests (Ricklefs, 1977a). Thus, an increase in parental feeding trips evidently has little effect on nest vulnerability. In addition, clutch sizes are just as low for tropical hole-nesting species and pendant-nesting species, even though their nests are less vulnerable to predation (Lack, 1966). If predation is the main factor, the trend toward lower clutch sizes in the tropics should not extend to these species.

As an alternative, Lack (1947–1948, 1954) maintained that clutch sizes are limited in the tropics by the maximum rate at which parents can feed nestlings. Skutch (1949, 1967) questioned Lack's views because tropical birds feed young at much slower rates than temperate birds, they often spend considerable periods in apparent idleness instead of feeding nestlings, and they are invariably capable of stepping up their feeding rate when broods are unusually large (see also Foster, 1974). Moreover, brood sizes are generally the same regardless of whether one or both parents feed the young, even though two parents should be able to feed the young twice as fast as one. Thus, Lack's hypothesis also appears inadequate.

A recent revision of Lack's hypothesis provides one plausible explanation for low clutch sizes in tropical birds (Snow and Lill, 1974; see also Charnov and Krebs, 1974; Ricklefs, 1977a, b). Lack's hypothesis was based on maximizing annual reproductive rates rather than lifetime reproductive output. Since increased reproductive effort is likely to detract from survival prospects (Goodman, 1974; Pianka and Parker, 1975), smaller clutch sizes can evolve if the lower annual reproductive effort leads to a sufficient increase in expected longevity. Future reproductive output would then compensate for the reduction in immediate effort. Since most tropical birds are apparently longer-lived than temperate species (Snow and Lill, 1974), their lower clutch sizes may well represent a shift in their optimal life-history strategies.

A second plausible hypothesis is also a modification of Lack's views. Owen (1977) suggested that higher species diversity of food items makes foraging more difficult in the tropics than in temperate regions, thus reducing the number of young that parent birds can support. This hypothesis is built on the assumption that the formation of search images augments foraging efficiency in birds. Greater prey diversity in the tropics would necessitate more frequent changing of search images and hence reduce foraging efficiency. Owen suggested that the periods of apparent idleness spent by tropical birds represent periods of uncertainty caused by rapidly changing search images. This argument is unconvincing, as these periods are often prolonged rather than transitory ones within feeding bouts, so

Owen's hypothesis cannot account for clutches that are apparently less than the maximum supportable by the parents.

While neither hypothesis has been proved, both imply that any loss of male parental assistance would be costly to females. According to the first hypothesis, females would either lose part of their annual reproductive success or they would have to compensate for lost male assistance at the expense of reduced future survival prospects. According to the second hypothesis, females would suffer an immediate reduction in reproductive output. In addition, clutch sizes of promiscuous tropical frugivores are no lower than those of related monogamous insectivores, so special dietary constraints such as protein deficiencies cannot explain why the loss of male help might be less costly in frugivores than in insectivores. The male-emancipation hypothesis seems invalid, and a new hypothesis is needed.

Promiscuity can theoretically evolve despite its being detrimental to female fitness if selection favors male desertion following copulation. A deserted female has the choice of either raising the brood by herself or seeking a new mate. In an ancestral population where most males are not deserters, a deserted female would have difficulty finding a new mate other than another desertion-prone male, because more faithful males would be busy caring for the broods of their own mates. Deserted females should therefore rear their broods instead of seeking new mates. Thus, conditions favoring male desertion could lead to promiscuity.

Males should desert their mates when opportunities for new matings lead to greater reproductive success than can be achieved by helping a current mate care for offspring. When food resources are economically defensible, selection favors male territory defense (Brown, 1964, 1975). A deserting male would then have to abandon his territory as well as his mate, and he would have to establish a new territory elsewhere before he could hope to mate again. Since establishing a new territory would be difficult, especially in the tropics where few suitable habitats are ever vacant, deserting males would have few opportunities to mate again. Promiscuity is therefore unlikely when food resources are defensible, and in fact few species with multipurpose territories are promiscuous.

Fruit resources are often spatiotemporally clumped and therefore economically indefensible (cf. Brown, 1964; Horn, 1968; Klein and Klein, 1975). In addition, suitable nest sites of noncolonial birds generally appear unlimited in availability and hence not worth defending. This combination removes a major constraint that ordinarily precludes male desertion, namely, the necessity to control resources required by females in order to attract mates. Because males of many tropical frugivorous birds need not defend any resources required by females, a deserting male would have little difficulty finding a place where he can profitably advertise for new mates. Males of tropical frugivores also have a good chance of attracting new mates because nests frequently fail and females generally breed several times each season (e.g., D. W. Snow, 1962a; B. K. Snow, 1970). Females have no way of distinguishing between males prone to desert and those prone to feed nestlings, so they cannot enforce monogamy through their mating preferences. Thus, the combination of indefensible resources and long breeding seasons could favor male desertion and hence promiscuity among tropical frugivores.

If this hypothesis is valid, it should also explain why some tropical frugivores are monogamous. Several tropical birds are monogamous even though they feed fruit to nestlings and do not defend their food resources.

The oilbird *(Steatornis caripensis)* is colonial and nests deep in caves (D. W. Snow, 1961–1962). Young oilbirds develop slowly and cannot thermoregulate until they reach 3 weeks of age. The low ambient temperatures inside nesting caves make continuous brooding by a parent necessary for nestling survival. Desertion by a male would therefore lead to almost certain nest failure.

Male parental care also appears essential to nestling survival in hornbills *(Bycanistes brevis)*. Females remain inside the nest cavity throughout the incubation and nestling periods, evidently as a defense against predation (Moreau, 1937; Moreau and Moreau, 1940). Males plaster the nest hole nearly shut with mud and single-handedly feed both the females and their nestlings. The unanswered question here is why this predator-defense tactic has evolved in hornbills but not in other hole-nesting birds.

In frugivorous toucans (Rhamphastidae), both sexes are required to maintain possession of a nesting hole (Van Tyne, 1929; Skutch, 1944, 1958, 1971; Wagner, 1944; Bourne, 1974). Suitable nest holes are extremely scarce, and each pair usually returns to the same hole every year. Defense of the hole begins well in advance of the breeding season, and continuous defense is necessary to retain occupancy. A deserted female would soon be evicted from her hole by a competing pair, and a deserting male would have little opportunity for breeding again with a new mate.

Several tropical tanagers and the blue honeycreeper *(Cyanerpes cyaneus)* are also monogamous despite feeding some fruit to nestlings, but they apparently defend multipurpose territories (Skutch, 1954, 1969, 1972). Why these species defend resources when other birds with partially or wholly frugivorous diets do not is unknown, but the fact that they do limits mating opportunities for deserting males.

A few temperate birds that feed fruit to nestlings and do not defend food resources are monogamous, too. In waxwings *(Bombycilla)*, mated pairs often raise two broods in a season (Putnam, 1949), and males can evidently be more successful by helping their mates feed each brood than they can by deserting. The reasons for this are unknown, but one important factor may be the apparent unavailability of mates once breeding begins. Pairing occurs in winter flocks and is rapidly completed early in the nesting season. Hence, few unmated females are present after that time, and a deserting male would have little opportunity to mate with another female.

Some promiscuous altricial birds do not fit the above hypothesis. In plain brown woodcreepers *(Dendrocincla fuliginosa)* and most hummingbirds, males and females defend individual territories against intruders of both sexes, and matings generally occur between occupants of adjacent territories or between territorial males and visiting females (Willis, 1972; Stiles, 1973). Individual territories generally evolve when energetic constraints make larger shared territories unfeasible (Gill and Wolf, 1975). These species are probably promiscuous because females suffer more by sharing a territory with a male than they do by giving up male parental assistance. Their mating systems appear comparable to the system discussed earlier for tree squirrels (see Smith, 1968).

Male orange-rumped honeyguides *(Indicator xanthonotus)* defend beehives where females forage (Cronin and Sherman, 1976). Males court foraging females and copulate after a brief courtship period. Since honeyguides are brood parasites, neither sex must contribute parental care to the young, and forgoing male parental assistance is of little or no consequence to females. Male village indigobirds *(Vidua chalybeata)* defend dispersed calling sites that are not associated with and copulate after a brief courtship period. Since honeyguides are brood parasites, neither sex must contribute parental care to the young, and forgoing male prolonged periods of time.

LEKS

The evolution of leks has been a difficult problem, partly because it has not been viewed from a female perspective. Most hypotheses have tried to explain lek behavior on the basis of benefits derived by males. Lack (1939) and D. W. Snow (1962a, 1963) suggested that group displays may have a stronger stimulating effect on females and hence increase each male's copulatory success. This hypothesis is at best a proximate explanation because it does not explain why females should benefit by responding more strongly to group stimulation. A related hypothesis is that males can be more conspicuous and thereby attract more females by displaying in groups (Chapman, 1935; Lack, 1939; Hjorth, 1970). However, several studies have failed to find a positive correlation between lek size and average male copulatory success, so males do not seem to benefit from this effect (Koivisto, 1965; Hogan-Warburg, 1966; Lill, 1976; but see also Hamerstrom and Hamerstrom, 1960). Since dispersed males also display on traditional perches, females should have little difficulty locating males regardless of how males are distributed (D. W. Snow, 1962a; Hjorth, 1970). Why, then, should females prefer visiting males on leks in some species but not in others?

Females could benefit from male lek behavior if mating within a group of males reduces their vulnerability to predation. In open habitats, mutual vigilance by males and other visiting females should be especially important, and in fact lek behavior is often associated with open environments. Promiscuous grouse that breed in open habitats all display on leks, while those that breed in forests all display from dispersed perches (Koivisto, 1965; Hjorth, 1970; Wiley, 1974; Wittenberger, 1978a). This correlation even holds among populations of the same species. Blue grouse display alone when breeding in dense underbrush but in groups when breeding in more open areas (Hoffmann, 1956; Blackford, 1958, 1963). Grouse leks are usually, though not always, situated in the most open, elevated terrain available (reviewed by Hjorth, 1970), where visibility of surrounding areas is greatest. This finding again suggests that lekking species depend on mutual vigilance for protection.

Lek behavior is also associated with open grasslands in the ruff, the great bustard, the little bustard, Jackson's whydah *(Coliuspasser jacksoni)*, and the Uganda kob *(Kobus kob)* (Van Someren, 1945; Gewalt, 1959; Buechner and Schloeth, 1965; Hogan-Warburg, 1966; Leuthold, 1966; Dement'ev and Gladkov, 1967; Buechner and Roth, 1974). However, the leks of Jackson's whydah are on the ground in tall grass, and the visibility of surrounding areas seems low (see Van Someren,

1945). Leks of the greater bird of paradise *(Paradisidaea apoda)* are usually in iso-lated trees within forest clearings, and those of the lesser bird of paradise *(P. minor)* are in isolated groves of trees on open savanna or in the tops of trees emerg-ing above the forest canopy (Gilliard, 1969). Leks of male cock-of-the-rocks *(Rup-icola rupicola)* are on the ground in especially open parts of tropical rain forests, where there is little understory vegetation (Gilliard, 1962; D. W. Snow, 1971b).

Females of many species behave in a manner that should reduce their vulnerability to predation while visiting a lek. In grouse, ruffs, and Uganda kob, females usually congregate on the most central territories (Hogan-Warburg, 1966; Hjorth, 1970; Wiley, 1973; Floody and Arnold, 1975; Shepard, 1975). Central territories should be less vulnerable to attack by terrestrial predators than periph-eral ones (cf. Tenaza, 1971), and because they are more tightly clustered, they contain more alternative targets for any attacking predator. Central territories are also held by superior males, so the female preference to mate on central territories can be (and usually is) interpreted as a preference for superior males. Quite pos-sibly, females choose central males because both advantages are important. Females also tend to congregate in groups while on a lek (e.g., Buechner and Schloeth, 1963; Hogan-Warburg, 1966; Wiley, 1973; Shepard, 1975), thereby using other individuals as a shield against terrestrial predators (cf. Hamilton, 1971). Finally, females usually visit leks for relatively short periods each day, thus minimizing their period of vulnerability.

In manakins and cock-of-the-rocks, females do not show a preference for central males (Gilliard, 1962; Lill, 1974a, 1976), but they are apparently attracted to particular territories rather than particular males. Lill (1974a) experimentally removed the most successful males from a lek of white-bearded manakins *(Man-acus manacus)* and found that females continued visiting the same territories even though the male occupants had changed. Females were evidently attracted to par-ticular site characteristics of the display court, but Lill could not identify any fac-tors making one court more attractive than others, despite an exhaustive analysis. The hypothesis that subordinate male long-tailed manakins *(Chiroxiphia linearis)* participate in group displays because they anticipate inheriting the display perch (Foster, 1977; D. W. Snow, 1977) also implies that display perches vary in their inherent attractiveness to females. Perhaps some positions on the lek offer better protection from surprise attacks by predators than others, or perhaps the advan-tages of displaying at a traditional site rather than displaying at a previously unused site are sufficient to make the wait worthwhile.

Despite this evidence, the predation hypothesis does not seem adequate for explaining all instances of lek behavior. Manakin leks are often in dense forest understory or in dense canopy foliage where visibility of approaching predators is low (D. W. Snow, 1962a, b, 1963; Sick, 1967; Lill, 1974b, 1976). The leks of Guy's hummingbirds *(Phaethornis guy)* are also in thick underbrush (D. W. Snow, 1968; B. K. Snow, 1974). These are associated with especially favorable foraging sites that attract females, but this is not the case for manakin leks. The recently described leks of hammerhead bats *(Hypsignathus monstrosus)* are situated in ripar-ian forest along streams and are found in both closed and open canopy forests (Bradbury, 1977b). It is difficult to believe that lekking behavior could evolve in bats as a defense against predation, especially since many other bats in the same forests inhabited by *Hypsignathus* do not display on leks. Bat leks are not associated with locally concentrated food resources and therefore cannot be explained by food distribution. The evolution of lek behavior in these species is not yet understood, but predation pressure does not seem implicated.

Whether male success will be higher at leks or at solitary display courts depends on the relative attractiveness of each type of display site to females. From the female point of view, vulnerability to predation should be an important factor. Females may also find it easier to identify superior males by visiting leks (Alexander, 1975). However, this factor cannot explain why lek behavior has evolved in some species but not in others. Lek behavior in open environments seems adaptive as a defense against predation, but why it has sometimes evolved in forests remains a mystery.

MONOGAMY

THEORY

The evolution of monogamy was left for last because it is easier to understand in light of the conditions favoring polygamy. A thorough review of the problem will be presented elsewhere, and only a summary will be given here.

Nonmonogamous mating systems evolve when they are advantageous to both sexes or when one sex, usually the male, can impose polygamy on the other. Similarly, monogamy evolves when it is advantageous to both sexes or when one sex, usually the female, can impose its best interests on the other. The polygyny-threshold model suggests two preconditions necessary for monogamy to evolve, while the theories for polyandry and promiscuity suggest a third precondition.

Precondition 1: Monogamous pair bonding must provide females with benefits that are not otherwise obtainable. Females may acquire nonshareable male parental assistance (see Figure 10) or avoid competition with other females for resources on the male's territory. When this precondition is not met, monogamy can evolve only when males impose it on females by actively sequestering them from other males.

Precondition 2: Females must be able to distinguish between unmated and already mated males while choosing their mates. This precondition precludes monogamy only in the rare cases when males are polyterritorial or otherwise prevent females from assessing their true mated status.

Precondition 3: Monogamy cannot evolve unless neither sex is prone to desert the other following fertilization. The only exception to this precondition occurs when prolonged pair bonds are maintained prior to fertilization, as in ducks. Males should not be predisposed to desert when mating seasons are short or when resource-based territories are a prerequisite to mating, because deserting males would then have little opportunity for attracting new mates. Females may reduce male proclivities to desert by requiring more prolonged courtship prior to accepting copulations, but this tactic would be effective only if mating seasons are relatively short. Female desertion should not be advantageous when females depend on social groups for protection, male defense of resources to alleviate competition, or biparental care to help rear young. Hence, female desertion is rare and occurs only under unusual environmental conditions.

When these preconditions are met, monogamy can evolve. The polygyny-threshold model and its underlying assumptions suggest five situations that would favor monogamy. These five hypotheses should not be viewed as mutually exclusive, but they should be comprehensive.

Hypothesis 1: Monogamy should evolve when male parental care is both nonshareable and crucial to offspring survival (cf. Lack, 1968; Orians, 1979). Males may still solicit promiscuous matings with other females, but they should maintain prolonged pair bonds with only a single mate. This hypothesis implies that monogamy is advantageous to both sexes.

Hypothesis 2: Monogamy should evolve in territorial species when differences between territories do not exceed the polygyny threshold (cf. Orians, 1969; Brown, 1975). As a corollary, monogamy cannot evolve unless the costs of competing for resources on a shared territory exceed any benefits potentially gained from female cooperation. This hypothesis implies that monogamy is advantageous for females but not necessarily for males.

Hypothesis 3: Monogamy should evolve in nonterritorial species when males are most successful by defending exclusive access to single females (cf. Emlen and Oring, 1977). Males might sequester individual females when sex ratios are skewed toward excess males if opportunities for additional matings are absent following insemination. When sex ratios are skewed, the majority of males could average more mates per year by sequestering a single female than they could by taking their chances in a promiscuous "lottery" system, but skewed sex ratios may not be a necessary prerequisite for this hypothesis to apply.

Hypothesis 4: Monogamy should evolve if the aggressiveness of mated females prevents males from obtaining additional mates (cf. Wittenberger, 1976a). In territorial species, female aggression may prevent polygyny even when the polygyny threshold is exceeded. It may also reinforce pair bonding in conjunction with Hypotheses 1 and 2. In social species, female dominance over other females may prevent polygyny if dominant females obtain substantial nonshareable parental assistance from the male or if breeding by other females in the group intensifies competition for resources.

Hypothesis 5: Monogamy should evolve if male reproductive success is less with two mates than with one (cf. Trivers, 1972). This might occur when the acquisition of a second female greatly reduces the reproductive success of the first female. Hypothesis 5 might hold in conjunction with Hypothesis 1, but it may not explain monogamy in any instance when unmated females would be willing to accept mated males as their mates.

Altricial Birds

Male parental assistance in feeding young is probably crucial whenever both parents combined can rear only one chick to independence at a time. This is the case in crab plovers *(Dromas ardeola)*, passenger pigeons *(Ectopistes migratorius)* (now extinct), gannets and boobies (Sulidae), petrels (Hydrobatidae and Pelecanoididae), albatrosses (Diomedeidae), shearwaters (Procellaridae), frigate birds (Fregatidae), and tropicbirds (Phaethontidae)(Meinertzhagen, 1954; Schorger, 1955; Nelson, 1966a, b, 1967a, b, 1970, 1977, 1978; Lack, 1968; Kepler, 1969), all of which are colonial. In tropicbirds, nest sites are extremely scarce and most chicks are killed during disputes over nest sites, so both parents are also necessary for defending the nest (Stonehouse, 1962). Frigate birds steal food from other colonial seabirds by midair piracy, a specialized hunting technique that makes food gathering more difficult (Nelson, 1967b). Both parents are necessary for feeding a single chick in most of these species because the large size of colonies severely depletes food resources near the colony site (see Hamilton and Watt, 1970) or because the species specializes on offshore food resources (see Lack, 1967; Nelson, 1970, 1977, 1978; Ashmole, 1971). Colonies are relatively small in crab plovers, but the reason for their one-egg clutches has not been investigated.

Parental contributions by both parents are required in some birds because nests must be attended continuously in order for the young to fledge. Herons and storks incubate eggs continuously from the day the first egg is laid until all eggs hatch and then brood the young continuously for another three weeks (Haverschmidt, 1949; Lowe, 1954; Cottrille and Cottrille, 1958; Palmer, 1962; Dusi and Dusi, 1968, 1970; Dickerman and Garino, 1969; Pratt, 1970; Scott, 1975). Continuous nest attendance is essential for preventing depredations by corvids and other predators, as well as for preventing interference by conspecifics. Pelicans must also attend eggs and young continuously to prevent predation (Palmer, 1962; Lamba, 1963; Burke and Brown, 1970). Most of these species are again colonial, and none is agile enough to mob predators hunting near the colony. Their large size probably makes nest guarding a better tactic for thwarting predators than mobbing.

When brood sizes are larger than one, male provisioning of nestlings is probably not crucial for the survivial of at least some young to independence. Females could theoretically reduce their clutch sizes in anticipation of lost male assistance, as occurs in the polygynous bobolink (Martin, 1974). The numerous instances of females' rearing broods alone following the mortality of their mate show that male assistance is not essential. These species are probably monogamous because differences between territories do not reach the polygyny threshold (Hypothesis 2).

Monogamy in brood-parasitic birds has always seemed anomalous because neither sex cares for eggs or nestlings. In fact, monogamy is well documented only in the cowbirds *(Molothrus)* (Friedmann, 1929; Darley, 1971), and even there not all matings are monogamous (Payne, 1973; Gochfeld, 1977, personal communication). Some males display in groups that attract females and mate promiscuously, while others maintain monogamous associations by defending access to individual females, generally in conjunction with territory defense. Sex ratios are skewed toward excess males, presumably because the energetic drain of egg production reduces female survival, so Hypothesis 3 is the most likely explanation for monogamous matings in cowbirds.

Current evidence indicates that cuckoos are not monogamous, despite the earlier conclusion of Lack (1968)(see Payne, 1967, 1971, 1977; Jensen and Jensen, 1969; Jensen and Vernon, 1970; Liversidge, 1971; Jensen and Clinning, 1974; Wyllie, 1975). The best evidence is for the African jacobin cuckoo *(Clamator jacobinus)*, in which females visit several male territories in succession and lay one egg on each (Liversidge, 1971; see also Payne, 1971; Jensen and Clinning, 1974; Gaston, 1976). Territorial males associate continuously with visiting females and sequester them from other males. The system is not monogamous in the usual sense of the term, but day-long pair bonds are formed as a result of males excluding other males from the vicinity of females that visit their territories.

Males of a few other altricial songbirds also defend females rather than territories (Hypothesis 3). This behavior is associated with male-biased sex ratios in black rosy finches *(Leucosticte atrata)*(Twining, 1938; French, 1959), probably gray-crowned rosy finches *(C. tephrocotis)* and other cardueline finches (Thompson, 1960; Johnson, 1965; Newton, 1972; Samson, 1976), and Hawaiian honeycreepers (Drepaniidae)(Amadon, 1950; Baldwin, 1953; Berger, 1972), but the reasons that sex ratios are skewed have not been studied. Males defend females instead of territories in Smith's longspurs *(Calcarius pictus)* as well (Jehl, 1968), but nothing is known of the sex ratio in this species.

To summarize, present evidence implicates Hypotheses 1–3 for explaining monogamy in altricial birds. Exclusion of unmated females from territories by resident females (Hypothesis 4) seems unlikely in birds because territory defense would conflict with incubation duties (see Orians, 1979). Female aggression may be important when both sexes help defend multipurpose territories, but whether any species are monogamous for this reason cannot be ascertained as yet. There is currently no evidence that any altricial birds are monogamous solely because males would be less successful with two mates than with one (Hypothesis 5), but experimental studies designed to test this possibility have yet to be performed.

PRECOCIAL AND SEMIPRECOCIAL BIRDS

A common misconception is that precocial young require relatively little parental care once they hatch and that females can incubate eggs adequately without assistance. Semiprecocial and some precocial young must be fed by their parents, and nearly all precocial young must be brooded and guarded from predators. Males contribute substantially to incubating eggs, feeding young, brooding young, and/or guarding young in virtually all species other than ducks, grouse, and bustards. The extensive literature on this topic will be reviewed elsewhere. Males may be able to help guard more than one brood at a time, but merging two or more broods may be more attractive to predators and hence may be disadvantageous to females. It is therefore unclear whether male guarding of young is a shareable or nonshareable type of parental investment. Because males can contribute substantial parental care, monogamous pair bonding can benefit females in nearly all precocial and semiprecocial birds.

Continuous nest attendance and hence male parental care is crucial for preventing predation losses (Hypothesis 1) in murres (Alcidae)(Penneycuik, 1956;

Tschanz, 1959), flamingos (Phoenicopteridae)(Brown and Root, 1971; Brown, Powell-Cotton, and Hopcraft, 1973), avocets (Recurvirostridae)(Gibson, 1971), and cranes (Gruidae)(Walkinshaw, 1965). In many gulls, nests must be continually protected from encroaching conspecific neighbors, which may cannibalize eggs or attack chicks (e.g., Drury and Smith, 1968; Vermeer, 1970; Parsons, 1971, 1975; Hunt, 1972; Hunt and Hunt, 1976). The need for continuous nest attendance is again associated with colonial nesting, except in cranes. Cranes are too large to depend on nest concealment even though nests are dispersed. Instead, they depend on their large size to actively thwart predators threatening their nest.

Nests must be attended continuously to prevent eggs from overheating in desert or tropical species of pratincoles (Glareolidae), skimmers (Rhynchopidae), doves (Columbidae), and terns (Sterninae)(Moreau and Moreau, 1937; Howell and Bartholomew, 1962; Modha and Coe, 1969; Russell, 1969). Since these species are all colonial or loosely colonial, predation pressure may also be an important factor. In penguins (Speniscidae), continuous incubation is necessary to prevent chilling of eggs, and both parents are required to feed the young (Lack, 1966, 1968). Finally, both parents are necessary for feeding a single chick in tropical terns and probably in most semiprecocial alcids (Lack, 1968).

Since males of most other precocial birds defend territories and make a substantial parental contribution, the costs of polygynous status are relatively high for females, and monogamy probably prevails because the polygyny threshold is not reached (Hypothesis 2) or possibly because resident females exclude unmated females from their territories (Hypothesis 4). Case by case analyses will be needed before any general conclusions can be reached.

The prevalence of monogamy in many species where males contribute little or no parental care has especially perplexed previous theorists (e.g., Selander, 1972). In monogamous grouse, males defend resources attractive to females, so they have little prospect for mating again should they desert, and laying females gain increased foraging time by relying on male vigilance for protection (Wittenberger, 1978a). Males continuously accompany females after pairing and may actually defend females rather than territories once they have attracted a mate (Hypothesis 3). The fact that sex ratios are always skewed toward excess males (e.g., Choate, 1963; Watson, 1965; Jenkins, Watson, and Miller, 1967; Bergerud, 1970) fits this interpretation. Nevertheless, monogamy may be prevalent largely because territory quality usually does not vary enough to reach the polygyny threshold (Hypothesis 2). Polygyny does occur regularly, though in low frequencies, among all three species of monogamous ptarmigan (Choate, 1963; Watson and Jenkins, 1964; MacDonald, 1970; Watson and Miller, 1971; Weeden and Theberge, 1972).

Monogamy in ducks results from males' defending individual females (Hypothesis 3; cf. McKinney, 1965; Lack, 1968). Males of migratory species generally pair with females on the wintering grounds and remain with them until incubation begins the following summer (Johnsgaard, 1975). During this time, males accompany their mates continuously and repulse any unmated males that approach too closely. Early pairing is probably a response to intense competition for mates, which arises because males outnumber females by about 60 to 40

(Johnsgaard and Buss, 1956; Bellrose, Scott, Hawkins, and Low, 1961; Aldrich, 1973). This skew in sex ratios probably results from the higher reproductive costs incurred by females while incubating eggs and accompanying broods (Lack, 1954). Females also benefit from pair bonding in ducks, since they are subjected to repeated harassment and even forcible copulation attempts by unmated males (Johnsgaard, 1975). The universal basis of pair formation in ducks is female "inciting" behavior, which induces males to attack nearby rivals, and in early stages of courtship, a female indicates her choice of mates by inciting a particular courting male to attack the other males in her vicinity (Johnsgaard, 1960, 1965). By avoiding harassment, female common eiders *(Somateria mollissima)* and perhaps females of other ducks increase their food intake rates during the critical laying period (Milne, 1974; Ashcroft, 1976).

Thus, monogamy has evolved in precocial birds for much the same reasons as in altricial birds. Hypotheses 1–3 appear especially applicable; Hypothesis 4 may be relevant when females help defend territories; and Hypothesis 5 appears inapplicable except in conjunction with Hypothesis 1.

Mammals

The evidence for most monogamous mammals is relatively sketchy compared to that for birds, and only tentative hypotheses are possible for many species. Monogamy is suspected but not yet proven in a number of species, and little can be said about the evolution of these species until more information becomes available. Kleiman (1977a) has reviewed the evidence for monogamy in mammals, along with the parental contributions made by males of these and various nonmonogamous species. Monogamy is nearly always associated with male defense of resources. Wolves *(Canis lupus),* Cape hunting dogs *(Lycaon pictus),* and to some extent tamarins *(Saguinus)* are exceptions (Kruuk and Turner, 1967; Mech, 1970; Schaller, 1972; Dawson, 1976).

Male parental contributions do not seem crucial to female reproductive success in any mammals. Male beavers *(Castor fiber* and *C. canadensis)* provide help in constructing dams and lodges, both important as safeguards against predation, and they help females cache food for winter use (Bradt, 1938; Tevis, 1950; Wilsson, 1968, 1971), but this help is probably not crucial because females do a majority of the work anyway (Hodgdon and Larson, 1973). Dividing male contributions may be deleterious to a resident female because space inside the lodge is limited or because competition for food hoards or food resources near the pond edge would reduce her survival or reproductive success. Thus, the male's parental contributions are largely nonshareable. Both males and females are aggressive toward intruders, but females take the more active role in territory defense (Wilsson, 1968, 1971; Hodgdon and Larson, 1973). Female aggression therefore appears responsible for maintaining monogamous pair bonding (Hypothesis 4). Muskrats *(Ondatra zibethicus)* also build lodges, though not dams, and both sexes are again highly aggressive (O'Neil, 1949; Banfield, 1974; Lowery, 1974), so muskrats are probably monogamous for a similar reason.

Male parental contributions are substantial but probably not essential in most canids, and the majority of canids are monogamous (Kleiman, 1977a). Both parents bring food to the young, and in foxes and jackals, differences in territory quality may never increase a female's hunting capability enough to make up for reduced or lost male parental assistance (Hypothesis 2). Since false vampire bats *(Vampyrum spectrum)* hunt mice and small birds (Goodwin and Greenhall, 1961; Greenhall, 1968), they may be monogamous for a similar reason, although male provisioning of the young has not been documented for this species.

Monogamous pair bonds are maintained in the canids by the aggressiveness of resident or dominant females (Hypothesis 3). In jackals and foxes, resident females regularly scent-mark territory boundaries and keep out intruding females (Kleiman, 1966, 1977a; Golani and Keller, 1975). In wolves, coyotes *(Canis latrans),* and probably Cape hunting dogs, the dominant female in each pack prevents breeding by subordinate females (Mech, 1970; Van Lawick and Van Lawick-Goodall, 1971; Schaller, 1972; Ryden, 1974; Gier, 1975; Frame and Frame, 1976).

Canid mating systems apparently differ from those of felids because conditions preclude male canids from deserting. Male foxes and jackals cannot desert because they would have to find a new territory before they could mate again. Male wolves and Cape hunting dogs probably cannot desert because they depend on pack hunting for capturing prey efficiently (see Estes and Goddard, 1967; Mech, 1970; Kleiman and Eisenberg, 1973; Bekoff, 1975). In Cape hunting dogs, male-biased sex ratios may be an additional factor limiting male mating opportunities away from the pack (see Schaller, 1972; Frame and Frame, 1976). Finally, female canids are usually monoestrus and hence are receptive for only limited periods each year (Kleiman and Eisenberg, 1973).

Males make a substantial though not essential parental contribution in several primates as well. Males help to carry infants in all monogamous marmosets *(Callithrix)* and tamarins studied to date (see Kleiman, 1977a, b), as well as in the monogamous night monkey *(Aotus trivirgatus)*(Moynihan, 1964), bearded sakis *(Chiropotes)*(Napier and Napier, 1967), and titi monkeys *(Callicebus)*(Mason, 1966, 1968; Kinzey, Rosenberger, Heisler, Prowse, and Trilling, 1977). Male carrying of infants may be partially responsible for the prevalence of twinning in female marmosets and tamarins, and it may enable females to become pregnant sooner than would otherwise be possible. Differences in territory quality may never compensate unmated females sufficiently for the loss of male parental assistance to favor polygyny, but aggressiveness by resident females is also involved. Female tamarins and marmosets live as social groups on more-or-less nonoverlapping territories, and the dominant female prevents other females in the group from breeding (DuMond, 1971; Epple, 1972, 1975; Rothe, 1975; Dawson, 1976). In titi monkeys, only one female resides on each territory, and her aggressiveness toward intruding females serves to reinforce monogamous pair bonding (Mason, 1966, 1968, 1971; Kinzey *et al.,* 1977).

Monogamy may also be advantageous for females of these and other primates because a second breeding female on the territory would intensify competition for food, especially when prior offspring remain on the territory through several breeding cycles. This factor may be particularly important in gibbons *(Hylobates),* where males contribute no nonshareable parental care (Carpenter, 1940; Ellefson, 1968; Tenaza, 1975), and possibly also in siamangs *(Symphalangus syndactylus),* where males only carry infants older than 12 months of age (Chivers, 1972, 1975). Females help defend territories in both gibbons and siamangs, and in Kloss's gibbons *(H. klossii),* their aggression is directed specifically at other conspecific females (Carpenter, 1940; Ellefson, 1968, 1974; Tenaza, 1975, 1976; Tilson, personal communication). Thus, female aggression may be a major factor in maintaining monogamy in these species.

Female aggression appears less important in the monogamous Mentawai langur *(Presbytis potenziani)*(Tilson and Tenaza, 1976). Tilson (personal communication) suggested that this species is monogamous because it evolved in an environment lacking important predators, reducing the potential benefits of mutual vigilance and hence making sociality less advantageous. Under such conditions, competition for food could override selection for the social behaviors typifying other langurs.

Female aggressiveness appears important in several other monogamous mammals. Microgales *(Microgale talazaci;* Insectivora) live as pairs in a common burrow, and pair bonds are maintained by the aggressiveness of both sexes toward like-sexed intruders (Eisenberg and Gould, 1970). Nothing is known of why the territorial behavior of each sex is adaptive. Meerkats *(Suricata suricatta)* live as social groups in burrows, often ones usurped from squirrels, but only the dominant female breeds in each group (Ewer, 1963, 1973; Wemmer and Flemming, 1975). Deermice *(Peromyscus californicus)* and grasshopper mice *(Onychomys)* live as monogamous pairs on territories, and both sexes are highly aggressive toward intruders (Egoscue, 1960; Eisenberg, 1962; Ruffer, 1965; Horner and Taylor, 1968). The territorial behavior of deermice is related to the hoarding of seeds. The ecology of all these species is poorly known, and further studies are needed before the environmental factors favoring female aggressiveness and monogamous pair bonding can be understood.

In some monogamous mammals, female aggression does not play a major role in maintaining monogamy. This is especially evident in antelope. Monogamy in antelope is associated with the exploitation of highly nutritious browse foods and male defense of foraging areas (Jarman, 1974). In klipspringers *(Oreotragus oreotragus),* Kirk's dikdik *(Madoqua kirki),* and southern reedbucks *(Redunca arundinum),* all of which live in habitats with relatively sparse cover, members of each pair are always together and depend on each other for vigilance (Tinley, 1969; Hendrichs and Hendrichs, 1971; Jungius, 1971; Dunbar and Dunbar, 1974; Hendrichs, 1975a). Trios consisting of one male and two females or two males and one female are often reported, but at least in klipspringers, these always consist of an adult pair and a full-grown subadult offspring (Tilson, unpublished data). Females depend on male vigilance for protection while foraging and escape up rock escarpments or into dense thickets when predators are near. These species seem to fit the cooperative version of the polygyny-threshold model (Figure 2), with polygynous matings precluded on most or all territories by food scarcity (Hypothesis 2). In effect, selection favoring sociality is countered by competition for food, leading to an optimal group size of only one female and one male on each territory.

Red duikers *(Cephalophus natalensis),* bush duikers *(Sylvicapra grimmia),* suni *(Neotragus moschatus),* steenbok *(Raphicerus campestris),* and grysbok *(R. melanotis)* inhabit densely vegetated forests or riverine thickets, and females spend much of their time apart from their mates even though a male and a female usually share a common territory (Wilson and Clarke, 1962; Heinichen, 1972; Dunbar and Dunbar, 1974; Manson, 1974; Cohen, 1977; Tilson, personal communication). Females depend on cryptic behavior and concealment rather than male vigilance for protection, apparently making continuous association with a male disadvantageous. Monogamy may prevail because males are capable of defending the home range of only a single female, but data are insufficient as yet for reaching a definite conclusion. In comparison, male northern reedbucks defend the overlapping home ranges of one to five solitary females and hence are polygynous (Hendrichs, 1975b). The difference between this species and monogamous duikers may be related to higher food availability or a lower dependence on concealment as an antipredator tactic in the reedbuck.

Males defend individual females for prolonged periods of time (Hypothesis 3) in relatively few mammals, presumably because desertion following the end of female receptivity is usually a better strategy. Maras *(Dolichotis patagonia;* Caviidae) are colonial burrowing rodents that breed as monogamous pairs (Dubost and Genest, 1974). All pairs roam freely throughout the colony and share all burrow systems. Territoriality is absent, and monogamy evidently results from males' defending their mates from other males. There was some indication of an excess of males in the colonies, as many males were unmated, but a skewed sex ratio was not explicitly documented. Male defense of females may also be responsible for monogamy in seals, as males closely attend their mates during the breeding season (Stirling, 1975).

To summarize, Hypotheses 2–4 appear capable of explaining all cases of monogamy in mammals. Lack of evidence makes detailed explanations difficult for most species, but a general picture is beginning to emerge. Monogamy in most mammals appears related to a lack of sufficient variability between territories to exceed the polygyny threshold (Hypothesis 2) and to female aggressiveness (Hypothesis 4). Female aggression appears to play a much greater role in maintaining monogamy in mammals than in birds, probably because female mammals are not constrained by time-intensive, site-specific parental activities such as the incubation of eggs. Male parental care does not appear crucial to female success in any mammals (Hypothesis 1), and males defend individual females for prolonged periods in only a few species (Hypothesis 3). At present, no evidence suggests that male mammals are ever less successful with two mates than with one (Hypothesis 5).

Conclusion

The evolution of animal mating systems can be greatly clarified by analyzing the fitness costs and benefits of each reproductive option open to individual males and females. The environmental factors affecting each option can then be identified, and the constraints placed on the mating behavior of each sex by the adoption of particular options can be evaluated.

The interests of each sex are never congruent, but the conflict of interests intensifies as females gain increased opportunities for exploiting the time and energy of males. Since female fecundity is limited by energetics, females should exploit male contributions to the fullest extent possible. The reproductive biology of females determines how much females can potentially gain from male assistance, while the propensity for males to desert following fertilization determines whether females can tap that potential.

When environmental conditions do not favor male desertion, females gain the option of acquiring or forgoing male assistance. The options chosen by unmated females and the subsequent responses made by already mated females then depend on the distribution and abundance of resources that affect female fitness and on the defenses adopted by females to avoid predation. The outcome of these female decisions determines which options remain available to males and hence the extent to which males actually contribute to female success.

When environmental conditions do favor male desertion, female options are severely constrained. Females are then prevented from tapping male contributions of time and energy, although their mating preferences still determine how males can best attract mates. Thus, the options taken by each sex limit the options left open to the other sex, until finally no options remain for either sex. The result is an animal's "mating system."

No simple hypothesis or theory can be expected to explain the great diversity of animal mating systems, but a reasonably comprehensive body of theory can be devised from relatively few general principles. Patchiness of crucial resources, opportunities for receiving male parental assistance, and male desertion strategies are seen as major factors affecting female reproductive options, while female sociality, female choice of breeding situations, and female desertion strategies are seen as major factors affecting male reproductive options. An understanding of how animal mating systems evolve requires knowledge of both the principles relating environmental conditions to individual reproductive strategies and the biological details underlying those principles.

Acknowledgments

My thinking on animal mating systems has especially profited from discussions with Gordon H. Orians, William J. Hamilton III, Ronald L. Tilson, Sarah Lenington, and Stuart A. Altmann. I thank Gordon H. Orians, Ronald L. Tilson, Peter Marler, William A. Searcy, Michael Gochfeld, and several anonymous reviewers for critically reviewing the manuscript and offering many helpful comments.

REFERENCES

Aldrich, J. W. Disparate sex ratios in waterfowl. In D. S. Farner (ed.), *Breeding Biology of Birds.* National Academy of Sciences, Washington, D.C., 1973, pp. 482–489.

Alexander, R. D. The evolution of social behavior. *Ann. Rev. Ecol. System.,* 1974, *5*, 325–383.

Alexander, R. D. Natural selection and specialized chorusing behavior in acoustical insects. In D. Pimentel (ed.), *Insects, Science, and Society.* Academic Press, New York, 1975, pp. 35–77.

Alexander, R. D., Hoogland, J. L., and Sherman, P. W. Sexual dimorphism in primates, ungulates, pinnipeds and humans. In N. A. Chagnon and W. G. Irons (eds.), *Sociobiology and Human Social Organization.* Duxbury Press, North Scituate, Mass., 1978.

Altmann, M. Patterns of herd behavior in free-ranging elk of Wyoming, *Cervus canadensis. Zoologica,* 1956, *41*, 65–71.

Altmann, S. A. Baboons, space, time, and energy. *Am. Zool.,* 1974, *14*, 221–248.

Altmann, S. A., Wagner, S. S., and Lenington, S. On the evolution of polygyny. *Behav. Ecol. Sociobiol.,* 1977, *2*, 397–410.

Amadon, D. The Hawaiian honeycreepers (Aves: Drepaniidae). *Bull. Am. Mus. Nat. Hist.,* 1950, *95*, 151–262.

Amadon, D. The significance of sexual difference in size among birds. *Proc. Am. Philosoph. Soc.,* 1959, *103*, 531–536.

Andersen, D. C., Armitage, K. B., and Hoffman, R. S. Socioecology of marmots: Female reproductive strategies. *Ecology,* 1976, *57*, 552–560.

Angst, W., and Thommen, D. New data and a discussion of infant killing in Old World monkeys and apes. *Folia Primatol.,* 1977, *27*, 198–229.

Anthony, R. Ecology and reproduction of California quail in southeastern Washington. *Condor,* 1970, *72*, 276–287.

Armitage, K. B. Social behavior of a colony of the yellow-bellied marmot *(Marmota flaviventris). Anim. Behav.,* 1962, *10*, 319–331.

Armitage, K. B. Vernal behaviour and territoriality in the yellow-bellied marmot *(Marmota flaviventris). Anim. Behav.,* 1965, *13*, 59–68.

Armitage, K. B., and Downhower, J. F. Demography of yellow-bellied marmot populations. *Ecology,* 1974, *55*, 1233–1245.

Armstrong, E. A. *The Wren.* Collins, London, 1955.

Armstrong, E. A., and Whitehouse, H. L. K. The behaviour of the wren. *Biol. Rev.,* 1977, *52*, 235–294.

Ashcroft, R. E. A function of the pairbond in the common eider. *Wildfowl,* 1976, *27*, 101–105.

Ashmole, N. P. Sea bird ecology and the marine environment. In D. S. Farner and J. R. King (eds.), *Avian Biology,* Vol. 1. Academic Press, New York, 1971, pp. 224–286.

Bailey, A. M., and Niedrach, R. J. *Birds of Colorado,* Vol. 1. Denver Museum of Natural History, Denver, 1965.

Baldwin, P. H. Annual cycle, environment and evolution in the Hawaiian honeycreepers (Aves: Drepaniidae). *Univ. Calif. Publ. Zool.,* 1953, *52*, 285–392.

Banfield, A. W. F. *The Mammals of Canada.* University of Toronto Press, Toronto, 1974.

Barash, D. P. The social biology of the Olympic marmot. *Anim. Behav. Monogr.,* 1973, *6*, 171–249.

Barash, D. P. The evolution of marmot societies: A general theory. *Science,* 1974a, *185*, 415–420.

Barash, D. P. Social behavior of the hoary marmot *(Marmota caligata). Anim. Behav.,* 1974b, *22*, 257–262.

Barash, D. P. Social behavior and individual differences in free-living alpine marmots *(Marmota marmota). Anim. Behav.,* 1976, *24*, 27–35.

Barash, D. P. *Sociobiology and Behavior.* Elsevier, New York, 1977.

Barlow, G. W. Contrasts in social behavior between Central American cichlid fishes and coral-reef surgeon fishes. *Am. Zool.,* 1974, *14*, 9–34.

Bartholomew, G. A. Reproductive and social behavior in the northern elephant seal. *Univ. Calif. Publ. Zool.,* 1952, *47*, 369–472.

Bartholomew, G. A. A model for the evolution of pinniped polygyny. *Evolution,* 1970, *24*, 546–559.

Bartholomew, G. A., and Hoel, P. G. Reproductive behavior of the Alaska fur seal, *Callorhinus ursinus. J. Mammal.,* 1953, *34*, 417–436.

Bateman, A. J. Intra-sexual selection in *Drosophila. Heredity,* 1948, *2*, 349–368.

Beebe, W. The variegated tinamou, *Crypturus variegatus variegatus* (Gmelin). *Zoologica,* 1925, *6*, 195–227.

Beebe, W. *Pheasants: Their Lives and Homes,* Vols. 1–2. Doubleday, Page, New York, 1926.

Bekoff, M. Social behavior and ecology of the African Canidae: A review. In M. W. Fox (ed.), *The Wild Canids: Their Systematics, Behavioral Ecology and Evolution.* Van Nostrand Rheinhold, New York, 1975, pp. 120–142.

Bell, R. H. V. A grazing ecosystem in the Serengeti. *Sci. Am.,* 1971, *225*, 86–93.

Bellrose, F. C., Jr., Scott, T. G., Hawkins, A. S., and Low, J. B. Sex ratios and age ratios in North American ducks. *Ill. Natur. Hist. Surv. Bull.,* 1961, *27,* 391–474.

Bendell, J. F., and Elliott, P. W. Habitat selection in blue grouse. *Condor,* 1966, *68,* 431–446.

Bendell, J. F., and Elliott, P. W. Behaviour and the regulation of numbers in blue grouse. *Wildl. Serv. Rep.,* 1967, *Series 4,* 1–76.

Bendell, J. F., King, D. G., and Mossop, D. H. Removal and repopulation of blue grouse in a declining population. *J. Wildl. Manage.,* 1972, *35,* 1153–1165.

Berger, A. J. *Hawaii Birdlife.* University of Hawaii Press, Honolulu, 1972.

Bergerud, A. T. Population dynamics of the willow ptarmigan *Lagopus lagopus alleni* L. in Newfoundland 1955 to 1965. *Oikos,* 1970, *21,* 299–325.

Bernstein, I. S. Dominance, aggression and reproduction in primate societies. *J. Theor. Biol.,* 1976, *60,* 459–472.

Bertram, B. C. R. The social system of lions. *Sci. Am.,* 1975, *232,* 54–65.

Blackford, J. L. Territoriality and breeding behavior of a population of blue grouse in Montana. *Condor,* 1958, *60,* 145–158.

Blackford, J. L. Further observations on the breeding behavior of a blue grouse population in Montana. *Condor,* 1963, *65,* 485–513.

Blaffer Hrdy, S. Male–male competition and infanticide among the langurs *(Presbytis entellus)* of Abu, Rahastan. *Folia Primatol.,* 1974, *22,* 19–58.

Blaffer Hrdy, S. Infanticide as a primate reproductive strategy. *Am. Sci.,* 1977, *65,* 40–49.

Boag, D. A., and Sumanik, K. M. Characteristics of drumming sites selected by ruffed grouse in Alberta, *J. Wildl. Manage.,* 1969, *33,* 621–628.

Boucher, D. H. On wasting parental investment. *Am. Natur.,* 1977, *111,* 786–788.

Bourne, G. R. The red-billed toucan in Guyana. *Living Bird,* 1974, *13,* 99–126.

Bradbury, J. W. Social organization and communication. In W. Wimsatt (ed.), *Biology of Bats,* Vol. 3. Academic Press, New York, 1977a.

Bradbury, J. W. Lek mating behavior in the hammer-headed bat. *Z. Tierpsychol.,* 1977b, *45,* 225–255.

Bradbury, J. W., and Emmons, L. Social organization of some Trinidad bats. I. Emballonuridae. *Z. Tierpsychol.,* 1974, *36,* 137–183.

Bradbury, J. W., and Vehrencamp, S. L . Social organization and foraging in Emballonurid bats. II. A model for the determination of group size. *Behav. Ecol. Sociobiol.,* 1976, *1,* 383–404.

Bradt, G. W. A study of beaver in Michigan. *J. Mammal.,* 1938, *19,* 139–162.

Braestrup, F. W. The function of communal displays. *Dan. Ornithol. Foren. Tidsskr.,* 1963, *57,* 133–142.

Brattstrom, B. H. The evolution of reptilian social behavior. *Am. Zool.,* 1974, *14,* 35–49.

Bray, O. E., Kennelly, J. J., and Guarino, J. L. Fertility of eggs produced on territories of vasectomized red-winged blackbirds. *Wilson Bull.,* 1975, *87,* 187–195.

Brown, J. L. The evolution of diversity in avian territorial systems. *Wilson Bull.,* 1964, *76,* 160–169.

Brown, J. L. Territorial behavior and population regulation in birds: A review and re-evaluation. *Wilson Bull.,* 1969, *81,* 293–329.

Brown, J. L. Alternate routes to sociality in jays—With a theory for the evolution of altruism and communal breeding. *Am. Zool.,* 1974, *14,* 63–80.

Brown, J. L. *The Evolution of Behavior.* W. W. Norton, New York, 1975.

Brown, J. L., and Balda, R. P. The relationship of habitat quality to group size in Hall's babbler *(Pomatostomus halli). Condor,* 1977, *79,* 312–320.

Brown, L. H., Powell-Cotton, D., and Hopcraft, J. B. D. The breeding of the greater flamingo and great white pelican in East Africa. *Ibis,* 1973, *115,* 352–374.

Brown, L. H., and Root, A. The breeding behaviour of the lesser flamingo *Phoeniconaias minor. Ibis,* 1971, *113,* 147–172.

Bruning, D. F. The greater rhea chick and egg delivery route. *Natur. Hist.,* 1973, *82,* 68–75.

Bruning, D. F. Social structure and reproductive behavior in the greater rhea. *Living Bird,* 1974, *13,* 251–294.

Buechner, R. K., and Roth, H. D. The lek system in Uganda kob antelope. *Am. Zool.,* 1974, *14,* 145–162.

Buechner, H. K., and Schloeth, R. Ceremonial mating behavior in Uganda kob *(Adenota kob thomasi* Neumann). *Z. Tierpsychol.,* 1965, *22,* 209–225.

Burke, V. E. M., and Brown, L. H. Observations on the breeding of the pink-backed pelican *Pelecanus rufescens. Ibis,* 1970, *112,* 499–512.

Caraco, T., and Wolf, L. L. Ecological determinants of group sizes of foraging lions. *Am. Natur.,* 1975, *109,* 343–352.

Carey, M. D. Aspects of the population dynamics of indigo buntings *(Passerina cyanea)* in two habitats: A test of the Verner–Willson–Orians model for the evolution of avian polygyny. Ph.D. thesis, Indiana University, Bloomington, 1977.

Carey, M., and Nolan, V., Jr. Polygyny in indigo buntings: A hypothesis tested. *Science*, 1975, *190*, 1296–1297.

Carl, E. A. Population control in arctic ground squirrels. *Ecology*, 1971, *52*, 395–413.

Carpenter, C. R. A field study in Siam of the behavior and social relations of the gibbon *(Hylobates lar)*. *Comp. Psychol. Monogr.*, 1940, *16*, 1–212.

Carrick, R. Ecological significance of territory in the Australian magpie, *Gymnorhina tibicen*. *Proc. XIII Int. Ornithol. Cong.*, 1963, pp. 740–753.

Carrick, R., Csordas, S. E., Ingham, S. E., and Keith, K. Studies on the southern elephant seal, *Mirounga leonina* (L.). *C.S.I.R.O. Wildl. Res.*, 1962, *7*, 119–197.

Chapman, F. M. The nesting habits of Wagler's oropendola *(Zarhynchus wagleri)* on Barro Colorado Island. *Bull. Am. Mus. Natur. Hist.*, 1928, *58*, 123–166.

Chapman, F. M. The courtship of Gould's manakin *(Manacus vitellinus vitellinus)* on Barro Colorado Island, Canal Zone. *Bull. Am. Mus. Natur. Hist.*, 1935, *68*, 471–525.

Charles-Dominique, P. Ecologie et vie sociale de *Galago demidovii* (Fischer 1808; Prosimii). *Z. Tierpsychol.*, 1972, *Suppl. 9*.

Charles-Dominique, P. Aggression and territoriality in nocturnal prosimians. In R. Holloway (ed.), *Primate Aggression, Territoriality, and Xenophobia: A Comparative Perspective*. Academic Press, New York, 1974, pp. 31–48.

Charles-Dominique, P., and Martin, R. D. Behaviour and ecology of nocturnal prosimians. *Z. Tierpsychol.*, 1972, *Suppl. 9*.

Charnov, E. L., and Krebs, J. R. On clutch-size and fitness. *Ibis*, 1974, *116*, 217–219.

Chivers, D. J. The siamang and the gibbon in the Malay Peninsula. *Gibbon and Siamang*, 1972, *1*, 103–135.

Chivers, D. J. The siamang in Malaya: A field study of a primate in tropical rain forest. *Contr. to Primatol.*, 1975, *4*, 1–335.

Choate, T. S. Habitat and population dynamics of white-tailed ptarmigan in Montana. *J. Wildl. Manage.*, 1963, *27*, 684–699.

Clutton-Brock, T. H. Primate social organisation and ecology. *Nature, London*, 1974, *250*, 539–542.

Clutton-Brock, T. H. Feeding behaviour of red colobus and black-and-white colobus in East Africa. *Folia Primatol.*, 1975, *23*, 165–207.

Cody, M. L. A general theory of clutch size. *Evolution*, 1966, *20*, 174–184.

Cohen, M. The steenbok—Hermit of the bush. *Fauna and Flora*, 1977, *30*, 16.

Collias, N. E., and Collias, E. C. Size of breeding colony related to attraction of mates in a tropical passerine bird. *Ecology*, 1969, *50*, 481–488.

Cottrille, W. P., and Cottrille, B. D. Great blue heron: Behavior at the nest. *Univ. Mich. Mus. Zool., Misc. Publ.*, 1958, *102*, 1–15.

Coulson, J. C., and Hickling, G. The breeding biology of the grey seal, *Halichoerus grypus* (Fab.), on the Farne Islands, Northumberland. *J. Anim. Ecol.*, 1964, *33*, 485–512.

Cox, C. R., and Le Boeuf, B. J. Female incitation of male competition: A mechanism in sexual selection. *Am. Natur.*, 1977, *111*, 317–335.

Crawford, R. D. Polygynous breeding of short-billed marsh wrens. *Auk*, 1977, *94*, 359–362.

Crome, F. H. J. Some observations on the biology of the cassowary in northern Queensland. *Emu*, 1976, *76*, 6–14.

Cronin, E. W., Jr., and Sherman, P. W. A resource-based mating system: The orange-rumped honeyguide, *Indicator xanthonotus*. *Living Bird*, 1976, *15*, 5–32.

Crook, J. H. The evolution of social organization and visual communication in the weaver birds (Ploceinae). *Behaviour*, 1964, *Suppl. 10*.

Crook, J. H. The adaptive significance of avian social organizations. *Symp. Zool. Soc. Lond.*, 1965, *14*, 181–218.

Crook, J. H. The socio-ecology of primates. In J. H. Crook (ed.), *Social Behaviour in Birds and Mammals: Essays on the Social Ethology of Animals and Man*. Academic Press, New York, 1970, pp. 103–166.

Crook, J. H. Sexual selection, dimorphism, and social organization in the primates. In B. Campbell (ed.), *Sexual Selection and the Descent of Man, 1871–1971*. Aldine, Chicago, 1972, pp. 231–281.

Darley, J. A. Sex ratio and mortality in the brown-headed cowbird. *Auk*, 1971, *88*, 560–566.

Darling, F. F. *A Herd of Red Deer*. Oxford University Press, London, 1937.

Darwin, C. *The Descent of Man and Selection in Relation to Sex*. John Murray, London, 1871.

Dawkins, R. *The Selfish Gene*. Oxford University Press, New York, 1976.

Dawkins, R., and Carlisle, T. R. Parental investment, mate desertion and a fallacy. *Nature, London,* 1976, *262*, 131–133.

Dawson, G. A. Behavioral ecology of the Panamanian tamarin, *Saguinus oedipus* (Callitrichidae, Primates). Ph.D. thesis, Michigan State University, East Lansing, 1976.

Delacour, J. *The Pheasants of the World.* Country Life, London, 1951.

Delacour, J. *The Waterfowl of the World.* Country Life, London, 1954–1964.

Dement'ev, G. P., and Gladkov, N. A. (eds.). *Birds of the Soviet Union,* Vol. 4. Israel Program of Scientific Translation, Jerusalem, 1967.

Denham, W. W. Energy relations and some basic properties of primate social organization. *Am. Anthropol.,* 1971, *73*, 77–95.

DeVore, I. Male dominance and mating behavior in baboons. In F. A. Beach (ed.), *Sex and Behavior.* Wiley, New York, 1965, pp. 266–289.

DeVore, I. The evolution of human society. In J. F. Eisenberg and W. S. Dillon (eds.), *Man and Beast: Comparative Social Behavior.* Smithsonian Institution Press, Washington, D.C., 1971, pp. 297–311.

Dickerman, R. W., and Garino, G. Studies of a nesting colony of green herons at San Blas, Nayarit, Mexico. *Living Bird,* 1969, *8*, 95–111.

Dixson, A. F., Everitt, G. F., Herbert, J., Rugman, S. M., and Scruton, D. M. Hormonal and other determinants of sexual attractiveness and receptivity in rhesus and talapoin monkeys. In C. H. Phoenix (ed.), *Primate Reproductive Behavior. Symposium of the 4th. International Congress of Primatology,* Vol. 2. Karger, Basel, 1973, pp. 36–63.

Downhower, J. F. An experimental analysis of the relationship between resource patterns and the structure of social systems. *Ann. Rep. Nat. S. Found., Washington, D.C.,* 1977.

Downhower, J. F., and Armitage, K. B. The yellow-bellied marmot and the evolution of polygamy. *Am. Natur.,* 1971, *105*, 355–370.

Drury, W. H., Jr. Breeding activities, especially nest building, of the yellowtail *(Ostinops decumanus)* in Trinidad, West Indies. *Zoologica,* 1962, *47*, 39–58.

Drury, W. H., Jr., and Smith, W. J. Defense of feeding areas by adult herring gulls and intrusion by young. *Evolution,* 1968, *22*, 193–201.

Dubost, G., and Genest, H. Le comportement social d'une colonie de maras *Dolichotis patagonum* Z. dans le Parc de Branfèrè. *Z. Tierpsychol.,* 1974, *35*, 225–302.

Duellman, W. E. Aggressive behavior in dendrobatid frogs. *Herpetologica,* 1966, *22*, 217–221.

Duellman, W. E. Social organization in the mating calls of some Neotropical anurans. *Am. Midl. Natur.,* 1967, *77*, 156–163.

DuMond, F. Comments on minimum requirements in the husbandry of the golden marmoset *(Leontopithecus rosalia).* *Lab. Primatol. Newsl.,* 1971, *10*, 30–37.

Dunbar, R. I. M., and Dunbar, E. P. Social organization and ecology of the klipspringer *(Oreotragus oreotragus)* in Ethiopia. *Z. Tierpsychol.,* 1974, *35*, 481–493.

Dunford, C. Kin selection for ground squirrel alarm calls. *Am. Natur.,* 1977, *111*, 782–785.

Dusi, J. L., and Dusi, R. T. Ecological factors contributing to nesting failure in a heron colony. *Wilson Bull.,* 1968, *80*, 458–466.

Dusi, J. L., and Dusi, R. T. Nesting success and mortality of nestlings in a cattle egret colony. *Wilson Bull.,* 1970, *82*, 458–460.

Eaton, G. G. Social and endocrine determinants of sexual behavior in simian and prosimian females. In C. H. Phoenix (ed.), *Primate Reproductive Physiology. Symposium of the 4th. International Congress of Primatology,* Vol. 2. Karger, Basel, 1973, pp. 20–35.

Eaton, R. L. *The Cheetah.* Van Nostrand Rheinhold, New York, 1974.

Eaton, R. L. Evolution of sociality in the Felidae. In R. L. Eaton (ed.), *The World's Cats,* Vol. 3, No. 2. Burke Museum, University of Washington, Seattle, 1976a, pp. 95–142.

Eaton, R. L. Why some felids copulate so much. In R. L. Eaton (ed.), *The World's Cats,* Vol. 3, No. 2. Burke Museum, University of Washington, Seattle, 1976b, pp. 73–94.

Egoscue, H. J. Laboratory and field studies of the northern grasshopper mouse. *J. Mammal.,* 1960, *41*, 99–110.

Eisenberg, J. F. Studies on the behavior of *Peromyscus maniculatus gambelli* and *Peromyscus californicus parasiticus. Behaviour,* 1962, *19*, 177–207.

Eisenberg, J. F. The social organization of mammals. *Handb. Zool.,* 1966, *8*, 1–92.

Eisenberg, J. F., and Gould, E. The tenrecs: A study in mammalian behavior and evolution. *Smithson. Contr. Zool.,* 1970, *27*, 1–137.

Eisenberg, J. F., and Lockhart, M. An ecological reconnaissance of Wilpattu National Park, Ceylon. *Smithson. Contr. Zool.,* 1972, *101*, 1–118.

Eisenberg, J. F., Muckenhirn, N. A., and Rudran, R. The relation between ecology and social structure in primates. *Science*, 1972, *176*, 863–874.

Ellefson, J. O. Territorial behavior in the common white-handed gibbon, *Hylobates lar* Linn. In P. C. Jay (ed.), *Primates: Studies in Adaptation and Variability.* Holt, Rhinehart, and Winston, New York, 1968, pp. 180–199.

Ellefson, J. O. A natural history of white-handed gibbons in the Malayan Peninsula. In D. M. Rumbaugh (ed.), *Gibbon and Siamang,* 1974, *3*, 1–136.

Elliott, P. F. Longevity and the evolution of polygamy. *Am. Natur.,* 1975, *109*, 281–287.

Ellison, L. N. Winter food selection by Alaskan spruce grouse. *J. Wildl. Manage.,* 1976, *40*, 205–213.

Eloff, F. Ecology and behavior of the Kalahari lion. In R. L. Eaton (ed.), *The World's Cats,* Vol. 1. World Wildlife Safari, Winston, Ore., 1973, pp. 90–126.

Emlen, J. T. Display and mate selection in the whydahs and bishop birds. *Ostrich,* 1957, *28*, 202–213.

Emlen, S. T. The evolution of cooperative breeding in birds. In J. Krebs and N. Davies (eds.), *Behavioural Ecology: An Evolutionary Approach.* Blackwell, London, 1978.

Emlen, S. T., and Oring, L. W. Ecology, sexual selection, and the evolution of mating systems. *Science,* 1977, *197*, 215–223.

Epple, G. Social communication by olfactory signals in marmosets, *Int. Zoo Yearb.,* 1972, *12*, 36–42.

Epple, G. The behavior of marmoset monkeys (Callitrichidae). In L. A. Rosenblum (ed.), *Primate Behavior: Developments in Field and Laboratory Research,* Vol. 4. Academic Press, New York, 1975.

Estes, R. D. The comparative behavior of Grant's and Thomson's gazelles. *J. Mammal.,* 1967, *48*, 189–209.

Estes, R. D. Territorial behavior of the wildebeest (*Connochaetes taurinus* Burchelli, 1823). *Z. Tierpsychol.,* 1969, *26*, 284–370.

Estes, R. D. Social organization of the African Bovidae. In V. Geist and F. Walther (eds.), *The Behaviour of Ungulates and its Relation to Management,* Vol. 1. I.U.C.N., Moreges, 1974, pp. 167–205.

Estes, R. D., and Goddard, J. Prey selection and hunting behavior of the African wild dog. *J. Wildl. Manage.,* 1967, *31*, 52–70.

Ewer, R. F. The behaviour of the meercat, *Suricata suricatta* (Schreber). *Z. Tierpsychol.,* 1963, *20*, 570–607.

Ewer, R. F. *The Carnivores.* Cornell University Press, Ithaca, N.Y., 1973.

Fautin, R. W. The establishment and maintenance of territories by the yellow-headed blackbird in Utah. *Great Basin Naturalist,* 1940, *1*, 75–91.

Federn, H. A. Hybridization between the Atlantic angelfishes, *Holacanthus isabelita* and *H. ciliaris. Bull. Mar. Sci.,* 1968, *18*, 351–382.

Feist, J. D., and McCullough, D. R. Social organization and reproduction in feral horses. *J. Reprod. Fertil.,* 1975, *Suppl. 23*.

Ferdinand, L. Display of the great snipe *(Gallinago media Latham). Dan. Ornithol. Foren. Tidsskr.,* 1966, *60*, 14–34.

Fiedler, K. Vergleichende Verhaltenstudien an Seenadeln, Schlangenadeln, und Seepferdchen. *Z. Tierpsychol.,* 1955, *11*, 358–416.

Fischer, C. A., and Keith, L. B. Population responses of central Alberta ruffed grouse to hunting. *J. Wildl. Manage.,* 1974, *38*, 585–600.

Fisher, R. A. *The Genetical Theory of Natural Selection,* 2nd Ed. Dover, New York, 1958.

Floody, O. R., and Arnold, A. P. Uganda kob *(Adenota kob thomasi):* Territoriality and the spatial distributions of sexual and agonistic behaviours at a territorial ground. *Z. Tierpsychol.,* 1975, *37*, 192–212.

Foster, M. S. Rain, feeding behavior, and clutch size in tropical birds. *Auk,* 1974, *91*, 722–726.

Foster, M. S. Odd couples in manakins: A study of social organization and cooperative breeding in *Chiroxiphis linearis. Am. Natur.,* 1977, *111*, 845–853.

Frädrich, H. Zur Biologie und Ethologie des Warzenschweines (*Phacochoeurus aethiopicus* Pallas), unter Berücksictigung des Verhaltens anderer Suiden. *Z. Tierpsychol.,* 1965, *22*, 328–374, 375–393.

Frädrich, H. A comparison of behaviour in the Suidae. In V. Geist and F. Walther (eds.), *The Behaviour of Ungulates and its Relation to Management,* Vol. 1. I.U.C.N., Moreges, 1974, pp. 133–143.

Frame, L. H., and Frame, G. W. Female African wild dogs emigrate. *Nature, London,* 1976, *263*, 227–229.

Francis, W. J. Double broods in California quail. *Condor,* 1965, *67*, 541–542.

Franklin, W. L., Mossman, A. S., and Doe, M. Social organization and home range of Roosevelt elk. *J. Mammal.,* 1975, *56*, 102–118.

French, N. R. Life history of the black rosy finch. *Auk,* 1959, *76*, 159–180.

Friedmann, H. *The Cowbirds: A Study in the Biology of Social Parasitism.* Thomas, Springfield, Ill., 1929.

Fry, C. H. The evolutionary significance of co-operative breeding in birds. In B. Stonehouse and C. M. Perrins (eds.), *Evolutionary Ecology.* Macmillan, London, 1977, pp. 127–135.

Gaston, A. J. Brood parasitism by the pied crested cuckoo *Clamator jacobinus. J. Anim. Ecol.,* 1976, *45,* 331–348.

Geist, V. *Mountain Sheep: A Study in Behavior and Evolution.* University of Chicago Press, Chicago, 1971.

Geist, V. On the relationship of social evolution and ecology in ungulates. *Am. Zool.,* 1974, *14,* 205–220.

Gewalt, W. *Die Grosstrappe (Otis tarda* L.). A. Ziemsen Verlag, Wittenberg Lutherstadt, 1959.

Gibson, F. The breeding biology of the American avocet *(Recurvirostra americana)* in central Oregon. *Condor,* 1971, *73,* 444–454.

Gier, H. T. Ecology and social behavior of the coyote. In M. W. Fox (ed.), *The Wild Canids: Their Systematics, Behavioral Ecology and Evolution.* Van Nostrand Rheinhold, New York, 1975, pp. 247–259.

Gill, F. B., and Wolf, L. L. Economics of feeding territoriality in the golden-winged sunbird. *Ecology,* 1975, *56,* 333–345.

Gilliard, E. T. On the breeding behavior of the cock-of-the-rock (Aves, *Rupicola rupicola). Bull. Am. Mus. Natur. Hist.,* 1962, *124,* 31–68.

Gilliard, E. T. *Birds of Paradise and Bower Birds.* The Natural History Press, New York, 1969.

Gochfeld, M. Social system and possible lek behavior in brown-headed cowbirds *(Molothrus ater).* Paper presented to the American Ornithological Union meetings, Berkeley, Calif., 1977.

Golani, I., and Keller, A. A longitudinal field study of the behavior of a pair of golden jackals. In M. W. Fox (ed.), *The Wild Canids: Their Systematics, Behavioral Ecology and Evolution.* Van Nostrand Rheinhold, New York, 1975, pp. 303–335.

Goodman, D. Natural selection and a cost ceiling on reproductive effort. *Am. Natur.,* 1974, *108,* 247–268.

Goodwin, D. Observations on voice and behaviour of the red-legged partridge *Alectoris rufa. Ibis,* 1953, *95,* 581–614.

Goodwin, G. G., and Greenhall, A. M. A review of the bats of Trinidad and Tobago. *Bull. Am. Mus. Natur. Hist.,* 1961, *122,* 195–301.

Gosling, L. M. The social behaviour of Coke's hartebeest, *Alcelaphus buselaphus* Gunther. In V. Geist and F. Walther (eds.), *The Behaviour of Ungulates and Its Relation to Management,* Vol. 1. I.U.C.N., Moreges, 1974, pp. 488–511.

Goss-Custard, J. D., Dunbar, R. I. M., and Aldrich-Blake, F. P. G. Survival, mating and rearing strategies in the evolution of primate social structure. *Folia Primatol.,* 1972, *17,* 1–19.

Gottfried, B. M., and Thompson, C. F. Experimental analysis of nest predation in an old-field habitat. *Auk,* 1978, *95,* 304–312.

Graul, W. D. Adaptive aspects of the mountain plover social system. *Living Bird,* 1973, *12,* 69–94.

Graul, W. D. Flood fluctuations and multiple clutches in the mountain plover. *Auk,* 1976, *93,* 166–167.

Graul, W. D., Derrickson, S. R., and Mock, D. W. The evolution of avian polyandry. *Am. Natur.,* 1977, *111,* 812–816.

Greenhall, A. M. Notes on the behavior of the false vampire bat. *J. Mammal.,* 1968, *49,* 337–340.

Gwynne, M. D., and Bell, R. H. V. Selection of vegetation components by grazing ungulates in the Serengeti National Park. *Nature, London,* 1968, *220,* 390–393.

Haartman, L. von. Successive polygamy. *Behaviour,* 1951a, *3,* 256–274.

Haartman, L. von. Der Trauerfliegenschnäpper. II. Populationsprobleme. *Acta Zool. Fenn.,* 1951b, *67,* 1–60.

Haartman, L. von. Territory in the pied flycatcher, *Muscicapa hypoleuca. Ibis,* 1956, *98,* 460–475.

Haartman, L. von. Nest-site and evolution of polygamy in European passerine birds. *Ornis Fenn.,* 1969, *46,* 1–12.

Hall, K. R. L. Behaviour and ecology of the wild patas monkey, *Erythrocebus patas,* in Uganda. In P. C. Jay (ed.), *Primates: Studies in Adaptation and Variability.* Holt, Rinehart and Winston, New York, 1968, pp. 32–119.

Hamerstrom, F. Comments relating to the paper given by R. Robel. *Proc. XV Int. Ornithol. Cong.,* 1972, p. 184.

Hamerstrom, F. N., Jr., and Hamerstrom, F. Comparability of some social displays of grouse. *Proc. XII Int. Ornithol. Cong.,* 1960, pp. 274–293.

Hamilton, W. D. The genetical theory of social behaviour, I, II. *J. Theor. Biol.,* 1964, *7,* 1–52.

Hamilton, W. D. Geometry for the selfish herd. *J. Theor. Biol.,* 1971, *31,* 295–311.

Hamilton, W. J., III, and Watt, K. E. F. Refuging. *Ann. Rev. Ecol. System.,* 1970, *1,* 263–286.

Harmeson, J. Breeding ecology of the dickcissel. *Auk,* 1974, *91,* 348–359.

Hausfater, G. Dominance and reproduction in baboons *(Papio cynocephalus). Contr. Primatol.,* 1975, 7, 1–150.

Haverschmidt, F. *The Life of the White Stork.* E. J. Brill, Leiden, 1949.

Hays, H. Polyandry in the spotted sandpiper. *Living Bird,* 1972, *11,* 43–57.

Heinichen, I. G. Preliminary notes on the suni, *Neotragus moschatus,* and the red duiker, *Cephalophus natalensis. Zool. Afr.,* 1972, 7, 157–165.

Hendrichs, H. Changes in a population of dikdik, *Madoqua (Rhynchotragus) kirki* (Günther 1880). *Z. Tierpsychol.,* 1975a, *38,* 55–69.

Hendrichs, H. Observations on a population of Bohor reedbuck, *Redunca redunca* (Pallas 1767). *Z. Tierpsychol.,* 1975b, *38,* 44–54.

Hendrichs, H., and Hendrichs, U. Freilanduntersuchungen zur Ökologie und Ethologie der Zwergan- tilope *Madoqua (Rhynchotragus) kirki,* Günter 1880. In H. Hendrichs and U. Hendrichs (eds.), *Dikdik and Elephanten.* Piper-Verlag, München, 1971, pp. 9–75.

Hildèn, O. Habitat selection in birds. A review. *Ann. Zool. Fenn.,* 1965a, 2, 53–75.

Hildèn, O. Zur Brutbiologie des Temminckstrandläufers, *Calidris temminckii* (Leisl.). *Ornis Fenn.,* 1965b, *42,* 1–5.

Hildèn, O., and Vuolanto, S. Breeding biology of the red-necked phalarope *Phalaropus lobatus* in Fin- land. *Ornis Fenn.,* 1972, *49,* 57–85.

Hjorth, I. Reproductive behavior in Tetraonidae, with special reference to males. *Viltrevy,* 1970, 7, 183–596.

Hladik, C. M. Ecology, diet, and social patterning in old and new world primates. In R. H. Tuttle (ed.), *Socio-ecology and Psychology of Primates.* Mouton, The Hague, 1975, pp. 3–35.

Hodgdon, H. E., and Larson, J. S. Some sexual differences in behaviour within a colony of marked beavers *(Castor canadensis). Anim. Behav.,* 1973, *21,* 147–152.

Hoffmann, A. Über die Brutpflege des polyandrischen Wasserfasans, *Hydrophasianus chirurgus* (Scop.). *Zoologisches Jahrbuch Abteilung Systematik, Ökol., Geog. Tiere,* 1949, *78,* 367–403.

Hoffman, A. Zur Brutbiologie des Wasserfasans. *Ornithol. Ber.,* 1950, *2,* 119–126.

Hoffman, R. S. Observations on a sooty grouse population at Sage Hen Creek, California. *Condor,* 1956, *58,* 321–337.

Hogan-Warburg, A. J. Social behavior of the ruff *Philomachus pugnax* (L.). *Ardea,* 1966, *54,* 109–229.

Höhn, E. O. Observations on the breeding biology of Wilson's phalarope *(Steganopus tricolor)* in central Alberta. *Auk,* 1967, *84,* 220–244.

Holm, C. H. Breeding sex ratios, territoriality, and reproductive success in the red-winged blackbird *(Agelaius phoeniceus). Ecology,* 1973, *54,* 356–365.

Hoogland, J. L. The evolution of coloniality in white-tailed and black-tailed prairie dogs (Sciuridae; *Cynomys leucurus* and *C. ludovicianus*). Ph.D. thesis, University of Michigan, Ann Arbor, 1977.

Horn, H. S. The adaptive significance of colonial nesting in the Brewer blackbird, *Euphagus cyanoce- phalus. Ecology,* 1968, *49,* 682–694.

Horner, B. E., and Taylor, J. M. Growth and reproductive behavior in the southern grasshopper mouse. *J. Mammal.,* 1968, *49,* 644–660.

Howe, M. A. Behavioral aspects of pair bond in Wilson's phalarope. *Wilson Bull.,* 1975a, *87,* 248–270.

Howe, M. A. Social interactions in flocks of courting Wilson's phalaropes *(Phalaropus tricolor). Condor,* 1975b, *77,* 24–33.

Howell, T. R., and Bartholomew, G. A. Temperature regulation in the sooty tern *Sterna fuscata. Ibis,* 1962, *104,* 98–105.

Hunt, G. L. Influence of food distribution and human disturbance on the reproductive success of herring gulls. *Ecology,* 1972, *53,* 1051–1061.

Hunt, G. L., and Hunt, M. W. Gull chick survival: The significance of growth rates, timing of breeding and territory size. *Ecology,* 1976, *57,* 62–75.

Huxley, J. S. The present standing of the theory of sexual selection. In G. R. De Beer (ed.), *Evolution: Essays to E. S. Goodrich.* Clarendon Press, Oxford, 1938, pp. 11–42.

Jarman, P. J. The social organisation of antelope in relation to their ecology. *Behaviour,* 1974, *48,* 215–267.

Jarman, P. J., and Jarman, M. V. Impala behaviour and its relevance to management. In V. Geist and F. Walther (eds.), *The Behaviour of Ungulates and Its Relation to Management,* Vol. 2. I.U.C.N., Moreges, 1974. pp. 871–881.

Jehl, J. R. The breeding biology of Smith's longspur. *Wilson Bull.,* 1968, *80,* 123–149.

Jenkins, D. The breeding of the red-legged partridge. *Bird Study,* 1957, *4,* 97–100.

Jenkins, D., Watson, A., and Miller, G. R. Population fluctuations in the red grouse, *Lagopus lagopus scoticus* (Lath.) in northeast Scotland, *J. Anim. Ecol.*, 1967, *36*, 97–122.

Jenni, D. A. Evolution of polyandry in birds. *Am. Zool.*, 1974, *14*, 129–144.

Jenni, D. A., and Betts, B. J. Sex differences in nest construction, incubation, and parental behaviour in the polyandrous American jacana (*Jacana spinosa*). *Anim. Behav.*, 1978, *26*, 207–218.

Jenni, D. A., and Collier, G. Polyandry in the American jacana (*Jacana spinosa*). *Auk*, 1972, *89*, 743–765.

Jensen, R. A. C., and Clinning, C. F. Breeding biology of two cuckoos and their hosts in South West Africa. *Living Bird*, 1974, *13*, 5–50.

Jensen, R. A. C., and Jensen, M. K. On the breeding biology of southern African cuckoos. *Ostrich*, 1969, *40*, 163–181.

Jensen, R. A. C. and Vernon, C. J. On the biology of the didric cuckoo in southern Africa. *Ostrich*, 1970, *41*, 237–246.

Johns, J. E. Field studies of Wilson's phalarope. *Auk*, 1969, *86*, 660–670.

Johnsgaard, P. A. Pair-formation mechanisms in *Anas* (Anatidae) and related genera. *Ibis*, 1960, *102*, 616–618.

Johnsgaard, P. A. *Handbook of Waterfowl Behavior.* Cornell University Press, Ithaca, N.Y., 1965.

Johnsgaard, P. A. *Grouse and Quails of North America.* University of Nebraska Press, Lincoln, 1973.

Johnsgaard, P. A. *Waterfowl of North America.* Indiana University Press, Bloomington, 1975.

Johnsgaard, P. A., and Buss, I. O. Waterfowl sex ratios during spring in Washington State and their interpretation. *J. Wildl. Manage*, 1956, *20*, 384–388.

Johnson, R. E. Reproductive activities of rosy finches, with special reference to Montana. *Auk*, 1965, *82*, 190–205.

Jolly, A. *The Evolution of Primate Behavior.* Macmillan, New York, 1972.

Joubert, E. The social organization and associated behaviour in the Hartmann zebra, *Equus zebra hartmannae. Madoqua*, 1972, *1*, 17–56.

Jungius, H. The biology and behaviour of the reedbuck (*Redunca arundinum* Boddaert, 1785) in the Kruger National Park. *Mammalia Depicta*. Verlag Paul Parey, Hamburg, 1971.

Kale, H. W., II. Ecology and bioenergetics of the long-billed marsh wren in Georgia salt marshes. *Publ. Nuttall Ornithol. Club*, 1965, *5*, 1–142.

Kaufmann, J. H. Ecology and social behavior of the coati, *Nasua narica*, on Barro Colorado Island, Panama. *Univ. Calif. Publ. Zool.*, 1962, *60*, 95–222.

Kelsall, J. P. *The Migratory Barren-Ground Caribou of Canada.* Department of Indian Affairs and Northern Development, Ottawa, 1968.

Kendeigh, S. C. Territorial and mating behavior of the house wren. *Ill. Biol. Monogr.*, 1941, *18*, 1–120.

Kenyon, R. F. Polygyny among superb lyrebirds in Sherbrook Forest Park, Kallista, Victoria. *Emu*, 1972, *72*, 70–76.

Kepler, C. B. Breeding biology of the blue-faced booby on Green Island, Kure Atoll. *Publ. Nuttall Ornithol. Club*, 1969, *8*, 1–97.

Kiley-Worthington, M. The waterbuck (*Kobus defassa* Ruppel 1835 and *K. ellipsyprymnus* Ogilby 1833) in East Africa: Spatial distribution. A study of the sexual behaviour. *Mammalia*, 1965, *29*, 177–204.

Kilgore, D. L., Jr., and Armitage, K. B. Energetics of yellow-bellied marmot populations. *Ecology*, 1978, *59*, 78–88.

King, J. A. Social behavior, social organization, and population dynamics in a black-tailed prairiedog town in the Black Hills of south Dakota. *Contributions of the Laboratory of Vertebrate Biology.* University of Michigan, Ann Arbor, 1955.

Kinzey, W. G., Rosenberger, A. L., Heisler, P. S., Prowse, D. L., and Trilling, J. S. A preliminary field investigation of the yellow-handed titi monkey, *Callicebus torquatus torquatus*, in northern Peru. *Primates*, 1977, *18*, 159–181.

Kistchinski, A. A. Breeding biology and behavior of the grey phalarope, *Phalaropus fulicarius*, in east Siberia. *Ibis*, 1975, *117*, 285–301.

Kitchen, D. W. Social behavior and ecology of the pronghorn. *Wildl. Monogr.*, 1974, *38*, 1–96.

Kleiman, D. G. Scent marking in the Canidae. *Symp. Zool. Soc. Lond.*, 1966, *18*, 167–177.

Kleiman, D. G. Monogamy in mammals. *Q. Rev. Biol.*, 1977a, *52*, 39–69.

Kleiman, D. G. (ed.). *Biology and Conservation of the Callitrichidae.* Smithsonian Press, Washington, D.C., 1977b.

Kleiman, D. G., and Eisenberg, J. F. Comparisons of canid and field social systems from an evolutionary perspective. *Anim. Behav.*, 1973, *21*, 637–659.

Klein, L. L., and Klein, D. J. Social and ecological contrasts between four taxa of neotropical primates. In R. H. Tuttle (ed.), *Socio-ecology and Psychology of Primates.* Mouton, The Hague, 1975, pp. 60–85.

Klingel, H. A comparison of the social behaviour of the equidae. In V. Geist and F. Walther (eds.), *The Behaviour of Ungulates and Its Relation to Management*. I.U.C.N., Moreges, 1974a, pp. 125–132.

Klingel, H. Soziale Organisation und Verhalten des Grevy-Zebras *(Equus grevyi)*. Z. Tierpsychol., 1974b, *36*, 37–70.

Klingel, H. Observations on social organization and behaviour of African and Asiatic wild asses *(Equus africanus* and *E. hemiosus)*. Z. Tierpsychol., 1977, *44*, 323–331.

Klomp, H. The determination of clutch-size in birds: A review. *Ardea*, 1970, *58*, 1–124.

Klopfer, P. F. *Habitats and Territories: A Study of the Use of Space by Animals*. Basic Books, New York, 1969.

Koford, C. B. The vicuña and the puna. *Ecol. Monogr.*, 1957, *27*, 153–219.

Koford, C. B. Prairie dogs, white faces, and blue grama. *Wildl. Monogr.*, 1958, *3*, 1–78.

Koivisto, I. Behaviour of the black grouse, *Lyrurus tetrix* (L.), during the spring display. *Pap. Game Res., Helsinki*, 1965, *26*, 1–60.

Kruuk, H. *The Spotted Hyena: A Study in Predation and Social Behavior*. University of Chicago Press, Chicago, 1972.

Kruuk, H., and Turner, M. Comparative notes on predation by lion, leopard, cheetah and wild dog in the Serengeti area, East Africa. *Mammalia*, 1967, *31*, 1–27.

Kummer, H. *Social Organization of Hamadryas Baboons*. University of Chicago Press, Chicago, 1968.

Kummer, H. *Primate Societies*. Aldine–Atherton, Chicago, 1971.

Lack, D. Habitat selection in birds. *J. Anim. Ecol.*, 1933, *2*, 239–262.

Lack, D. The display of the black cock. *Br. Birds*, 1939, *32*, 290–303.

Lack, D. Ecological aspects of species-formation in passerine birds. *Ibis*, 1944, *86*, 260–282.

Lack, D. The significance of clutch size, I, II. *Ibis*, 1947–1948, *89*, 302–352; *90*, 25–45.

Lack, D. *The Natural Regulation of Animal Numbers*. Clarendon Press, Oxford, 1954.

Lack, D. *Population Studies of Birds*. Clarendon Press, Oxford, 1966.

Lack, D. Interrelationships in breeding adaptations as shown by marine birds. *Proc. XIV Int. Ornithol. Cong.*, 1967, pp. 3–42.

Lack, D. *Ecological Adaptations for Breeding in Birds*. Methuen, London, 1968.

Lack, D., and Emlen, J. T. Observations on breeding behavior in tricolored redwings. *Condor*, 1939, *41*, 225–230.

Lamba, B. S. Nidification of some common Indian birds. VII. The spottedbilled or grey pelican *(Pelecanus philippensis* Gmelin). *Pavo*, 1963, *1*, 110–119.

Lancaster, D. A. Biology of the brushland tinamou, *Nothoprocta cinerascens*. *Bull. Am. Mus. Natur. Hist.*, 1964a, *127*, 269–314.

Lancaster, D. A. Life history of the Boucard tinamou in British Honduras. *Condor*, 1964b, *66*, 165–181, 253–276.

Lanyon, W. The comparative biology of the meadowlarks *(Sturnella)* in Wisconsin. *Publ. Nuttall Ornithol. Club*, 1957, *1*, 1–67.

Le Boeuf, B. J. Sexual behavior in the northern elephant seal *Mirounga angustirostris*. *Behaviour*, 1972, *41*, 1–26.

Le Boeuf, B. J. Male–male competition and reproductive success in elephant seals. *Am. Zool.*, 1974, *14*, 163–176.

Le Boeuf, B. J., and Briggs, K. T. The cost of living in a seal harem. *Mammalia*, 1977, *41*, 167–195.

Le Boeuf, B. J., Whiting, R. J., and Gantt, R. F. Perinatal behavior of northern elephant seal females and their young. *Behaviour*, 1972, *43*, 121–156.

Lenington, S. The evolution of polygyny in red-winged blackbirds. Ph.D. thesis, University of Chicago, Chicago, 1977.

Lent, P. C. Rutting behavior in a barren-ground caribou population. *Anim. Behav.*, 1965, *13*, 259–264.

Leuthold, W. Variations in territorial behavior of Uganda kob *(Adenota kob thomasi)*(Neumann, 1896), *Behaviour*, 1966, *27*, 215–258.

Leuthold, W. Observations on the social organization of impala *(Aepyceros melampus)*. Z. Tierpsychol., 1970, *27*, 215–258.

Leuthold, W. *African Ungulates: A Comparative Review of Their Ecology and Behavioral Ecology*. Springer–Verlag, New York, 1977.

Lill, A. Sexual behavior of the lek-forming white-bearded manakin *(Manacus manacus trinitatis* Hartert). Z. Tierpsychol., 1974a, *36*, 1–36.

Lill, A. Social organization and space utilization in the lek-forming white-bearded manakin, *M. manacus trinitatis* Hartert. Z. Tierpsychol., 1974b, *36*, 513–530.

Lill, A. Lek behavior in the golden-headed manakin, *Pipra erythrocephala* in Trinidad (West Indies). Z. Tierpsychol., 1976, *Suppl. 18*, 1–83.

Lindburg, D. Mate selection in rhesus monkey *(Macaca mulatta). Am. J. Phys. Anthropol.,* 1975, *42*, 315 (Abstract).

Liversidge, R. The biology of the jacobin cuckoo *Clamator jacobinus. Proceedings of the 3rd Pan-African Ornithological Congress, Ostrich Supplement,* 1971, *26*, 18–27.

Löhrl, H. Polygynie, Sprenung der Ehegemeinshaft und Adoption beim Halsbandfliegenschnäpper *(Muscicapa a. albicollis). Die Vogelwarte,* 1949, *15*, 94–100.

Löhrl, H. Weitere Fälle von Polygynie und Adoption beim Halsbandschnäpper *(Ficedula albicollis). Die Vogelwarte,* 1959, *20*, 33–34.

Low, R. M. Interspecific territoriality in a pomacentrid reef fish, *Pomacentrus flavicauda* Whitley. *Ecology,* 1971, *52*, 648–654.

Lowe, F. A. *The Heron.* Collins, London, 1954.

Lowery, G. H., Jr. *The Mammals of Louisiana and Its Adjacent Waters.* Louisiana State University Press, Baton Rouge, 1974.

Lukschanderl, L. Zur Verbreitung und Ökologie der Grosstrappe *(Otis tarda* L.) in Österreich. *J. Ornithol. Berl.,* 1971, *112*, 70–93.

Lutz, B. Fighting and an incipient notion of territory in male tree frogs. *Copeia,* 1960, 61–63.

MacDonald, S. D. The breeding behavior of the rock ptarmigan. *Living Bird,* 1970, *9*, 195–238.

Manson, J. Aspects of the biology and behaviour of the Cape Grysbok, *Raphicerus melanotis* Thunberg. M.Sc. thesis, University of Stellenbosch, S.W.A., 1974.

Marshall, W. H. Ruffed grouse behavior. *Bioscience,* 1965, *15*, 92–94.

Martin, R. D. Adaptive radiation and behaviour of the Malagasy lemurs. *Phil. Trans. Roy. Soc. Lond., Series B.,* 1972, *264*, 295–352.

Martin, S. G. Polygyny in the bobolink: Habitat quality and the adaptive complex. Ph.D. thesis, Oregon State University, Corvallis, 1971.

Martin, S. G. Adaptations for polygynous breeding in the bobolink, *Dolichonyx oryzivorus. Am. Zool.,* 1974, *14*, 109–119.

Mason, W. A. Social organization of the South American monkey *Callicebus moloch:* A preliminary report. *Tulane Stud. Zool.,* 1966, *13*, 23–28.

Mason, W. A. Use of space by *Callicebus* groups. In P. C. Jay (ed.), *Primates: Studies in Adaptation and Variability.* Holt, Rinehart, and Winston, New York, 1968, pp. 200–216.

Mason, W. A. Field and laboratory studies of social organization in *Saimiri* and *Callicebus.* In L. A. Rosenblum (ed.), *Primate Behavior: Developments in Field and Laboratory Research,* Vol. 2. Academic Press, New York, 1971, pp. 107–137.

Mathew, D. N. Observations on the breeding habits of the bronze-winged jacana, *Metopidius indicus* (Latham). *J. Bombay Natur. Hist. Soc.,* 1964, *61*, 295–302.

Maynard Smith, J. *The Theory of Evolution.* Penguin, Harmondsworth, 1958.

Maynard Smith, J. Parental investment: A prospective analysis. *Anim. Behav.,* 1977, *25*, 1–9.

Maynard Smith, J., and Ridpath, M. G. Wife sharing in the Tasmanian native hen *(Tribonyx mortierii):* A case of kinship selection? *Am. Natur.,* 1972, *106*, 447–452.

McHugh, T. Social behavior of the American buffalo *(Bison bison bison). Zoologica,* 1958, *43*, 1–40.

McIlhenny, E. A. Life history of the boat-tailed grackle in Louisiana. *Auk,* 1937, *54*, 274–295.

McKinney, F. Spacing and chasing in breeding ducks. *Wildfowl Trust Ann. Rep.,* 1965, *16*, 92–105.

McLaren, I. A. Seals and group selection. *Ecology,* 1967, *48*, 104–110.

McLaren, I. A. Polygyny as the adaptive function of breeding territory in birds. *Trans. Conn. Acad. Sci.,* 1972, *44*, 189–210.

McMillan, I. I. Annual population changes in California quail. *J. Wildl. Manage.,* 1964, *28*, 702, 711.

Mech, L. D. *The Wolf: The Ecology and Behavior of an Endangered Species.* Natural History Press, Garden City, N.Y., 1970.

Meinertzhagen, Col. R. *Birds of Arabia.* Liver and Boyd, London, 1954.

Miller, A. H. Habitat selection among higher vertebrates and its relation to intraspecific variation. *Am. Natur.,* 1942, *76*, 25–35.

Milne, H. Breeding numbers and reproductive rate of eiders at the Sands of Forvic National Nature Reserve, Scotland. *Ibis,* 1974, *116*, 135–154.

Modha, M. L., and Coe, M. J. Notes on the breeding of the African skimmer *Rynchops flavirostris* on Cental Island, Lake Rudolf, *Ibis,* 1969, *111*, 593–598.

Moehlman, P. Behavior and ecology of feral asses. Ph.D. thesis, University of Wisconsin, Madison, 1974.

Monahan, M. W. Determinants of male pairing success in the red-winged blackbird *(Agelaius phoeniceus):* A multivariate and experimental analysis. Ph.D. thesis, Indiana University, Bloomington, 1977.

Moreau, R. E. The comparative breeding biology of the African hornbills (Bucerotidae). *Proc. Zool. Soc. Lond.*, 1937, *107a*, 331–346.

Moreau, R. E., and Moreau, W. M. Biological and other notes on some East African birds. *Ibis*, 1937, *1* (14), 152–174.

Moreau, R. E., and Moreau, W. M. Hornbill studies. *Ibis*, 1940, *82*, 639–656.

Morton, E. S. On the evolutionary advantages and disadvantages of fruit eating in tropical birds. *Am. Natur.*, 1973, *107*, 8–22.

Moss, R. A comparison of red grouse *(Lagopus l. scoticus)* stocks with the production and nutritive value of heather *(Calluna vulgaris)*. *J. Anim. Ecol.*, 1969, *38*, 103–122.

Moss, R., Watson, A., and Parr, R. Maternal nutrition and breeding success in red grouse *(Lagopus lagopus scoticus)*. *J. Anim. Ecol.*, 1975, *44*, 233–244.

Moynihan, M. Some behavior patterns of platyrrhine monkeys. I. The night monkey *(Aotes trivirgatus)*. *Smithson. Misc. Coll.*, 1964, *146*(5), 1–84.

Murray, B. G., Jr. A comparative study of the Le Conte's and sharp-tailed sparrows. *Auk*, 1969, *86*, 199–231.

Myrberg, A. A., Jr., and Thresher, R. E. Interspecific aggression and its relevance to the concept of territoriality in reef fishes. *Am. Zool.*, 1974, *14*, 81–96.

Napier, J. R., and Napier, P. H. *A Handbook of Living Primates*. Academic Press, New York, 1967.

Nel, J. A. J. Aspects of the social ethology of some Kalahari rodents. *Z. Tierpsychol*, 1975, *37*, 322–331.

Nelson, J. B. The breeding biology of the gannet *Sula bassana* on the Bass Rock, Scotland. *Ibis*, 1966a, *108*, 584–626.

Nelson, J. B. Clutch size in the Sulidae. *Nature, London*, 1966b, *210*, 435–436.

Nelson, J. B. The breeding behaviour of the white booby *Sula dactylatra*. *Ibis*, 1967a, *109*, 194–232.

Nelson, J. B. Etho-ecological adaptations in the great frigate-bird. *Nature, London*, 1967b, *214*, 318.

Nelson, J. B. The relationship between behaviour and ecology in the Sulidae with reference to other sea birds. *Oceanogr. Mar. Biol. Annu. Rev.*, 1970, *8*, 501–574.

Nelson, J. B. Some relationships between food and breeding in the marine Pelecaniformes. In B. Stonehouse and C. M. Perrins (eds.), *Evolutionary Ecology*. Macmillan, London, 1977, pp. 77–87.

Nelson, J. B. *The Sulidae: Gannets and Boobies*. Oxford University Press, New York, 1978.

Nero, R. W. A behavior study of the red-winged blackbird. *Wilson Bull.*, 1956, *68*, 5–37, 129–150.

Nero, R. W., and Emlen, J. T. An experimental study of territorial behavior in breeding red-winged blackbirds. *Condor*, 1951, *53*, 105–116.

Nethersole-Thompson, D. *The Dotterel*. Collins, London, 1973.

Newton, I. *Finches*. Taplinger, New York, 1972.

Nolan, V., Jr. An analysis of the sexual nexus in the prairie warbler. *Proc. XIII Inter. Ornithol. Cong.*, 1963, pp. 329–337.

Nolan, V., Jr. The ecology and behavior of the prairie warbler *(Dendroica discolor)*. *Am. Ornithol. Un. Monogr.*, 1978, No. 24.

Norton, D. W. Incubation schedules of four species of calidrine sandpipers at Barrow, Alaska. *Condor*, 1972, *74*, 164–176.

Oates, J. F. The social life of a black-and-white colobus monkey, *Colobus guereza*. *Z. Tierpsychol.*, 1977, *45*, 1–60.

Oliver, J. A. Reproduction in the king cobra, *Ophiophagus hannah* Cantor. *Zoologica*, 1956, *41*, 145–152.

O'Neil, T. The muskrat in the Louisiana coastal marshes. Louisiana Department of Wildlife and Fisheries, Baton Rouge, 1949.

Orians, G. H. The ecology of blackbird *(Agelaius)* social systems. *Ecol. Monogr.*, 1961, *31*, 285–312.

Orians, G. H. On the evolution of mating systems in birds and mammals. *Am. Natur.*, 1969, *103*, 589–603.

Orians, G. H. The adaptive significance of mating systems in the Icteridae. *Proc. XV Int. Ornithol. Cong.*, 1972, pp. 389–398.

Orians, G. H. *Adaptations of Marsh-Nesting Blackbirds. Princeton Monographs in Population Biology*. Princeton University Press, Princeton, N.J., 1979.

Orians, G. H., and Collier, G. Competition and blackbird social systems. *Evolution*, 1963, *17*, 449–459.

Orians, G. H., and Pearson, N. E. On the theory of central place foraging. In D. J. Horn (ed.), *Analysis of Ecological Systems*. Ohio State University Press, Columbus, 1978.

Orians, G. H., and Willson, M. F. Interspecific territories of birds. *Ecology*, 1964, *45*, 736–745.

Oring, L. W., and Knudson, M. L. Monogamy and polyandry in the spotted sandpiper. *Living Bird*, 1972, *11*, 59–73.

Oring, L. W., and Maxson, S. J. Instances of simultaneous polyandry by a spotted sandpiper *Actitus mucularia*. *Ibis*, 1978, *120*, 349–353.

Orr, R. T. Interspecific behavior among pinnipeds. *Z. Säugetierkd.*, 1965, *30*, 163–171.

Orr, R. T. The Galapagos sea lion. *J. Mammal.*, 1967, *48*, 62–69.

Orr, R. T., and Poulter, T. C. Some observations on reproduction, growth, and social behavior in the Steller sea lion. *Proc. Calif. Acad. Sci.*, 1967, *35*, 193–226.

Osbourne, D. R., and Bourne, G. R. Breeding behavior and food habits of the wattled jacana. *Condor*, 1977, *79*, 98–105.

Owen, D. F. Latitudinal gradients in clutch size: An extension of David Lack's theory. In B. Stonehouse and C. M. Perrins (eds.), *Evolutionary Ecology*. Macmillan, London, 1977, pp. 171–179.

Owen-Smith, N. On territoriality in ungulates and an evolutionary model. *Q. Rev. Biol.*, 1977, *52*, 1–38.

Owings, D. H., and Ross, V. A. Alarm calls of California ground squirrels *(Spermophilus beecheyi)*. *Z. Tierpsychol.*, 1978, *46*, 58–70.

Palmer, R. S. *Handbook of North American Birds*, Vol. 1. Yale University Press, New Haven, 1962.

Parker, G. A., Baker, R. R., and Smith, V. G. F. The origin and evolution of gamete dimorphism and the male-female phenomenon. *J. Theor. Biol.*, 1972, *36*, 529–553.

Parmelee, D. F. Breeding behavior of the sanderling in the Canadian high arctic. *Living Bird*, 1970, *9*, 97–146.

Parmelee, D. F., and Payne, R. B. On multiple broods and the breeding strategy of arctic sanderlings. *Ibis*, 1973, *115*, 218–226.

Parsons, J. Cannibalism in herring gulls. *Br. Birds*, 1971, *64*, 528–537.

Parsons, J. Seasonal variation in the breeding success of the herring gull: An experimental approach to pre-fledging success. *J. Anim. Ecol.*, 1975, *44*, 553–573.

Payne, R. B. Interspecific communication signals in parasitic birds. *Am. Natur.*, 1967, *101*, 363–376.

Payne, R. B. The breeding seasons and reproductive physiology of tricolored blackbirds and redwinged blackbirds. *Univ. Calif. Publ. Zool.*, 1969, *90*, 1–137.

Payne, R. B. Duetting and chorus singing in African birds. *Proc. 3rd Pan-African Ornithol. Cong., Ostrich Suppl.*, 1971, *9*, 125–146.

Payne, R. B. The breeding season of a parasitic bird, the brown-headed cowbird, in central California. *Condor*, 1973, *75*, 80–99.

Payne, R. B. The ecology of brood parasitism in birds. *Ann. Rev. Ecol. System.*, 1977, *8*, 1–28.

Payne, R. B., and Payne, K. Social organization and mating success in local song populations of village indigobirds, *Vidua chalybeata*. *Z. Tierpsychol.*, 1977, *45*, 113–173.

Peek, F. W. Seasonal change in the breeding behavior of the male red-winged blackbird. *Wilson Bull.*, 1971, *83*, 383–395.

Penneycuik, C. J. Observations on a colony of Brünnich's guillemot *Uria lomvia* in Spitzbergen. *Ibis*, 1956, *98*, 80–99.

Perrone, M., Jr. The relation between mate choice and parental investment patterns in fish who brood their young: Theory and case study, Ph.D. thesis, University of Washington, Seattle, 1975.

Perrone, M., Jr., and Zaret, T. M. Parental care patterns in fish. *Am. Natur.*, 1979, *113*, 351–361.

Peterson, R. S. Social behavior in pinnipeds. In R. J. Harrison (ed.), *The Behavior and Physiology of Pinnipeds*. Appleton-Century-Crofts, New York, 1968, pp. 3–53.

Peterson, R. S., and Bartholomew, G. A. *The Natural History and Behavior of the California Sea Lion. Special Publication No. 1.* American Society of Mammalogists, Stillwater, Okla., 1967.

Pianka, E. R. On *r*- and *K*- selection. *Am. Natur.*, 1970, *104*, 592–597.

Pianka, E. R., and Parker, W. S. Age-specific reproductive tactics, *Am. Natur.*, 1975, *109*, 453–464.

Picman, J. Destruction of eggs by the long-billed marsh wren *(Telmatodytes palustris)*. *Can. J. Zool.*, 1977a, *55*, 1914–1920.

Picman, J. Intraspecific nest destruction in the long-billed marsh wren, *Telmatodytes palustris palustris*. *Can. J. Zool.*, 1977b, *15*, 1997–2003.

Pitelka, F. A. Territoriality, display, and certain ecological relations of the American woodcock. *Wilson Bull.*, 1943, *55*, 88–114.

Pitelka, F. A. Numbers, breeding schedule, and territoriality in pectoral sandpipers of northern Alaska. *Condor*, 1959, *61*, 233–264.

Pitelka, F. A., Holmes, R. T., and MacLean, S. F., Jr. Ecology and evolution of social organization in arctic sandpipers. *Am. Zool.*, 1974, *14*, 185–204.

Pleszczynska, W. K. Microgeographic prediction of polygny in the lark bunting. *Science*, 1978, *201*, 935–937.

Popp, J. L., and DeVore, I. Aggressive competition and social dominance theory. In D. A. Hamburg and J. Goodall (eds.), *Perspectives on Human Evolution*, Vol. 6: *Behavior of Great Apes*. Staples Press/ W. A. Benjamin, Menlo Park, Calif., 1979.

Pratt, H. M. Breeding biology of great blue herons and common egrets in central California. *Condor,* 1970, *72*, 407–416.

Putnam, L. S. The life history of the cedar waxwing. *Wilson Bull.,* 1949, *61*, 141–182.

Ralls, K. Sexual dimorphism in mammals: Avian models and unanswered questions. *Am. Natur.,* 1977, *111*, 917–938.

Rand, A. L. Social feeding behavior of birds. *Fieldiana Zool.,* 1954, *36*, 1–71.

Raner, L. Förekommer polyandri hos smalnäbbad simsnäppa *(Phalaropus lobatus)* och svartsnäppa *(Tringa erythropus). Fauna Flora,* 1972, *3*, 135–138.

Reese, E. A comparative field study of the social behavior and related ecology of reef fishes of the family Chaetodontidae. *Z. Tierpsychol.,* 1975, *37*, 37–61.

Rhoades, D. F., and Cates, R. G. Toward a general theory of plant antiherbivore chemistry. In J. W. Wallace and R. L. Mansell (eds.), *Biochemical Interaction between Plants and Insects.* Plenum Press, New York, 1976, pp. 168–213.

Ricklefs, R. E. An analysis of nesting mortality in birds. *Smithson. Contr. Zool.,* 1969, *9*, 1–48.

Ricklefs, R. E. A note on the evolution of clutch size in altricial birds. In B. Stonehouse and C. M. Perrins (eds.), *Evolutionary Ecology.* Macmillan, London, 1977a, pp. 193–214.

Ricklefs, R. E. On the evolution of reproductive strategies in birds: Reproductive effort. *Am. Natur.,* 1977b, *111*, 453–461.

Ridpath, M. G. The Tasmanian native hen, *Tribonyx mortierii.* II. The individual, the group, and the population. *CSIRO Wildl. Res.,* 1972, *17*, 53–90.

Rippin, A. B., and Boag, D. A. Recruitment to populations of male sharp-tailed grouse. *J. Wildl. Manage.,* 1974, *38*, 616–621.

Robertson, R. J. Optimal niche space of the red-winged blackbird *(Agelaius phoeniceus).* I. Nesting success in marsh and upland habitat. *Can. J. Zool.,* 1972, *50*, 247–263.

Robinson, A. The annual reproductive cycle of the magpie, *Gymnorhina dorsalis* Campbell, in southwestern Australia. *Emu,* 1956, *56*, 233–336.

Rohwer, S. Parent cannibalism of offspring and egg raiding as a courtship strategy. *Am. Natur.,* 1978, *112*, 429–440.

Rohwer, S., Fretwell, S. D., and Niles, D. M. Delayed maturation in passerine plumages and the deceptive acquisition of resources. *Am. Natur.,* in press.

Roseberry, J. L., and Klimstra, W. D. The nesting ecology and reproductive performance of the eastern meadowlark. *Wilson Bull.,* 1970, *82*, 243–267.

Rothe, H. Some aspects of sexuality and reproduction in groups of captive marmosets *(Callithrix jacchus). Z. Tierpsychol.,* 1975, *37*, 255–273.

Rowley, I. Communal activities among white-winged choughs *Corcorax melanorhamphus. Ibis,* 1978, *120*, 178–197.

Rudnai, J. A. *The Social Life of the Lion. A Study of the Behaviour of Wild Lions (Panthera leomassica* (Newman)) *in the Nairobi National Park, Kenya.* Washington Square East, Wallingsford, Pa., 1973.

Ruffer, D. G. Sexual behaviour of the northern grasshopper mouse *(Onychomys leucogaster). Anim. Behav.,* 1965, *13*, 447–452.

Rusch, D. H., and Keith, L. B. Seasonal and annual trends in numbers of Alberta ruffed grouse. *J. Wildl. Manage.,* 1971, *35*, 803–822.

Russell, S. M. Regulation of egg temperature by incubating white-winged doves. In C. C. Hoff and M. L. Ridesel (eds.), *Physiological Systems in Semiarid Environments.* University of New Mexico Press, Albuquerque, 1969, pp. 107–112.

Ryden, H. The "lone" coyote likes family life. *Nat. Geog.,* 1974, *146*(2), 279–294.

Ryves, H. H., and Ryves, B. H. The breeding habits of the corn-bunting as observed in North Cornwall: With special reference to its polygamous habit. *Br. Birds,* 1934, *28*, 2–26.

Samson, F. B. Territory, breeding density and fall departure in the Cassin's finch. *Auk,* 1976, *93*, 477–497.

Sauer, E. G. F., and Sauer, E. M. The behavior and ecology of the South African ostrich. *Living Bird,* 1966, *5*, 45–75.

Schäfer, E. Les conotos. *Bonn. Zool. Beitr.,* 1954, *5*, 1–148.

Schaller, G. B. *The Serengeti Lion.* University of Chicago Press, Chicago, 1972.

Schemnitz, S. D. Ecology of the scaled quail in the Oklahoma panhandle. *Wildl. Monogr.,* 1961, *8*, 1–47.

Schorger, A. W. *The Passenger Pigeon: Its Natural History and Extinction.* University of Wisconsin Press, Madison, 1955.

Scott, J. A. Observations on the breeding of the woollynecked stork. *Ostrich,* 1975, *46*, 201–207.

Searcy, W. A. The effect of sexual selection on male red-winged blackbirds *(Agelaius phoeniceus)*. Ph.D. thesis, University of Washington, Seattle, 1977.

Selander, R. K. On mating systems and sexual selection. *Am. Natur.,* 1965, *99*, 129–141.

Selander, R. K. Sexual selection and dimorphism in birds. In B. Campbell (ed.), *Sexual Selection and the Descent of Man.* Aldine, Chicago, 1972, pp. 180–230.

Seyfarth, R. M. Social relationships among adult male and female baboons. I. Behaviour during sexual consortship. *Behaviour,* 1978, *64*, 204–226.

Sharma, I. K. Habitat et comportement du paon *(Pavo cristatus). Alauda,* 1969, *37*, 219–223.

Sharma, I. K. Analyse écologique des parades du paon *(Pavo cristatus). Alauda,* 1970, *38*, 290–294.

Sharma, I. K. Etude écologique de la reproduction du paon, *Pavo cristatus. Alauda,* 1972, *40*, 378–384.

Sheldon, W. G. *The Book of the American Woodcock.* University of Massachusetts Press, Amherst, 1967.

Shepard, J. M. Factors influencing female choice in the lek mating system of the ruff. *Living Bird,* 1975, *14*, 87–111.

Sherman, P. W. Nepotism and the evolution of alarm calls. *Science,* 1977, *197*, 1246–1253.

Sick, H. Courtship behavior in the manakins (Pipridae): A review. *Living Bird,* 1967, *6*, 5–22.

Sinclair, A. R. E. The social organization of the East African buffalo *(Syncerus caffer* Sparrman). In V. Geist and F. Walther (eds.), *The Behaviour of Ungulates and Its Relation to Management.* I.U.C.N., Moreges, 1974, pp. 676–689.

Sinclair, A. R. E. *The African Buffalo: A Study of Resource Limitation of Populations.* University of Chicago Press, Chicago, 1977.

Skutch, A. F. Life history of the blue-throated toucanet. *Wilson Bull.,* 1944, *56*, 133–151.

Skutch, A. F. Do tropical birds rear as many young as they can nourish? *Ibis,* 1949, *91*, 430–455.

Skutch, A. F. *Life Histories of Central American Birds,* Vol. 1: *Pacific Coast Avifauna No. 31.* Cooper Ornithological Society, Berkeley, Calif., 1954.

Skutch, A. F. Roosting and nesting of aracari toucans. *Condor,* 1958, *60*, 201–219.

Skutch, A. F. Adaptive limitation of the reproductive rate of birds. *Ibis,* 1967, *109*, 579–599.

Skutch, A. F. *Life Histories of Central American Birds,* Vol. 3: *Pacific Coast Avifauna No. 35.* Cooper Ornithological Society, Berkeley, Calif., 1969.

Skutch, A. F. Life history of the keel-billed toucan. *Auk,* 1971, *88*, 381–396.

Skutch, A. F. Studies of tropical American birds. *Bull. Nuttall Ornithal. Club,* 1972, *10*, 1–223.

Smith, C. C. The adaptive nature of social organization in the genus of tree squirrels *Tamiasciurus. Ecol. Monogr.,* 1968, *38*, 31–63.

Smith, W. J., Smith, S. L., Oppenheimer, C. C., de Villa, J. G., and Ulmer, F. A. Behavior of a captive population of blacktailed prairie dogs: Annual cycle of social behavior. *Behaviour,* 1973, *46*, 189–220.

Smythe, N. Relationships between fruiting seasons and seed dispersal methods in a neotropical forest. *Am. Natur.,* 1970, *104*, 25–35.

Snow, B. K. A field study of the bearded bellbird in Trinidad. *Ibis,* 1970, *112*, 299–329.

Snow, B. K. Lek behaviour and breeding of Guy's hermit hummingbird *Phaethornis guy. Ibis,* 1974, *116*, 278–297.

Snow, D. W. The natural history of the oilbird *Steatornis caripensis. Zoologica,* 1961–1962, *46*, 27–47; *47*, 199–221.

Snow, D. W. A field study of the black and white manakin, *Manacus manacus,* in Trinidad. *Zoologica,* 1962a, *47*, 65–104.

Snow, D. W. A field study of the golden-headed manakin, *Pipra erythrocephala,* in Trinidad, W. I. *Zoologica,* 1962b, *47* 183–198.

Snow, D. W. The evolution of manakin displays. *Proc. XIII Int. Ornithol. Congr.,* 1963, pp. 553–561.

Snow, D. W. The singing assemblies of little hermits. *Living Bird,* 1968, *7*, 47–55.

Snow, D. W. Evolutionary aspects of fruit-eating by birds. *Ibis,* 1971a, *113*, 194–202.

Snow, D. W. Notes on the biology of the cock-of-the-rock *(Rupicola rupicola). J. Ornithol.,* 1971b, *112*, 322–333.

Snow, D. W. Duetting and other synchronised displays of the blue-backed manakins, *Chiroxiphia* spp. In B. Stonehouse and C. M. Perrins (eds.), *Evolutionary Ecology.* Macmillan, London, 1977, pp. 239–251.

Snow, D. W. and Lill, A. Longevity records for some neotropical birds. *Condor,* 1974, *76*, 262–267.

Sowls, L. K. Social behaviour of the collared peccary *Dicotyles tajacu* L. In V. Geist and F. Walther (eds.), *The Behaviour of Ungulates and Its Relation to Management.* I.U.C.N., Moreges, 1974, pp. 144–165.

Spinage, C. A. Territoriality and social organization of the Uganda defassa waterbuck. *J. Zool.,* 1969, *159*, 329–361.

Stamps, J. A. Social behavior and spacing patterns in lizards. In C. Gans and D. W. Tinkle (eds.), *Biology of the Reptilia*, Vol. 7: *Ecology and Behavior, A*. Academic Press, New York, 1977, pp. 265–334.

Stearns, S. C. Life-history tactics: A review of ideas. *Q. Rev. Biol.*, 1976, *51*, 3–47.

Stiles, F. G. Food supply and the annual cycle of the Anna hummingbird. *Univ. Calif. Publ. Zool.*, 1973, *97*, 1–109.

Stirling, I. Studies on the behaviour of the South Australian fur seal, *Arctocephalus forsteri* (Lesson), 1, 2, *Austral. J. Zool.*, 1971, *19*, 243–273.

Stirling, I. Observations on the Australian sea lion, *Neophoca cinerea* (Peron). *Austral. J. Zool.*, 1972, *20*, 271–279.

Stirling, I. Factors affecting the evolution of social behaviour in the Pinnipedia. *Procès-Verbaux Réunions Conseil International Exploration de Mer*, 1975, *169*, 205–212.

Stobo, W. T., and McLaren, I. A. *The Ipswich Sparrow*. Nova Scotian Institute, Halifax, Canada, 1975.

Stonehouse, B. The tropic birds *(G. phaethon)* of Ascension Island. *Ibis*, 1962, *103b*, 124–161.

Strawn, K. Life history of the pigmy seahorse, *Hippocampus zosterae* Jordan and Gilbert, at Cedar Key, Florida. *Copeia*, 1958, 16–22.

Struhsaker, T. T. Correlates of ranging behavior in a group of red colobus monkeys *(Colobus badius tephrosceles)*. *Am. Zool.*, 1974, *14*, 177–184.

Struhsaker, T. T. *The Red Colobus Monkey*. University of Chicago Press, Chicago, 1975.

Struhsaker, T. T., and Oates, J. F. Comparison of the behavior and ecology of red colobus and black-and-white colobus monkeys in Uganda: A summary. In R. H. Tuttle (ed.), *Socio-Ecology and Psychology of Primates*. Mouton, The Hague, 1975, pp. 103–123.

Svärdson, G. Competition and habitat selection in birds. *Oikos*, 1949, *1*, 157–174.

Svendsen, G. E. Behavioral and environmental factors in the spatial distribution and population dynamics of a yellow-bellied marmot population. *Ecology*, 1974, *55*, 760–771.

Swanberg, P. O. Great snipe. *British Birds*, 1965, *58*, 504–508.

Takai, T., and Mizokami, A. On the reproduction, eggs, and larvae of the pipefish, *Syngnathus schlegeli* Kaup. *J. Shimonoseki Coll. Fish.*, 1959, *8*, 85–89.

Tashian, R. E. Nesting behavior of the crested oropendola *(Psarocolius decumanus)* in northern Trinidad, B. W. I. *Zoologica*, 1957, *42*, 87–97.

Tenaza, R. R. Behavior and nesting success relative to nest location in Adélie penguins *(Pygoscelis adeliae)*. *Condor*, 1971, *73*, 81–92.

Tenaza, R. R. Territory and monogamy among Kloss' gibbons *(Hylobates klossii)* in Siberut Island, Indonesia. *Folia Primatol.*, 1975, *24*, 60–80.

Tenaza, R. R. Songs, choruses and countersinging of Kloss' gibbons *(Hylobates klossii)* in Siberut Island, Indonesia. *Z. Tierpsychol.*, 1976, *40*, 37–52.

Tevis, L. Summer behavior of a family of beavers in New York State. *J. Mammal.*, 1950, *31*, 40–65.

Thompson, W. L. Agonistic behavior in the house finch. I. Annual cycle and display patterns. *Condor*, 1960, *62*, 245–271.

Tilson, R. L., and Tenaza, R. R. Monogamy and duetting in an Old World monkey, *Presbytis potenziani*. *Nature, London*, 1976, *263*, 320–321.

Tinley, K. L. Dikdik, *Madoqua kirki*, in South West Africa: Notes on ecology and behavior. *Madoqua*, 1969, *1*, 7–35.

Trivers, R. L. Parental investment and sexual selection. In B. Campbell (ed.), *Sexual Selection and the Descent of Man, 1871–1971*. Aldine, Chicago, 1972, pp. 136–179.

Trivers, R. L. Foreword. In R. Dawkins, *The Selfish Gene*. Oxford University Press, New York, 1976.

Tschanz, B. Zur Brutbiologie der Trottellumme *(Uria aalge aalge* Pont.). *Behaviour*, 1959, *14*, 1–100.

Twining, H. The significance of combat in male rosy finches. *Condor*, 1938, *40*, 246–247.

Tyler, S. The behaviour and social organization of the New Forest ponies. *Anim. Behav. Monogr.*, 1972, *5*, 85–196.

Van Lawick, H., and Van Lawick-Goodall, J. *Innocent Killers*. Houghton, Mifflin, Boston, 1971.

Van Someren, V. D. The dancing display and courtship of Jackson's whydah *(Coliuspasser jacksoni* Sharpe). *J. E. Afr. Natur. Hist. Soc.*, 1945, *18*, 131–141.

Van Tyne, J. Life history of the toucan *Ramphastos brevicarinatus*. *Univ. Mich. Mus. Zool. Misc. Publ.*, 1929, *19*, 5–43.

Vehrencamp, S. L. Relative fecundity and parental effort in communally nesting anis, *Crotophaga sulcirostris*. *Science*, 1977, *197*, 403–405.

Vermeer, K. Breeding biology of California and ring-billed gulls: A study of ecological adaptation to the inland habitat. *Can. Wildl. Serv. Rep.*, 1970, *Series 12*, 1–52.

Verner, J. Evolution of polygamy in the long-billed marsh wren. *Evolution,* 1964, *18*, 252–261.

Verner, J. Breeding biology of the long-billed marsh wren. *Condor,* 1965, *67*, 6–30.

Verner, J., and Willson, M. F. The influence of habitats on mating systems of North American passerine birds. *Ecology,* 1966, *47*, 143–147.

Vernon, C. J. Polyandrous *Actophilornis africana. Ostrich,* 1973, *44*, 85.

Wagner, H. O. Notes on the life history of the emerald toucanet. *Wilson Bull.,* 1944, *56*, 65–76.

Walkinshaw, L. H. Attentiveness of cranes at their nests. *Auk,* 1965, *82*, 465–476.

Walther, F. Verhalten studien an der Grantgazelle (*Gazella granti* Brooke, 1872) im Ngorongoro Krater. *Z. Tierpsychol.,* 1965, *22*, 167–208.

Waring, G. H. Sound communications of black-tailed, white-tailed, and Gunnison's prairie dogs. *Am. Midl. Natur.,* 1970, *83*, 167–185.

Watson, A. A population study of ptarmigan *(Lagopus mutus)* in Scotland. *J. Anim. Ecol.,* 1965, *34*, 135–172.

Watson, A., and Jenkins, D. Notes on the behaviour of the red grouse. *Br. Birds,* 1964, *57*, 137–170.

Watson, A., and Miller, G. R. Territory size and aggression in a fluctuating red grouse population. *J. Anim. Ecol.,* 1971, *40*, 367–383.

Watson, A., and Moss, R. A current model of population dynamics in red grouse. *Proc. XV Int. Ornithol. Cong.,* 1972, pp. 134–149.

Weatherhead, P. J., and Robertson, R. J. Harem size, territory quality, and reproductive success in the redwinged blackbird *(Agelaius phoeniceus). Can. J. Zool.,* 1977, *55*, 1261–1267.

Weeden, R. B., and Theberge, J. B. The dynamics of a fluctuating population of rock ptarmigan in Alaska. *Proc. XV Int. Ornithol. Cong.,* 1972, pp. 90–106.

Wells, K. D. The social behaviour of anuran amphibians. *Anim. Behav.,* 1977, *25*, 666–693.

Welsh, D. A. Savannah sparrow breeding and territoriality on a Nova Scotia dune beach. *Auk,* 1975, *92*, 235–251.

Welter, W. A. The natural history of the long-billed marsh wren. *Wilson Bull.,* 1935, *47*, 3–34.

Wemmer, C., and Fleming, M. J. Management of meercats, *Suricata suricatta,* in captivity. *Int. Zoo Yearb.,* 1975, *15*, 73–77.

Wiley, R. H. Territoriality and non-random mating in sage grouse, *Centrocercus urophasianus. Anim. Behav. Monogr.,* 1973, *6*, 87–169.

Wiley, R. H. Evolution of social organization and life-history patterns among grouse. *Q. Rev. Biol.,* 1974, *49*, 201–227.

Williams, G. C. *Adaptation and Natural Selection: A Critique of Some Current Evolutionary Thought.* Princeton University Press, Princeton, N.J., 1966.

Williams, G. C. *Sex and Evolution. Monographs in Population Biology 8.* Princeton University Press, Princeton, N.J., 1975.

Williams, L. Breeding behavior of the Brewer blackbird. *Condor,* 1952, *54*, 3–47.

Willis, E. O. The behavior of plain brown woodcreepers *Dendrocincla fuliginosa. Wilson Bull.,* 1972, *84*, 377–420.

Willis, E. O., Wechsler, D., and Oniki, Y. On behavior and nesting of McConnell's flycatcher *(Pipromorpha macconnelli):* Does female rejection lead to male promiscuity? *Auk,* 1978, *95*, 1–8.

Willson, M. F. The breeding ecology of the yellow-headed blackbird. *Ecol. Monogr.,* 1966, *36*, 51–77.

Willson, M. F., and Orians, G. H. Comparative ecology of red-winged and yellow-headed blackbirds during the breeding season. *Proc. XVI Int. Cong. Zool.,* 1963, *3*, 342–346.

Wilson, E. O. *Sociobiology: The New Synthesis.* Belknap Press of Harvard University Press, Cambridge, 1975.

Wilson, H. The life history of the western magpie (*Gymnorhina dorsalis). Emu,* 1946, *45*, 233–244, 271–286.

Wilson, V. J., and Clarke, J. E. Observations on the common duiker, *Sylvicapra grimmia* Linn., based on material collected from a tsetse control game elimination scheme. *Proc. Zool. Soc. Lond.,* 1962, *138*, 487–497.

Wilsson, L. *My Beaver Colony.* Doubleday, Garden City, N.Y., 1968.

Wilsson, L. Observations and experiments on the ethology of the European beaver (*Castor fiber* L.). *Viltrevy,* 1971, *8*, 115–266.

Wittenberger, J. F. The ecological factors selecting for polygyny in altricial birds. *Am. Natur.,* 1976a, *110*, 779–799.

Wittenberger, J. F. Habitat selection and the evolution of polygyny in bobolinks (*Dolichonyx oryzivorus).* Ph.D. thesis, University of California, Davis, 1976b.

Wittenberger, J. F. The breeding biology of an isolated bobolink population in Oregon. *Condor,* 1978a, *80*, 355–371.

Wittenberger, J. F. The evolution of mating systems in grouse. *Condor,* 1978b, *80*, 126–137.

Wittenberger, J. F. Group size and polygamy in social mammals. *Am. Natur.,* in press, a.

Wittenberger, J. F. A model for delayed reproduction in iteroparous animals. *Am. Natur.,* in press, b.

Wyllie, I. Study of cuckoos and reed warblers. *Br. Birds,* 1975, *68*, 369–378.

Yasukawa, K. Male quality in the redwinged blackbird *(Agelaius phoeniceus).* Ph.D. thesis, Indiana University, Bloomington, 1977.

Yeaton, R. I. Social behavior and social organization in Richardson's ground squirrel *(Spermophilus richardsonii)* in Saskatchewan. *J. Mammal.,* 1972, *53*, 139–147.

Zimmerman, J. L. Polygyny in the dickcissel. *Auk,* 1966, *83*, 534–546.

Zimmerman, J. L. The territory and its density dependent effect in *Spiza americana. Auk,* 1971, *88*, 591–612.

Zwickel, F. C. Removal and repopulation of blue grouse in an increasing population. *J. Wildl. Manage.,* 1972, *36*, 1141–1152.

Zwickel, F. C., and Bendell, J. F. Early mortality and the regulation of numbers in blue grouse. *Can. J. Zool.,* 1967, *45*, 817–851.

Zwickel, F. C., and Bendell, J. F. Blue grouse, habitat, and populations. *Proc. XV Int. Ornithol. Cong.,* 1972, pp. 150–169.

7

The Roles of Individual, Kin, and Group Selection in the Evolution of Sociality

SANDRA L. VEHRENCAMP

INTRODUCTION

The main intent of this chapter is to develop a general framework in which to answer the question: What are the roles of individual, kin, and group selection in the evolution of social behavior? Evolution occurs when the gene frequencies in a population or species change. Natural selection in response to environmental conditions is the primary source of genetic change in most populations. But what is the unit of selection? Classically, the differential survival and reproduction of individuals, or individual selection, are regarded as the major cause of genic evolution. More recently, units larger than the individual have been proposed. The feasibility of the differential survival and reproduction of groups such as families, demes, trait groups, populations, and species has been examined qualitatively and quantitatively in theory, but few field data exist yet that prove the occurrence of these selection processes in nature.

Students of social behavior have precipitated a controversy over selection processes by identifying certain social systems in which some individuals appear to sacrifice their own personal reproduction for the reproductive benefit of another individual. Such apparently "altruistic" behavior cannot be easily explained by traditional individual selection. The theory of kin selection has been invoked to explain the occurrence of aid-giving behavior toward relatives. This theory recog-

SANDRA L. VEHRENCAMP Department of Biology, University of California at San Diego, La Jolla, California 92093.

nizes that individuals may selfishly enhance the spread of their genes by promoting the reproduction of kin possessing the same genes. Group selection theory focuses on the deme or population as the unit of selection and explains altruistic behavior as a beneficial act promoting the survival of a group of unrelated individuals. Individual, kin, and group selection are often considered alternative hypotheses, and the study of the evolution of social behavior provides a means for testing various selection models.

The approach taken here is not to expel two of the hypotheses in favor of a third, but rather to recognize the potential existence of all three and to determine the relative importance of each in the evolution of social organization. A vast array of social systems occurs in the animal kingdom. In particular, groups of animals differ markedly in the degree to which aid-giving or sacrificial behavior is apparent. Some animal groups may be more aptly called *passive aggregations,* in which individuals group around clumped resources, and where the reproductive success of an individual is not enhanced by the presence of neighboring individuals. Other species form *cooperative groups,* characterized by mutual giving and receiving of aid and the sharing of tasks such as predator defense, foraging, and brood care. In still other types of societies, a *division of labor* exists among cooperating individuals, and the tasks of defense, foraging, and reproduction are divided unequally among group members. It is in this third type of society that the greatest potential for altruistic behavior exists, because the reproductive success of some individuals appears to be much greater than that of others. While the potential importance of kin and/or group selection is greatest in these societies with a division of labor, it is far from clear whether social living entails a net sacrifice to the less successful individuals, or whether there is some hidden benefit to helping others.

In the following sections, I attempt to (1) develop an operational definition of *fitness* with which to compare the evolutionary success of different behavioral strategies; (2) differentiate individual, kin, and group selection and identify the types of "altruism" that can evolve via each process; (3) develop indices for the relative importance of individual, kin, and group selection; (4) survey the major groups of social animals to examine similarities in their evolutionary pathways to sociality; (5) summarize the ecological factors that select for different types of sociality; and (6) develop an alternative model for the evolution of societies with a division of labor that does not require altruism.

INDIVIDUAL, KIN, AND GROUP SELECTION DEFINED

Recently, the distinctions between individual, kin, and group selection have been blurred to the point where these terms are almost meaningless. Dawkins (1976) argued that parental behavior toward offspring is really extreme kin selection, where offspring are to be regarded as merely the most closely related relatives. Wilson (1975) merged the concepts of kin and group selection by placing them in a "continuum of selection on ever enlarging nested sets of related individuals" from the nuclear family to the clan, tribe, deme, and species. D. S. Wilson (1975) proposed a group selection model that Maynard Smith (1976) claimed is actually a kin selection model and that is identical to an individual selection model developed by Charnov and Krebs (1975). Obviously, the actual unit undergoing selection is not always evident. Instead of categorizing individual, kin, and group selection according to demographic patterns, I suggest that they be distinguished on the basis of their effects on individual fitness. The fitness of an individual is defined here as the rate at which its genes are propagated relative to the genes of other individuals in the population. All three selection processes can potentially contribute to the spread of an individual's genes. In an extension of the notion of inclusive fitness developed by Hamilton (1964), three components of fitness can be differentiated: (1) the component due to the offspring produced by the individual, or the personal component (P); (2) the component due to contemporary relatives, or the kinship component (K); and (3) the contribution due to future generations (grandchildren, great-grandchildren, etc.), or the future component (F). Inclusive fitness is therefore a function of the combined variables P, K, and F. While individuals should strive to maximize all three components of fitness, this may not always be possible, and one component may be increased only at the expense of others to maximize inclusive fitness. Kin selection is a process that increases the kinship component, usually at the expense of the personal component. Group selection is a process that maximizes the future component, usually at the expense of the personal component. Finally, behaviors that increase the personal component of fitness are classified as having evolved via individual selection.

Evolution occurs when individuals with different genetic makeups exhibit differential rates of gene propagation, that is, differential inclusive fitnesses. While we can measure changes in the frequency of single genes in a population, following the spread of the particular genes that affect social behavior is currently beyond our reach. Thus, fitness, although defined as relative gene propagation, is operationally measured as relative production of offspring, relatives, and descendants. Offspring can be counted much more easily than genes, and in substituting reproductive rates for gene propagation, it is implicitly assumed that genes cause phenotypic differences in reproductive behavior and that these genes are inherited with known probabilities by each offspring, relative, and descendant. Inclusive fitness can therefore be measured precisely if the number of young produced in a lifetime by all relevant individuals is known. Lifetime fitness is a function of the chances of survival and the rate of offspring production and is conveniently calculated by use of the equation for net reproductive output, R_o:

$$R_o = \sum_{x=0}^{\text{max age}} l_x m_x$$

where l_x is the probability of surviving to age x and m_x is the fertility at age x. Use of R_o as an index of fitness assumes a stable population size. Where populations are growing or declining, the Euler–Lotka equation can be substituted and the reproductive rate, r, may be used:

$$1 = \sum_{x=0}^{\text{max age}} l_x m_x e^{-rt}$$

where t = max age $- x$ and the age structure of the population is stable. Throughout this chapter, I will assume stable populations for simplicity, and lifetime fitness will be indicated by W, where $W = R_0$.

INDIVIDUAL SELECTION

Natural selection of individuals results from the differential reproduction and survival of the smallest gene-carrying unit, the individual. Any behavior that increases the personal component of fitness—that is, offspring production—of an individual, without affecting the kinship or future components, will spread in a population via individual selection. Lifetime fitness can be maximized by improving either survival or fecundity. Survival and fertility are frequently inversely related, since an increase in energy expended on eggs or offspring usually results in a decreased survival rate, and survival increases with a reduction in the number of offspring raised. Organisms therefore cannot maximize both l_x and m_x, and a compromise is reached that maximizes R_0 (Williams, 1966; Pianka, 1974).

Grouping is an important social strategy by which animals can increase their chances of survival and/or their reproductive success in certain ecological contexts. Group formation is, of course, a prerequisite for sociality, yet not all groups are inherently social. It is important to distinguish active groups, in which animals actively cooperate to their mutual advantage, from passive groups or aggregations in which the presence of nearby animals does not benefit the group joiner. A simple experiment can differentiate these two types of groups: a comparison of the fitness (R_0 or r) of an individual or pair in a group to its fitness when all other group members are removed. Passive groups tend to form as a result of a patchy distribution of resources, such as rich food clumps, sparse water holes, or a limited occurrence of safe refugia or nest sites. Therefore, the removal of all but one individual in the group should lead to no change in fitness, or perhaps an increase in fitness if there was excessive competition for the limited resources. If, on the other hand, the removal of all but one individual leads to a lower fitness, then grouping confers a positive benefit and constructive social interaction is implied. Cooperative behavior and certain types of altruism can therefore arise by individual selection, and these can be classified into two categories: mutualism and reciprocal altruism.

Mutualism is the cooperation of two or more individuals in a joint activity. It evolves by individual selection when an individual can benefit others while benefiting itself. This type of altruism or giving of aid is therefore incidental to the pursuit of personal reproductive success. It is likely to happen only when the altruistic act simultaneously affects the donor and the recipients. One example is the joint defense of a crèche of young belonging to different parents, where each individual improves the chances of its own young's surviving at the same time as the neighbors' young (Tener, 1954; Kruuk, 1972; Michener, 1969). A second example is the improved capture rate of large prey by predators that hunt in groups (Caraco and Wolf, 1975; Schaller, 1972; Mech, 1970). Finally, Hamilton (1971) and Treisman (1975) demonstrated mathematically how herding can reduce encounter rates with predators to the benefit of the average herd member.

The moment a time delay occurs between the benefit received by the recipient and the benefit received by the donor, a short-term cost to the donor can be shown, and the cooperative system that arises is called *reciprocal altruism* (Trivers, 1971). Reciprocal altruism involves truly altruistic acts, where the donor, at some cost to himself, helps another individual and where the recipient at some later date repays the debt by altruistically helping the original donor. When altruistic acts are always reciprocated, all cooperating individuals increase their overall fitness; an individual is transiently altruistic only in order to receive aid later. However, the delay between an altruist's help and the recipient's repayment sets the stage for invasion by "cheaters" that never repay the aid given.

Reciprocal altruism can evolve only when (1) the benefit of altruistic acts is much greater than the cost, so that there is a net gain in fitness from a reciprocal exchange; (2) individuals are exposed to many altruistic opportunities in a lifetime; and (3) the costs and benefits are constant for successive acts, that is, giving and receiving are symmetrical. Two types of reciprocal altruism can be recognized. First, in the most sophisticated form of reciprocal altruism, a method exists for discriminating against cheaters. Altruists dispense favors only to reciprocators, withholding aid from individuals they know to be nonreciprocators. Cheaters are therefore at a disadvantage and cannot invade the exchange system. Elaborate mechanisms evolve for the detection of potential reciprocators and nonreciprocators, and Trivers (1971) has described how such an elaborate system may have developed in humans. Second, if the altruist cannot regulate who the recipients of his act will be (e.g., he gives a food location signal or an alarm call that is detected by all members of his group), a reciprocal system can develop if the fitness of all group members increases as the number of altruists in the group increases (Charnov and Krebs, 1975). Thus groups with many altruists are more successful than groups with one or no altruists, and altruists also benefit from the presence of other altruists in the group. Altruism will spread in such a situation if the cost to each altruist is less than the benefit to the group of adding one more altruist. The problem of cheaters is avoided here because the average fitness of altruists in the population is greater than the average fitness of nonaltruists. The conditions for this type of reciprocal altruism may be met for some potentially altruistic behaviors. Large groups of alarm-calling birds can react much faster to a predator than small groups (Hoogland and Sherman, 1976; Powell, 1974). Food localization signals are given only when the patch of food is very rich (i.e., the cost of calling in other animals is small) in chimpanzees (Reynolds and Reynolds, 1965), lion-tailed macaque (Green, personal communication), and vultures (personal observation). Hard evidence for the operation of reciprocal altruism in animals is still lacking because of the paucity of critical, quantitative studies.

Some cases of aid-giving behavior are difficult to categorize as either mutualism or reciprocal altruism. These are reciprocal systems in which the existence of a short-term cost has not been demonstrated. The hypothesized exchange of food location information in refuging foraging colonies of bats and birds is perhaps an example of such zero-cost reciprocation (Hamilton and Watt, 1970; Ward and Zahavi, 1973; Fleming, Heithaus, and Sawyer, 1977; Emlen and Demong, 1975). It will be necessary to show whether individuals that join the colony to cash in on the food finds of others actually suffer a cost when they are themselves followed by roostmates. Thus, the line between mutualism and reciprocal altruism may be very fine.

Kin Selection

The family is the actual unit of selection according to kin selection theory. But instead of measuring the differential rate of survival and offspring production among family groups (which may be difficult to define), kin selection measures the spread of genes throughout a group of variously related individuals. The calculation of R_o or r takes into account the number of gene replicates an individual produces in the form of offspring. But relatives other than offspring also possess a certain fraction of genes that are common by descent. It follows that a more accurate measure of fitness should also include the spread of genes by relatives as well as offspring, and this concept has been termed *inclusive fitness* (Hamilton, 1964). Inclusive fitness adds the contribution of fitness by relatives, devalued by the probability that the relative possesses the same gene(s), to the individual's own production of offspring. If we denote the lifetime fitness of an individual A by W_A ($W = R_o$ in a stable population), the lifetime fitness of A's relative R_i by W_{R_i}, the coefficient of relatedness between A and its own offspring by r_{Ay}, and the coefficient of relatedness between A and R_i's offspring by r_{AR_iy}, then the inclusive fitness of A (IF_A) is the simple sum of all offspring produced by A and its relatives, each weighted by the degree of relatedness between the offspring and A:

$$IF_A = W_A r_{Ay} + \sum_{i=1}^{\text{all relatives}} W_{R_i} r_{AR_iy}$$

A's inclusive fitness therefore depends upon the fitness of his relatives. If A behaves in such a way as to affect the offspring production of his relatives, A's inclusive fitness becomes:

$$IF_{AR} = W_{AR} r_{Ay} + \sum_{i=1}^{\text{all relatives}} W_{R_iA} r_{AR_iy}$$

where W_{AR} is the offspring production of A when he is influencing R_i's fitness, and W_{R_iA} is the offspring production of the ith relative when A is influencing its fitness. This behavior toward relatives will increase A's inclusive fitness if IF_{AR} is greater than IF_A, or $IF_{AR} - IF_A \equiv \Delta IF_A > 0$:

$$\Delta IF_A = (W_{AR} - W_A) r_{Ay} + \sum_{i=1}^{\text{all affected relatives}} (W_{R_iA} - W_{R_i}) r_{AR_iy}$$

A may affect his relatives in two ways, positively or negatively. Whatever the effect on R's fitness, the effect on A's fitness is likely to be the inverse. If A selfishly increases his own personal fitness at the expense of a relative, his own inclusive fitness may be decreased. Similarly, if A's behavior toward R is altruistic, and the increase in the kinship component is greater than the decrease in the personal component, A's inclusive fitness is improved. Such altruistic behavior toward relatives that increases the kinship component of fitness is called *kin altruism*. In the case of kin altruism, the above equation is simplified and rearranged. ($W_{RA} - W_R$) becomes the benefit to R, and $-(W_{AR} - W_A)$ the cost to A. For ΔIF_A to be positive:

$$\text{Benefit}_R \, r_{ARy} > \text{Cost}_A \, r_{Ay}$$

or, in the more familiar form of the equation:

$$\frac{\text{Benefit}_R}{\text{Cost}_A} > \frac{r_{Ay}}{r_{ARy}}$$

(Wilson, 1975; West-Eberhard, 1975). In general, altruistic behavior should increase as the coefficient of relatedness increases, and selfish behavior should increase as the coefficient of relatedness decreases.

Since the identification of inclusive fitness by Hamilton (1964) and its subsequent development into the theory of kin selection by Maynard Smith (1964), Hamilton (1972), and others, kin selection has become a panacea for explaining not only altruistic behavior but all types of cooperative behavior in animals and man. In particular, kin selection seemed to have solved the problem of sterile female workers in Hymenoptera. Because of the haplodiploid genetic system in these insects, in which males are haploid and produced by unfertilized eggs and females are diploid and produced by fertilized eggs, a female hymenopteran is more closely related to her sisters than to her own offspring. Given that a female could raise sisters as well as offspring at the same cost per larva (i.e., cost = benefit), inclusive fitness would be higher by helping the mother produce sisters, since $r_{Ay} = 1/2$ and $r_{ARy} = 3/4$:

$$\frac{\text{Benefit}_R}{\text{Cost}_A} > \frac{1/2}{3/4}$$

$$1 > 2/3$$

Letting Benefit = Cost preserves the inequality, and hence altruism will evolve in this context. If $r_{ARy} = 1/2$ or less, as in most other taxa, the inequality is not preserved unless $\text{Benefit}_R > \text{Cost}_A$.

Five major problems suggest that this simple relation is not sufficient to explain the evolution of sociality in Hymenoptera:

1. Many haplodiploid hymenopteran species and other known haplodiploid insects are completely solitary.

2. Termites, which are diplodiploid, have achieved the same high level of sociality as the Hymenoptera.

3. If the queen mates with even two males, the relatedness of sisters is reduced to 1/2 (or less if more than two males are involved), which increases the right side of the equation above the left side.

4. For hymenopteran species in which two or more full sisters found nests but only one breeds, the maximum r_{ARy} to the recipient's offspring would be 3/8.

5. Since a female is related to a brother by only 1/4, the mean relatedness to all reproductive sibs is 1/2, as in most organisms (Alexander, 1974; Alexander and

Sherman, 1977; Evans, 1977; Lin and Michener, 1972; Trivers and Hare, 1976). Therefore, while haplodiploidy may encourage the evolution of sterile workers in Hymenoptera, it cannot be the only factor involved.

More recently, the emphasis on high coefficients of relatedness has been lessened in favor of an emphasis on high benefit/cost ratios (West/Eberhard, 1975). Even with r_{ARy} on the order of 1/4 to 1/8, kin altruism can evolve if the benefit greatly exceeds the cost, and the left-hand side of the equation is greater than the right side. West-Eberhard argued that environmental factors primarily affect the values of benefit and cost and dictate whether kin altruism will evolve or not. Altruism is likely when (1) the benefit is great (e.g., in emergency situations where a relative has a high chance of dying if not helped); (2) the cost is very low (e.g., the donor will not reproduce successfully on its own or is in control of an abundant resource); and (3) if many relatives can be aided at the same time (e.g., alarm calls). West-Eberhard provided examples of a wide variety of social behaviors, including food sharing, antipredation responses, grooming, adoption, alarm calls, and social subordinance, which may have evolved via kin selection. Trivers and Hare (1976), capitalizing on the differential relatedness to brothers and sisters in Hymenoptera, have shown that a conflict of interest between the queen and the workers regarding the optimal sex ratio of the brood is resolved in favor of the workers. These authors concluded that this is positive evidence of the action of kin selection, but Alexander and Sherman (1977) have offered an alternative explanation for sex-ratio differences.

For kin selection to operate, individuals must be able to dispense aid selectively to relatives. In many animals, dispersal is so low that an individual can assume that all neighbors living nearby are relatives. Such animals may not discriminate exact degrees of relatedness and dispense aid equally to all group members (e.g., elephants, Douglas-Hamilton, 1973). Other animals may remember very close relatives with which they have grown up. Sherman (1977) has shown that in ground squirrel populations where females usually breed near their parents and males always disperse, females are more altruistic when they have young or sisters in the vicinity and less altruistic if they are new immigrants in the population; adult males rarely give alarm, but predispersal juvenile males call as frequently as juvenile females (Dunford, 1977). That humans are keenly aware of familial relationships suggests that kin selection has played a role in human evolution.

Kin selection theory claims to explain the evolution of altruism by demonstrating a net advantage to the altruist. However, three critical assumptions that are often overlooked by proponents of this theory must be met. The first assumption is that the altruistic gene must initially spread throughout a family without causing a great personal loss to its bearers. If the original mutant is an extreme altruist (i.e., produces no offspring himself), his genes will not spread because relatives do not possess the altruistic gene with a known probability. Low degrees of altruism must develop first, so that selection against the altruist in the first generation will be slight (see West-Eberhard, 1975). Thereafter, the gene will increase if mutant-carrying relatives help eath other. The second assumption of kin selection is that all relatives at a given level in the family tree (e.g., all full siblings) share the same fraction of genes, in this case 50%. Yet, this is an average figure, and in fact, there is considerable variation around the mean (Steven Hubbel, unpublished manuscript). Only direct descendants (offspring, grandchildren, etc.) possess precisely the fraction of identical genes given by r. Thus, if the number of relatives an individual aids is small and the cost is high, the uncertainty of true relatedness may increase the risk of helping relatives. The third assumption of kin selection is that recipient relatives must not carry alleles at the same or other loci that negate or compete with the altruistic allele(s). Even though the altruistic allele is increasing via kin selection, the alleles of recipients may be increasing faster. This effect will be lessened if the altruist dispenses his aid to several relatives instead of one, and if the altruist is not permanently sterile and can expect reciprocation later.

It is generally the case that the recipient benefits more from kin altruism than the donor, both personally and genetically. If the change in inclusive fitness for the altruist A is:

$$\Delta IF_A = (W_{AR} - W_A)r_{Ay} + (W_{RA} - W_R)r_{ARy}$$

then the change in inclusive fitness for the recipient R is:

$$\Delta IF_R = (W_{RA} - W_R)r_{Ry} + (W_{AR} - W_A)r_{RAy}$$

ΔIF_R is always greater than ΔIF_A, since $(W_{AR} - W_A)$ is negative, $(W_{RA} - W_R)$ is positive, and $r_{Ry} > r_{RAy}$. The possibility therefore exists that an altruistic act that improves the inclusive fitness of the recipient could decrease the inclusive fitness of the donor. The values of the cost and benefit at which A and R disagree over the performance of altruism can be specified precisely. We note that the cost to A of helping is $C_A = (W_{AR} - W_A)$, the benefit to R is $B_R = (W_{RA} - W_R)$, and that for most animals $r_{Ry} = r_{Ay} = 1/2$. This means that:

(a) $\Delta IF_A > 0$ if $B_R/C_A > \dfrac{1}{2r_{ARy}}$

$\Delta IF_A < 0$ if $B_R/C_A < \dfrac{1}{2r_{ARy}}$

(b) $\Delta IF_R > 0$ if $B_R/C_A > 2r_{RAy}$

$\Delta IF_R < 0$ if $B_R/C_A < 2r_{RAy}$

Thus, when $B_R/C_A > 2r_{RAy}$, both R and A benefit from A's altruistic act; for $B_R/C_A < \frac{1}{2}r_{ARy}$, both suffer as a result of the act. For $2r_{RAy} > B_R/C_A > \frac{1}{2}r_{ARy}$, R benefits while A suffers a loss in inclusive fitness. Is it possible for R to demand and receive aid from A in this situation? This question brings to light a different interpretation of kin altruism that might well be called *kin manipulation*. The behaviors that we view as altruistic on the part of the donor may in fact be manipulation and extreme selfishness on the part of the recipient.

The opportunity for the recipient to manipulate the donor is most likely to occur between parent and offspring, since the fitness of each is greatly dependent on the other. Trivers (1974) and Alexander (1974) have offered two opposing points of view on this issue, which can be reconciled with the framework established above. Trivers argued that the offspring can apply devious and psychological pressure on the mother to gain more parental care than the parent is optimally selected to give. Alexander countered that the parent, being larger and dominant, is in a better position to exert its will. Both Trivers and Alexander actually agreed that the recipient may be able to manipulate the donor, but Trivers envisioned the offspring as the potential recipient of parental aid, while Alexander suggested that the offspring may potentially aid the parent in the production of siblings. The argument therefore boils down to: Is the parent a donor or a recipient of aid? Under what circumstances will selection favor the parent, in what circumstances the offspring?

In summary, aid-giving behavior can be viewed as altruism that indirectly increases the fitness of the donor or as manipulation by a dominant individual. If manipulation is occurring, then how far can the dominant reduce the fitness of the subordinate for his own personal gain? The question of manipulation among kin and nonkin will be examined later.

GROUP SELECTION

The idea of group selection permeates the biological literature and predates Darwin (see Van Valen, 1975). Wright (1956) first applied the term *intergroup selection* to selection at the level of populations, demes, species, and higher taxa. Group selection is commonly invoked to explain the succession of major taxa through geological time, the evolution of genetic mechanisms, the widespread occurrence of sexual (versus asexual) reproduction, and the evolution of mechanisms for population regulation (Fisher, 1930; Darlington, 1939; Thoday, 1953; Van Valen, 1975; and others, see Wilson, 1975). Nonevolutionary biologists inadvertently invoke group selection when they view biological adaptations as "good for the species." Finally, the marriage of biology with computers and economic theory has led to a group-selection-type of logic in which "efficiency" is the primary goal of the system or group. Group selection was recently brought to the forefront of biology when it was applied to the evolution of social behavior and altruism by Wynne-Edwards (1962). Wynne-Edwards invoked interdemic selection to explain the apparent constraint exercised by animals in not overeating their food supply. He argued that those populations or demes that altruistically reduced their exploitation rate of the environment (and therefore their reproductive success) survived better than populations that consumed and reproduced selfishly, and he identified numerous behaviors as "epideictic" displays that evolved solely for the purpose of allowing individuals to assess the population density and decide whether or not to reproduce. Wynne-Edwards's thesis was the subject of much emotional criticism. Most critics felt that alternative hypotheses were ignored, that the behaviors could be explained on the basis of individual or kin selection, and that evolution by group selection was highly unlikely except in rare circumstances (Williams, 1966, 1971; Lack, 1966; Ghiselin, 1974).

More recently, the feasibility of group selection has been investigated with the use of mathematical models and computer simulations (Levins, 1970; Boorman and Levitt, 1973; Gadgil, 1975; Levin and Kilmer, 1974; see Wilson, 1975, for review). The goal of the models was to identify the demographic conditions under which selection on groups could lead to changes in gene frequencies. Groups composed of reproducing individuals are assigned death rates and birth rates. In order to distinguish the processes of group and individual selection, the models ask whether true altruism, a trait that cannot evolve by individual selection, can evolve via group selection in a population with mostly selfish individuals. Group selection must therefore be able to counteract individual selection. The initial conditions for the models are as follows: (1) altruistic genes exist initially at low frequencies in the population; (2) selfish individuals outreproduce altruistic individuals; and (3) the group extinction rate decreases as the proportion of altruists in the group increases.

The models depend on genetic drift and other stochastic processes to produce occasional groups with a high frequency of altruists. For altruism to spread throughout the population, the following conditions must be met: (1) groups are small and/or founded by a few individuals; (2) gene flow (immigration) is low after founding, so that altruistic groups are not infected by selfish genes; and (3) extinction rates are very high for selfish groups and very low for altruistic groups, with a nonlinear relationship between the percentage of altruists and survival rate (Boorman and Levitt, 1973). In order to maintain altruism in the population, the migration rate of selfish individuals between groups must be lower than that for altruistic individuals. Most of the above models at best resulted in a balanced polymorphism of altruistic and selfish genes, and even so, the population parameters required were stringent and not likely to occur widely in nature. The most likely ecological situation for group selection to occur may be island archipelagos, where populations are small and go extinct frequently, and where migration rates are low (MacArthur and Wilson, 1967; J. Diamond, personal communication).

It is generally agreed (Lewontin, 1970) that group selection can rarely counteract individual selection because of the former's slow rate of evolution. The speed of evolution depends on the rates of mortality and birth; the greater the birth rate, the greater the mortality rate, and this can lead to very rapid selection. Because the birth and extinction rates of groups are usually much less than the birth and death rates for individuals, selection on groups cannot proceed as fast and is usually swamped out by individual selection. Gilpin (1976), however, has shown that if groups do go extinct rapidly, group selection can occur even when the conditions of small group size and low migration rates are relaxed. The ecological situation envisioned by Gilpin that causes the rapid group extinction is predator/prey interaction. Predators that are too efficient overexploit their prey and rapidly go extinct. The evolution of predator prudence via group selection is precisely the situation envisioned by Wynne-Edwards. Mathematical models and laboratory experiments of predator–prey interactions often do lead to rapid extinction, and it is possible to "evolve" less efficient predators in the laboratory by using a group selection process (Pimentel, 1968). Whether such rapid turnover of predator and prey populations occurs in nature is still open to question. Gilpin's model works best for parasites specializing on a single prey species. To prove this or any other group selection model, it would be necessary to show that discrete groups of animals differ in their abilities to exploit food or in some other altruistic tendency, and that these groups survive differentially according to the fraction of altruists or lower consumers in the group.

In earlier sections, we saw that altruistic acts may lose their altruism when the more far-reaching effects of the act are considered. Altruism is therefore construed as selfish behavior that increases an individual's fitness either at a later point in his life or indirectly via close kin. Group selection is classically viewed as capable of producing purely altruistic acts, in which an individual sacrifices his fitness for the benefit of his species or a group of unrelated individuals. However, if such an altruistic individual can insure that future generations of his genetic line will benefit in the long run from his personal sacrifice, it may be possible to view group selection as ultimately selfish behavior where reciprocation occurs after the death of the individual. In a similar vein, Williams (1975) distinguished the short-term versus long-term advantages of reproductive strategies in his discussion of sexual versus asexual reproduction. If group selection operates at all, it must be the case that altruists are more fit than selfish individuals when viewed over a long enough period of time. It follows that a true measure of the spread of genes should include not only the contributions of personal offspring and contemporaneous kin but also the contribution of future generations. Alexander (1974) and Orlove (1975) pointed out that selection may operate on grandchildren and great-grandchildren in certain situations. This notion can also be extended to future generations beyond the lifetime of individuals. Thus, group selection occurs when a decrease in personal reproduction leads to an increase in the future component of fitness.

D. S. Wilson (1975, 1977) has proposed a type of group selection model in which groups with different proportions of altruists survive differentially, but that does not meet the condition of lower personal fitness–higher future fitness. Wilson envisioned a population divided into discrete groups, called *trait groups*, in which the proportion of altruists and nonaltruists varies randomly. Within each group, altruists have lower chances of survival than nonaltruists, but groups with many altruists survive better than groups with few or no altruists. The mean fitness of altruists in the population is higher than the mean fitness of nonaltruists if at least one of three conditions is met: (1) the altruist increases his own fitness as well as the fitness of other group members; (2) altruistic behavior lowers the fitness of the altruist but the cost is less than the benefit, and the fitness of recipients increases linearly as the number of altruists in the group increases; or (3) the distribution of altruists in the trait groups is greater than random. Situation 1 is essentially mutualism, Situation 2 is precisely the model of reciprocal altruism developed by Charnov and Krebs (1975), and Situation 3 is met either when altruists are attracted to each other or when kin associate (Maynard Smith, 1976). The basic effect of Wilson's complicatedly structured demes is to allow two or more altruists to interact mutualistically or reciprocally. Since benefits are received within the lifetime of an individual, the model may be better classified as a case of individual or kin selection.

INDICES FOR THE RELATIVE IMPORTANCE OF INDIVIDUAL, KIN, AND GROUP SELECTION

To summarize the preceding section, the different types of altruism can be defined as follows in their pure form. In each case, the fitness of individuals living in a cooperative group situation is compared to the fitness of individuals living solitarily or in groups lacking the cooperative or altruistic behaviors. In practice, the solitary or nonaltruistic condition may have to be created experimentally, since naturally occurring differences in group structure may be adapted to microhabitat differences. W_{AR}, W_{RA}, and W_{CA} refer to the fitness of individuals in groups, and W_A, W_R, and W_C refer to the fitness of the same individuals in the same place when all other group members are removed or when group members are prevented from cooperating. A refers to the altruist or aid giver, R refers to a relative of A, and C refers to a nonrelated colleague of A.

Case 1: Passive aggregation

$$W_A \geq W_{AC}$$

Case 2: Active cooperation (mutualism or reciprocal altruism)

$$W_{AC} > W_A \text{ and } W_{CA} > W_C$$

Case 3: Kin altruism

$$W_A > W_{AR} \text{ and } (W_{RA} - W_R)\, r_{ARy} > (W_A - W_{AR})\, r_{Ay} \qquad (\Delta IF_A \text{ positive})$$

Case 4: Manipulation

$$(W_{RA} - W_R)\, r_{Ry} > (W_A - W_{AR})\, r_{RAy} \qquad (\Delta IF_R \text{ positive})$$

$$\text{and}$$

$$(W_A - W_{AR})\, r_{Ay} > (W_{RA} - W_R)\, r_{ARy} \qquad (\Delta IF_A \text{ negative})$$

Case 5: Group altruism

$$\text{Both } \Delta IF_R \text{ and } \Delta IF_A \text{ are negative}$$

There is a great likelihood that individual, kin, and group selection act in conjunction with each other (see also Hamilton, 1975). For example, reciprocal altruism or mutualism among kin may bring benefits via both individual and kin selection, and altruism among kin may be enhanced by the action of family-group selection. Two indices have therefore been devised to determine the relative importance of these processes; the first rates the relative importance of individual versus kin selection, and the second rates the relative importance of individual versus group selection.

INDIVIDUAL VERSUS KIN SELECTION

The usual method of determining the feasibility of kin selection is to ask whether an altruistic gene will increase in a population, given a certain benefit to the recipient, cost to the altruist, and degree of relatedness between the two individuals:

$$\frac{\text{Benefit}_R}{\text{Cost}_A} > \frac{r_{Ay}}{r_{ARy}}$$

This sort of analysis does not permit us to evaluate the relative roles of the personal component and the kinship component of fitness for species in which altruists also produce some young. Furthermore, it cannot be applied to species in which aid giving leads to a positive personal benefit to the altruist, since the cost term $(W_{AR} - W_A)$ must be negative by definition. Thus, two types of aid giving among kin cannot be evaluated: (1) mutualistic behavior among kin, where both the personal and kinship components of fitness are simultaneously increased, and (2) temporary altruism between parent and offspring, where altruists become recipients at another time in life. When the equation is applied to mammals and birds, where altruists eventually become breeders, it is applied only to the altruistic period of life. Instead of using R_o (lifetime fitness), reproductive success per breeding attempt is substituted, and the important effects of survival and success of dispersal are therefore ignored. This approach overemphasizes the importance of the kinship component to the overall change in inclusive fitness.

Interaction patterns could be ranked on a continuum from selfish to altruistic behavior as follows:

$$\text{Manipulation} \rightarrow \begin{array}{c} \text{Mutualism or} \\ RA \text{ among nonkin} \end{array} \rightarrow \begin{array}{c} \text{Mutualism or} \\ RA \text{ among kin} \end{array} \rightarrow \text{Kin altruism}$$

The importance of individual selection decreases, and kin selection increases, along this scale from left to right. An index of the relative importance of kin selection could then be computed as follows:

$$I_k = \frac{(W_{RA} - W_R)r_{ARy}}{(W_{AR} - W_A)r_{Ay} + (W_{RA} - W_R)r_{ARy}}$$

where A is the actor of a selfish or altruistic strategy and R is the recipient. When the denominator (which is ΔIF_A) is ≤ 0, the index is undefined, and either the actor is being manipulated or group selection explains the observed behavior. These two processes can be distinguised by calculating ΔIF_R as described earlier; if ΔIF_R is positive, then A is being manipulated by R; if negative, then group selection is indicated. The above index essentially rates the relative fraction of the kinship component to the total change in inclusive fitness of pursuing the particular strategy. When $I_k > 1$, pure kin altruism is occurring, in which A sacrifices his own personal reproduction for the benefit of relatives. For I_k between 0 and 1, the relative importance of kin selection increases from 0% to 100%, where 0 is pure individual selection with no kinship component, 0.5 is equal contributions of kin and individual selection, and 1 implies that relatives are benefited at zero cost to the actor. When I_k is < 0, A is manipulating R, with the severity of manipulation increasing as the index becomes more negative.

To calculate this index, longitudinal studies must be made of individuals pursuing different social strategies. To measure R_o, data must be collected on rate of offspring production, survivorship, and dispersal success. For many animals, it is not possible to find the nonsocial (solitary) condition occurring in nature. In this case, small social units must be created experimentally in the field. The index would be most difficult to calculate for the highly eusocial Hymenoptera, where solitary individuals never occur because the reproductive individual is obligatorily dependent on the nonreproductive (sterile) workers. The success of a solitary queen would therefore be zero, and the cost to the worker of not reproducing would be $0 - 0 = 0$, resulting in a meaningless I_k. The importance of kin selection in Hymenoptera will therefore have to be calculated for facultatively social species in which queens are still capable of foraging. I have attempted to calculate the index of kin selection for three social organisms for which sufficient data are available: lions, Florida scrub jays, and a *Polistes* wasp.

Schaller (1972) and Bertram (1975, 1976) have managed to amass a great deal of information on the longevity, reproductive success, and kinship of lions in Serengeti Park. Female lions breed cooperatively in groups averaging seven individuals, but some females breed solitarily or peripherally. Group females produce an average of .18 adult young per year, solitary females produce .07 young per year, and females of both classes have a life expectancy of 12 years. The lifetime reproductive success of a group female is therefore 2.16 (= W_{AR} and W_{RA}), and for a solitary female, .84 (= W_A and W_R). Group females are related by an average r of .15, and assuming that seven female relatives always cooperate, the index of kin selection is .51; that is, about half of the advantage to grouping is accumulated via personal reproduction, and half is accumulated via relatives.

Woolfenden (1973, 1975) has spent many years observing the Florida scrub jay, a species in which youngsters may delay reproduction as long as three years to remain on the parental territory and assist their parents with subsequent broods. Unhelped pairs produce .5 independent young per season, while helped pairs produce 1.3 young. Annual survivorship is 87% for breeders and helpers in groups, 80% for solitary breeders. The probability of successful dispersal by juveniles can be estimated by assuming a stable population size and dividing the number of adult deaths per 100 adults by the number of juveniles produced per 100 adults (34%). Because dispersal success is lower than the survival rate of remaining on the parental territory, youngsters can afford to forgo reproduction for several years if they are then assured of obtaining a breeding territory. Interestingly, males have a greater tendency to remain as helpers, apparently because they are the dominant, territorial sex and have the opportunity to obtain a portion of the parental territory (Woolfenden and Fitzpatrick, 1978). R_o is higher for a juvenile that delays breeding for three years, then begins breeding itself (0.64 = W_{AR}), than if it disperses in its first year (0.33 = W_A and W_R). A helper that stays with its parents and assists with the care of its sibs (r_{ARy} = 1/2) for three years increases the R_o of its parents to 0.73 (= W_{RA}). The index of kin selection from the point of view of a juvenile who helps its parents for three years is +.55; that is, both the kinship and the personal components of fitness are increased.

With the recent work of Metcalf and Whitt (1977a,b) and previous studies by West-Eberhard (1969), data on the relatedness, reproductive success, longevity, and relative egg ownership of multiple foundress and solitary-foundress nests of a social wasp, *Polistes metricus*, are now available. Two-foundress nests produce 2.25 times more young than solitary queens and have a higher chance of succeeding (81% versus 59%). But the alpha queen of a duo produces 82.5% of the brood and forces the beta queen to do most of the risky foraging. The relative reproductive success of alpha and beta queens is 1.50 (W_{RA}) and .32 (W_{AR}), respectively, and solitary queens have a success of .59 (W_A and W_R). The queens of a group have a high probability of being full sisters, with an average r of .63. The index of kin selection from the point of view of the beta queen in a group is +1.89, meaning that she reduces her personal fitness for the benefit of her sister.

SANDRA L.
VEHRENCAMP

Group selection, as discussed earlier, results in a maximization of the future component of fitness, or the number of descendants n generations from now. Group selection could act either in conjunction with or in opposition to individual selection. An index of group selection must therefore evaluate the relative contribution of group selection to future fitness. One difficulty in developing an index of group selection is that future fitness is a multiplicative function of current, or personal fitness, and any change in personal fitness will result in a change in future fitness via individual selection. An increase in future fitness does not necessarily indicate group selection if it was caused by an increase in personal fitness. Group selection is occurring if future fitness increases more than would be expected by individual selection acting alone, or if there is an inverse relationship between personal fitness and future fitness.

A comprehensive measure of future fitness might be the geometric mean of all descendants over an infinite number of generations. But for the purposes of comparing social strategies and devising an index of group selection, future fitness can be defined as the number N of descendants in some subsequent generation n, times the coefficient of relatedness to those descendants $(1/2)^n$:

$$W_{F_n} = N_n\,(1/2)^n$$

The number of descendants is determined by the joint action of group and individual selection:

$$W_{F_n} = W_{I_n} + W_{G_n}$$

The contribution from individual selection could be measured in the field if group selection can be eliminated, but it could also be predicted from a knowledge of reproductive rates. If population growth is exponential, individual selection should lead to an exponential change in the number of descendants at each generation:

$$W_{I_n} = \left(\frac{W_P}{2}\right)^n$$

where W_P is the personal lifetime fitness of an individual in generation $n = 1$. The contribution due to group selection is therefore the observed future fitness at generation n minus the contribution due to individual selection at generation n:

$$W_{G_n} = N_n\,(1/2)^n - \left(\frac{W_P}{2}\right)^n$$

An index of group selection would therefore rate the relative contribution of W_G to total future fitness:

$$I_g = \frac{W_{G_n}}{W_{F_n}} = \frac{N_n\,(1/2)^n - \left(\dfrac{W_P}{2}\right)^n}{N_n\,(1/2)^n}$$

This index is 0 when there is no contribution of group selection to future fitness and increases to a maximum of 1 when group selection explains 100% of the gain in future fitness. A positive I_g indicates that group selection and individual selection are acting in conjunction with each other. The index becomes negative when group selection is selecting for altruism in opposition to individual selection.

While such a group selection index can be calculated in theory, in practice it may prove difficult to collect the appropriate data and estimate the individual selection component. The index is merely suggested as a possible approach to the problem. Unfortunately, no field data exist with which to attempt a computation of the index.

Evolutionary Routes to Sociality

The preceding sections have outlined methods by which the relative contributions of individual, kin, and group selection to a given level of sociality (e.g., mutualism, reciprocal altruism, true personal altruism) can be measured. To date, such quantitative methods have rarely been attempted. Instead, it has been the practice to correlate such factors as average relatedness ($\bar{r}$) and level of sociality in a variety of species and to infer an increasing importance of, in this case, kin selection, where a correlation exists (Barash, 1974; Wilson, 1975). Correlations always leave open the question of cause and effect: Is a high degree of relatedness the cause or a side effect of sociality? In the absence of detailed quantitative studies on lifetime fitness, the only way to estimate the relative roles of each type of selection is to reconstruct the probable evolutionary routes by which each social state evolved. Since social systems can rarely be determined from the fossil record, one can only array clusters of existing species from simple to complex and assume that existing simple stages are similar to those passed through by complex stages at an earlier epoch.

Although the shortcomings of this latter approach are obvious, it is instructive to note that independent attempts for the four most social groups of animals have all resulted in nearly identical conclusions: spiders (Shear, 1970), insects (Wilson, 1971), birds (Brown, 1974), and mammals (Eisenberg, 1966). Each taxon reviewed shows a span of sociality ranging from solitary breeding females to highly social or eusocial groups. *Eusociality* is a term originally coined by entomologists to denote insect societies characterized by: (1) cooperative brood care; (2) an overlap of generations within a colony; and (3) a reproductive division of labor. Given this general definition, *eusociality* can also be used to describe some vertebrate social systems as well. The key component of an eusocial society is a reproductive division of labor, and this deserves further clarification. A reproductive division of labor occurs when the ratio of work performed to offspring produced differs for group members of the same sex. If individuals that produce fewer offspring also work less (i.e., work load is positively correlated with reproductive success), then there is no true reproductive division of labor. It must be the case that some individuals perform more or less than their fair share of the labor relative to their reproductive output. Reproductive division of labor ranges from slight (some group members produce slightly fewer offspring and/or work a little harder than other group members) to extreme (one individual produces all the offspring and other group members perform all of the work), and from temporary (an individual is a worker or a reproducer during only a portion of its life) to permanent (lifetime sterility).

In all four taxa, two clear routes from solitary breeding toward eusociality can be discerned. They differ primarily in whether the initial formation of groups entails a preferential recruitment of kin or not. I shall call these the *familial route* and the *parasocial route,* respectively. I use the terminology of Wilson (1975) to outline the steps taken along each route. Each step, or stage of sociality, is represented by different species; that is, these are not ontogenetic stages. The familial route traverses the following stages of increasing social complexity:

1. *Solitary:* adults breed solitarily and provide no or minimal parental care to their offspring.

2. *Subsocial:* adults care for their own young for an extended period of time, creating an overlap of generations.

3. *Intermediate subsocial:* group members (all relatives from at least two generations) share and cooperate in labor. Some or all of the following activities may be shared: predator alarm and defense, construction and maintenance of a refuge or nest, communal foraging, and communal brood care. It is implied that all adults breed without a reproductive division of labor.

4. *Eusocial:* as in intermediate subsocial, but with a reproductive division of labor.

The parasocial route shows somewhat similar stages, but the sequential arrangement is different:

1. *Solitary:* adults breed solitarily.

2. *Communal:* adults of the same generation aggregate passively to form nonsocial groups. Aggregations may form around clumped, patchy resources such as rich food localities or refugia/nest sites of limited occurrence.

3. *Quasisocial:* passive group formation is replaced by the development of active cooperation benefiting all members of the group. Cooperative labors may include predator alarm and defense, construction of refugia or nests, communal foraging, and communal brood care.

4. *Semisocial:* as in quasisocial, but with a reproductive division of labor.

5. *Eusocial:* as in semisocial, but colonies persist long enough for members of two or more generations to overlap and to cooperate.

For both routes, the critical step to high levels of sociality is the third stage, where active cooperation between group members evolves. Cooperative behaviors such as predator alarm and defense, communal nest construction, communal foraging, and cooperative brood care may be mutualistic or reciprocally altruistic ventures, depending on the species. In the following section I shall outline the evolution of sociality in the spiders, insects, birds, and mammals with the following questions in mind:

1. What ecological or phylogenetic factors predispose a taxon to evolve sociality along the familial versus the parasocial route?
2. What adaptations facilitate the transitions between stages?
3. What types of cooperative behaviors are most likely to evolve among kin groups versus nonkin groups?
4. What types of cooperative behaviors are most likely to lead to a reproductive division of labor and eusociality?
5. To what degree are kin groups a prerequisite for the evolution of advanced sociality?

Spiders

Most spiders are solitary, build an exclusive web, deposit one or more egg sacs in a protected place, and either abandon the eggs or disperse the young immediately. However, a few web-building species are highly social and exhibit communal web construction, cooperative prey capture, and communal defense and care of spiderlings. The route taken correlates with whether the web is of the sheet-web type or of the colonial orb-web type.

FAMILIAL ROUTE. Spiders of the families Eresidae, Theridiidae, and Agelenidae are excellent examples of the familial route (Kullmann, 1972; Shear, 1970). These spiders build either sheetlike webs or tangled networks. Subsocial species show female parental care of spiderlings; this may take the form of regurgitation or the direct offering of prey, or in one exceptional case, the female sacrifices herself as prey. Examples of species in which the spiderlings remain longer and longer in the parental web can be found. Spiderling sibs may cooperate to capture and consume prey and to construct webs and retreats before eventually dispersing, providing a transition into the intermediate subsocial stage. In the intermediate subsocial species, related adults form colonies with large communal webs, in which web construction, prey capture, and defense are shared by all colony members. The primary advantage of the communal web appears to be the capture and subduing of prey much larger than a single individual could handle (Darchen, 1965; Kraft, 1970, 1971). Sheetlike webs appear to be more amenable to enlargement for this purpose than orb webs. The highest social level reached by spiders via the familial route is the cooperative care of eggs and spiderlings found in *Agelena consociata* and *Oecobius* sp. (Shear, 1970). Most adult females appear to breed in these colonies, and thus, there is no evidence for a reproductive division of labor.

PARASOCIAL ROUTE. Orb-web spiders of the family Araneidae are an example of the communal route (Buskirk, 1975; Lubin, 1974; Shear, 1970). None of these species exhibits parental care beyond the guarding of eggs, so no initial proximity of close relatives exists. Species at the communal level show a tendency to clump their webs, probably in particularly good food locations (e.g., *Nephila*).

Two types of quasisocial species occur. In *Araneus banderleiri,* females aggregate only to lay eggs and construct a large bag within which each female guards her own egg sac. The most common quasisocial system among araneid spiders is the aggregation of many individual orb webs into a cohesive colony (Figure 1). All members help to construct the support lines for the communal web, and in some species, a communal retreat is also constructed, but each spider builds, defends, and feeds in her own orb. Cooperative prey capture and feeding has not evolved among orb-web spiders. The adaptive significance of the colonial web appears to be the ability to span large open areas inaccessible to single spiders. Individual orb webs may not be amenable to expansion as with sheet webs or tangled networks, thus preventing the evolution of communal capture of larger prey. In addition, since parental care is minimal among orb spiders, cooperative brood care has not evolved, and no opportunity for a reproductive division of labor exists.

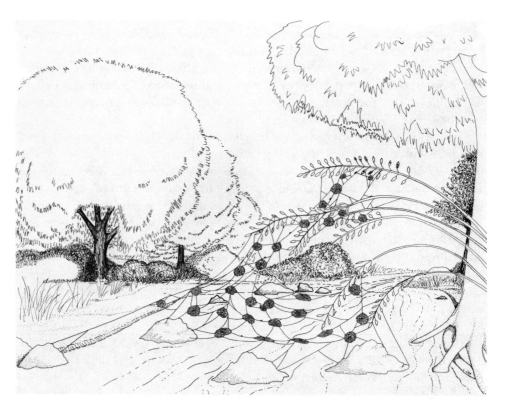

Fig. 1. A colony of the orb-weaving spider *Metabus gravidus* stretching out over a stream in Costa Rica. To form these colonies, 15–20 spiders aggregate at riparian sites where the stream is narrow, the current is steady, and insect abundance is high. The spiders cooperate only to build colony support lines extending out over the river; within this structure, each female constructs and feeds in her own web. The largest adult spiders build their orbs low over the water, where insect abundance is highest. Smaller spiders and juveniles build smaller orbs higher over the water. Egg cases are laid on leaves and branches overhanging the water. At night, all spiders retreat to sheltered areas under rocks and logs along the bank. Males do not construct webs but temporarily take over female webs. The advantage of coloniality in this species appears to be the reduction of web-building costs and the ability of groups of spiders to reach optimal foraging locations that are unattainable for single spiders. (Buskirk, 1975; original drawing by Lisa Üke, based on photographs by R. Buskirk.)

True eusociality therefore does not occur among spiders, and the most advanced levels of cooperation (communal prey capture and brood care) are reached only by species traversing the familial route.

INSECTS

Eusociality occurs among the Hymenoptera (ants, bees, and wasps) and Isoptera (termites). In addition, low levels of sociality are exhibited by numerous other insects. Since bees and wasps are the only groups showing intermediate stages from solitary to eusocial, they will be described in some detail.

FAMILIAL ROUTE. The familial route is characteristic of most wasps and allodapine bees (Wilson, 1971; Michener, 1969). The solitary species in all of these groups are either parasitoids (i.e., eggs are deposited into the larvae or nests of other organisms) or solitary nesters (i.e., a nest is constructed and mass-provisioned with food, eggs are deposited, and the chamber is sealed and abandoned before the young eclose). No overlap of generations therefore exists. In the subsocial species, the female associates longer with the nest, guarding it from predators and parasites and, in many cases, reopening the larval chambers to feed the young (progressive feeding). When the female is still present after the young eclose, an overlap of generations is achieved. With only a very few exceptions (see West-Eberhard, 1975), female offspring then cooperate with the mother to rear additional broods (reproductive division of labor). It is rare to find parent and offspring breeding together in the same nest. Thus, the intermediate subsocial stage along the familial route is frequently bypassed, and the overlap of generations leads directly to cooperative brood care, reproductive division of labor, and eusociality. In the more primitively eusocial species, the female helpers are still capable of reproducing and will do so if the mother disappears. In other species, the female "helpers" may lay many of the unfertilized male eggs. Among the highly advanced species, however, the majority of the female offspring produced are sterile workers that perform all of the foraging, guarding, and brood maintenance. Several other characteristics are correlated with the change from primitively eusocial to highly eusocial. Among primitive species, worker and reproductive caste distinctions are maintained by the aggressive dominance of the laying female; worker and queen do not differ greatly morphologically; and mature colony size is relatively small. In the more advanced species, nutritional and hormonal control over larval development by the queen determines caste; castes are well differentiated morphologically; and mature colony size is large.

All the ants and termites are eusocial, and it is argued that they have taken the familial route to sociality (Wilson, 1971). Both groups have progressively fed young, and therefore, an overlap of generations must have been an initial condition. Both also show the same progression as bees and wasps from primitively eusocial to highly eusocial species; that is, caste differentiation changes from behavioral to hormonal control, size differentiation of castes increases, and mature colony size increases. Termites differ from ants in having both male and female workers, whereas ants and other Hymenoptera have only female workers (Figure 2). It has been argued (Wilson, 1975) that the haplodiploidy of the Hymenoptera, which makes sisters more closely related to each other than brothers are to sisters, is the cause of this sexual bias in colony composition. Caste specialization is more extreme in ants and termites than in bees and wasps, with individuals being specialized for defense, foraging, or brood care.

PARASOCIAL ROUTE. The communal route has been described for many bees and polybiine wasps (Wilson, 1971). This route, outlined and championed by Michener (1969, 1974), is frequently taken by species that continue to mass-provision and abandon the larvae throughout the early stages, so there is no initial overlap of generations. In communal species, females of the same generation aggregate their nests in the same general location. In the quasisocial stage, females cooperate in building a communal nest with a single entrance, but each female lays eggs in her own cells, mass-provisions them, and seals them up. The benefit of this behavior is presumably mutual aid in predator and parasite defense. An advanced quasisocial stage is reached by species in which females rear their broods cooperatively. If a reproductive division of labor develops in which some females perform

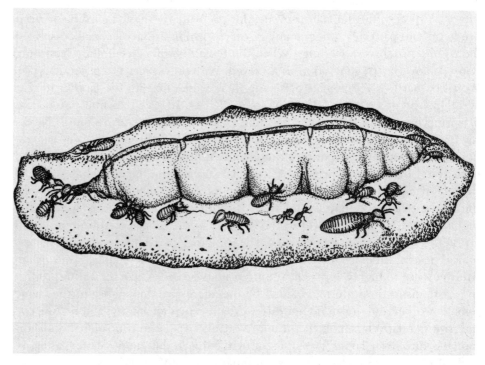

Fig. 2. A view into the reproductive cell of a *Macrotermes* sp. termite nest, showing the greatly enlarged queen, the male (lower right), and several types of workers and larvae. The mated male and female alates together find a nest site and burrow into the ground. They gradually begin to produce workers, and as the colony grows, soldiers and reproductives are eventually produced. Unlike in the Hymenoptera, the worker castes are composed of both sterile males and females. Since termites are diploid and the king and queen remain associated for many years, all of the colony members are full siblings related by 1/2. The nests of *Macrotermes* species are some of the largest and most complex known for termites. Fungus combs are cultivated in special gardens in the center of the nest; the fungi provide not only some of the food for the colony but may also aid in the ventilation system of the large nest. Many workers are required to produce the large and complex nests. Queens of these species are unusually productive, laying about 30,000 eggs per day or 10 million per year. Workers forage extensively for cellulose food outside the nest by marching in columns over exposed odor trails. (Grassé and Noirot, 1958a,b; original drawing by Lisa Üke, based on photographs by E. S. Ross.)

more of the egg laying and others more of the foraging, a semisocial stage is attained. Finally, an increased association between females and their young results when the adults live long enough to coexist in the same colony with their offspring. As with the familial route, an overlap of generations invariably leads to true eusociality, and offspring become the new source of workers. Such nests may continue to maintain several laying females, or one female may dominate the others to become the sole reproducer.

Outside of the Hymenoptera and Isoptera, numerous other insects have developed complex social behavior via the familial and parasocial paths, but none has become eusocial. Extended parental care (subsociality) occurs in a number of species and takes the form of guarding (many hemipterans), mass provisioning (scarabaeid dung beetles), and a form of progressive feeding in which the parent seals itself into a provisioned burrow with the eggs (some crickets; *Necrophorus* burying beetles) (Wilson, 1971). The highest level of sociality reached via the parasocial route is the quasisocial stage exhibited by the wood-boring scolytid beetles. Several adults cooperate to penetrate the bark of a tree; apparently more than one beetle is required to overcome the resistance of the host tree (Anderson, 1948). The first beetle to find an appropriate host releases an aggregation pheromone to attract conspecifics (Borden, 1974). Once inside, each female or male–female pair builds and maintains its own tunnel system. The larvae are sealed into side pockets of the tunnels, called *cradles,* and the parent regularly renews their food (Schedl, 1958). The newly emerged adults always disperse eventually and do not cooperate with the parent to raise subsequent broods.

Birds

Most birds breed as solitary monogamous pairs on defended, all-purpose territories (Lack, 1968). Most species exhibit parental care and overlap of generations but disperse their young when they reach independence.

Familial Route. In subsocial species, the young are retained longer than usual on the parental territory. If the parents attempt a second brood, these juveniles may help to feed the nestlings, their sibs. In some species, the helpers are not yet old enough to breed themselves, but in most cases, the helpers are potentially mature offspring suppressed from breeding by the dominant pair (e.g., scrub jay, Woolfenden, 1975; superb blue wren, Rowley, 1965). Many such "helper-at-the-nest" species have now been described (Skutch, 1961; Woolfenden, 1976; Rowley, 1976; Grimes, 1976; Zahavi, 1976). As in the Hymenoptera, the overlap of generations and the evolution of cooperative breeding lead directly to a reproductive division of labor and eusociality. Only two species are known in which closely related females breed together in a communal nest, the pukeko (Craig, 1974) and the white-winged chough (Rowley, 1978). While the reproductive division of labor in these helper species is extreme, eusociality is only a temporary condition as in some primitively eusocial insects, since the offspring frequently rise to reproductive status on their parent's or their own territory. They are never permanently sterile or intrinsically inferior to their parents as in the advanced eusocial species. One species, the Mexican jay (Brown, 1970, 1974), has taken an additional evolutionary step in which a family group develops into a small colony with several breeding females at individual nests. The majority of the individuals in the colony are still nonbreeding helpers that provide aid at all of the colony nests. Most of the "helper-at-the-nest" species are so-called *K*-selected species with high, stable population densities, high adult survival, delayed maturation, and a low probability of successful dispersal in suitable habitat for juveniles (Brown, 1974; Woolfenden, 1976; Grimes, 1976). Thus, juveniles may be forced by ecological conditions, not by their parents, to remain on the parental territory. It is argued that offspring greatly improve their chances of surviving and eventually breeding by remaining on the parental territory, and that the costs of feeding and caring for subsequent broods of sibs are offset by the gains from kin altruism and increased survival (Brown, 1978).

PARASOCIAL ROUTE. In the parasocial route, the territorial defense system of pairs is abandoned in favor of aggregations of individuals or nests and broadly overlapping home ranges. Brown (1974) suggested that the single most important factor that causes the abandonment of territorial behavior is an increase in home range size. Jays exhibit a series of species from small, nonoverlapping territories to larger, slightly overlapping home ranges to very large, completely overlapping ranges. Nesting aggregations could result from the fact that all individuals sharing

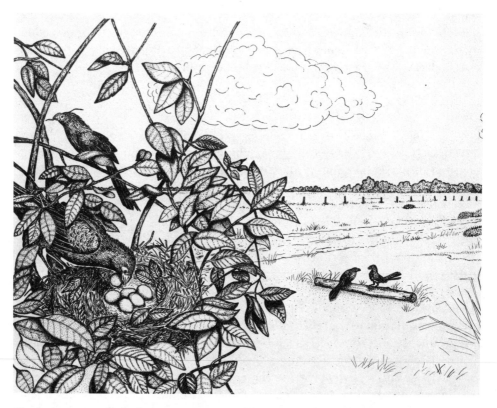

Fig. 3. A communally nesting group of groove-billed anis (*Crotophaga sulcirostris*) comprised of three monogamously mated pairs and a single juvenile from a previous brood (sitting on fence post). The alpha female is in the process of tossing out some of the eggs previously laid by the subordinate females, while her mate waits with a twig. Females do not recognize their own eggs but only toss out eggs they find in the nest before they themselves have begun to lay. The alpha female will then commence laying, and the subordinate females will continue laying, creating a skew in egg ownership of the joint clutch

a particular home range attempt to place their nests in the center of the range to reduce travel time (Horn, 1968). Alternatively, nesting colonies may form because there is a limited area of safe nesting sites close to the foraging area, as in sea birds (Ashmole, 1971; Erwin, 1977). Finally, birds may form feeding flocks as a result of patchily distributed food (Krebs, 1974). All of the above-mentioned groups are passive associations at the communal level of sociality, where nesting or foraging success is not affected directly by the presence of neighbors. But once groups form for passive reasons, active cooperation may quickly evolve (quasisociality). Two cooperative behaviors that frequently occur are active following of group members to currently available patches of food and concerted defense of the clumped nests against predators. In some colonial species, such as bee eaters (Fry, 1972), miners (Swainson, 1970; Dow, 1970), and long-tailed tits (Gaston, 1973), unrelated adult helpers are present that aid in the feeding and defense of offspring. Thus, cooperative brood care and a reproductive division of labor (semisociality) can arise among unrelated individuals in birds. The most advanced stage of sociality achieved by birds on the communal route is found in the anis of the New World tropics (D. E. Davis, 1942; Köster, 1971). In these birds, several unrelated adult pairs build a single communal nest and all females contribute eggs (Figure 3).

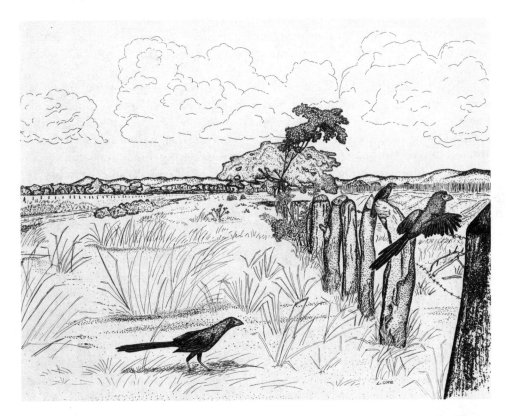

averaging 44% for the alpha pair, 30% for the beta pair, and 24% for the gamma pair. The two subordinate pairs are engaged in courtship (center) and foraging and basking (right). All group members will assist in incubation and care of the nestlings, but the alpha male will be the most attentive parent and the only bird to incubate at night. The primary advantage of such communal nesting appears to be increased adult survival as a result of sharing the risky incubation duties among more individuals. (Vehrencamp, 1978; original drawing by Lisa Üke, based on photographs by the author.)

SANDRA L.
VEHRENCAMP

Incubation and nestling care are shared by all members of the group. Although all females in the group breed, there is skew in reproductive success and an inverse relationship between the number of eggs each female owns and the amount of time spent incubating and feeding nestlings (Vehrencamp, 1977). Since the males in a group are frequently related and perform a great deal of the parental care, the anis border on having achieved a slight degree of eusociality.

Summarizing, it is extremely rare among birds for closely related females to breed together in the same nest. As in the Hymenoptera, the familial route to sociality leads directly to eusociality without an intermediate social step. The communal route is common among birds and usually leads to quasisocial colonies in which each pair retains its own nest but cooperates with neighboring pairs. Cooperative brood care also evolves via the communal route but never leads to extreme eusociality as in the insects.

MAMMALS

Like birds, all mammals exhibit some parental care, but unlike birds and other taxa discussed so far, only the reproductively active female can suckle the young. In those species in which parental care terminates with weaning, cooperative feeding of the young by nonreproductives, and hence true division of labor, are not possible. In spite of this constraint, mammals have shown the evolution of complex sociality by both routes and, in a few species, true eusociality by the familial route.

FAMILIAL ROUTE. The familial route occurs more commonly among mammals than the communal route. Complex sequences of the familial route can be found in squirrels, cervids, primates, and carnivores (see Eisenberg, 1966; Wilson, 1975). The smallest social units in all of these groups consist of solitary females and recent young or, more rarely, a single adult pair and recent young. Subsociality occurs with the prolongation of parental care. Most typically, there is a bias in favor of retention of female offspring (rodents, ungulates, and primates), but in some canids, male offspring are favored. A variety of cooperative behaviors usually evolve simultaneously with the retention of young. Colony formation in ground squirrels results in a predator alarm system that benefits all colony members (King, 1955; Smith, Oppenheimer, De Villa, Jill, and Ulmer, 1973). Active predator defense appears to be one benefit of family groups in cervids (Hirth and McCullough, 1977). All of the social carnivores form cooperative groups composed primarily of kin that can capture larger prey more efficiently than solitary individuals (Schaller, 1972; Kruuk, 1975). In hyenas, each female still cares only for her own offspring, and no obvious reproductive division of labor exists (Lawick and Lawick-Goodall, 1971; Kruuk, 1972). One advantage of primate groups appears to be a reciprocally altruistic broadcasting of rich food locations (Reynolds and Reynolds, 1965; Green, personal communication). A few species have evolved communal suckling and brood care. Communal suckling can evolve in mammals only if either (1) all females synchronize parturitions, or (2) the lactation period is so long that there is a high probability of overlap between several females. Lions (Bertram, 1975) are an example of the first case, and elephants (Laws, Parker, and Johnstone, 1975; Douglas-Hamilton, 1973) are an example of the second. The first signs of a slight division of labor can be seen in the elephants and a few primates (Hrdy and Hrdy, 1976) in which older females reduce their personal reproduction and provide aid in the form of food location and predator defense for younger, related females in the group. Thus, unlike most eusocial species, the altruistic period in these mammals is toward the end of life rather than the beginning. The final step to eusociality has occurred only among two families of the order Carnivora, the social canids and some mustelids. In both taxa, a monogamous pair and their successive offspring live in a cohesive group. The offspring are retained in the parental group past sexual maturity and are prevented from breeding by the dominant pair. In wolves (Mech, 1970; Zimen, 1976), Cape hunting dogs (Lawick and Lawick-Goodall, 1971; Lawick, 1973), coyotes, and jackals (Kleiman and Eisenberg, 1973), both the male parent and the nonbreeding subordinates provision the mother and the pups. In some colonial mongooses (Rasa, 1977; Ewer, 1973), the breeding male and the subordinates guard the young while the mother forages and provision the young as well. The resulting inverse relationship between reproductive effort and success is thus a true division of labor analogous to the helpers-at-the-nest in birds. As with birds, subsequent evolution into permanent nonreproductive castes has not been observed in mammals, with the possible exception of a few human societies.

PARASOCIAL ROUTE. The communal route is more difficult to trace out in mammals. The communal stage in which unrelated adults aggregate because of limited refugia or patchy resources or as an antipredation mechanism is quite common among savanna antelopes (Jarman, 1974), pinnipeds (Bartholomew, 1970), and the majority of bat species (Bradbury, 1977). Active cooperation among unrelated mammals appears to be rare. Several species of bats (Figure 4) form stable colonies of unrelated females (Bradbury and Vehrencamp, 1976a, 1977; McCracken and Bradbury, 1977; McCracken, personal communication). Each colony possesses a group-specific, sometimes defended, territory, but group members appear to forage independently within this area. Since group stability is affected by the stability of the food supply within the territory, grouping clearly evolves as a result of a structured group-foraging territory. Large savanna antelopes, such as buffalo, form large stable groups that actively defend themselves against predators (Sinclair, 1970). While some female young are retained within the parental unit, the extremely large size of these herds makes it unlikely that the average relatedness among group members is appreciable. The most advanced quasisocial stage to evolve in mammals via the communal route is the supposedly communal or indiscriminate suckling in several bat species (R. B. Davis, Herreid, and Short, 1962; Brosset, 1962). Thousands of synchronously breeding females place their young in a central crèche; although each female gives birth to only one young, females suckling several young at once are frequently observed. The number of females present makes it extremely unlikely that all are closely related. These species thus constitute a possible mammalian case in which cooperative brood care may have evolved among unrelated females via reciprocal altruism, but further investigation is greatly needed. A reproductive division of labor and true eusociality apparently have not evolved in mammals via the parasocial route.

SANDRA L.
VEHRENCAMP

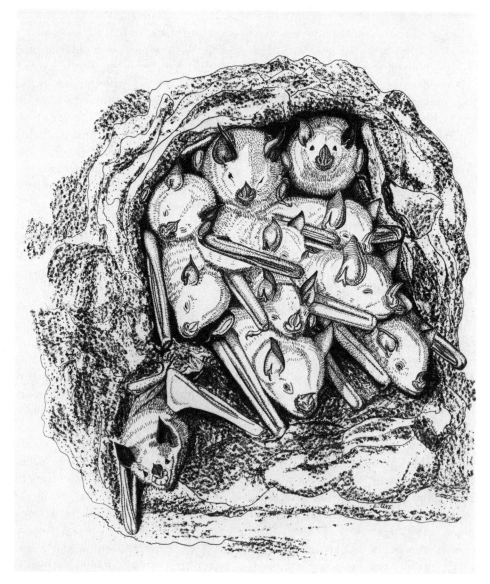

Fig. 4. A harem group of the neotropical fruit bat *Phyllostomus hastatus* with its single harem male (lower left). Females in this species form cohesive, stable groups that cluster tightly in the potholes of limestone caves in Trinidad. Each female group possesses its own relatively exclusive foraging area, within which the harem females usually feed in individual beats. When a particularly rich food source is located, females apparently vocalize and draw in their roost-mates. New female groups are assembled from the ousted youngsters of all the harems in the cave; once such a group finds an available foraging area, it remains stable in composition for many years. Thus, the females in a group are unrelated but all are similar in age. A single male defends the female roost group from other males in the cave for up to two years. The harem male does not forage in the same area as the females and therefore has no control over either resources or the foraging females, but his reproductive control over the females is nonetheless very high. The other males in the cave cluster in bachelor groups and replace harem males when they disappear. (McCracken and Bradbury, 1977, and McCracken, personal communication; original drawing by Lisa Üke, based on photographs by F. F. McCracken and L. Emmons.)

The preceding review of the four major taxa showing advanced sociality suggests a number of generalizations about social evolution:

1. Advanced sociality requires the existence of cohesive groups.

2. Cooperative labor—that is, the performance of acts that benefit other group members—is a necessary condition for advanced sociality. Mechanisms leading to cooperative behavior include mutualism, reciprocal altruism, kin altruism, and manipulation.

3. The opportunity for dominants to influence the distribution both of cooperative labor and of reproductive success is a necessary condition for the evolution of eusociality.

4. The existence of the parasocial route to eusociality argues that the preferential recruitment of kin into groups is not a necessary condition for reproductive division of labor.

5. The fact that all eusocial species with a relatively strong reproductive division of labor do show recruitment of kin into groups suggests that kin selection accelerates or modulates the factors that permit the formation of weakly eusocial groups regardless of composition.

These generalizations permit the asking of more specific questions concerning the ecological conditions that lead to advanced sociality. These critical questions include:

1. What environmental factors facilitate greater cohesiveness and stability of groups?

2. What environmental factors facilitate the evolution of cooperative labor?

3. Which forms of cooperative labor are most likely to lead to an inverse correlation between effort and reproductive success?

4. What environmental factors permit dominants to manipulate subordinates to generate skews in labor and reproductive success? Why don't manipulated subordinates leave such groups? How much skew is possible?

5. How does the opportunity to preferentially recruit kin enhance or diminish the fitness benefits of the preceding factors: cohesive groups, cooperative labor, and skews in labor and reproductive success? What factors limit the opportunities for preferential recruitment of relatives?

Some possible answers to these questions are attempted below.

Factors Affecting Group Stability

Two types of environmental factors encourage the formation of groups: active factors and passive factors. Active factors are those that draw individuals together for the express purpose of cooperation (see below). Passive factors lead to aggregations of individuals for reasons other than cooperation. For taxa exhibiting the parasocial route to sociality, passive factors may be responsible for the initial step. The further advancement of sociality will then depend on the stability of these passive aggregations. Advanced sociality generally means more complex interactions between individuals, greater dependency on group members, and greater costs of cooperative acts. The greater the cost of cooperation, the more important it becomes to give aid only to known individuals who will reciprocate. Unstable groups such as bird flocks and antelope herds can evolve refuging foraging strategies and even alarm calling, both of which appear to be low-cost–high-gain behaviors. But development of presumably higher-cost cooperation, such as predator defense, cooperative prey capture, and cooperative brood care, occurs only among stable groups. Stable group composition may therefore provide a milieu in which more complex cooperation can evolve. Environmental conditions that increase the stability of passive aggregations include:

1. *Long-term attachment to a nesting site:* In animals with parental care that deposit eggs or young in a nest or burrow (e.g., insects, birds, some mammals), stable groups are created when nests are clumped in a common site.

2. *Long-term attachment to a foraging site:* In web-building spiders and some territorial birds and mammals, attachment to a fixed foraging site may lead to stable groups if webs or territories are clumped.

3. *Centrally located roost site:* Stable groups may be created when many individuals with the same home range roost in a centrally located site, à la Horn (1968).

4. *Migration between successively available food patches:* If many individuals with the same annual home range move en masse between predictable successively available food patches, mobile but stable groups will result (Bradbury and Vehrencamp, 1976b).

5. *Active group formation:* Active cooperation, of course, may also be the cause of group stability as well as the result. Environmental conditions leading to cooperative behavior are discussed below.

FACTORS LEADING TO COOPERATIVE BEHAVIOR

Some of the environmental conditions that lead to a fitness advantage for individuals that cooperate actively are listed for each of the four major categories of cooperation.

COMMUNAL CONSTRUCTION OF NESTS OR RETREATS.

1. Cold weather coupled with otherwise adequate breeding conditions may select for large communal nests that conserve heat (e.g., sociable weavers; White, Bartholomew, and Howell, 1975).

2. Breeding sites are difficult for a solitary individual to construct or penetrate (e.g., scolytid beetles; Borden, 1974).

ANTIPREDATION.

1. Open habitat is one of the most important conditions leading to grouping for the purpose of improved predator detection (Jarman, 1974; King, 1955; Pulliam, 1973).

2. Large body size (e.g., antelopes; Geist, 1974) and possession of formidable weapons (antlers, teeth, claws, poisonous stings, etc.) may lead to group formation for the purpose of cooperative defense against predators.

1. The availability of large prey that can only be captured by a coordinated hunting group (e.g., social carnivores, sheet-web spiders).
2. The opportunity to exploit new habitats unavailable to solitary individuals (e.g., orb-web spiders).
3. Highly cryptic prey that are more effectively flushed up by foraging groups (e.g., bird flocks; Brosset, 1969; Bell, 1970; Moynihan, 1962).
4. Patchy and unpredictable food, which may lead to the sharing of food location information (e.g., refuging birds and bats; Krebs, this volume).
5. Reduced path overlap of individuals in foraging flocks (Cody, 1971).

COOPERATIVE BROOD CARE.

1. Predation on young by large predators that can be warded off more effectively by a group of adults (e.g., musk oxen, Tener, 1954).
2. Adults spend a long time away from the young while foraging, so that the alternation of guard duty by several adults leaves the young better protected (e.g., bees; Lin, 1964).
3. Young are more efficiently fed by groups of parents (e.g., lions; Bertram, 1975).
4. Parental care is more efficient if shared among group members, leading to an increase in adult survivorship (e.g., anis; Vehrencamp, 1978).

WHAT COOPERATIVE BEHAVIORS ARE MOST LIKELY TO LEAD TO A REPRODUCTIVE DIVISION OF LABOR?

While cooperative brood care is part of the definition of eusociality among entomologists, any cooperative behavior could potentially be skewed to create an inverse relationship between effort and reproductive success and a complex "altruistic" society. For example, the age-specific division of labor in monkeys and elephants, where older females do more searching for food and take more risks in defense of the group, is analogous to primitive eusociality. Nevertheless, cooperative brood care is the primary cooperative labor that produces this inverse relationship between effort and fitness. Very few cases of a reproductive division of labor are known for cooperative predator alarm, predator defense, or cooperative foraging, except where these also involve cooperative brood care. This could be due to a lack of knowledge rather than a rarity of existence. An inverse relationship between effort and fitness may be more difficult to discover where the cooperative behaviors affect primarily adult survivorship rather than the number of offspring produced. But the lack of a division of labor for cooperative behaviors not involving brood care may be due to the fact that at least among species with extensive parental care, much greater skews in fitness can be produced where cooperative brood care is unequally divided than when predator alarm, defense, or cooperative foraging is unequally divided. A second explanation may lie in the dynamics of the different types of cooperative behavior. The benefits of predator alarm, defense, and cooperative foraging may increase directly with the number of participants, so that the individual who tries to skew these cooperative efforts by declining to participate reduces his own fitness in the process. Cooperative brood care involves primarily the cooperative feeding of young. The advantages of cooperative brood care may depend less on the number of individuals and more on the amount of time and effort spent by each individual. Parental effort can be increased for some individuals and decreased for others in the group without changing the total output of effort for the group.

Not only is cooperative brood care a requirement for a strong reproductive division of labor, but the form of parental care is also an important factor. Most eusocial species share in common the parental care strategy of nourishing the young by gathering food at some distance from the nest and bringing it back in many foraging trips. Many hymenopterans are renowned for their foraging strategy of collecting tiny, widely scattered food items (R. Carroll, personal communication; Wilson, 1971). Among birds, helper-at-the-nest systems are restricted to altricial species and semiprecocial species that bring food to immobile young in a nest. (For an extreme case of this, see Dow, 1977.) Canids are among the few mammals in which nonreproductives and males can feed the young by bringing bits of food back to the den (Kleiman and Eisenberg, 1973); otherwise, mammals feed their young by lactation. Web spiders do not forage for food for the young but wait for food to arrive in the web. Thus, the taxa that lack this particular foraging strategy also lack eusociality. However, there are many Hymenoptera and birds that do feed their young in this manner but do not show eusociality. This form of parental care may therefore be a necessary, but not a sufficient, prerequisite for eusociality. This parental care strategy may lead to group formation and eusociality for several reasons: (1) it is extremely energy- and time-consuming; (2) it may increase the conspicuousness of the nest to predators; and (3) it requires that adults be away from the nest for long periods of time. Therefore, some forms of parental care may not be amenable to skewing. Reasons for this will become apparent in the following sections.

How Much Skew Is Possible?

Given that natural selection always selects for individuals that can dominate and increase their fitness above that of others, a skew in reproductive success should always be generated where domination is possible, and an inverse correlation between reproductive success and effort should also evolve when the form of cooperative brood care allows it. What is the maximum differentiation in reproductive success that can occur? Or in other words, what is the maximum skew a dominant individual can demand from subordinates?

A simple model is outlined below that clarifies some of the factors involved in domination and that defines the maximum amount of skew that a dominant can demand from a subordinate (Vehrencamp, in press). There are several necessary conditions that must be met for my model to apply. These are:

1. That group living and/or cooperative nesting confers some overall benefit to all group members compared to solitary pair breeding. Specifically, the mean fitness of all group members ($\overline{W}$ = total combined fitness of the group, divided by the number of individuals in the group) is greater than solitary breeding (W_1). I assume that $\overline{W}$ first increases with increasing group size, plateaus at some optimal group size, then declines with larger group sizes.

2. That dominance hierarchies will form once groups form. (See Wilson, 1975, for a general discussion of dominance.)

3. That dominants will try to skew the reproductive success in their favor as much as possible. Selection on dominants to dominate will occur as long as the benefits of dominating outweigh the costs.

4. That the ultimate defense of the subordinate against domination and skewing is to leave the group. Subordinates will leave when their fitness in the group goes below what their fitness would be as solitary breeders, devalued by the costs of dispersal. Since it is to the advantage of the dominant to maintain the group, it should skew only to the point where the subordinate's fitness in the group is equal to or slightly better than that of a solitary breeder.

5. That for every unit of fitness by which the dominant can reduce the reproductive success of a subordinate, the dominant's fitness increases one unit. For example, if the dominant can prevent each subordinate from laying one egg, then the dominant can usurp the subordinate's parental potential and produce one more of its own offspring for each subordinate in the group. Units of survival can be skewed in the same way. In other words, there is a fixed output for the group equal to $\overline{W}$ times the group size, and the fraction of this that belongs to subordinates and dominants changes with differing degrees of skew.

6. That all subordinates are skewed by the same amount, and that there is only one dominant in the group.

In the simplest case of a group of unrelated animals, the maximum amount of skew in reproductive success that can be generated is illustrated in Figure 5A. Average fitness $\overline{W}$ increases to a peak, then declines with increasing group size. W_1 is the fitness of a solitary individual or pair, and a horizontal line intersecting W_1 is W_ω, the lowest point that the dominant can push the fitness of subordinates. The dominant's enhanced fitness is then calculated from these two lines and is the difference between $\overline{W}$ and W_ω times the number of subordinates, or $W_\alpha = \overline{W} + (\overline{W} - W_\omega)(k - 1)$, where k = group size. The greater the difference in reproductive success for groups and solitary individuals, the greater the skew can be. If $\overline{W}$ is equal to W_1, as at the group size c, groups without skew might form. Where $\overline{W}$ is less than W_1, no groups can form. Notice that the optimum group size that a dominant would prefer (b) may not be the same as the optimum group size of a nonskewed group(a).

Environmental conditions that permit dominants to manipulate subordinates are therefore: (1) an increase in the mean fitness of group members compared to solitary breeders and no vacant territories or (2) a subordinate that is intrinsically or temporarily less fit if it breeds alone. Condition 1 is most likely to occur in stable, high-density populations at their carrying capacity. Several studies of eusocial species have verified this condition. Brown (1970, 1974) and Woolfenden (1975) have argued for jays that populations with extensive juvenile retention and helping at the nest are habitat-limited and at much higher densities compared to populations with fewer or no helpers. Mech (1977) found that in an area where the wolf population was drastically reduced by man, many individuals from adjacent groups dispersed into the area and formed solitary breeding pairs. In a comparison of two sibling species of *Polistes* wasps, Metcalf (personal communication) found that the high-density species exhibited a higher fraction of multiple-foundress–solitary-foundress nests than the lower-density (parasite-susceptible)

SANDRA L.
VEHRENCAMP

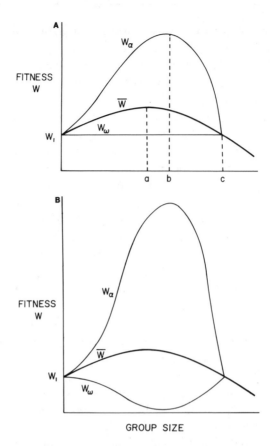

Fig. 5. The maximum amount of skew in fitness that can be generated between dominants and subordinates in groups containing (A) unrelated animals and (B) individuals related by $r = 1/4$. $\bar{W}$ is the average fitness of a group member. W_α is the fitness of the dominant, and W_ω is the fitness of the subordinates. See text for further explanation.

species. Thus, for K-selected species, potential dispersers may be forced to remain in their natal groups and submit to manipulation. Condition 2 may occur in several situations. In colonial birds, where nesting synchrony is critical to breeding success, a late arrival may be more successful by nesting as a subordinate with another pair than by attempting to build its own nest (Emlen and Demong, 1975, and personal communication). Among Hymenoptera, small individuals may be much less fit than larger individuals; their success may be much greater when nesting near or with these superior individuals than alone (Lin and Michener, 1972). Finally, young individuals may gain experience by breeding as subordinate members in a group before attempting to breed alone (Woolfenden, 1975).

THE EFFECTS OF COOPERATION AND MANIPULATION AMONG KIN

If a dominant individual has the option of recruiting kin into its group, should it reduce the reproductive skew to zero, or should it increase the skew? The maximum amount of skew the dominant can impose on relatives related by $\bar{r}$ (the mean relatedness of all group members) can be determined in the same way as for unrelated individuals using inclusive fitness. Subordinates leave the group only when their *inclusive fitness* in the group falls below what their *inclusive fitness* would be if all the group members bred solitarily (see Appendix A). Figure 5B illustrates the maximum amount of skew in personal fitness that could be demanded by the dominant relative. The $\overline{W}$ line is the same as in the previous case, but here, the group members are related by an r of .25. The subordinate's *personal fitness* is line W_ω; at each point along this line, inclusive fitness for subordinates in the group is equal to their inclusive fitness when solitary. For the case of related individuals, therefore, W_ω can go below W_1, and the greater the degree of relatedness, the lower W_ω can be pushed. W_ω can even be pushed to zero among close relatives, depending once again on the difference between $\overline{W}$ and W_1. The fitness of the dominant is calculated in the same way as before. Because the difference between $\overline{W}$ and W_ω is greater, the dominant gains a rather large benefit, and the skew in this case is very great. One of the most interesting predictions of this model is that even among close relatives, the dominant cannot manipulate subordinates and force group formation unless the average personal fitness of group members, $\overline{W}$, is greater than the personal fitness derived from solitary breeding, W_1. Parental manipulation of offspring is a special case of this model. The fitness of some offspring is reduced in order to produce more total offspring. The equations require a correction factor to account for the cost to the parent of producing the initial set of helpers. If this cost is great, it has the effect of reducing the amount of skew the parent can demand.

Several questions follow from the model. The most obvious is: What determines whether groups contain relatives or not? Let us take the point of view of a dominant individual trying to decide whether to recruit relatives or nonrelatives as subordinates into its group, and whether or not to skew them to the maximum allowable. Using straightforward equations for inclusive fitness, the relative success of these options can be compared (see Appendix B). Given that $\overline{W} > W_1$, skewing is always better than not skewing. But whether to skew relatives or nonrelatives is a complicated issue and depends on two factors: (1) the magnitude of the difference in reproductive success of groups and pairs and (2) the probability of successful dispersal. These two factors are components of lifetime fitness, so that $W = s \cdot R$ (s = the probability of dispersing successfully, and R = total output of young after successful dispersal). Holding all other variables constant, and increasing the relative reproductive success of groups ($\overline{R}/R_1$), the optimal strategy changes from recruiting and skewing kin (when the group benefit is small) to dispersing kin and skewing nonkin (when the advantage of grouping is large). The reason for this reversal of strategies is that for large group benefits, the advantage gained by the dominant in allowing the kin to breed in low-skew, non-kin groups (where some may even be dominant) far outweighs the loss of skewing only nonkin.

The probability of successful dispersal, s, is particularly relevant to the case of parental manipulation of young, since s is applied only to the individual that leaves the kin group in which it was born. Holding all else constant and varying s between 0 and 1 also leads to shifts in the optimal dispersal strategy. If dispersal survival is high, a parent (or dominant relative) gains by dispersing its offspring (kin). The lower the probability of dispersing successfully, the greater the advantage gained from retaining and skewing the offspring (kin). Dispersal survival and the relative advantage of grouping over solitary breeding interact in complicated ways to determine whether kin or nonkin groups should form. When s is high and $\overline{R}$ is much greater than R_1, nonkin groups should form. When s is low and $\overline{R}$ is not much larger than R_1, kin groups should form. The other mixed possibilities depend on the relative values of s and $\overline{R}/R_1$.

Another question arises from the model: Is the dominant always able to skew the reproduction to the predicted maximum? The skew may be less than predicted for several reasons.

1. If the skew is less than predicted for the case of related animals but not for unrelated animals, then we might suspect some problem with kin theory, for which this model is a test. If the skew is less for both related and unrelated groups, then one of the following explanations may be applicable.

2. If the cost of parental care is small compared to the cost of eggs, then it may not be worth skewing. This may explain the failure of precocial birds and spiders to evolve cooperative systems with high degrees of skew.

3. The dominant may not have the opportunity to skew the reproduction. For example, in rheas, females may attempt to roll eggs out of the nest but are usually prevented from doing so by the parental male (Bruning, 1974).

4. Subordinates may have effective strategies for reducing the skew. In the anis, subordinate females have adopted three strategies for reducing the skew caused by the dominant female's egg tossing (see Vehrencamp, 1977).

5. Hormonally, animals may have to breed before they can perform parental care. This may explain why avian helpers don't incubate, and why helping in mammals is very rare.

6. Finally, behavioral domination may be too costly in terms of time and energy. For example, if the optimal group size is very large, the dominant may not be able to effectively control all of the subordinates.

Since it is *a priori* always to the advantage of the dominant to impose the maximum skew, species that breed cooperatively without skew must fall into one or more of the above categories.

How do existing data support these models? Survival and lifetime fitness are rarely determined for cooperative nesting species, but some species appear to fit the model well. Data on anis support well the case for unrelated group members (Vehrencamp, 1978). Groups of two to three pairs form largely in the optimal, high-density habitat, but dispersing birds have available to them vast areas of suboptimal breeding habitat. Thus, all females disperse from their parental groups. In the optimal area, groups of two to three pairs are slightly more successful than single pairs, and a small skew in egg ownership is generated by the dominant's egg tossing. The fitness curve for subordinates in groups forms a very nearly straight horizontal line with W_1, as predicted by the model. The data of Metcalf and Whitt (1977b) on a facultatively social wasp, *Polistes metricus*, support well the case of related group members. Two-female sib groups ($r \approx .63$) are more successful than single females, but the skew in offspring production is high, 82% − 18%. The beta female's personal fitness is about half that of a solitary female. However, inclusive fitness for the beta female is slightly higher in the group than if both sisters bred solitarily, again supporting the model.

In conclusion, this model of manipulation by dominants seems to rest on quite reasonable assumptions and is consistent with available data. It places in perspective the varied tendency for certain taxa to exhibit eusociality and greatly clarifies the parasocial route to eusociality in the Hymenoptera. Finally, it may be applicable to other social groupings, such as foraging flocks and male–male interactions.

The interaction of close kin clearly modulates the form of social behavior. The final question involving the role of relatives in social evolution is: Does the proximity of kin facilitate the evolution of cooperative behaviors, or is the evolution of cooperation followed by the recruitment of kin? For species following the parasocial route, it was clear that cooperation could evolve first and might be followed by the recruitment of kin. For species taking the familial route, there has been a tendency to conclude that increased sociality between mother and offspring provides a milieu in which cooperation can evolve. But for most species following the familial route, recuitment of kin and cooperative behavior evolve simultaneously, and it is not possible to determine cause and effect. A case in point is a study by Barash (1974) on the evolution of sociality in marmots. Barash found a correlation among marmot species between the degree of sociality (solitary to colonial), the altitude at which the species resides, and the duration of maternal care. He argued that the increased duration of interaction between mother and offspring leads to stronger social tendencies and is followed by daughters settling close to their mothers to breed. However, there are other alternative explanations for these correlations. Svendsen (1974) and Andersen, Armitage, and Hoffman (1976) have shown that the quality of the winter burrow greatly affects the survival of adults and young. Colonies tend to form in the better burrow sites and solitary individuals in the poorer sites for the middle-elevation species, the yellow-bellied marmot. Therefore, at higher altitudes, not only is the growing season shorter and the maturation period longer, but the quality of the winter burrow is much more important and probably more variable. Altitude may therefore affect sociality via the distribution of burrows, and the correlation with duration of maternal care is a side effect of the inverse correlation between length of the growing season and harshness of the winter season. It should not be forgotten that cooperative behavior can evolve only when ecological conditions lead to increased fitness for groups, regardless of the relatedness among individuals. Whenever grouping leads to a positive advantage, inclusive fitness is always increased when cooperative acts are bestowed on relatives rather than nonrelatives.

Some forms of cooperation could probably not evolve among unrelated individuals. Reciprocal altruism may be one such case. A form of reciprocal altruism, drawing attention to rich food patches, does occur between unrelated individuals, but only when the cost is very small (the food patch is very rich). Reciprocal altruism that is more costly, such as communal suckling and cooperative predator defense, occurs primarily among related individuals. It can be shown mathematically that related individuals can support a higher cost for reciprocal altruism. Charnov and Krebs (1975) have shown that alarm calling can evolve among unrelated individuals only when the fitness of group members increases linearly as the number of callers in the group increases, and the cost of calling is less than the benefit of adding one more caller, or:

$$\alpha/\beta < 1$$

where α is the decrease in fitness due to calling and β is the increase in fitness due to the addition of a caller. This same calculation can be made for groups of related individuals. In this case, the cost–benefit ratio can be greater than 1:

$$\alpha/\beta < 1 + \bar{r}\,(k - 1)$$

where $\bar{r}$ is the mean relatedness of group members and k is the group size (D. S. Wilson, 1977). Thus, the more expensive the altruistic behavior, the more likely it is to evolve only among related individuals. Alarm calling for many birds is probably not very expensive, since it frequently does occur among unrelated individuals and between different species. Charnov and Krebs (1975) have even argued that the caller may benefit most of all. But for mammals such as ground squirrels, a definite cost to the caller has been shown (Sherman, 1977), and ground squirrel colonies that form in open habitats for the purpose of predator detection are always composed of related females.

Ecological Factors Affecting Group Selection

In the last sections of this chapter, I have concentrated heavily on the factors affecting individual and kin selection. Group selection has been slighted, not because it is potentially less important but because essentially no field data exist on the survival rates of groups, demes, or populations and the parameters that affect group survival. In tracing out the routes to sociality and the ecological factors that help to promote social evolution, we saw that subdivision of the population into groups because of passive ecological factors was an important initial step along the parasocial route. It is tempting to suggest that group selection might be important in the evolution of active cooperation and advanced sociality via this route. However, there is at this point no evidence indicating that the other two requirements for group selection—high group mortality rates and low migration rates between groups—are also met. One obvious place to look for group selection would be in species living on oceanic or ecological islands, where all of the requirements may actually be met (Diamond, personal communication). Mutualistic cooperation and close associations of kin may also lead to cohesive group structure, where intergroup migration rates are low and groups survive differentially. Thus, group selection may frequently act in conjunction with individual and kin selection. One of the greatest problems with group selection is that the ecological factors that promote it also promote kin selection (Levin and Kilmer, 1974). The perspective of group selection presented earlier—that is, current versus long-term fitness—points out the close relationship between the two processes.

One of the most important ecological conditions leading to advanced sociality is a K-selected population structure. Populations at their carrying capacity exhibit increased stability, increased adult longevity, and increased parental care, which in turn promote cohesive groups, retention of offspring, and kin selection. Population stability has another effect on breeding strategies, which is to increase the relative importance of current and future generations to lifetime fitness (Orlove, 1975). In growing populations, the offspring produced earliest in life are more important to total fitness than young produced later; in stable populations, all young contribute equally to lifetime fitness; and in declining populations, the last young produced are more important. To extend this idea, current offspring production (individual selection) ought to be more important for species with growing populations, but future generations (group selection) should be promoted in species with slowly declining populations. Since r-selected populations probably pass more time in growing phases and K-selected populations are more likely to experience periods of slow decline, both group selection and kin selection may be more important in relatively K-selected species. Therefore, not only do similar ecological conditions lead to kin and group selection, but kin selection should facilitate evolution via group selection and vice versa. The current use of the term *kin-group* selection attests to the likelihood that the most important role of group selection is in conjunction with kin (and individual) selection (Brown, 1974; Wilson, 1976).

Humans are probably an example of kin-group selection par excellence. Early human populations apparently consisted of small, fairly cohesive groups composed primarily of kin (Alexander, 1974). Competition between such kin groups caused antagonism and probably rapid extinction of many such groups. Human history is replete with the rise and fall of many distinct groups and civilizations. The strong tendency toward warfare between tribes and the within-group chauvinism found in many societies even today suggest that group selection did play an important role in human social evolution (Hamilton, 1975). The role of kin selection is undeniable in view of our ability to recognize and categorize kin according to degree of relatedness, with certain types of altruistic behavior given differentially to close relatives. The long-term association of close kin probably also facilitated the evolution of reciprocal altruism in humans. Individual, kin, and group selection can therefore act in the same direction and in conjunction with each other, and sorting out the relative importance of each is a current challenge for sociobiology.

Acknowledgments

I am grateful to J. W. Bradbury, G. C. Williams, P. W. Sherman, and M. C. Baker for their critical appraisals of earlier drafts of this chapter and to M. E. Gilpin and K. Fristrup for their advice on some mathematical formulations. L. Üke artfully depicted scenes of animal social life from photographs kindly provided by G. F. McCracken, L. Emmons, R. Buskirk, and E. S. Ross.

REFERENCES

Alexander, R. D. The evolution of social behavior. *Ann. Rev. Ecol. Syst.*, 1974, *5*, 325–384.

Alexander, R. D., and Sherman, P. W. Local mate competition and parental investment in social insects. *Science*, 1977, *196*, 494–500.

Andersen, D. C., Armitage, K. B., and Hoffman, R. S. Socioecology and marmots: Female reproductive strategies. *Ecology*, 1976, *57*, 552–560.

Anderson, R. F. Host selection by the pine engraver, *J. Econ. Entomol.* 1948, *41*, 596–602.

Ashmole, N. P. Sea bird ecology and the marine environment. In D. S. Farner and J. R. King (eds.), *Avian Biology*, Vol. 1. Academic Press, New York, 1971, pp. 223–286.

Barash, D. P. The evolution of marmot societies: A general theory. *Science*, 1974, *185*, 415–420.

Bartholomew, G. A. A model for the evolution of pinniped polygyny. *Evolution*, 1970, *24*, 546–559.

Bell, R. H. V. The use of the herb layer by grazing ungulates in the Serengeti. In A. Watson (ed.), *Animal Populations in Relation to Their Food Resources*. Blackwell Scientific Publications, Oxford, 1970.

Bertram, B. C. R. Social factors influencing reproduction in wild lions. *J. Zool. Lond.*, 1975, *177*, 463–482.

Bertram, B. C. R. Kin selection in lions and in evolution. In P. P. G. Bateson and R. A. Hinde (eds.), *Growing Points in Ethology*. Cambridge University Press, Cambridge, 1976.

Boorman, S. A., and Levitt, P. R. Group selection at the boundary of a stable population. *Theor. Pop. Biol.*, 1973, *4*, 85–128.

Borden, J. H. Aggregation pheromones in the Scolytidae. In M. C. Birch (ed.), *Pheromones*. American Elsevier, New York, 1974, pp. 135–160.

Bradbury, J. W. Social organization and communication. In W. A. Wimsatt (ed.), *Biology of Bats III*. Academic Press, New York, 1977, pp. 1–73.

Bradbury, J. W., and Vehrencamp, S. L. Social organization and foraging in emballonurid bats. I. Field studies. *Behav. Ecol. Sociobiol*, 1976a, *1*, 337–381.

Bradbury, J. W., and Vehrencamp, S. L. Social organization and foraging in emballonurid bats. II. A model for the determination of group size. *Behav. Ecol. Sociobiol*. 1976b, *1*, 383–404.

Bradbury, J. W., and Vehrencamp, S. L. Social organization and foraging in emballonurid bats. IV. Parental investment patterns. *Behav. Ecol. Sociobiol.*, 1977, *2*, 19–29.

Brosset, A. The bats of central and western India, Pt. 3. *J. Bombay Nat. Hist. Soc.*, 1962, *59*, 707–746.

Brosset, A. La vie sociale des oiseaux dans une forêt équatoriale du Gabon. *Biol. Gabonica*, 1969, *5*, 26–69.

Brown, J. L. Cooperative breeding and altruistic behavior in the Mexican jay, *Aphilocoma ultramarina*. *Anim. Behav.*, 1970, *18*(2), 366–378.

Brown, J. L. Alternate routes to sociality in jays. *Amer. Zool.*, 1974, *14*, 63–80.

Brown, J. L. Avian communal breeding systems. *Ann. Rev. Ecol. Syst.*, 1978, *9*, 123–156.

Bruning, D. Social structure and reproductive behavior in the Argentine gray rhea, Ph.D. thesis, University of Colorado, 1974.

Buskirk, R. E. Coloniality, activity patterns and feeding in a tropical orb-weaving spider. *Ecol.*, 1975, *56*, 1314–1328.

Caraco, T., and Wolf, L. L. Ecological determinants of group sizes of foraging lions. *Amer. Nat.*, 1975, *109*, 343–351.

Charnov. E. L., and Krebs, J. R. The evolution of alarm calls: Altruism or manipulation? *Amer. Nat.* 1975, *109*, 107–112.

Cody, M. L. Finch flocks in the Mohave Desert. *Theor. Pop. Ecol.*, 1971, *2*, 142–158.

Craig, J. L. The social organization of the pukeko, Ph.D. thesis, Massey University, New Zealand, 1974.

Darchen, R. Etholgie d' une araignée sociale, *Agelena consociata*. *Biol. Gabonica*, 1965, *1*, 117–146.

Darlington, C. D. *The Evolution of Genetic Systems*. University Press, Cambridge, 1939.

Davis, D. E. The phylogeny of social nesting habits in the Crotophaginae. *Quart. Rev. Biol.*, 1942, *17*, 115–134.

Davis, R. B., Herreid, C. F., and Short, H. L. Mexican free-tailed bat in Texas. *Ecol. Monogr.*, 1962, *32*, 311–346.

Dawkins, R. *The Selfish Gene*. Oxford University Press, New York, 1976.

Douglas-Hamilton, I. On the ecology and behavior of the Lake Manyara elephants. *East African Wild. Jour.*, 1973, *11*, 401–403.

Dow, D. D. Communal behavior of nesting noisy miners. *Emu*, 1970, *72*, 131–134.

Dow, D. D. Indiscriminate interspecific aggression leading to almost sole occupancy of space by a single species of bird. *Emu*, 1977, *77*, 115–121.

Dunford, C. Kin selection for ground squirrel alarm calls. *Amer. Nat.*, 1977, *111*, 782–785.

Eisenberg, J. F. The social organization of mammals. *Handbuch der Zool.*, 1966, *10*, 1–92.

Emlen, S. T., and Demong, N. J. Adaptive significance of synchronized breeding in a colonial bird: A new hypothesis. *Science*, 1975, *188*, 1029–1031.

Erwin, R. M. Foraging and breeding adaptations to different food regimes in three seabirds. *Ecology*, 1977, *58*, 389–397.

Evans, H. E. Extrinsic versus intrinsic factors in the evolution of insect sociality. *Bioscience*, 1977, *27*, 613–617.

Ewer, R. F. *The Carnivores.* Cornell University Press, Ithaca, N.Y., 1973.

Fisher, R. A. *The Genetical Theory of Natural Selection.* Clarendon Press, Oxford, 1930.

Fleming, T. H., Heithaus, E. R., and Sawyer, W. B. An experimental analysis of the food location behavior of frugivorous bats. *Ecology,* 1977, *58*, 619–627.

Fry, C. H. The social organization of Bee-eaters (Meropidae) and cooperative breeding in hot-climate birds. *Ibis,* 1972, *114*, 1–14.

Gadgil, M. Evolution of social behavior through interpopulation selection. *Proc. Nat. Acad. Sci. USA,* 1975, *72*, 1199–1201.

Gaston, A. J. The ecology and behavior of the long-tailed tit. *Ibis,* 1973, *115*, 330.

Geist, V. On the relationship of social evolution and ecology in ungulates. *Amer. Zool.,* 1974, *14*, 205–220.

Ghiselin, M. T. *The Economy of Nature and the Evolution of Sex.* University of California Press, Berkeley, 1974.

Gilpin, M. E. Group selection in predator–prey communities. *Monographs in Population Biology,* Princeton University Press, Princeton, N.J., 1976.

Grassé, P. P., and Noirot, C. La meule des termites champignonnistes et sa signification symbiotique. *Annales des Sciences Naturelles,* 1958a, *20*, 113–128.

Grassé, P. P., and Noirot, C. Construction et architecture chez les termites champignonnistes (Macrotermitinae). *Proc. 10th Internat. Congr. Entomol. Montreal,* 1958b, *2*, 515–520.

Grimes, L. G. Cooperative breeding in African birds. *Proc. Internat. Ornithol. Cong.,* 1976, *16*, 667–673.

Hamilton, W. D. The genetical evolution of social behavior, I and II. *J. Theor. Biol.,* 1964, *7*, 1–52.

Hamilton, W. D. Geometry for the selfish herd. *J. Theor. Biol.,* 1971, *31*, 295–311.

Hamilton, W. D. Altruism and related phenomena, mainly in social insects. *Ann. Rev. Ecol. Syst.,* 1972, *3*, 193–232.

Hamilton, W. D. Innate social aptitudes of man: An approach from evolutionary genetics. In R. Fox (ed.), *Biosocial Anthropology.* Wiley, New York, 1975.

Hamilton, W. J., and Watt, K. E. F. Refuging. *Ann. Rev. Ecol. Syst.,* 1970, *1*, 263–286.

Hirth, D. H., and McCullough, D. R. Evolution of alarm signals in ungulates with special reference to cervids. *Amer. Nat.,* 1977, *111*, 31–42.

Hoogland, J. L., and Sherman, P. W. Advantages and disadvantages of bank swallow (*Riparia riparia*) coloniality. *Ecol. Monogr.,* 1976, *46*, 33–58.

Horn, H. S. The adaptive significance of colonial nesting in the Brewer's blackbird (*Euphagus cyanocephalus*). *Ecology,* 1968, *49*, 682–694.

Hrdy, S. B., and Hrdy, D. B. Hierarchical relations among female Hanuman langurs (Colobinae, *Presbytis entellus*), *Science,* 1976, *193*, 913–915.

Jarman, P. J. The social organization of antelope in relation to their ecology. *Behavior,* 1974, *58*, 215–267.

King, J. A. Social behavior, social organization, and population dynamics in a black-tailed prairiedog town in the Black Hills of South Dakota. *Contr. Lab. Vert. Zool., Univ. of Michigan,* 1955, *67*, 1–123.

Kleiman, D. G., and Eisenberg, J. F. Comparisons of canid and felid social systems from an evolutionary perspective. *An. Beh.,* 1973, *21*, 637–659.

Köster, F. Zum Nistverhalten des Ani. *Bonn. Zool. Beit,* 1971, *22*, 4–27.

Kraft, B. Contribution à la biologie et à l'éthologie d'*Agelena consociata* Denis (Araignée sociale du Gabon). *Biol. Gabonica,* 1970, *6*, 199–367.

Kraft, B. Contribution à la biologie et à l'éthologie d'*Agelena consociata. Biol. Gabonica,* 1971, 7, 2–56.

Krebs, J. R. Colonial nesting and social feeding as strategies for exploiting food resources in the great blue heron (*Ardea herodias*). *Behavior,* 1974, *51*, 99–134.

Kruuk, H. *The Spotted Hyena—A Study of Predation and Social Behavior.* University of Chicago Press, Chicago, 1972.

Kruuk, H. Functional aspects of social hunting by carnivores. In G. Baerends, C. Beer, and A. Manning (eds.), *Function and Evolution in Behavior.* Clarendon Press, Oxford, 1975.

Kullmann, E. Evolution of social behavior in spiders. *Amer. Zool.,* 1972, *12*, 419–426.

Lack, D. *Population Studies of Birds.* Oxford University Press, Oxford, 1966.

Lack, D. *Ecological Adaptations for Breeding in Birds.* Methuen and Co., London, 1968.

Lawick, H. van. *Solo: The Story of an African Wild Dog Puppy and Her Pack.* Collins, London, 1973.

Lawick, H. van, and van Lawick-Goodall, J. *Innocent Killers.* Houghton, Mifflin, Boston, 1971.

Laws. R. M., Parker, I. S. C., and Johnstone, R. C. B. *Elephants and Their Ecology: The Ecology of Elephants in N. Bunyoro, Uganda.* Clarendon Press, Oxford, 1975.

Levin, B. R., and Kilmer, W. L. Interdemic selection and the evolution of altruism: A computer simulation study. *Evolution,* 1974, *28*, 527–545.

Levins, R. Extinction. In M. Gerstenhaber (ed.), *Some Mathematical Questions in Biology.* American Mathematical Society, Providence, R.I., 1970, pp. 77–107.

Lewontin, R. C. The units of selection. *Ann. Rev. Ecol. Syst.,* 1970, *1*, 1–18.

Lin, N. Increased parasitic pressure as a major factor in the evolution of social behavior in halictine bees. *Insectes Sociaux,* 1964, *11*, 187–192.

Lin, M., and Michener, C. Evolution of sociality in insects. *Quart. Rev. Biol.,* 1972, *47*, 131.

Lubin, Y. D. Adaptive advantages and the evolution of colony formation in *Cyrtophora* (Araneae:Araneidae). *Zool. J. Linn. Soc.,* 1974, *54*, 321–339.

MacArthur, R. A., and Wilson, E. O. *The Theory of Island Biogeography.* Princeton University Press, Princeton, N.J., 1967.

Maynard Smith, J. Group selection and kin selection. *Nature,* 1964, *201*, 1145–1147.

Maynard Smith, J. Group selection. *Quart. Rev. Biol.,* 1976, *51*, 277–283.

McCracken, G. F., and Bradbury, J. W. Paternity and genetic heterogeneity in the polygynous bat, *Phyllostomus hastatus. Science,* 1977, *198*, 303–306.

Mech, L. D. *The Wolf: The Ecology and Behavior of an Endangered Species.* Natural History Press, New York, 1970.

Mech. L. D. Productivity, mortality, and population trends of wolves in northeastern Minnesota. *J. Mammal.,* 1977, *58*, 559–574.

Metcalf, R. A., and Whitt, G. S. Intra-nest relatedness in the social wasp, *Polistes metricus. Behav. Ecol. Sociobiol.,* 1977a, *2*, 339–352.

Metcalf, R. A., and Whitt, G. S. Relative inclusive fitness in the social wasp *Polistes metricus. Behav. Ecol. Sociobiol.,* 1977b, *2*, 353–360.

Michener, C. D. Comparative social behavior of bees. *Ann. Rev. Entomol.,* 1969, *14*, 299–342.

Michener, C. D. *The Social Behavior of Bees.* Belknap Press, Cambridge, 1974.

Moynihan, M. The organization and probable evolution of some mixed species flocks of neotropical birds. *Smithson, Misc. Coll.,* 1962, *143*, 1–140.

Orlove, M. J. Some further insights into kin selection. *J. Theor. Biol.,* 1975, *55*, 547–551.

Pianka, E. R. *Evolutionary Ecology.* Harper and Row, New York, 1974.

Pimentel, D., Population regulation and genetic feedback. *Science,* 1968, *159*, 1432–1437.

Powell, G. V. N. Experimental analysis of the social value of flocking by starlings (*Sturnus vulgaris*) in relation to predation and foraging. *Anim. Behav.,* 1974, *22*, 501–505.

Pulliam, H. R. On the advantages of flocking. *J. Theor. Biol.,* 1973, *38*, 419–422.

Rasa, O. A. E. The ethology and sociology of the dwarf mongoose (*Helogale undulata rufula*). *Z. Tierpsychol.,* 1977, *43*, 337–406.

Reynolds, V., and Reynolds, F. Chimpanzees of the Budongo Forest. In I. DeVore (ed.), *Primate Behavior.* Holt, Rinehart and Winston, New York, 1965, pp. 368–424.

Rowley, I. The life history of the superb blue wren (Malurinae). *Emu,* 1965, *64*, 251–297.

Rowley, I. Cooperative breeding in Australian birds. *Proc. 16th Internatl. Ornithol. Congr.,* 1976, *657*, 666.

Rowley, I. Communal activities among white-winged choughs *Corcorax melanorhamphus. Ibis,* 1978, *120*, 178–197.

Schaller, G. B. *The Serengeti Lion: A Study of Predator–Prey Relations.* University of Chicago Press, Chicago, 1972.

Schedl, K. W. Breeding habits of arboricole insects in Central Africa. *Proc. 10th Internat. Congr. Entomol.,* 1958, *1*, 183–197.

Shear, W. A. The evolution of social phenomena in spiders. *Bull. Br. Arachnol. Soc.,* 1970, *1*, 65–76.

Sherman, P. W. Nepotism and the evolution of alarm calls. *Science,* 1977, *197*, 1246–1253.

Sinclair, A. R. E. Studies of the ecology of the East African buffalo, Ph.D. thesis, Oxford University, 1970.

Skutch, A. F. Helpers among birds. *Condor,* 1961, *63*, 198–226.

Smith, W. J., Oppenheimer, S. L., De Villa, E. C., Jill, G., and Ulmer, F. A. Behavior of a captive population of black-tailed prairiedogs: Annual cycle of social behavior. *Behavior,* 1973, *46*, 189–153.

Svendsen, G. E. Behavioral and environmental factors in the spatial distribution and population dynamics of a yellow-bellied marmot population. *Ecol.,* 1974, *55*, 760–771.

Swainson, G. W. Cooperative rearing in the bell miner. *Emu,* 1970, *70*, 183–188.

Tener, J. S. A preliminary study of the musk-oxen of Fosheim Peninsula, Ellesmere Island, N.W.T., Canada Wildlife Service, Wildlife Management Bulletin, 1st ser., No. 9, 1954.

Thoday, J. M. Components of fitness. *Symp. Soc. Exp. Biol.,* 1953, *7*, 96–113.

Treisman, M. Predation and the evolution of gregariousness. I. Models for concealment and evasion. *Anim. Behav.*, 1975, *23*, 779–800.

Trivers, R. L. The evolution of reciprocal altruism. *Quart. Rev. Biol.*, 1971, *46*, 35–57.

Trivers, R. L. Parent–offspring conflict. *Amer. Zool.*, 1974, *14*, 249–264.

Trivers, R. L., and Hare, H. Haplodiploidy and the evolution of the social insects. *Science,* 1976, *191*, 249–263.

Van Valen, L. Group selection, sex, and fossils. *Evolution,* 1975, *29*, 87–94.

Vehrencamp, S. L. Relative fecundity and parental effort in communally nesting anis, *Crotophaga sulcirostris. Science,* 1977, *197*, 403–405.

Vehrencamp, S. L. The adaptive significance of communal nesting in groove-billed anis (*Crotophaga sulcirostris*). *Behav. Ecol. Sociobiol.,* 1978, *4*, 1–33.

Vehrencamp, S. L. To skew or not to skew? *Proc. 12th Internat. Ornithol. Congr.,* in press.

Ward, P., and Zahavi, A. The importance of certain assemblages of birds as "information-centres" for food-finding. *Ibis,* 1973, *115*, 517–534.

West-Eberhard, M. J. The social biology of Polistine wasps. *Misc. Pub. Mus. Zool.,* Univ. Michigan, 1969, *140*, 1–101.

West-Eberhard, M. J. The evolution of social behavior by kin selection. *Quart. Rev. Biol.,* 1975, *50*, 1–34.

White, F. N., Bartholomew, G. A., and Howell, T. R. The thermal significance of the nest of the sociable weaver *Philetairus socius:* Winter observations. *Ibis,* 1975, *117*, 171–179.

Williams, G. C. *Adaptation and Natural Selection.* Princeton University Press, Princeton, N.J., 1966.

Williams, G. C. *Group Selection.* Aldine Atherton, New York, 1971.

Williams, G. C. Sex and evolution. *Monographs in Population Biology.* Princeton University Press, Princeton, N.J., 1975.

Wilson, D. S. A theory of group selection. *Proc. Nat. Acad. Sci. USA,* 1975, *72*, 143–146.

Wilson, D. S. Structured demes and the evolution of group-advantageous traits. *Amer. Nat.,* 1977, *111*, 157–185.

Wilson, E. O. *The Insect Societies.* Belknap Press, Cambridge, 1971.

Wilson, E. O. *Sociobiology: The New Synthesis.* Belknap Press, Cambridge, 1975.

Wilson, E. O. The central problems of sociobiology. In R. May (ed.), *Theoretical Ecology: Principles and Applications.* W. B. Saunders, Philadelphia, 1976.

Woolfenden, G. E. Nesting and survival in a population of Florida scrub jays. *Living Bird,* 1973, *12*, 25–49.

Woolfenden, G. E. Florida scrub jay helpers at the nest. *Auk,* 1975, *92*, 1–15.

Woolfenden, G. E. Cooperative breeding in American birds. *Proc. Internat. Ornithol. Congr.,* 1976, *16*, 674–684.

Woolfenden, G. E., and Fitzpatrick, J. W. The inheritance of territory in group-breeding birds. *Biosci.,* 1978, *28*, 104–108.

Wright, S. Modes of selection. *Amer. Nat.,* 1956, *90*, 5–25.

Wynne-Edwards, V. C. *Animal Dispersion in Relation to Social Behavior.* Oliver and Boyd, Edinburgh, 1962.

Zahavi, A. Cooperative breeding in Eurasian birds. *Proc. Internat. Ornithol. Congr.,* 1976, *16*, 685–694.

Zimen, E. On the regulation of pack size in wolves. *Z. Tierpsychol.,* 1976, *40*, 300–341.

Appendix A

Calculation of maximum possible skew for related and unrelated groups. In the case of unrelated individuals:

$$W_\omega = W_1$$
$$W_\alpha = \overline{W} + (k - 1)(\overline{W} - W_1) \qquad k = \text{group size}$$

In the case of related individuals:
Inclusive fitness if all k individuals breed solitarily:

$$IF_{sol} = W_1 + (k - 1)W_1 r$$

Inclusive fitness of a subordinate in a group:

Let X = amount by which dominant lowers the personal fitness of each subordinate below $\overline{W}$; $X \leqslant \overline{W}$

$$IF_\omega = \underbrace{(\overline{W} - X)}_{\substack{\text{personal} \\ \text{component}}} + \underbrace{r[\overline{W} + (k - 1)X]}_{\substack{\text{component due to} \\ \text{dominant's offspring}}} + \underbrace{(k - 2)(\overline{W} - X)r}_{\substack{\text{component due to other} \\ \text{subordinate's offspring}}}$$

Setting $IF_\omega = IF_{sol}$ and solving for X:

$$X = \frac{(\overline{W} - W_1)[1 + r(k - 1)]}{1 - r}$$

Therefore: $W_\omega = \overline{W} - X$

$$W_\alpha = \overline{W} + (k - 1)(\overline{W} - X)$$

APPENDIX B

Calculation of inclusive fitness for several alternative social strategies for a group of $k = 5$ relatives. Three components of inclusive fitness, s, R, and r, are varied to show how they affect the relative success of these strategies. s and R refer to the dispersal success and reproductive success components of personal fitness W ($W = sR$), and r is the coefficient of relatedness between group members. NP = skew not possible because $\overline{W} < W_1$.

Social strategy	IF	$R_1 = 1$ $R = 3$ $s = .95$ $r = .5$	$R_1 = 1$ $R = 1.2$ $s = .4$ $r = .25$	$R_1 = 2$ $R = 1$ $s = .4$ $r = .5$	$R_1 = 2$ $R = 1$ $s = .95$ $r = .5$
All breed solitarily	$R_1 + (k - 1)sR_1r$	3.0	0.8	2.4	5.7
All k relatives breed in a group without skew	$\overline{R} + (k - 1)\overline{R}r$	9.0	2.4	3.0	3.0
The dominant relative imposes maximum skew on other relatives	$\overline{R} + (k - 1)X + (k - 1)(\overline{R} - X)r$	15.0	4.0	5.0	NP
The dominant recruits 4 nonrelatives and breeds without skew; all other relatives disperse and join similar nonskewed groups	$\overline{R} + (k - 1)s\overline{R}r$	8.8	1.7	1.8	2.9
The dominant recruits 4 nonrelatives and imposes maximum skew; all other relatives disperse and randomly become dominants or subordinates in similar skewed groups	$\overline{R} + (k - 1)(\overline{R} - R_1)s + (k - 1)s\overline{R}r$	16.4	1.8	NP	NP

Index

Acimonyx jubatus, 175
Aconitum, nectar extraction from, 262
Actitus macularis, 305
Active defense
  versus aggression, 60–61
  defined, 61
Activity fields
  spacing patterns and, 161–167
  spatial relationships of, 169
Actophilornis africana, 310
Adaptive potential, versus goodness of fit,
    11–12
Adélie penguins, territory size versus
    aggression in, 186
Advertisement or threat, communication of,
    191–196
Advertising behavior, spacing mechanisms
    and, 191
Aepyceros melampus, 294
Affective attack, defined, 57
Affective defense, in cats, 58
Agelaius icterocephalus, 180
Agelaius phoeniceus, 181, 238
Agelaius tricolor, 283
Agelena consociata, 369
Aggression, 56–64. *See also* Agonistic
    tendencies
  active defense against, 60–61
  attacks in, 58
  defense against, 60
  defensive, 60, 64
  den or localized food as referent in,
    181
  eating and, 58–59
  endocrine basis of, 57
  flight and, 58

Aggression *(cont.)*
  food availability and, 181, 185
  glandular poisons released in, 61
  hunger and, 185–186
  in isolated animals, 184
  kinds of, 57–58
  location effects in, 178–180
  neurally defined components of, 59–60
  neural organization and, 57–58
  patterning mechanisms in, 59
  predatory, 57
  proximity and, 176
  responses to, 60–64
  sensorimotor mechanisms in, 59–60
  sex and, 56–65
  sex/age contacts in, 183
  territory and, 180–181
Aggression field
  agonistic tendencies and, 172–182
  defined, 178
  nests and, 181–182
Aggression gradient, 178
Aggressiveness, measurement of, 178
Aggressive tendencies, versus aggressive
    encounters, 173. *See also* Agonistic
    tendencies
Agonistic behavior. *See also* Aggression;
    Agonistic tendencies
  in animals, 174–182
  external referents for, 180
  food availability and, 185–186
  individual and population differences in,
    182–187
  social interaction and, 184
  spacing behavior and, 183
  spatial variation in, 177

Agonistic behavior *(cont.)*
  steroid hormone administration and, 182–183
  territory size and, 186–187
  in tree squirrels, 180
Aid-giving behavior, as mutualism or reciprocal altruism, 354–355
Alarm signals
  in animal communication, 127–128
  symbolic signaling as, 130–133
Alcelaphus buselaphus, 295
Alectoris rufa, 307
Alouatta, 160
Altricial birds. *See also* Birds
  clutch sizes in, 317–318
  frugivorous, 317
  monogamy in, 324–326
  versus precocial, 285
Altruism
  coefficient of relatedness and, 357
  group selection and, 361–362
  kin selection and, 358–359
  reciprocal, 355
Amakihis, foraging of, 252
American robin, agonistic behavior of, 187
American woodcock, promiscuity in, 316
Analog information, in signal coding, 96–97
Animal communication. *See also*
    Communication; Signal; Signaling
  affect plus indexing in, 127
  alarm signals in, 127–128, 131–133
  analysis of, 73–143
  arbitrary signals in, 97–98
  arousal, emotion, and external referents in, 129–130
  artificial communication systems and, 133–134
  in birds, 110–112, 124
  categorical and continuous perception in, 99–103
  click-train repertoire in, 92–94
  communicative familiarity and social organization in, 136–137
  deictic signals in, 125
  digital versus analog coding in, 96–97
  discontinuous or discrete signals in, 103–106
  enemy specifications in, 127–129
  "familiar groupings" in, 137
  forgetting as, 123
  game theory in, 200
  graded systems and, 103–106
  iconic signals in, 97–98
  imperfect information in, 200
  information in, 127, 200
  input and output values in, 85
  internal and external triggering in, 135–136
  just noticeable difference in, 95

Animal communication *(cont.)*
  kinship relations and, 122–123
  model action pattern in, 91
  new directions in, 137–143
  nominal addressing in, 125
  open and closed systems in, 106–107
  "receiving" animals in, 95–96
  rule transmission and, 107
  selective addressing in, 125–126
  shared procedures for production and perception in, 109–110
  signal address in, 125–126
  signaler identity recognition in, 120–125
  signaler output categories in, 91–95
  signaling, sensation, and perception in, 108–109
  signal intensity in, 129
  signals and individual referents in, 134–136
  signals with continuous variations in, 101–102
  signal variation in, 89–107
  spacing signals in, 192–194
  specific transformation in, 86–87
  stereotyping and variability in, 90–91, 96
  strangeness, familiarity, and kin recognition in, 122–123
  strangers' signals in, 122–123
  variability in, 96
  voice-onset-time in, 99–100
Animal movements
  computer simulation of, 166–167
  estimation of, 161–167
  information about, 170
  radio tracking in, 166
  recording of, 161–162
Animals
  agonistic behavior in, 174–182
  familiarity of with area, 204–205
  home range sizes for, 163
  isolation effects in, 183–184
  isolation fields of, 171
  proximity of, 174–176
  spacing in. *See* Spacing
  spatial relations between, 167–173
Anolis segreyi, 293
Anser caerulescens, 230
Antbirds, spacing behavior of, 159, 177, 202
Antelopes, harem polygyny in, 304
Antiaggression mechanisms, evolutionary development of, 62–64
Antilocapra americana, 294
Ants, eusociality in, 371–372
Aotus trivirgatus, 329
Apheloria corrugata, 61
Apistogramma ramirezi, 171
Arbitrariness, in animal communication, 97–98
"Arbitrary" behavior, motivation and, 54

Arboreal primates, territories of, 160–161
Arctic shorebirds, clutch size in, 308
Arctocephalus, 292
Ardea herodias, 242
Assessments, in signal processing, 84
Ateles belzebuth, 203
Attack
    affective. *See* Affective attack
    hypothalamic stimulation in, 59
    predatory, 60
    quiet, biting, 57
Auditory capability, signal direction and, 79
Australian bell-magpies, 283

Baboons
    aggressive interactions in, 181
    dominance and tail position in, 121
Barnacle geese, foraging of, 252
Bats, harem group of, 378
Beachbirds, foraging time for, 238. *See also*
        Birds
Beavers, male parental care in, 328
Bee dance, as communication, 98
Bees, "specialist" versus "generalist" types of,
        262
Beetles
    chemical attraction in, 117
    chemical defense discharges in, 61–62
Behavior
    aggressive. *See* Aggression; Agonistic
        behavior
    "arbitrary," 54
    biological mechanisms in, 29
    developmental plasticity in, 5–7
    evolutionary-genetic cause of, 30
    proximal mechanisms in, 30
    sexual. *See* Sexual behavior
    signal perception and, 140–143
    social. *See* Social behavior
    tabula rasa in, 14
Behavioral depression, 204
Behavioral development, retardation in rate
        of, 14
Behavioral science
    mechanistic view in, 2–3
    organismic view in, 3
Behavior analysis, distal factors in, 52
Behavior modification, spacing signals and,
        192–193
Behavior pattern, development of, 30
Benefit/cost ratios, in individual and kin
        selection, 354–357, 363–364
Biological clock
    circadian, 37
    photically inducible and noninducible
        phases of, 39
    reproduction and, 38
    tuning of, 40
Biology, behavior and, 29–30

Bird of paradise, leks of, 322
Birds
    adoption of, 87, 88
    alarm calls of, 131
    altricial versus precocial, 285, 314–321,
        324–328
    brood-parasitic, 325
    deserted clutches of, 306–308
    familial evolutionary route of, 373–374
    female aggressiveness in, 281, 393
    female desertion in, 275
    flock-feeding, 243
    foraging behavior in, 208–209, 242–243
    frequency sensitivity of, 78
    "helper-at-the-nest" species of, 373
    "ideal free distribution" of, 245
    increased foraging efficiency of, 261–262
    learning in, 110–111
    male parental care in, 283
    and mated status of prospective mates, 303
    mating system evolution in, 271–332
    monogamous females in, 281
    optimal clutch size for, 265
    optimal return times after searching by,
        250–254
    parasocial route of, 374–376
    passerine. *See* Passerine birds
    pitch differences in calls of, 118–119
    polygamy in, 285
    polygynous-polyandrous systems of, 305–
        307
    polygyny in, 301–303
    precocial versus altricial, 285, 314–321,
        324–328
    precopulating posturing and courtship
        feeding in, 89
    predation pattern form, 234
    prior territorial ownership of, 199–200
    promiscuity in, 311–312
    sampling as aid to foraging in, 240
    semiprecocial, 326–328
    sex role reversal in, 275
    spacing behavior in, 190, 201–203
    territorial behavior of, 198
    territorial defense among, 188
    territorial polygyny in, 278–280
    ventriloquial sound in, 79
    vocal communication in, 110–112. *See also*
        Birdsong
    vocalizations of, 121
Birdsong
    dialects in, 124
    pitch differences in, 118–119
    playbacks to, 190–191
    production and perception of, 110–112
    sensorimotor interplay in, 110
    sex, age, and, 124
    as spacing signals, 194
Birgus latro, 181

Bitterling, 141
Bison bison, 314
Biziura lobata, 317
Blackbirds. *See also* Birds
  Brewer's, 283, 303
  foraging of, 230
  habitat heterogeneity for, 286
  marsh nestings of, 301–302
  nesting and food access of, 201
  polygyny in, 286, 301
  search path modification by, 250
Black-capped chickadees, foraging of, 235
Black-headed gulls, territories of, 176
Blue geese, foraging of, 230
Blue honeycreeper, diet and defense of, 320
Blue monkeys, foraging behavior of, 207–208
Blue tit, 141
Bobolinks
  male parental behavior in, 283
  polygyny in, 302
Bobwhite quail, aggression in, 190
Bombycilla, 320
Bonasa umbellus, 35, 315
Boobies, monogamy in, 325
Brachinus genus, aggression-discharges in, 62
Brain changes, immaturity syndrome and, 16
Brain size, information processing and, 15
Branta bernicla, 252
Branta leucopsis, 252
Breeding. *See also* Copulatory behavior;
    Mating; Reproduction
  proper time and place for, 37–40
  temporal factors in, 37–40
Brewer's blackbirds, 283, 303
Brood-parasitic birds, monogamy and, 325
Brood pouches, in male seahorses, 274
Brown woodcreeper, defense in, 330
Bullfrogs
  signals of, 124
  spacing behavior in, 190
  vocalizations of, 34
Bumblebees
  flower nectar content and, 234, 248, 262
  individual recognition in, 120
Buntings, hunger and aggression in, 185
Butterfly, monarch, 62–63
Bycanistes brevis, 320

Calamospiza melanocorys, 283
Calcarius pictus, 326
Calidris alba, 307
Calidris melanotos, 317
Callicebus moloch, 160, 168, 189
Callipepla squamata, 307
Callithrix, 189
Campylorhynchus nuchalis, 191
Canada geese, 121
Canids
  monogamous pair bonds in, 189, 329
  olfactory discrimination in, 121

Canis latrans, 128, 329
Canis lupus, 328
Cape buffalo, dominance hierarchies of, 313
Cape hunting dogs, monogamy of, 328
Capreolus capreolus, 33
Cassidix mexicanus, 242
Castor fiber, 328
Casuarius casuarius, 274
Cats
  affective defense in, 57–58
  copulatory behavior of, 30
  hypothalamic stimulation in, 59–60
Centrocercus urophasianus, 187
Cephalophus natalensis, 331
Ceratotherium simum, 184
Cercocebus albigena, 167
Cercopithecus monkeys, 124
Cercopithecus ascanius, 160, 194
Cercopithecus mitis, 160, 194
Cervus canadensis, 304
Cervus elephas, 304
Chaffinch
  alarm calls of, 131
  foraging of, 255
  mutual avoidance in, 174
  optimal diet of, 255
Chaffinch song, territorial aspects of, 119
Change, Heraclitean, 13
Cheetahs
  mutual avoidance in, 175
  promiscuity of, 313
Chemical defense, in beetles, 61–62
Chemical noise, in olfactory signaling, 81
Chickadees
  foraging success of, 242, 244
  "giving up time" for, 235–236
Chimpanzee
  artificial communication in, 133–134
  food calls of, 130
  imitation in, 113
  pant hooting of, 121
Chipmunks, site-dependent dominance in,
    177–178
Chiroxiphia linearis, 322
Chiroxiphia pareola, 33
Cichlids, aggression in, 171, 183, 190
Cichlasoma nigrofasciatum, 190
Cicadas, long-distance calls of, 194
Circadian rhythm
  photoperiodism and, 39
  in sexual activity, 37
Clamator jacobinus, 326
Clibanarius, 183
Click-train repertoire, in animal
    communication, 92–94
Clock, biological. *See* Biological clock
Closed communication system, defined, 106–
    107. *See also* Animal communication;
    Communication
Clutch sizes, in altricial birds, 317–319

Coal tit, feeding habits of, 220
Coatimundis, harem polygyny of, 304–305
Cocks-of-the-rock, leks of, 322
Coconut crabs, agonistic behavior, 181
Coke's hartebeest, territory defense of, 295
Cognition, communication and, 73
Colinus virginianus, 190
Coliuspasser jacksoni, 321
Colobus badius, 252, 294
Colobus guereza, 136, 181, 294
Colobus monkeys
  overlap of territories in, 181
  territorial polygyny in, 294
  threat display of, 136
Colobus, resource foraging by, 206–207
Coloniality, defined, 288
"Colonial" passerine birds. *See also* Birds;
    Passerine birds
  habitat distributions for, 299–300
  polygyny in, 295–296
Colonial rodents, polygyny-threshold model
    for, 288–292
Color, communication and, 74
Columba palumbus, 226
Communication. *See also* Animal
    communication; Human
    communication
  of advertisement or threat, 191–196
  and auditory capacity of birds and
    mammals, 79
  categorical perception in, 102–103
  defined, 73
  distance traveled by signal in, 82
  evolution of, 106–107
  heredity and ontogeny of, 107–114
  in insects, 120
  internal processing of, 75
  learning in, 113
  motor theory of speech perception in,
    112–113
  noise and, 80–81
  odor-trail laying and, 80
  open and closed systems in, 106–107
  responses in, 75
  sensory templates and schemata in, 113–
    114
  signal direction in, 78–80
  signaling organ in, 73
  signal nonconstancy in, 74
  signal production in, 76–83
  signal sender in, 76–77
  signal structure and function in, 114–120
  spatial characteristics and, 80
  specialization and, 74
  transmission versus environment in, 82–83
Communication systems
  artificial, 133–134
  discrete and graded, 103–106
  operation of without complementation of
    other sensory modalities, 105–106

Communication systems *(cont.)*
  overall characteristics of, 75
  scientific disciplines in, 73
  social organization and, 136–137
Conditioning, socialization as, 21–22
Connochaetus taurinus, 180, 313
Coolidge effect, 36
Cooperation, among kin, 384–388
Cooperative behavior
  factors leading to, 380–382
  and reproductive division of labor, 381–
    382
Copulation mechanisms, 40–44
Copulatory behavior
  "darting and hopping" in, 56
  lordosis in, 55
  multiple intromissions in, 46–47
  postejaculatory refractory period in, 50
  "reproductive memory" in, 41
  sexual motivation in, 40–41
Copulatory patterns, adaptive, 50–51
Copulatory reflexes, integration of, 43
Copulatory stimulation
  neuroendocrine reflex and, 47
  parturition facilitation through, 47–
    48
  sperm transport and, 49–50
  storage and, 48
Corophium, 243, 245
Corticosteroids, in insect chemical defense,
    62
Cost–benefit model, in feeding dispersion,
    263–265
Courting song, in copulatory behavior, 41.
    See also Birdsong
Cowbirds
  brood parasitism of, 302
  monogamy in, 325
Crab plovers, monogamy in, 325
Crickets
  body size and song, 118
  signal production and perception in, 109–
    110
Crickets, tree, songs of, 109
Critical period, defined, 6
Crocuta crocuta, 313
Cross-species signal recognition, 116–117
Crypturellus variegatus, 274
Cuckoldry, 52
Cuckoos, monogamy and, 326
Cyanocitta stelleri, 171, 177

Damselfish chirps, temporal patterning of,
    117
Danaus plexippus, 62
Dance language, of honeybees, 98
Daphnia magna, 257
Deer, antler size and dominance, 121
Deermice, monogamy in, 330
Defassa waterbuck, territories of, 295

Defensive aggression
    defined, 64
    versus predatory attack, 60
Dendragapus obscurus, 315
Dendrocincla fuliginosa, 320
Dendroica discolor, 283
Development. *See also* Behavior; Social
        behavior
    concept of in behavioral science, 2–5
    environment and, 16–17
    experience in, 21
    general systems theory and, 19
    macroevolutionary view of, 16
    microevolutionary view of, 16
    orthogenesis in, 20
    plasticity in, 5–7
    in social context, 16–23
    social environment and, 16–17, 20
Developmental plasticity, 5–7
Dickcissels, nesting failures in, 302
Digital information, in signal coding, 96–98
Directionality, in foraging strategy, 246–247
Discrete communication systems, just
            noticeable differences in, 105. *See also*
            Communication systems
Dispersal, among kin, 385
Distance-increasing behavior, 191
Division of labor, reproductive, 381–382
Dolichonyx oryzivorus, 283
Dominant-subordinate relationships
    among kin, 386
    skew in, 382–384
Dromas ardeola, 325
Drosophila melanogaster, 41, 50
    fast- and slow-mating, 42–43
Drosophila pseudoobscura, 34–35
Duikers, monogamy in, 331
Dungflies, copulation time for, 236–237
Dytiscus marginalis, 62
Dytiscus plexippus, 63

Eating, aggression and, 58–59
Ectopistes migratorius, 325
Effective environment, defined, 21
Eggs, fertilization of in sexual reproduction,
        271–272
Eider, food intake of common, 318
Electric fish, signals among, 117
Elephant seals, polygyny in, 292
Elephantulus rufescens, 188
Elodes stink beetle, defense reaction in, 64
Emberiza calandra, 283
Emotional states, signals and, 129
Encounter site, location effects in, 178–180
Enemy specifications, in animal
            communication, 127–129
Environment
    effective, 21
    predator's "memory window" and, 233
    social. *See* Social environment

Environmental factors, detection of rivals
        through, 192
Environmental feedback, valence or hedonic
        tone in, 19
Environmental variables, characterizations of,
        20–23
Ephestia cantella, 239
Epideictic displays, 360
Equus africanus, 314
Equus grevi, 314
Equus hemionus, 314
Erithacus rubecula, 188
Erythrocebus patas, 198
Estrous cycle, behavioral control in, 45
Eulampis jugularis, 192
Eumetopias, 292
Eupatorium capillifolium, 63
Euphagus cyanocephalus, 201
Eupoda montana, 307
European robin, aggression in, 188
European warblers, body weight versus song
        pitch in, 118
Eusocial insects, 371
Eusociality
    defined, 367
    in Hymenoptera, 371–372
Evolution
    genetic factors in, 353
    sociality and, 367–378
    spacing behavior and, 196–197
Experience, modification by, 5
Exploitation depression, 204
Eye spots, as "frightening device," 64

Facilitation functions, 21, 25
Falco parverius, 64
Familial route, for spiders, 369
Feeding dispersion, cost–benefit analysis in,
        262–265
Feeding places, social learning and, 242. *See
        also* Foraging behavior
Felis concolor, 176
Female
    novel, 35–36
    properties of in mate selection, 35–36
    sexual behavior of, 41–42
Female aggression
    reproductive success and, 289–290
    in territorial polygyny, 281
Female animal
    abandonment of first clutch by, 306
    harem polygyny and, 304
Female competition
    and male choice in mating systems, 274–
        276
    sex role reversal and, 275–276
Female copulation signal, as communication,
        126
Female-defensive monogamy, 277
Female desertion, 275, 306

Female fecundity, promiscuity and, 311
Female fitness, in territorial polygyny, 280
Female groups, male defense of, 304
Ficedula albicollis, 303
Ficedula hypoleuca, 283
Ficus, 206
Fiddler crabs, claw waving by, 175
Field dominance, site-dependent, 177
Field orientation, in socialization, 21, 24
Finches
    call modification of, 122
    foraging efficiency of, 261
    male defense in, 326
    male parental care in, 283
    vocal sexual solicitation in, 135
Fireflies, 120
Fish
    chemical signals in, 79
    electrical communication of, 81, 117
    male quality in, 279
Fitness
    foraging behavior and, 226
    future, 366
    inclusive, 356
    lifetime, 353
    operational definition of, 352
Flexibility, change and, 13
Flight, aggression and, 58–59
Florida scrub jay, juvenile aid in, 365
Flycatchers
    foraging of, 245
    male parental care in, 283
    polygyny in, 285, 303
Food. *See* Foraging behavior
Food availability, aggression and, 185–186
Food deprivation, aggression and, 185
Food source, nest aggregation and, 201–202
Foraging animal, "resource" knowledge of, 204
Foraging behavior. *See also* Foraging time
    of bees, 261–262
    and cost of alternative foraging activities, 260–261
    directionality in, 246
    feeding dispersion in, 262–265
    fitness and, 226
    "group" versus "individual" optimization in, 238, 241–245
    optimal diets in, 255–259
    prey length in, 256
    prey size and, 253
    prey types in, 254–259
    sampling in, 259–260
    search paths in, 246–254
    social learning in, 242
    social significance of, 225–265
    specialists and generalists in, 261–262
Foraging-decision rules, 225
Foraging strategies, resting in, 226

Foraging time, allocation of between areas, 228–246
Forest monkeys, loud calls of, 119
Foxes, aggression in, 190
Fringilla coelebs, 174, 255
Frog songs
    frequency structure of, 78
    responses to, 109
Frugivorous birds, resource defense by, 317–319. *See also* Birds
Fruit bat, harem group of, 378
Fur seals, polygyny in, 292
Future fitness, defined, 366

Galerita janus, 61
Gallinago media, 316
Gallus gallus, 304
Game theory, in animal communication, 200
Gannets, monogamy in, 325
Gasterosteus aculeatus, 177
Gazella granti, 295
Geese, recognition in Canadian, 121
Generalist, versus specialist, 13, 261–262
Generality-specificity, stimulus effects in, 22
Genes, in evolution, 353
Genetic variability, reduction of, 13
Genital reflexes, in rat, 43
Gestation times, life spans and, 16
Gibbon
    monogamy in, 329
    spacing behavior in, 189
"Giving-up time," in foraging, 235–238
Glaucidium pygmy owl, 64
Glycosides, in insect chemical defense, 62
Goodness of fit, versus adaptive potential, 11–12
Grackles
    aggression in, 182
    male parental care in, 283
Graded communication system, 105. *See also* Communication; Communication systems
Grant's gazelles, male defenders in, 295
Grasshoppers, defensive secretions of, 63
Great bustard, 321
Great snipe, promiscuity in, 316
Great-tailed grackles, mating seasons of, 283
Great tit
    age and residence in, 199
    foraging behavior of, 236, 241–242
Grevy's zebra, social groups in, 314
Ground squirrels
    alarm calls in, 128–129, 289
    territory defense in, 291
Group cooperative behavior, factors leading to, 380–381
Group foraging, time allocation and, 241–245. *See also* Foraging behavior
Grouping, as social strategy, 354

Group memberships, promiscuity and, 313–314

Group selection
altruism and, 361–362
defined, 360
ecological factors affecting, 388–389
relative importance of, 362–367
in sociality evolution, 351–389

Group stability, factors affecting, 379–380

Grouse
male removal in, 315
sexual selection of, 33, 35

Growth, as "evolution of immaturity," 8–9. *See also* Development

Grus canadensis, 167

Guppy, prey choice in, 241

Guy's hummingbird, leks of, 322

Gymnopithys bicolor, 171, 177

Gymnorhina, male parental behavior in, 283

Habitat heterogeneity, polygyny and, 285–286

Habitat quality, foraging time and, 231–232

Halichoerus grypus, 292

Hamadryas baboon, 182

Hammerhead bats, leks of, 322

Hamster
reproductive behavior in, 39–40
reproductive storage in, 48

Hanuman langur, groups of, 294

Haplochromis burtoni, 183, 190

Harem polygyny, 304–305

Harem size, female reproductive success and, 286–287

Hawaiian honeycreeper, feeding territory of, 264

Hedonic tone, environmental feedback and, 19

Helper-at-the-nest species, 373

Hemichromis bimaculatus, 179

Hermit crab
isolation of, 183
signal perception in, 141

Hippocampus zosterae, 274

Home range size, estimation of, 163–165

Honeybee, dance language of, 98

Honeyguides, beehive defense by, 321

Hornbills, male parental care in, 320

Horses, harem polygyny in, 304

Houseflies, foraging of, 230

House wrens
male parental care in, 283–284
mate's activity fields in, 189

Human communication, categorical perception in, 102–103

Humans, as kin-group selection example, 389. *See also* Primates

Hummingbird
diet choice of, 255
visual spacing signal from, 192

Humpbacked whales, song transmission of, 82

Hunger, aggression and, 185–186. *See also* Foraging behavior

Hybrid crickets, shared production and perception of signals from, 109–110

Hydrophasianus chirurgas, 310

Hyenas, hunting of, 313

Hylobates, hunting of, 160, 189

Hylobates klossii, 329–333

Hypothalamus, attack patterns and, 59–60

Hypsignathus monstrosus, 322

Iconicity, in animal communication, 97–98

Immaturity
"evolution" of, 7–16
goodness-of-fit versus adaptive-potential orientation in, 11–12
versus learning, 9–10
life-history pattern of, 9–10
prolongation of, 8–9

Immaturity syndrome, 23–24
brain changes in, 16
as "escape from specialization," 13

Impala, 125, 295

Inclusive fitness
altruistic behavior and, 357
defined, 356

Indicator xanthonotus, 321

Individual selection
defined, 354
relative importance of, 362–367
in sociality evolution, 351–389

Indigo bunting, polygyny of, 286

Induction functions, 21, 25

Infants, phonemes and, 112

Information
central processing and, 6
from central receiver, 114
social environment as source of, 17–19

Information processing, brain size and, 15

Insect defenses, origination of in plants, 61–63

Insect hormones, use of by plants, 62–63

Insects
familial evolutionary route of, 371–372
parasocial evolutionary route of, 372
visual communication in, 120

Intention, in communication, 75

Interaction, in social life, 22–23

Interdependence, in social life, 22–23

Intergroup selection, defined, 360

Internal transformations
in signal processing, 83–88
uniqueness and specificity of, 88

Intruders, territorial defense and, 198

Isolated animals, aggression in, 184

Isolation fields, 171–173

Isolation ratio, 171

Jacana
    polyandry in, 305, 308, 310
    polygyny-polyandry in, 305
    sex role reversal in, 274–275
Jacana jacana, 311
Jacana spinosa, 275
Jackson's whydah, 321
Japanese quail, copulatory behavior in, 55
Jewelfish, novel environments and, 179
JND. *See* Just noticeable difference
Junco hyemalis, 185
Jungle fowl, harem polygyny in, 304
Just noticeable difference (JND)
    in animal communication, 95–96
    in discrete and graded communication
        systems, 105

Kin altruism, 358–359
Kin, cooperation and manipulation among,
    384–388
Kin group selection, humans as example of,
    389
Kin manipulation, defined, 359
Kin selection
    altruism and, 358–359
    defined, 352, 356
    relative importance of, 362–367
    selective aid dispensing in, 358
    in sociality evolution, 351–389
Kinship, communicative familiarity and, 123
Kirk's dikdik, monogamy in, 330
Kobus defassa, 295
Kobus kob, 321

Lagopus lagopus, 185
Langurs, territorial polygyny in, 294
Lark buntings
    male parental care in, 283
    nesting success of, 285
Larus atricilla, 177
Larus ridibundus, 176
Lattice hierarchy, 55
Laughing gulls, territories of, 177
Learning
    in birdsong production and perception,
        110–111
    in communication, 113
    versus immaturity, 9–10
    schemata in, 15
    signaling behavior and, 113–114
Lebistes reticulata, 240
Leks
    evolution of, 321
    male and female behavior in, 321–322
Leonotis, 264
Lepomis macrochirus, 257
Leptasterias, 256
Lepus americanus, 165
Leucosticte atrata, 326
Life spans, gestation times and, 16

Lifetime fitness, defined, 353
Limosa lapponica, 242
Limpet, grazing pattern of, 252–253
Lions
    defense of pride by males of, 304
    familiar groupings of, 304
    harem polygyny in, 304
    males as "family" defenders of, 293, 304
    reproductive success of, 365
    territorial polygyny of, 293
Lobipes lobatus, 307
Location, aggression and, 178–180
Lophortyx californicus, 183, 307
Lordosis
    in copulatory pattern, 55
    estrogen and, 56
    neonatal, 55
Lottia gigantea, 252–253
Loxops vireus, 252
Lycaon pictus, 328
Lynx rufus, 128
Lyrebird, female aggression in, 293

Madoqua kirki, 330
Maintenance functions, in socialization, 21–
    22, 25
Male aggression, in mate selection, 32–33. *See
    also* Aggression
Male attractiveness, in mate selection, 32
Male cooperation, in mate selection, 33–34
Male parental behavior
    in monogamy, 329–331
    in polygyny, 282–284
Male quality, polygyny threshold and, 279
Males, reproductive strategy of, 273. *See also*
        Copulatory behavior; Sexual behavior
Mammals
    defensive aggression in, 60–61
    familial evolutionary route for, 376–377
    intrasexual spacing in, 188
    mating system evolution in, 271–332
    monogamy in, 328–331
    parasocial evolutionary route for, 377–379
Manacus manacus, 322
Manakins
    behavior of male, 33
    long-tailed, 322
    parental visitation of, 318
Mangabey
    aggression with food in, 181
    group location of gray-cheeked, 167–168,
        175
    resource foraging in, 206–227
    spacing calls of, 195
Manipulation, among kin, 384–388
Marmosets
    male parental contributions in, 329
    monogamy in, 329
Marmota caligata, 293
Marmota flaviventris, 286

Marmota marmota, 293
Marmota olympus, 293
Marmota sp., 11
Marmots
  as single-family group, 293–294
  play of, 11
  spacing of, 174
  yellow-bellied, 286–290
Marsh-breeding blackbirds, polygyny in, 301–302. *See also* Birds
Marsh wrens
  female aggression in, 281
  killing of blackbirds by, 301
Mate changing, Coolidge effect in, 36
Mate, choice of, 32–36. *See also* Mating behavior
Maternal behavior, maintenance functions in, 21–22
Mate selection. *See also* Mating behavior; Mating systems
  female properties in, 35–36
  frequency-dependent mating and, 34
  intraspecific, 32–36
Mating behavior. *See also* Copulatory behavior; Mating systems; Sexual behavior
  frequency-dependent, 34
  pituitary-gonadal secretions and, 38
Mating systems. *See also* Copulatory behavior
  classification of, 277
  economic decisions compared to, 271–272
  evolution of in birds and mammals, 271–332
  female competition and male choice in, 274–276
  harem polygyny in, 304–305
  male competition and female choice in, 273–274
  monogamous, 52, 277
  options in, 272
  polyandry as, 277, 305–311
  polygyny as, 277
  promiscuity and, 277, 311–323
  simultaneous polyandry in, 309–311
Meadowlarks, male parental care in, 284
Mechanistic view, in behavioral science, 2–5
Meerkats, monogamy in, 330
Memory, communication and, 73
"Memory window," of optimal predator, 233
Menura novaehollandiae, 293
Mesocricetus auratus, 196
Metabus gravidus, 370
Metopidius indicus, 310
Metrosideros, 264
Mice
  aggressive behavior in, 181
  monogamy in, 330
  reproductive blocking in, 50
Microgalus, 330

Micropathodon chrysurus, 183
Millipedes, 61
Miopithecus talapoin, 174
Molothrus ater, 302
Monias benschi, 274
Monkeys
  alarm calls of, 125, 126, 131
  foraging behavior of, 206–208
  rhesus, 119
Monogamous animals, spacing behavior in, 188–189
Monogamy
  in altricial birds, 324–326
  in brood-parasitic birds, 325
  evolution of, 323–324
  female aggressiveness in, 330
  hypotheses concerning, 324
  male defense of females in, 327–328
  male parental care in, 326–327, 331
  in mammals, 328–331
  as mating system, 52, 277, 323–331
  nest attendance and, 327
  preconditions of, 323–324
  in primates, 329
Motacilla alba, 185
Motacilla flava, 253
Moths, receptor systems of, 81
Motivation, in social behavior, 53–54
Motor behavior, in hierarchical analysis, 55
Mountain plovers, polygyny and polyandry in, 307–308
Multiple intromissions, in rat copulatory behavior, 46–47
Musicapa striata, 245
Muskrats, female aggression in, 328
Mutualism, defined, 354
Myrica cerifera, 63

Narceus gordanus, 61
Nasua narica, 304
Natural selection, spacing behavior and, 196–197
Nectarinia kilimensis, 255
Nectarinia reichenowi, 264
Nemeritis, parasitism of *Ephestia cantella* by, 239–240
Neotragus moschatus, 331
Nephthys, 258
Nereis, 258
Nest aggregates, spacing behavior and, 200–202
Nests, aggression field and, 181–182
Neural organization, aggression and, 57–58
Neuroendocrine reflex
  copulatory stimulus and, 47–48
  multiple intromissions in, 47–49
Noise, communication and, 80–81
Nominal addressing, defined, 125

"Noncolonial" passerine birds, breeding habits of, 299–300. *See also* Birds; Passerine birds
Nothocercus bonapartei, 306
Nothoprocta cinerascens, 306
Notonecta glauca, 236

Oilbird, nesting habits of, 320
Olfaction, communication identity and, 120–121
Olympic marmot syndrome, 11
Onchomys, 330
Ondatra zibethicus, 328
Ontogeny
  broad variations in, 7–16
  learning during, 15
  phylogeny and, 8
Open communication system, defined, 106. *See also* Animal communication; Communication
Openness
  age-related, 7
  constraints on, 6
  defined, 5
  special sensitivity and, 6
Operant response, arbitrary nature of, 54
Opponent, proximity of, 174–176
Optimal diet models
  in foraging strategy, 255–259
  polychaete worms in, 258
Optimal foraging models, alternative foraging activities and, 260–261
Optimal foraging, sampling and, 259–260
Optimal predator, 227
  cumulative net intake of, 232
  "fixed giving-up time" for, 234
  foraging time of, 228–246
  goal of, 226–227
  habitat quality and, 231–232
  "memory window" of, 233
  optimal diet models and, 255–259
  prey types chosen by, 254–259
  profitable foraging areas for, 228–230
  selection threshold of, 258
Optimal return time, in searching or foraging strategy, 250–254
Optimal time allocation, 234–241
Orange-rumped honeyguide, beehive defense by, 321
Orb-web spiders, 369–370
Organic odorants, as signals, 117
Organismic view, in behavioral science, 3–5
Orthoptera, songs of, 118, 194
Ostrich, male parental care in, 306
Ovarian cycle, sexual activity and, 37
Ovenbirds. *See also* Birds
  foraging behavior of, 205, 241–242
  "giving-up time" for, 237–238
  insect densities in habitat of, 185

Ovenbirds *(cont.)*
  spacing behavior of, 202
  trespassing by, 171–172
Overlap promiscuity, 312–313
Ovulators, "induced" versus "spontaneous," 45–46

Pagurus samuelis, 183
Panaus plexippus, 62
Panthera leo, 293
Papio cynocephalus, 314
Paradisidaea apoda, 322
  P. minor, 322
Parasocial evolutionary route, of spiders, 369–371
Parental behavior
  as maintenance function, 21–22
  and trophic requirements of young, 17
Parental investment, in mating system evolution, 273
Parrotfish, spacing behavior of, 187
Partridge, double clutching in, 307. *See also* Birds
Parus ater, 226
Parus atricapillus, 235
Parus major, 199
Passenger pigeons, monogamy in, 325. *See also* Birds
Passerculus sandwichensis princeps, 284
Passer domesticus, 243
Passerina cyanea, 283
Passerine birds. *See also* Birds
  "colonial" versus "noncolonial," 295–296
  sexual roles in territorial defense among, 188
  territorial polygyny in, 295–303
  unpredictability of male mating prospects in, 297–299
Patas monkeys. *See also* Monkeys
  harem polygyny in, 304
  spacing behavior in, 198
Patterning mechanisms, in aggression, 59
Pavo cristatus, 304
Peafowl, harem polygyny in, 304–306
Pedioectes phasianellus, 315
Pelage color, in individual identity, 74
Penguins
  incubation in, 327
  territoriality in, 186
Perception
  in animal communication, 108–109
  opportunities in social environment for, 18
Peromyscus californicus, 330
Phaethornis guy, 322
Phalaropes. *See also* Birds; Sandpipers
  mate finding by, 275
  polygynous-polyandrous system in, 307
Phenotypic variability, reduction of, 13

Pheromones
  "active space" of, 83
  species-specificity of, 117
Philohela minor, 316
Philomachus pugnax, 316–317
Phonemes, infants' interpretation of, 112
Photoperiodism, sexual activity and, 39
Phylogeny, as succession of ontogenies, 8
Phyllostomus hastatus, 378
Pipefish, sex role reversal in, 274
Pituitary-gonadal secretions, sexual activity
  and, 38
Plants, use of insect hormones by, 62–63
Plasticity
  general, 7
  ontogeny and, 7–16
Ploceus cucullatus, 34
Pogonomyrmex, 257
Polistes metricus, 365
Polistes wasps
  individual recognition in, 120
  nests of, 383–384
Polyandry, 305–311. *See also* Mating
  behavior; Mating system
  as mating system, 277
  simultaneous, 309–311
Polychaete worms, selection of in optimal
  diets, 258
Polygamy. *See also* Mating behavior; Mating
  system
  male parental behavior and, 282–284
  serial, 305
Polygyny. *See also* Mating behavior; Mating
  system
  in birds. *See* Birds
  harem, 304–305
  and heterogeneity of habitat quality, 285–
    286
  in marsh-breeding blackbirds, 301
  as mating system, 277
  territorial. *See* Territorial polygyny
  in wrens, 303
Polygyny threshold concept, 278
Polygyny threshold model, 288–303
  colonial rodents and, 288–292
  competitive version of, 290
  evidence for, 284–288
  exceptions to, 303–304
  for seals and sea lions, 292–293
Polygynous-polyandrous systems, 305–308
Postejaculatory refractory period, in rat, 50
Prairie dogs, female aggression in, 292
Prairie warbler, double brooding of, 283
Precocial birds. *See also* Birds
  monogamy in, 326–328
  promiscuity in, 314–317
Predator
  foraging-decision rules for, 225–226
  optimal. *See* Optimal predator

Predator *(cont.)*
  time allocation by, without prey depletion,
    245–246
Predator-prey interactions, group selection
  and, 361
Predatory attack, defensive aggression and,
  60
Prediction, in social environment, 18
Pregnancy, behavioral induction of, 44–51
Presbytis potenziani, 330
Presbytis senex, 294
Prey types
  in foraging strategy, 254–259
  optimal choice and, 254–255
  predator and, 361
Primate calls, long-distance, 194
Primates. *See also* Monkeys
  foraging behavior of, 206–208
  imitation in, 113
  monogamy in, 329
Prior ownership, in territorial defense, 199–
  200
Progestational hormone secretion, behavioral
  induction of, 46–48
Promiscuity
  evolution of, 311–312
  food availability and, 316
  fruit resources and, 317–319
  in mammals, 312–314
  mating system and, 277
  overlap, 312–313
  in precocial versus altricial birds, 314–321
  sexual bimaturism and, 315
Pronghorn antelopes, territorial polygyny in,
  294–295
Proximity, versus spacing, 174–176
Ptarmigan, polygyny in, 327
Pukebo, 373
Pygoscelis adeliae, 186

Quadrat grid method, in home range size
  estimation, 164–166
Quail. *See also* Birds
  double clutching in, 307
  food calls of, 130
  Japanese, sexual reflexes of, 55
Quasisociality, defined, 375
Quiet biting attack, 57. *See also* Aggression
Quiscalus mexicanus, 283
Quiscalus quiscula, 152

Raccoons, aggression in, 190
"Radius of repulsion," defined, 167
Rana catesbeiana, 34, 110
Rape, as molar category, 52
Rats
  adaptive copulatory patterns in, 50–51
  aggressive behavior in, 181
  cervical stimulation, effects of, 42

Rats (*cont.*)
  circadian cycles of female, 39
  copulatory behavior in, 43, 46
  female sexual receptivity in, 47–51
  hormonal priming in, 56
  mating sequence of, 43
  motivated behavior of, 54
  multiple intromissions by, 46–47
  neuroendocrine reflex in, 47
  progestational female behavior in, 47–48
  reproductive behavior in, 38–39
  reproductive process blocking in, 49–50
  as spontaneous ovulator, 45–46
  "tonic immobility" pattern in, 50
Rattus norvegicus, 36, 181
Reactor glands, in *Alephoria* system, 61
Reciprocal altruism, 355
Red colobus, food types of, 206, 252
Red deer
  harem polygyny in, 304
  male dominance in, 33
  roe deer versus, 33
Red duikers, monogamy in, 331
Red grouse, territory size in, 185–186
Red jungle fowl, harem polygyny in, 304–305
Red-tailed monkey, foraging behavior of,
      207–208
Redunca redunca, 293
Red-winged blackbirds
  female aggressiveness, 281
  foraging of captive, 238
  habitat heterogeneity of, 286
  male quality in, 279
  mating season of, 283
  nests and aggression in, 181
Relatedness coefficient, altruistic behavior
      and, 357
Reproduction, biological clock and, 38–39.
      See also Copulatory behavior; Mating
      behavior; Sexual behavior
Reproductive division of labor, 381–382
Reproductive processes, blocking of in rat,
      49–50
Reproductive storage, in hamster, 48
Reproductive strategy, of males, 273–274
Reproductive success
  female aggression and, 289–290
  harem size and, 286–287
Resource
  defendability of, 263
  spacing behavior in relation to, 200–209
Response
  in communication, 75
  goal-oriented, 54
Response sequence, four stages in, 54
Retardation, selective, 14
Rhea, in polygynous-polyandrous system,
      304–305
Rheinartia pheasants, 317

Rhyncocyon chrysopygus, 188
Ring-billed gulls, sounds of, 122
Robin, spacing behavior of, 187. *See also*
      Birds
Rodents, isolation and aggression in, 183
Romalea microptera, 63
Ruff, promiscuity in, 316–317. *See also* Birds
Rule transmission, in animals, 107

Saccopteryx bilineata, 293
Sage grouse, male territories in, 187
Salix nigra, 63
Sampling, in optimal foraging, 259–260
Sanderlings, polygynous-polyandrous system
      of, 307
Sandpipers
  foraging behavior of, 209
  parental care in, 330
  promiscuity among, 317
  sex role reversal in, 275
  true polygyny of, 305
Savanna baboons, promiscuity of, 314
Scarus croicensis, 187
Scatophaga stercoraria, 236
Schemata
  concept of, 5–7
  learning and, 15
  sensory templates and, 113
Scrub jay
  familial evolutionary route of, 373
  parental territory of, 365
Seahorses, sex role reversal in, 274
Sea lions, colonies of, 292
Seals, polygyny-threshold model in, 292–293
Search images, for foraging animals, 205
Search paths
  in foraging behavior, 246–254
  modification of by experience, 248–250
  optimal, 246–248
  optimal return times for, 250–254
Seiurus aurocapillus, 171, 237
Selective addressing, 125–126
Self-instruction, openness and, 5
Sensation, in animal communication, 108–
      109
Sensitive period, defined, 6
Sensorimotor mechanisms, aggression and,
      59–60
Sensory templates, imitation and, 113
Sequestering, in sexual behavior, 52
Sex. *See also* Copulatory behavior; Mating
      system; Sexual behavior
  aggression and, 29–64
  evolution of, 271–332
Sex role reversal
  evolution of, 274
  female competition versus male choice in
      relation to, 275–276
  female desertion and, 275

Sexual activity
  daily rhythms in, 37
  ovarian cycle and, 37–38
  seasonal rhythms in, 39–40
Sexual behavior. *See also* Breeding;
    Copulatory behavior; Mating systems
  copulation mechanisms in, 40–44
  defined, 31
  estrous cycle and, 45
  female mechanisms in, 41–42
  large-scale motor movement in, 52
  mate selection in, 32–36
  mechanisms of, 31–51
  motivation and, 53–54
  progestational hormone secretion in, 46–
    48
Sexual bimaturism hypothesis, 315
Sexual bond, establishment of, 32
Sexual differentiation, rationale of, 31
Sexual dimorphism, 274
Sexual drive, mechanism of, 41–42. *See also*
    Sexual behavior
Sexuality
  behavioral mechanisms in, 45–46
  as evolutionary strategy, 31
Sexual receptivity, in female rat, 47–51
Sexual reflexes. *See also* Sexual behavior
  hormonal control of, 56
  spinally programmed, 43–44
Sexual reproduction, evolution of, 271–332
Sexual synchronization, problems of, 51
Shorebirds, polygynous-polyandrous systems
  of, 306–308. *See also* Birds;
    Sandpipers
Siamang, territory range of, 210
Signal(s)
  in animal communication, 76
  arbitrary, 97
  background and, 81
  deictic, 125
  distance traveled by, 82–83
  emotion-based, 129
  faint odor as, 115
  iconic, 97
  internal referents and, 134–136
  memory and, 115
  organic odorants as, 117
  production and perception of, 109–110,
    139–140
  repetition of, 115
  sequential versus syntactical, 143
  shared procedures in, 109–110
  spacing. *See* Spacing signals
  structure and function in, 114–120
Signal address, in animal communication,
  125–126
Signal direction, auditory capacity and, 79
Signal elements, temporal order of, 143

Signaler identity
  "familiar" discrimination in, 121–122
  individual recognition in, 120–121
  recognition modes in, 120–125
Signaler output categories, in animal
  communication, 91–95
Signaler species, identification of, 116–117
Signal indexing, in enemy specification, 127–
  128
Signaling. *See also* Signal(s)
  as alarm calls, 130–133
  in animal communication, 108–109
  emotion-based, 129
  food specification in, 130
  learning and, 113
  phylogeny of, 107–108
  selective pressures and description in, 138–
    139
  sex and age factors in, 124–125
  specification of conditions for production
    of, 138
  of strangers, 122
  symbolic, 130–133
Signal patterns, change of during
  transmission, 103–104
Signal perception
  behavior and, 140–143
  signal production and, 139–140
Signal processing
  assessments in, 83–84
  internal transformations in, 83–88
  transformation rules in, 83–84
Signal production
  in communication, 74, 76–83
  rules governing, 138–140
  sender and receiver in, 76–78
  signal direction in, 78–80
Signal receiver
  context and past experience in relation to,
    114–115
  information from, 114
  sender and, 76–78
Signal recognition, cross-species, 116–117
Signal repertoire, species-specificity in, 117–
  120
Signal structures, digital versus analog coding
  in, 96–97
Signal variation, 89–107. *See also* Animal
  communication
  arbitrariness versus iconicity in, 97–99
  categorical and continuous perception in,
    99–103
  digital versus analog coding in, 96–97
  discontinuous or discrete signals and, 103
  stereotyping and variability in, 90–91
Site-dependent dominance, 127–128
Smith's longspur, male defense in, 326
Snipe, promiscuity of, 316

Social agents
  information and, 17–18
  mothers and fathers as, 20
Social behavior. *See also* Behavior; Behavioral
      science; Mating behavior
  aggression and, 56–64
  development of, 2–5
  developmental plasticity in, 5–7
  general properties and mechanisms of, 51–
      56
  hierarchical organization in, 54–56
  kin interaction and, 386–387
  ontogeny of, 1–25
  openness in, 5
  physiological bases of, 29–64
Social development, special features of, 1
Social environment
  gross demographic variables and, 20
  as information service, 17–19, 24
  prediction in, 18
  social agents and, 17–18
Social experience, spacing behavior and, 183
Social insects, evolutionary routes of, 371–
      372. *See also* Bees; Social wasps
Social interactions, contingencies in, 199–200
Sociality. *See also* Socialization
  evolutionary routes to, 367–378
  individual, kin, and group selection in
      evolution of, 351–389
  parasocial evolutionary route to, 368
Socialization
  conditioning as, 21–22
  field orientation in, 21
  maintenance functions in, 21–22
  multiplicity of stimulus effects in, 21
  transactions in, 22–23
Social life, interaction and interdependence
      in, 22–23
Social objects, activity and, 18
Social ontogeny, defined, 1. *See also*
      Ontogeny
Social organization, communicative
      familiarity and, 136–137
Social wasps, nests of, 365
Solitary habits, promiscuity and, 313
Somateria mollissima, 328
Song sparrows, territoriality in, 179
Sound attenuation, physical nature of, 195–
      196
Sound, distortion of, 82
Sound transmission, spacing signals and, 195
Spacing. *See also* Spacing behavior
  activity fields and movement patterns in,
      161–167
  aggression and, 184
  behavioral mechanisms of, 173–191
  constraints on, 174
  defined, 159

Spacing *(cont.)*
  intrasexual, 188
  literature on, 159
  mechanisms and evolution of, 159–212
  versus proximity, 174–176
Spacing behavior. *See also* Spacing
  aggregations as factor in, 209–210
  categories of individuals engaging in, 187–
      191
  costs and benefits of, 197–199
  evolution of, 196–210
  examples of, 206–209
  of foraging animals, 204–205
  kinship factor in, 209–210
  in monogamous animals, 188–189
  optimal spacing in, 210–212
  resources and, 200–209
  territorial defense and, 197–198
Spacing patterns, quantitative description of,
      161–173
Spacing signals. *See also* Spacing; Spacing
      behavior
  behavior modification and, 192
  channels for, 193–194
  direction and distance factors in, 195–196
  modality of, 193–194
  modifying effects of, 192
  range of, 194–195
  sound attenuation and, 195
Sparrows
  double-brooding of, 284
  foraging of, 243
  song and hormones in, 111
Spatial relations, between animals, 167–173.
      See also Spacing behavior
Spatial variation, ethology and, 173
Specialist, versus generalist, 13, 261–262
Specialization, "escape" from, 13
Special sensitivity, concept of, 6
Species specificity, in signal repertoire, 117–
      120
Specificity
  in animal transformation, 86–87
  stimulus effects and, 22
Speech, imitation in, 113
Speech perception, motor theory of, 112–
      113
Spermophilus richardsonii, 291
Spermophilus undulatus, 289
Sperm transport, in female rats, 49–50
Spider monkeys, spacing behavior in, 203
Spiders, familial and parasocial evolutionary
      routes of, 369–371
Spiza americana, 283
Squirrels
  alarm calls in, 131
  range for seed collection in, 201
Starfish, foraging strategy of, 256

Starlings, foraging behavior of, 238. *See also*
Birds
Steatornis caripensis, 320
Stereotypy, in animal communication, 90–91,
96
Steroids. *See* Corticosteroids
Sticklebacks, search efficiency of, 248
Stimulus effects
multiplicity of, 21–25
specificity-generality problems in, 22
Stripe-backed wren, group territories of, 191
Strix aluco, 205
Sturnus vulgaris, 238
Subordinate-dominant relationships, 382–
384
among kin, 386–387
Sula bassana, 265
Sunbird, optimal diet of, 255, 264. *See also*
Birds
Suricata suricatta, 330
Sylvicapra grimmia, 331
Symphalangus syndactylus, 210, 330
Syncerus caffer, 313
Systems theory, development and, 19

Taeniopygia guttata, 181
Tamiasciurus squirrels, nonoverlapping
territories of, 180, 263, 313
Tamias striatus, 177–178
Tasmanian native hens, polyandrous mating
of, 305, 309–310
Tawny owls, prey selection by, 205
Telmatodytes palustris, 281
Temminck's stint, polygyny and polyandry in,
307–308
Termites, eusociality in, 371
Territorial behavior
intruders and, 198–199
prior ownership and, 199
Territorial defense
economics of, 263–264
spacing behavior and, 197–198
territorial size and, 198
Territorial monogamy, 277
Territorial neighbors, relationships between,
200
Territorial polygyny, 278–304. *See also*
Polygyny
female aggressiveness in, 281
"female fitness" in, 280
male parental behavior and, 282–284
in passerine birds, 295–303
theory of, 278–282
in ungulates and primates, 294
Territory size, agonistic tendencies and, 186–
187
Threat
versus attack behavior, 192
communication of, 191–196

Three-spined stickleback, neighbor
interactions in, 190
Tiaris olivicea, 244
Tinamou, polygynous-polyandrous system of,
306–307
Tit, blue, 141
Titmice
foraging of, 232
resident dominance in, 179
Toucans, frugivorous, 320. *See also* Birds
Towhees, abnormal song of, 191
Trait groups, defined, 362
Transactions, taxonomy of, 22–23, 25
Transformation
in animal communication, 86–87
in signal processing, 83–88
unique determination of, 87–88
Treculia, 181
Tree sparrow, spacing behavior of, 160
Tree squirrel
agonistic responses to referents in, 180
nonoverlapping territories of, 263, 313
Tribonyx mortierii, 305
Trichogaster trichopterus, 179
Tricolored blackbird, male parental care in,
283
Triggering, internal and external, 135–136
Troglodytes aedon, 189, 283
Troglodytes troglodytes, 283
Tropical birds, parental care in, 318–319
Tryngites subruficollis, 317
Turdus merula, 230
Turdus migratorius, 187
Turkeys, 142
Tympanuchus cupido, 315

Uca terpsichores, 175
Uganda Kob, lek behavior of, 321
Umwelt. See Effective environment

Valence, environmental feedback and, 19
Valley quail, effect of male hormones on,
182–183
Vampire bats, monogamy of, 329
Vampyrum spectrum, 329
Ventriloquial sound, in communication, 79
Vertebrate mating systems, selective nature
of, 272. *See also* Mating systems
Vervet monkeys. *See also* Monkeys
aggressive interactions in, 181
alarm calls in, 131–133
Vestinaria coccinea, 264
Village indigo birds, male calling of, 321
Village weavers, colonies of, 34
Voice-onset-time, in animal communication,
99–100
Vulpes fulva, 190
Vulpes vulpes, 188

Wapiti, harem polygyny in, 364
Wasps, nests of, 365, 371, 385–386
Waxwings, food resource defense by, 320. *See also* Birds; Passerine birds
Weaver finches, nesting sites of, 283, 301. *See also* Birds
Weber-Fechner law, 95
White-bearded manakin, lek of, 322
White-crowned sparrow, 124, 191
White-lined bats, territory defense of, 293
White rhinoceros, spacing of, 184
White wagtail, changing aggressions of, 185
Wildebeest, exclusive areas of, 183, 313
Wolves
    howling of, 121
    monogamy in, 328
Woodcock, promiscuity in, 316
Wood pigeon, feeding behavior of, 226
World, mechanistic perspective on, 2
Wrens. *See also* Birds
    male parental care in, 283–284
    polygyny in, 303

Xanthocephalus xanthocephalus, 279
Xiphophorus, 178

Yellow-bellied marmots
    female reproductive success in, 286–289
    hibernation of, 289
    polygyny-threshold model of, 290
Yellow-hooded blackbird
    female aggressiveness in, 281
    mating season of, 283
    polygyny in, 296
    territories of, 181
    vasectomies in, 279
Young, parental behavior affected by trophic requirements of, 17

Zebra finch, 181
Zebras, harem polygyny in, 304
Zonotrichia albicollis, 191
Zonotrichia leucophrys, 124, 191